Driving and Community Mobility:

Occupational Therapy Strategies Across the Lifespan

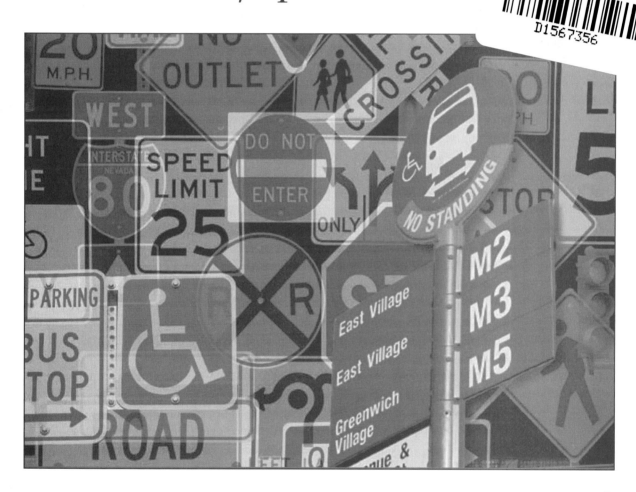

Edited by

Mary Jo McGuire, MS, OTR/L, FAOTA,
and **Elin Schold Davis,** OTR/L, CDRS

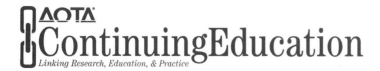

AOTA
ContinuingEducation
Linking Research, Education, & Practice

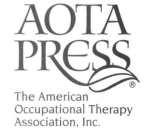

AOTA
PRESS

The American
Occupational Therapy
Association, Inc.

AOTA Centennial Vision
We envision that occupational therapy is a powerful, widely recognized, science-driven, and evidence-based profession with a globally connected and diverse workforce meeting society's occupational needs.

Mission Statement
The American Occupational Therapy Association advances the quality, availability, use, and support of occupational therapy through standard-setting, advocacy, education, and research on behalf of its members and the public.

AOTA Staff
Frederick P. Somers, *Executive Director*
Christopher M. Bluhm, *Chief Operating Officer*
Maureen Peterson, *Chief Professional Affairs Officer*

Chris Davis, *Director, AOTA Press*
Sarah Hertfelder, *Continuing Education Program Manager*
Ashley Hofmann, *Development/Production Editor*
Victoria Davis, *Production Editor/Editorial Assistant*

Beth Ledford, *Director, Marketing*
Amanda Fogle, *Marketing Specialist*
Emily Zhang, *Technology Marketing Specialist*
Jennifer Folden, *Marketing Specialist*

American Occupational Therapy Association, Inc.
4720 Montgomery Lane
Bethesda, MD 20814
301-652-AOTA (2682)
TDD: 800-377-8555
Fax: 301-652-7711
www.aota.org
To order: 1-877-404-AOTA or store.aota.org

Disclaimers
This publication is designed to provided accurate and authoritative information in regard to the subject matter covered. It is sold or distributed with the understanding that the publisher is not engaged in rendering legal, accounting, or other professional service. If legal advice or other expert assistance is required, the services of a competent professional person should be sought.

—From the Declaration of Principles jointly adopted by the
American Bar Association and a Committee of Publishers and Associations

It is the objective of the American Occupational Therapy Association to be a forum for free expression and interchange of ideas. The opinions expressed by the contributors to this work are their own and not necessarily those of the American Occupational Therapy Association/AOTA Press.

ISBN: 978-1-56900-335-0

Library of Congress Control Number: 2012935510

Cover Design by Debra Naylor, Naylor Design, Inc., Washington, DC
Composition by Maryland Composition, Laurel, MD
Printed by Automated Graphic Systems, Inc., White Plains, MD

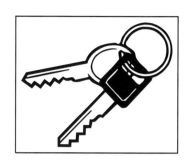

Contents

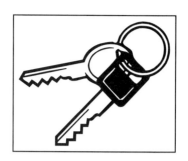

Acknowledgments

The editors acknowledge and thank the following professionals who served as invited content reviewers, providing an in-depth review of all the chapter manuscripts.

Donna Costa, DHS, OTR/L, FAOTA
Professor (Clinical) and Director of the Post-Professional OTD Program
Division of Occupational Therapy
University of Utah
Salt Lake City

Gayle J. San Marco, OTR/L, CDRS
Program Coordinator Driver Preparation Program
Northridge Hospital Medical Center
Northridge, CA

Jennifer Radloff, MHS, OTR, CDRS
Assistant Professor
School of Occupational Therapy
University of Indianapolis
Indianapolis

Karin Bonfils-Kleinhans, OTR/L
Occupational Therapy–Neurorehabilitation and Driving
Sierra Nevada Memorial Hospital
Grass Valley, CA

Robyn Y. Ogawa, OTR/L
Clinical Operations Manager
Rehabilitation Therapies
Long Beach Memorial Medical Center
Long Beach, CA

The editors thank the following professionals who provided critiques of early chapter manuscript drafts, providing input and encouragement:

C. Dan Allison

Carolyn Bousfield

Felicia Chew

Jami Dalchow

Anne Dickerson

Colleen Durkin

Michael D. Justiss

Michele Luther-Krug

Brenda Marvel

Dennis P. McCarthy

Robyn Ogawa

Christine Raber

Susan Shah

Nina Silverstein

Amy Smith

Wendy Stav

Donna Stressel

Meredith Sweeney

Michelle Tipton-Burton

Susan Touchinsky

Fay Tripp

Marie VanDevere

Sandra Winter

The editors acknowledge and thank the following individual for creating the driving assessment table that is part of Chapter 9:

Sandra Winter, PhD, OTR/L

Research Coordinator, Institute for Mobility, Activity, and Participation

Department of Occupational Therapy

College of Public Health and Health Professions

University of Florida

Gainesville

I want to first thank God for the joy of serving Him as an occupational therapist, and for the challenging experience of serving as one of the editors of this American Occupational Therapy Association (AOTA) Self-Paced Clinical Course and AOTA Press text. Co-editor Elin Schold Davis has done a magnificent job in her role as coordinator of the AOTA Older Driver Initiative, networking with stakeholders across the nation (and world) to advance the visibility and role of occupational therapy in the field of driving and community mobility, and promoting the role of generalists in serving the driving and community mobility needs of society. I cannot thank Elin enough for her amazing work, wonderful mentorship, and friendship.

Thank you to the National Highway Traffic Safety Administration, and particularly to Essie Wagner, the Older Driver Analyst, for the support they have given to AOTA to advance the role of occupational therapy in serving society's driving and community mobility needs.

Finally, with tears of gratitude, I thank my family for sacrificing many hours of family time so that I could work on this book. Thank you to my dear husband, Jim, and to my four wonderful children—Mike, Sara, Dan, and Beth. You all own my heart.

—*Mary Jo McGuire, MS, OTR/L, FAOTA*

I want to thank my fellow editor, Mary Jo McGuire, for her vision, dedication, and commitment to ensuring that occupational therapy practitioners have the knowledge and skills needed to listen when driving is in question to ensure the highest-caliber service within their scope of practice. I thank each author for his or her commitment to increasing our profession's capacity to provide evaluation and intervention, integrating evidence-based practice with their expertise, experience, and clinical reasoning to provide client-centered care as we address this highly valued and complex instrumental activity of daily living so critical to "living life to its fullest."™

—Elin Schold Davis, OTR/L, CDRS

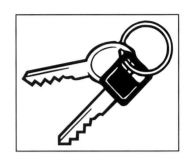

About the Editors

Mary Jo McGuire, MS, OTR/L, FAOTA, is the founder and director of a group of occupational therapists in private practice in Akron, Ohio, who serve clients in the home and community as Medicare Part B providers. Their clinical work focuses on older adults who are aging in place and on survivors of traumatic brain injury. Ms. McGuire is a 1976 graduate of the Ohio State University; she earned her master's 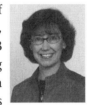 in health sciences education and evaluation from State University of New York at Buffalo in 1981. She has served as a clinical supervisor and then as the clinical education specialist at the Rehabilitation Institute of Chicago; she was on faculty at the University of North Carolina at Chapel Hill; and from 1995 to 2005, she and her husband, Jim, operated Rehab Educators, a continuing education company serving occupational therapists across the nation.

Ms. McGuire was awarded AOTA's Cordelia Myers Writer's Award in 1987. Her writings have been published in the *American Journal of Occupational Therapy, OT Practice*, and several book chapters; she authored the final chapter in *Strategies to Advance Gerontology Excellence: Promoting Best Practice in Occupational Therapy*. Her awards include the Continuing Education Award, the Model Practice Award and the Passion Award from the Ohio Occupational Therapy Association and an Award for Excellence from the Summit County Traumatic Brain Injury Collaborative. In 2009, she received a mini-grant from AOTA, funded by the National Highway Traffic Safety Administration, that focused on advancing the role of the generalist in addressing the driving and community mobility needs of clients. In 2012, she was selected by AOTA to represent the profession as *CPT™ (Current Procedural Terminology)* advisor to the American Medical Association's Health Care Professionals Advisory Committee, which represents the interests of non-physician practitioners.

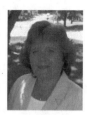

Elin Schold Davis, OTR/L, CDRS, is the Older Driver Initiative project coordinator for AOTA. She earned her bachelor of science in occupational therapy from the University of Minnesota and became a Certified Driver Rehabilitation Specialist through the Association for Driver Rehabilitation Specialists. Her experience in long-term care and adult rehabilitation at the Sister Kenny Rehabilitation Institute in Minneapolis, Minnesota, led Schold Davis to her current position.

Since 2003, the projects of the AOTA Older Driver Initiative have been building awareness of occupational therapy's role in senior safe mobility while increasing the capacity of occupational therapy programs to address driving as an instrumental activity of daily living. Under her guidance, AOTA holds cooperative agreements with the National Highway Traffic Safety Administration to develop education and awareness-building materials, the Massachusetts Institute of Technology Age Lab to explore collaborative research, and the Hartford Advance 50 Team to develop an educational brochure. Schold Davis is a member of the American Society on Aging's DriveWell Speakers Bureau; a member of the Transportation Research Board's Safe Mobility for Older Persons Committee; a member of the National Older Driver Safety Advisory Council; and AOTA's national liaison–instructor for CarFit, a program that offers older adults the opportunity to check how well their personal vehicles "fit" them to increase safety.

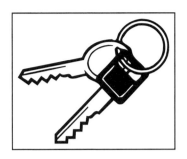

About the Authors

Rosanna Arnold, MS, OTR/L, graduated from Towson University in 2011 with a combined bachelor's and master's degree in occupational therapy and as a member of the Honors College. At Towson, she was a research assistant to Dr. Wendy Stav and researched community mobility and older driver safety. She was also involved with a team that created a transition and orientation program for students 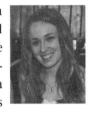 with autism spectrum disorders. She currently works at MedStar Union Memorial Hospital in Baltimore, focusing on physical dysfunction acute and comprehensive inpatient rehabilitation.

Peggy P. Barco, MS, BSW, OTR/L, received her master of science in occupational therapy and her bachelor's degree in occupational therapy from Washington University. She also has a bachelor's degree in social work from the University of Missouri at Columbia. She is currently pursuing her doctorate degree in occupational therapy at Washington University Medical School in St. Louis. Her areas of 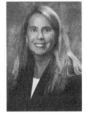 clinical interest are awareness deficits after brain injury, the assessment and treatment of cognitive disorders, and driving assessment in medically impaired individuals. She is an instructor at the Program in Occupational Therapy at Washington University and teaches courses in cognitive assessment and intervention. Ms. Barco also is a driving rehabilitation specialist, having performed driving assessments and trainings for more than 15 years. In collaboration with David Carr, MD, she is studying medical fitness-to-drive in various populations, including older adults with dementia, stroke, Parkinson's disease, and visual disorders. Their work has been funded by the Missouri Department of Transportation for the past 5 years. She has mentored occupational therapists in driving rehabilitation; assisted in the start of two driving programs at major medical centers, including Driving Connections at the Rehabilitation Institute of St. Louis; and presented at local and national conferences on medical fitness and driving.

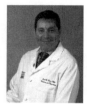

David B. Carr, MD, is a professor in the Department of Medicine and Neurology at Washington University at St. Louis. He is a board-certified internist and geriatrician who completed his fellowship training in geriatrics at Duke University in 1990. Dr. Carr accepted a position as clinical director in the Division of Geriatrics and Nutritional Science at Washington University in 1994. He has been a clinician in the Memory and Aging Project in the Alzheimer's Disease Research Center for the past 15 years. He is the director of the geriatric fellowship program, which educates general internal medicine physicians for careers in geriatric medicine. Dr. Carr is medical director of the Rehabilitation Institute of St. Louis, where he has assisted in the development of the Driving Connections clinic, which opened in January 2008. He maintains an outpatient consultative practice at the Memory Diagnostic Center in the Department of Neurology, and he is medical director of Parc Provence, a long-term-care facility for dementia care in the greater St. Louis area. His research interests are in medical conditions that affect driving, especially issues of assessing driving safety and cessation in older drivers with dementia and stroke.

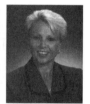

Sherrilene Classen, PhD, MPH, OTR/L, FAOTA, is an associate professor in the Department of Occupational Therapy and director of the University of Florida's Institute for Mobility, Activity and Participation, and she holds a position as extraordinary professor at the University of Stellenbosch in South Africa. Dr. Classen is a nationally funded prevention-oriented scientist, who uses a public health and rehabilitation science perspective to research the screening, evaluation, and intervention processes for at-risk older drivers, drivers with neurological conditions (Parkinson's disease, mild traumatic brain injury, epilepsy), and adolescent pre-drivers. She studies the use of clinical (off-road) tests, simulated driving technology, on-road driving assessments, and alternative transportation options to driving. She has 50 peer-reviewed publications, six book chapters, and three special journal issues related to driving and community mobility options. Dr. Classen serves on two national Transportation Research Board committees, is an editorial board member of the *Canadian Journal for Occupational Therapy*, and is a fellow of AOTA and the Gerontological Society of America. She mentors junior faculty, postdoctoral fellows, graduate students, and undergraduates in occupational therapy, rehabilitation science, public health, and epidemiology.

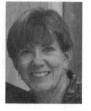

Anne Dickerson, PhD, OTR/L, FAOTA, is a professor and project director of ROADI—Research for the Older Adult Driving Initiative in the Occupational Therapy Department at East Carolina University. Dr. Dickerson has been an occupational therapist for more than 30 years, has a PhD in developmental psychology, is a fellow of AOTA, and has been honored with awards from professional organizations and universities in research, teaching, and service. She is a well-known leader among transportation experts through her translational research between driving research and occupational therapy's commitment to driving and community mobility. She has numerous publications in occupational therapy, psychology, and gerontology journals.

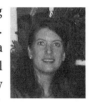

Jennifer Elgin, OTR/L, CDRS, is the clinic coordinator of the Driving Assessment Clinic at the University of Alabama at Birmingham (UAB). She obtained a bachelor of arts degree at the University of Alabama in 1992, majoring in psychology; a master of science in occupational therapy degree at UAB in 2002; and a graduate certificate in low vision in 2004. Ms. Elgin is a Certified Driver Rehabilitation Specialist. She has provided driving assessment and rehabilitation services to hundreds of clients for more than a decade. Her research interests include low-vision rehabilitation, vision impairment driving, mobility in older adults, and predictors of fitness-to-drive for persons with neurological impairment or vision impairment.

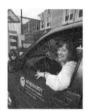

Anne Hegberg, MS, OTR/L, CDRS, is a Certified Driver Rehabilitation Specialist and a Certified Driving Instructor (CDI). She has been at Marianjoy Rehabilitation Hospital for more than 20 years and is a master clinician for the driver rehabilitation program. Under Ms. Hegberg, the program has grown to one of the largest in the country, with six highly qualified registered occupational therapists who are all CDIs. The Marianjoy driving program addresses the needs of a wide client population. Specialties include adolescents, low vision, and the elderly as well as drivers needing to drive from their wheelchair. In 2010, Ms. Hegberg obtained a grant to fund a van equipped with state-of-the-art driving equipment. With this high-tech van, she serves clients throughout the Midwest. She is a past president of the Association for Driver Rehabilitation Specialists and remains active in the organization. She also is involved in AOTA as well as the National Mobility Equipment Dealers Association. She was a consultant for the second edition of the *Physician's Guide to Assessing and Counseling Older Drivers*. Ms. Hegberg has presented nationally and internationally on the topic of driver rehabilitation.

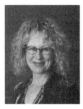

Linda A. Hunt, PhD, OTR/L, FAOTA, is a professor in the School of Occupational Therapy and director of the Graduate Certificate in Gerontology for Healthcare Professionals at Pacific University in Oregon. Her research and numerous publications focus on the effects of aging, dementia, and disease on driving capacity. Her most recent research explores driving and the outcomes of getting lost for drivers who are in the early stages of dementia. She has received research funding from the National Institute on Aging, General Motors, the State of Missouri, and other institutions. In addition, Dr. Hunt explores how vision affects cognitive processing in everyday occupations and abilities. Furthermore, she explores mindfulness practice for those who work in health care to hopefully help them provide better care to clients through stress reduction and the practice of enhanced empathy. She received her degree in occupational therapy from the University of Kansas, a master in health care services from Washington University School of Medicine in St. Louis, and a PhD in physiological optics/vision science from the Optometry School at the University of Missouri–St. Louis.

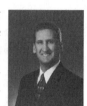

Michael D. Justiss, PhD, OTR, is an assistant professor and director of research in the Department of Occupational Therapy within the Indiana University (IU) School of Health and Rehabilitation Sciences. He received his PhD from the University of Florida in rehabilitation sciences with a minor and a graduate certificate in gerontology from the university's Center for Gerontological Studies. He received his master of occupational therapy from Duquesne University in Pittsburgh and holds bachelor of science degrees in neuroscience and medical technology from the University of Pittsburgh. Dr. Justiss is the director of the Driving Safety and Rehabilitation Research Laboratory in the IU School of Health and Rehabilitation Sciences. He is the associate director for the Transportation Active Safety Institute Driving Simulator Laboratory located within the Purdue School of Engineering and Technology (Indianapolis). His current research efforts focus on cognitive aging and human factors; assessment strategies to identify deficits in driving-related skills and driving performance; rehabilitation and intervention strategies to maintain driving independence; and alternative transportation strategies to maintain community mobility and participation when driving is no longer a safe option.

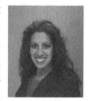

Desiree N. Lanford, MOT, OTR/L, CDRS, is an occupational therapist and a Certified Driver Rehabilitation Specialist with 10 years of experience in driving evaluation and rehabilitation. She coordinates three Independence Drive offices located in North Florida. She serves clients enrolled in the University of Florida Institute for Mobility, Activity and Participation's research programs; those referred for clinical services in a large retirement community at the Villages, Florida; and those referred for clinical services at Shands Rehab at Magnolia Parke in Gainesville. Ms. Lanford is a trained CarFit event coordinator, she presents content knowledge related to driving and community mobility on local and national levels, and she often is invited to participate in expert panels for driving rehabilitation specialists. She mentors driving rehabilitation specialists in training and supervises the Level II fieldwork activities of master's-level students in occupational therapy.

Michele Luther-Krug, COTA/L, SCADCM, CDRS, ROH, has practiced as an OTA for 31 years and in the field of driver rehabilitation for 21 years. She specializes in driver training and assessment at the Shepherd Center in Atlanta, for those with physical, neurological, and visual dysfunction. She has earned credentials in the field of driving and community mobility from AOTA and the Association for Driver Rehabilitation Specialists (ADED). She has contributed to the development of competencies for specialty certification in driver rehabilitation for AOTA and served as the certification chair for ADED in 2003. She is currently serving as the OTA representative to the AOTA Representative Assembly. Ms. Luther-Krug earned the AOTA Roster of Honor in 2010 for OTA leadership and service. She also earned the 2010 Georgia Occupational Therapy Association Award for Outstanding Practitioner for advocacy and service. She was most recently awarded the Terry Brittell OTA/OT Partnership award in 2011 for pioneering roles in the field of driver rehabilitation. She has coauthored textbook chapters, journal articles, and courses related to driving and community mobility for ADED and AOTA.

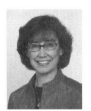

Mary Jo McGuire, MS, OTR/L, FAOTA, is the founder and director of a group of occupational therapists in private practice in Akron, Ohio, who serve clients in the home and community as Medicare Part B providers. Their clinical work focuses on older adults who are aging in place and on survivors of traumatic brain injury. Ms. McGuire is a 1976 graduate of the Ohio State University; she earned her master's in health sciences education and evaluation from State University of New York at Buffalo in 1981. She has served as a clinical supervisor and then as the clinical education specialist at the Rehabilitation Institute of Chicago; she was on faculty at the University of North Carolina at Chapel Hill; and from 1995 to 2005, she and her husband, Jim, operated Rehab Educators, a continuing education company serving occupational therapists across the nation. Ms. McGuire was awarded AOTA's Cordelia Myers Writer's Award in 1987. Her writings have been published in the *American Journal of Occupational Therapy*, *OT Practice*, and several book chapters; she authored the final chapter in *Strategies to Advance Gerontology Excellence: Promoting Best Practice in Occupational Therapy*. Her awards include the Continuing Education Award, the Model Practice Award and the Passion Award from the Ohio Occupational Therapy Association, and an Award for Excellence from the Summit County Traumatic Brain Injury Collaborative. In 2009, she received a mini-grant from AOTA, funded by the National Highway Traffic Safety Administration, that focused on advancing the role of the generalist in addressing the driving and community mobility needs of clients. In 2012, she was selected by AOTA to represent the profession as *CPT™ (Current Procedural Terminology)* advisor to the American Medical Association's Health Care Professionals Advisory Committee, which represents the interests of non-physician practitioners.

Miriam Monahan, MS, OTR/L, CDRS, CDI, is an occupational therapist, Certified Driver Rehabilitation Specialist, and Vermont-licensed driving school instructor. She is currently a research therapist at the University of Florida studying adolescents with special needs and driving. Ms. Monahan has been practicing in the field of driver rehabilitation since 1998 in a variety of settings including hospitals and private practice. She founded the nonprofit Driver Rehabilitation Institute to further research, education, and innovation in the field of driver rehabilitation. She lectures and consults extensively on the topic of driver rehabilitation, both locally and nationally, to medical professionals, law enforcement, educational institutions, and others. She has authored several textbook chapters on various aspects of driver rehabilitation. She also authored three courses for AOTA on the topic of driving and community mobility for adolescents with special needs and was awarded the 2005 Clinical Practice Award by the Vermont Occupational Therapy Association. Ms. Monahan has served as public relations chair for the Association for Driver Rehabilitation Specialists. She has participated in National Highway Traffic Safety Administration–funded projects to educate law enforcement personnel about the impact of medical conditions on driving and on guidelines for state motor vehicles departments on medical conditions and driving.

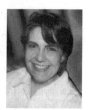

Pat Niewoehner, OTR/L, CDRS, is a staff occupational therapist at the VA Medical Center in St. Louis. She is a certified driver rehabilitation specialist and treats patients with a wide variety of diagnoses in the driver rehabilitation clinic. She is a member of the St. Louis Consortium for Older Driver Education and Research team, an interdisciplinary research group that focuses on the older driver. Ms. Niewoehner's main area of research interest is the older driver with dementia. In addition, she provides occupational therapy services for the mental health division at the St. Louis VA Medical Center.

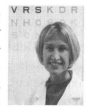

Cynthia Owsley, PhD, MSPH, is the Nathan E. Miles Chair, professor, and vice chair for clinical research in the Department of Ophthalmology, School of Medicine, at the University of Alabama at Birmingham (UAB). She is a Phi Beta Kappa graduate of Wheaton College, Massachusetts; received her PhD in experimental psychology from Cornell University, where she was a National Science Foundation predoctoral fellow; and completed a master of science in public health in epidemiology at the UAB School of Public Health. Dr. Owsley's research program focuses on aging-related eye disease and vision impairment and on improving the quality of and access to eye care in underserved adult populations. One of her research foci is vision impairment and driving. She has been continuously funded by the National Institutes of Health since 1983. Her research program embodies many approaches including methodologies from psychophysics, epidemiology, clinical trials, HRQoL questionnaire development, and health services research. Dr. Owsley has served on three panels for the National Research Council of the National Academies, is a Research to Prevent Blindness senior scientific investigator, and is on the Board of Directors for Prevent Blindness America. She is an inaugural fellow of the Association for Research in Vision and Opthalmology and the recipient of the Glenn A. Fry Award from the American Optometric Foundation and the Bartimaeus Award from the Detroit Institute of Ophthalmology.

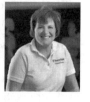

Christine Raber, PhD, OTR/L, is an associate professor in the master of occupational therapy program at Shawnee State University, where she has taught for more than 16 years. She received a PhD in health-related sciences from Virginia Commonwealth University in 2007 in addition to a post-professional master's degree in occupational therapy and a bachelor's degree in occupational therapy from the Ohio

State University, in 1992 and 1984, respectively. Her clinical background includes a broad range of mental health and older adult practice settings, and she currently supervises Level I and service-learning experiences with these populations in multiple settings. Dr. Raber's research focuses on understanding the dynamics of volition in persons experiencing dementia, and she has presented on this topic as well as other biopsychosocial topics at state, national, and international conferences. Her publications include contributions to *Model of Human Occupation, 4th Edition;* the *British Journal of Occupational Therapy;* and *Physical and Occupational Therapy in Geriatrics.* Dr. Raber is an Eden Alternative Associate and advocate of person-centered care and culture change in long-term care. The psychosocial core of occupational therapy is of critical importance to driving and community mobility, and she is passionate about helping students and clinicians value and own their unique role in this area.

Elin Schold Davis, OTR/L, CDRS, is the Older Driver Initiative project coordinator for AOTA. She earned her bachelor of science in occupational therapy from the University of Minnesota and became a Certified Driver Rehabilitation Specialist through the Association for Driver Rehabilitation Specialists. Her experience in long-term care and adult rehabilitation at the Sister Kenny Rehabilitation Institute in 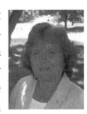 Minneapolis, Minnesota, led Schold Davis to her current position. Since 2003, the projects of the AOTA Older Driver Initiative have been building awareness of occupational therapy's role in senior safe mobility while increasing the capacity of occupational therapy programs to address driving as an instrumental activity of daily living. Under her guidance, AOTA holds cooperative agreements with the National Highway Traffic Safety Administration to develop education and awareness-building materials, the Massachusetts Institute of Technology Age Lab to explore collaborative research, and the Hartford Advance 50 Team to develop an educational brochure. Schold Davis is a member of the American Society on Aging's DriveWell Speakers Bureau; a member of the Transportation Research Board's Safe Mobility for Older Persons Committee; a member of the National Older Driver Safety Advisory Council; and AOTA's national liaison–instructor for CarFit, a program that offers older adults the opportunity to check how well their personal vehicles "fit" them to increase safety.

Nina M. Silverstein, PhD, is a professor of gerontology at the University of Massachusetts Boston, College of Public and Community Service. She received her PhD in 1980 from Brandeis University. Since 1984, she has worked closely with the Alzheimer's Association on projects relating to the association's Helpline, its Safe Return Pro- gram, respite care, support groups for family caregivers, home safety adaptations, and environmental and behavioral issues in special care units for people with dementia. She is a fellow of the Gerontological Society of America and in 2010 was elected chair-elect of the Social Research Planning and Practice Section. In 2007 she was honored as the person of the year by the Alzheimer's Association, Massachusetts/New Hampshire Chapter. In 2008 she received the Louis Lowy Award from the Massachusetts Gerontology Association and was honored as the Foley Lecturer by the Alzheimer's Association, Cleveland Chapter. In 2010 she received the David A. Peterson Award for best article in volume for her paper on exploring livable communities from the journal *Gerontology & Geriatrics Education.* Dr. Silverstein has coauthored two books, *Dementia and Wandering Behavior: Concern for the Lost Elder* and *Improving Hospital Care for Persons with Dementia.* Recent publications have appeared in *The Gerontologist, Gerontology and Geriatrics Education, Alzheimer's and Dementia, American Journal of Alzheimer's Disease,* and *Transportation Research Record.* She has written several technical research reports on transportation available through the Gerontology Institute, University of Massachusetts Boston. She spent a sabbatical in Washington, DC, for the 2004–2005 academic year, where she divided her time between the Department of Transportation and the Alzheimer's Association Public Policy Division. Recently, she was a coinvestigator on an Alzheimer's Association–funded study: *Fitness to Drive in Early Stage Dementia: An Instrumented Vehicle Study.*

Deborah Yarett Slater, MS, OT/L, FAOTA, has more than 38 years of experience in clinical and administrative positions in a broad variety of organizational settings. Her clinical specialty area is hand rehabilitation, but for more than 20 years she focused on management roles overseeing large single and multidisciplinary departments in both inpatient and outpatient settings. She has developed start-up off-site satellite clinics for several organizations, including new program development, and has extensive experience in financial management, as well as reimbursement. Ms. Slater also has been active in a variety of volunteer leadership positions for her state occupational therapy association and AOTA, including Administration and Management Special Interest Section (SIS) committee member and chair, Special Interest Section Council chair, practice representative to the Ethics Commission, member of the AOTA Board of Directors, and chair of the ad hoc committee on scope of practice. Since June 2003, she has worked for AOTA as a practice associate and staff liaison to the Ethics Commission and the SISs. She has done numerous presentations on ethics at state and national conferences and also has published book chapters and continuing education products on this subject. In addition, she coedits the AOTA *Scope of Practice Issues Update* newsletter and has done conference workshops and a continuing education presentations. Ms. Slater is a fellow of AOTA and has received numerous service awards for various volunteer leadership positions. In 2002 she received the Herbert Hall Award for outstanding service to the occupational therapy profession from the Massachusetts Association for Occupational Therapy. In May 2005 she received the Distinguished Alumna Award from Columbia University in New York.

Wendy B. Stav, PhD, OTR/L, SCDCM, FAOTA, is an associate professor in the Department of Occupational Therapy and Occupational Science at Towson University. Her work has addressed driving and community mobility specific to the examination of assessments, determining fitness-to-drive, driver–vehicle fit, injury prevention in 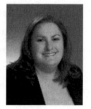pedestrian travel and child passenger safety, and exploration of clinical practice in the area. She has been involved in several key projects in the practice area, including coauthoring AOTA official documents and fact sheets, development of the AOTA specialty certification in driving and community mobility, contribution to the older-driver evidence-based literature review, and coauthorship of AOTA practice guidelines. Dr. Stav's participation in driving and community initiatives has extended beyond AOTA to the American Medical Association, the American Automobile Association, the National Highway Traffic Safety Administration, state motor vehicles administrations, and the U.S. Department of Defense. She was named to the AOTA Roster of Fellows for her advancement of practice in driving and community mobility.

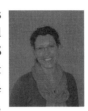

Susan Martin Touchinsky, OTR/L, is a clinical specialist with Genesis Rehabilitation Services (GRS) and a master clinician in driving and dementia. She has 11 years of experience and has worked for GRS and with the Johns Hopkins Driving Program. She has presented at the AOTA Annual Conference 2010 and 2011, presented at the 2004 Association for Driver Rehabilitation Specialists Annual Conference, coauthored a chapter in *Driver Rehabilitation and Community Mobility* (2006), was a contributing author in the *GRS Community and Transportation Guide*, and completed her training as a CarFit instructor. Ms. Touchinsky has been instrumental in bringing driving and community mobility into the forefront at GRS. She is passionate about providing comprehensive care, working to continually evolve her own practice, advocating for occupational justice for all patients, and sharing her knowledge with others.

Jennifer L. Womack, MA, MS, OTR/L, SCDCM, is a clinical associate professor in the Division of Occupational Science and Occupational Therapy at the University of North Carolina. Her clinical background includes work in neurorehabilitation, long-term care, and community-based aging services. She has addressed community mobility issues from the perspective of both individual and organizational clients, working to help nondrivers with disabilities to access alternate transportation and with an urban paratransit system to develop eligibility determination processes for paratransit. She was a member of the inaugural AOTA board for specialty certification in driving and community mobility. At the time of this publication, she serves on the transportation consolidation committee for Chapel Hill and Orange County, North Carolina, and on the transportation planning subcommittee of the Orange County Master Aging Plan.

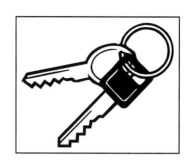

List of Figures, Tables, Exhibits, Appendixes, Case Examples, and Practitioner's Reflections

Figures

Tables

Exhibits

Appendixes

Case Examples

Practitioner's Reflections

Foreword

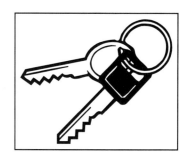

As a geriatric neurologist who has made her career in academia and caring for people with various dementias, I have relied often on occupational therapists to maximize my patients' independence. My first exposure to occupational therapy was during my neurology training on a wonderful interdisciplinary in-patient unit at the Veterans' Affairs Medical Center in Gainesville, Florida. Since I learned of the profession's existence, I have marveled at the difference it can and has made in the lives of my patients. I did not anticipate just how big a role occupational therapy would play as my career unfolded.

I first thought about issues of medically at-risk drivers while caring for a patient on the VA Neurology Unit who was having daily seizures: without warning and during waking hours. When I spoke with him about the risk, he said, "I have to work, and I have to drive. I will not stop until someone takes my driver's license away."

This was the VA. The rules are quite different between federal and state agencies. The VA is not required to adhere to state laws. And in this case, the state laws were vague as well. So I had to get clearance from the VA Legal Department to contact the state's Department of Motor Vehicles (DMV). When I did, the DMV indicated that I should send a letter to them and they would look into it. I responded that I needed them to come to the hospital and take his license, because I would not discharge him until I was assured that he would not drive. It may have been the first and last time the state sent a representative to a hospital, but it worked. Amazingly the patient accepted this action with grace.

Little did I realize that this episode so early in my training would influence my career path. My clinical interests have always been tied to the relationship between cognition and function. I specialized in behavioral and geriatric neurology. The most memorable conversations I had with my patients were around the issue of driving. It was not uncommon for them to say they would rather be dead than not drive. Sometimes they would become angry and even threaten me. Driving is so critical to community mobility and impacts the ability to access care and activities that enrich our lives.

I decided that this was too important an issue to ignore. But I could find little guidance in the literature or from my mentors on how to deal with this issue. I decided to work on it. I developed a standardized road test with significant input from occupational and kinesio therapists (perhaps unique in the VA). I compared the scoring by the experienced driver rehabilitation specialist (DRS) with the clinical measures I use in the office setting. I learned just how complex this process can be.

The further I got down this road the more I depended on occupational therapists for guidance. I was delighted to be invited to speak at regional occupational therapy meetings and at a national VA conference for VA DRSs. I now teach physicians and medical students all over the United States about this difficult issue and urge them to consider DRSs the gold standard of driving assessment.

DRSs are my most important allies when I need help determining which of my patients are too dangerous to be behind the wheel. They can assess and sometime train my patients to be safer drivers. Although DRSs are usually occupational therapists, I was dismayed to learn that driver-related training is not standard in all occupational therapy programs. I am excited to be part of a growing emphasis on this training for occupational therapy professionals. The need is tremendous.

One of my missions is now to encourage occupational therapy practitioners to get more involved in driving-related decisions. We physicians are depending on you. The other mission is to get physicians to appreciate the rich resource of occupational therapy practitioners and refer to them more liberally.

I am delighted to have the opportunity to voice my support of this book, for this very important field, and for the growth of DRSs. As the U.S. population ages, medically at-risk drivers are going to overwhelm us. Occupational therapy as a field is the best positioned to take the lead in this arena.

What do I tell my medical audiences? Call occupational therapy!

—Germaine L. Odenheimer, MD
Associate Professor of Geriatric Neurology
Clerkship Director of the Geriatrics Rotation for 4th-Year Medical Students
University of Oklahoma College of Medicine
Donald W. Reynolds Department of Geriatrics
Oklahoma City

Introduction

Mary Jo McGuire, MS, OTR/L, FAOTA, and
Elin Schold Davis, OTR/L, CDRS

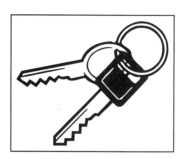

An important tool of the occupational therapy process is the evaluation of the actual performance of an activity in the natural context in which it occurs. "Dry runs" of certain tasks, such as bathing, can provide some but not all of the information an occupational therapist needs to determine safety or the need for intervention. Stepping out of a tub while warm, dry, fully clothed, and with nonslip shoes on one's feet is very different from exiting a tub after exhausting one's energy while bathing and attempting the task while wet, cool, tired, and undressed. Actual performance evaluations are valuable tools, as they often uncover issues not uncovered during dry runs.

However, the actual performance evaluation of driving a vehicle requires training beyond the occupational therapy professional curriculum. Such performance evaluation of driving also is related to the behavior of other drivers, the conditions of the road, and the route selected. This text provides occupational therapists with a knowledge base to determine if, when, and why an on-road evaluation is indicated in a client's plan of care.

The scope of driving and community mobility includes readiness to drive to competence to drive to the transition to alternative modes of transportation. The issues are complex, and the consequences related to changes in independence in driving and community mobility are life-altering.

The field of driving and community mobility is a dynamic area to capture. This text, in both organization and scope, illustrates that clients must be examined as a whole and that intervention must involve an understanding of and access to a range of services. Providers ranging from licensing agencies to health care facilities to physicians in practice are all seeking a simple "test" to make driving decisions, and they often defer the responsibility for licensing action to the "score."

This text and Self-Paced Clinical Course (the test materials are in a separate packet) gathers researchers and clinicians in a team effort to offer expert guidance for occupational therapy's work in the ever-developing practice area of driving and community mobility. It is published with great hope in the power of occupational therapy to increasingly and meaningfully serve the needs of society and in the ability of every occupational therapist to contribute to the achievement of the *Centennial Vision* of the American Occupational Therapy Association (AOTA) that occupational therapy is "a powerful, widely recognized, science-driven, and evidence-based profession with a globally connected and diverse workforce meeting society's occupational needs" (AOTA, 2007, p. 613). This resource captures an impressive depth of knowledge and range of tools.

About This Publication

Specialty Certification

The development of this text began with the competencies established by AOTA for meeting the requirements for Specialty Certification in Driving and Community Mobility (SCDCM) in which experts had worked to clarify what distinguishes an occupational therapist or assistant as a specialist. This text guides occupational therapy professionals to recognize driving and community mobility as an instrumental activity of daily living (IADL) within their scope of practice, promotes the professional obligation to address it, and expands their understanding of specialized content related to driving and community mobility. Practitioners can find updated information related to AOTA's SCDCM at www.aota.org/Practitioners/ProfDev/Certification.aspx.

Authors

The authors of this text are from across the United States and are leaders in research and clinical practice, addressing the spectrum of driving concerns with diverse clients such as those with cognitive impairments (e.g., dementia); are experts in visual impairments; and are practitioners who offer hope, adaptation, strategies, and compensation for the physical limitations that require the complex and highly skilled incorporation of equipment, vehicle modification, and training. Some authors focus on the details of the comprehensive driving evaluation; others offer content analyzing the challenges and benefits of using simulators. The outcome is a group of chapters that provide guidance for generalist clinicians, highly experienced clinicians, or researchers seeking to increase their knowledge of the importance of community mobility and driving.

Scope

It is impossible to talk about the complex IADL of driving and community mobility without acknowledging or referring to other issues. For instance, when discussing how visual impairments affect driving, it is impossible to avoid the topic of cognition. Visual input informs cognition. Moreover, when authors are asked to plumb the literature and provide guidance to therapists on the topic of cognition, the issue of visual attention, critical to gathering salient information to make informed decisions, is of paramount importance.

No effort was made to prevent one author from providing insights, developed over years of clinical practice, related to their primary content area to another content area. Each chapter has its own authors and focus, but readers can expect appropriate overlap and linking of content to ensure a clear understanding of the relationships that exist among the various factors analyzed. In the chapters, the authors have prioritized and expanded on content they deemed to be critical as a foundation for the topic they were asked to address.

Format

Each chapter contains a variety of table, figures, case examples, and exhibits, as well as key words, learning objectives (see below), and callouts of important points. The text begins with a general introduction to driving and community mobility (Chapter 1) and comprehensive community mobility options (Chapter 2). Chapter 3 discusses the various stakeholders in driving and community mobility. Chapter 4 examines the psychosocial issues that can affect driving and how occupational therapists can address them.

Chapter 5 discusses the unique ethical questions that can arise when occupational therapy professionals are obligated to help their clients as well as protect the safety of the public at large. Chapter 6 deconstructs and analyzes the complex components that make up the IADL of driving and community mobility.

Chapters 7 and 8 thoroughly explore how cognition and vision affect driving and community mobility. Chapter 9 provides extensive examples of evidence-based screening, assessment, and evaluation tools to best serve the medically at-risk driving population. Chapter 10 focuses on the wide range adaptive equipment vehicle modification options and includes myriad photographs.

Chapter 11 examines the clinical reasoning process during the comprehensive driving evaluation, and Chapter 12 discusses possible interventions that result from it. Finally, as this work addresses driving across the life span, Chapter 13 discusses how to evaluate and instruct younger drivers, an often-overlooked population.

The epilogue and Appendix A delineate the importance of advocating on behalf of clients on driving and community mobility issues, as well as understanding the critical importance of driving and community mobility as IADLs, both now and in the future.

Learning Objectives

The overall learning objectives and breadth of content offer a comprehensive view of the complexity of driving and community mobility and support the importance of the role of occupational therapy.

After reading this material, readers will be able to do the following:

- Recognize why it is important for all occupational therapists to address community mobility and driving across the life span and in different practice settings;
- Recognize the imperative to broaden the focus from driving rehabilitation toward a more comprehensive consideration of community mobility at the individual, community, and societal levels;
- Recognize that addressing driving and community mobility as a routine part of occupational therapy practice cannot be accomplished working in isolation and identify a range of stakeholders who may play a role in this important practice area;

- Recognize that there are often unspoken psychosocial issues related to one's sense of autonomy and self-determination that are associated with issues related to driving and community mobility;
- Recognize that occupational therapists have an ethical responsibility, through the evaluation process, to identify impairments in occupational performance that may correlate with driving risks and to inform clients (and caregivers or significant others if applicable), even if they do not have a legal responsibility to report them to the state;
- Identify occupational therapists' unique contribution as a health care professional to be able to take everyday tasks and analyze their components and to relate this to the occupational areas of driving and community mobility;
- Delineate how cognition involves organizing, assimilating, and integrating new information with prior experiences and the need to apply this information to plan and structure behavior for safe driving and community mobility performance in unpredictable and dynamic conditions;
- Recognize that the visual demands of driving are intricate and important for the ability to detect, discriminate, recognize, and identify objects and events during driving and that these abilities are not exclusively sufficient for understanding the role of vision in driving;
- Delineate the distinctions among the different assessments and types of assessments, the domains of functional performance assessed, and the evidence supporting the use of individual assessments as they relate to driving;
- Identify physical factors in driving and how the appropriate equipment can make driving possible;
- Identify how the clinical reasoning process along with other assessment data are used throughout the entire comprehensive driving process to provide recommendations and counseling about driving fitness;
- Identify the role of intervention in determining driving and community mobility outcomes;
- Identify the principles that are essential for driver training when working with youth with special needs and the essential evaluation components for assessing a student's readiness to learn to drive and to independently access the community; and
- Identify collaboration as a key attribute for the continued successful development of occupational therapists in the areas of driving and community mobility.

Terminology

The terminology used to describe the needs and services related driving and community mobility is varied among a diverse group of stakeholders.

Emerging Definitions of Terms: A Multidisciplinary Challenge

The use of various terms among many stakeholders in driving and community mobility presents a complicated issue. *Stakeholders* include legal professionals (e.g., licensing authorities, law enforcement officials, reporting laws), medical professionals (e.g., physicians, medical insurance, clinicians), and clients and their families.

Some terminology decisions had to be made for consistency and ease in reading. Readers can expect a certain amount of variance in terminology across the different chapters. Some terms are used with confidence in certain regions or areas of practice, while the same terms are altered and used with the same level of confidence in other areas. Key words at the beginning of each chapter help guide readers through the chapter.

Consider the following terms: *behind-the-wheel evaluation, behind-the-wheel assessment, behind-the-wheel testing, on-the-road evaluation, on-road evaluation, on-the-road assessment, on-road assessment, on-the-road testing,* and *on-road testing.* In some chapters, the authors have chosen to use *behind-the-wheel evaluation* rather than *on-road evaluation.* The terms chosen may reflect the specificity of intervention, distinguishing, in some instances, simulated driving from in-vehicle, on-the-road driving.

Because this text is a compilation of various authors' works, the editors have chosen not to force one set of terms into use across all of the chapters. As much as possible, the editors have attempted to move the occupational therapy profession toward a more uniform use of the term *comprehensive driving evaluation (CDE).* The editors have chosen to continue advancing the work incorporating terminology used within the *Occupational Therapy Practice Guidelines for Driving and Community Mobility for Older Adults* (Stav, Hunt, & Arbesman, 2006) and the Online Course *Driving and Community Mobility for Older Adults: Occupational Therapy Roles, Revision* (Pierce & Schold Davis, 2010; see "Key Terms," p. 11), which provides the profession with the following definitions:

- *Comprehensive driving evaluation*—An in-depth evaluation of driving performance skills and client factors related to driving. The CDE is made up of two parts, a *clinical evaluation* and an *on-road evaluation* (Pierce & Schold Davis, 2010, p. 11).
- *Clinical evaluation*—A part of CDE process during which the occupational therapist interviews the client to identify his or her specific assets, problems, or potential problems. The therapist considers the client's performance skills, performance patterns, context, activity demands, and client factors through a battery of assessment tools that look at these aspects related to driving skills and demands (Pierce & Schold Davis, 2010, p. 11).
- *On-road evaluation*—A part of the CDE performed in an evaluation vehicle with a specialist in driving. As the client drives through a structured traffic route, the specialist assesses whether performance skill impairments or contextual or environmental concerns impede safe driving. The on-road portion of the CDE is essential for recommending adaptive equipment or driving aids, vehicle modification, and the need for lessons and training. In some instances, the outcome of the on-road evaluation supports the recommendation for driving cessation because of the driver's high risk for harm to self or others while driving (Pierce & Schold Davis, 2010, p. 11).
- *Medical fitness-to-drive*—While this concept is applicable to all age groups, it is particularly salient for older adults. As a group, older adults are at a greater risk for health conditions that may impair driving ability and increase crash risk, especially after age 70 (Li, Braver, & Chen, 2003). The "medically fit" driver is one with sufficient vision, alertness, cognition,

joint range of motion, and motor skills to manage the operational, tactical, and strategic demands of driving (Carr, Schwartzberg, Manning, & Sempek, 2010). Health conditions that detract meaningfully from these key abilities may increase crash risk and thus require focused evaluation and intervention by health professionals (Dobbs, 2005).

- *Medically at-risk driver*—The increasingly preferred and more accurately descriptive term, over *older driver* or *aging driver*, and is used to describe the driver with impairments that result from medically related changes that may interfere with the ability to drive a vehicle safely (in contrast to driving concerns for the well elderly or related to typical aging; Dobbs, 2005).

Credentials and Certifications

This text is directed toward occupational therapy assistants as well as occupational therapists. However, in this book, the text may refer to *occupational therapists* rather than to *occupational therapy practitioners, occupational therapy professionals,* or *occupational therapy assistants.* This choice no way negates or diminishes the contribution of occupational therapy assistants in the evaluation and service delivery process, as outlined in the *Guidelines for Supervision, Roles, and Responsibilities During the Delivery of Occupational Therapy Services* (AOTA, 2009). The occupational therapy assistant delivers occupational therapy services under the supervision of and in partnership with the occupational therapist in accordance with state regulations, the AOTA *Standards of Practice for Occupational Therapy* (AOTA, 2010d), the *Occupational Therapy Code of Ethics and Ethics Standards (2010)* (AOTA, 2010a), the *Standards for Continuing Competence* (AOTA, 2010c), and the *Scope of Practice* (AOTA, 2010b).

Occupational therapy driving and community mobility generalists are occupational therapists and occupational therapy assistants with the education, training, and credentials necessary to practice occupational therapy but who do not possess the level of specialized training, experience in driver evaluation or driver rehabilitation, or the credentials to fully administer the comprehensive driving evaluation on which to base the determination of driving competence (Pierce & Schold Davis, 2010, p. 10).

Occupational therapy driver rehabilitation specialists (DRSs) are occupational therapists and occupational therapy assistants who have advanced education and training specifically in the field of driver evaluation and driver rehabilitation (including intervention, vehicle modification, and adapted driving equipment). DRSs are encouraged to seek specialty certification and recommended credentials. Both state and reimbursement guidelines vary nationally; some states specify the credentials required to practice as a DRS (Pierce & Schold Davis, 2010, p. 10).

The editors recognize that occupational therapists and occupational therapy assistants who are generalists in driving are often specialists in areas other than driver rehabilitation, such as hand or brain injury rehabilitation, gerontology, or pediatrics. Although the terms are admittedly somewhat artificial, we hope that distinguishing the roles of *generalist in driving* and *specialist in driving* will be useful in helping therapists and assistants define and expand their own skills and practices. However, because this dimension of practice is changing rapidly, these and other terms will likely be refined during the next few years. In addition, these terms are intended to be used descriptively and not as professional titles (Pierce & Schold Davis, 2010, p. 10).

Table I.1. Professionals Involved in Driving and Community Mobility

Term	Regulated or Credentialed by	Role in Driving Rehabilitation	Role in Community Mobility
Occupational therapist	State	Yes*	Yes*
Occupational therapy assistant	State	Yes*	Yes*
AOTA Specialty Certification in Driving and Community Mobility	AOTA	Yes	Yes
Certified driving instructor	State	Yes	No
Certified driver rehabilitation specialist (CDRS)	ADED	Yes	Sometimes, not required
Driving rehabilitation specialist (DRS)	Some states define standards; otherwise, no	Yes	No

Note. AOTA = American Occupational Therapy Association; ADED = Association for Driver Rehabilitation Specialists.
* Within the limits of training and competence (see Chapter 5 on ethics).

A *certified driver rehabilitation specialist (CDRS)* is an individual who meets the educational and experiential requirements and successfully completes the certification exam provided by the Association for Driver Rehabilitation Specialists (ADED, 2011). *Specialty Certification in Driving and Community Mobility* and *Specialty Certification Assistant in Driving and Community Mobility* credentials are awarded to occupational therapy specialists who meet standards established by AOTA (see www.aota.org/Practitioners/ProfDev/Certification.aspx).

Table I.1 provides a general comparison of various professionals involved in this multidisciplinary field; the role delineations may vary in actual practice.

In addition to the terms described above, additional stakeholders who may work with occupational therapists include the following:

- *Driver educator*—A professional with a college degree in education and specialized study in driver education or traffic safety (Stav et al., 2006, p. 101).
- *Driving instructor*—As required by many states, an individual with a high school degree and a clear legal and driving record who has completed a driver education training program and has been licensed as a driving instructor by the state motor vehicle administration (Stav et al., 2006, p. 101).

The following definitions of terms from the *Standards of Practice for Occupational Therapy* (AOTA, 2010d) are used in this text:

- *Assessment*—Specific tools or instruments that are used during the evaluation process.
- *Evaluation*—The process of obtaining and interpreting data necessary for intervention. This includes planning for and documenting the evaluation process and results.
- *Screening*—Obtaining and reviewing data relevant to a potential client to determine the need for further evaluation and intervention. (p. S107)

Supplemental Materials

This publication includes a flash drive with supporting content. The flash drive offers active links organized to promote continued learning and to promote (without endorsement) easy access to an ever-growing array of important tools that can advance the quality of care in clinics across the United States.

 The **flash drive** is organized by chapter and includes additional information, Web sites, and documents discussed in individual chapters. In the text, items mentioned that also appear on the flash drive are indicated in **bold** and with a car key icon

Conclusion

This text should be considered only a snapshot of what was known and how it was being applied at the time it was written. Even well-accepted standards for licensing drivers, such as assessing visual acuity, are in flux in U.S. society. For example, as this text was prepared for final production, the State of New York made the decision to not continue to assess visual acuity as part of the relicensing process.

This text strengthens occupational therapy's commitment to providing holistic evaluations that recognize a person's need to participate in community-based occupations; community mobility, which includes driving, is an occupational area that is of critical importance to all clients. Too often, questioning whether someone can drive triggers the search for a test and a score, but occupational therapists can respond by addressing the complex IADL that driving represents.

Stakeholders who recognize the dynamic complexity of driving and the critical importance of driving in an individual's life are increasingly seeking evaluation and intervention approaches that serve clients at risk. Just as the newly injured client with paraplegia presents with the clearly stated goal "to walk," an occupational therapist's intervention would not serve the client if it focused only on "failure to walk." Instead, skilled therapy transitions toward mobility provided by the "new" and appropriate transportation option, allowing time for the client to realize a wheelchair's benefits.

By addressing the occupation of driving and community mobility that includes, for some, the transition to modes that are alternatives, more clients might benefit from occupational therapy's person-centered intervention and "live life to its fullest."

References

American Occupational Therapy Association. (2007). AOTA's *Centennial Vision* and executive summary. *American Journal of Occupational Therapy, 61*, 613–614. doi:10.5014/ajot.61.6.613

American Occupational Therapy Association. (2009). Guidelines for supervision, roles, and responsibilities during the delivery of occupational therapy services. *American Journal of Occupational Therapy, 63*, 797–803. doi: 10.5014/ajot.63.6.797

American Occupational Therapy Association. (2010a). Occupational therapy code of ethics and ethics standards (2010). *American Journal of Occupational Therapy, 64*(Suppl.), S17–S26. doi:10.5014/ajot.2010.64S17

American Occupational Therapy Association. (2010b). Scope of practice. *American Journal of Occupational Therapy, 64*(Suppl.), S70–S77. doi:10.5014/ajot.2010.64S70

American Occupational Therapy Association. (2010c). Standards for continuing competence. *American Journal of Occupational Therapy, 64*(Suppl.), S103–105. doi:10.5014/ajot.2010.64S103

American Occupational Therapy Association. (2010d). Standards of practice for occupational therapy. *American Journal of Occupational Therapy, 64*(Suppl.), S106–S111. doi:10.5014/ajot.2010.64S106

Association for Driver Rehabilitation Specialists. (2011). *Definition of a driver rehabilitation specialist.* Retrieved April 12, 2011, from http://www.driver-ed.org/i4a/pages/index.cfm?pageid=507

Carr, D. B., Schwartzberg, J. G., Manning, L., & Sempek, J. (2010). *Physician's guide to assessing and counseling older drivers.* Washington, DC: National Highway Traffic Safety Administration.

Dobbs, B. (2005). *Medical conditions and driving: A review of the literature (1960–2000)* (Report No. DOT HS 809 690). Retrieved April 12, 2012, from http://www.nhtsa.gov/people/injury/research/Medical_Condition_Driving/pages/TRD.html

Li, G., Braver, E. R., & Chen, L. H. (2003). Fragility versus excessive crash involvement as determinants of high death rates per vehicle-mile of travel among older drivers. *Accident Analysis and Prevention, 35,* 227–235.

Pierce, S., & Schold Davis, E. (2010). *Driving and community mobility for older adults: Occupational therapy roles* (rev., Online Course). Bethesda, MD: American Occupational Therapy Association.

Stav, W. B., Hunt, L. A., & Arbesman, M. (2006). *Occupational therapy practice guidelines for driving and community mobility for older adults.* Bethesda, MD: AOTA Press.

CHAPTER 1

Introduction to Community Mobility and Driving

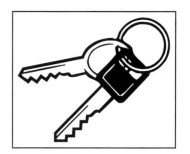

Wendy B. Stav, PhD, OTR/L, SCDCM, FAOTA, and Mary Jo McGuire, MS, OTR/L, FAOTA

Learning Objectives

At the completion of this chapter, readers will be able to

- Identify all areas of occupational therapy practice, and all Special Interest Sections, as having a role in addressing issues of community mobility;
- Recognize community mobility as an "occupational enabler";
- Recognize driving as an important aspect of community mobility that occupational therapists have a right and a responsibility to explore as a part of the general occupational therapy process; and
- Recognize driving and community mobility as instrumental activities of daily living to be addressed as part of a client's occupational profile.

Key Words

- **community mobility**
- **consultation**
- **evaluation**
- **intervention**
- **occupation**
- **occupation enabler**

Defining *Community Mobility*

The *Occupational Therapy Practice Framework: Domain and Process, 2nd Edition* (*Framework–II*), created by the American Occupational Therapy Association (AOTA; 2008), recognizes community mobility as an area of occupation within the scope of occupational therapy practice. More specifically, *community mobilty* is categorized as an instrumental activity of daily living (IADL) and is defined as "moving around in the community and using public or private transportation, such as driving, walking, bicycling, or accessing and riding in buses, taxi cabs, or other transportation systems" (AOTA, 2008, p. 631).

Therapeutic attention to community mobility by occupational therapists takes into account client factors that may affect performance, the activity demands of the various modes of community mobility, the performance skills used to engage in community mobility, the performance patterns that shape how humans engage in community mobility, and the multiple contexts and environments in which community mobility takes place (AOTA, 2008). Supporting the safe and effective engagement of community mobility by clients in spite of health or contextual issues is therefore under the purview of occupational therapists regardless of the mode of that movement.

The Centers for Disease Control and Prevention (CDC) also recognizes the health focus of community mobility, as evidenced by the presence of transportation topics in its focus on injury, violence, and safety. Specifically, the CDC (2011) identifies child passenger safety, seat belts, teen drivers, older adult drivers, impaired driving, distracted driving, pedestrian safety, and global road safety as areas of concern. These areas of concern are individually addressed in Healthy People 2020, which maintains national health goals and includes objectives to decrease motor vehicle crash–related deaths and injuries, increase seat-belt use, increase use of child vehicle restraint systems, reduce pedestrian fatalities and injuries, reduce pedal-cyclist fatalities, and increase helmet use when riding bicycles and motorcycles (Healthy People, 2010).

On an international level, the World Health Organization (WHO) acknowledges community mobility from a health perspective, as the occupation is classified as *Driving and Using Transportation* in a category titled "Moving Around Using Transportation" in the domain of "Mobility" in the *International Classification of Functioning, Disability and Health* (WHO, 2001). It is evident that health organizations of all sizes, both within and external to our discipline, recognize community mobility as integral to the health of society and within the scope of health care practice.

Contributions of Community Mobility to Life

Community mobility is first and foremost a means of transporting oneself from Point A to Point B within the community; however, there are more complex considerations related to how that mobility contributes to daily life. It has been several decades since individuals took "Sunday drives" and traveled within the community solely for the sake of getting out of the house. In fact, our daily lives are so busy that community mobility currently is performed primarily to arrive at a destination for a specific purpose. The use of community mobility to travel from a location to a destination allows members of society to access health care, go shopping, and participate in socialization and leisure pursuits.

The mode of transportation used to travel to destinations varies considerably depending on the community and can range from a subway, taxi, or bus in an urban city; to a private motor vehicle in the suburbs; and to walking or biking in a rural area. Whatever the mode of travel, engaging in community mobility allows individuals, groups, and communities to do far more than transport themselves from Point A to Point B; it allows for engagement in a broad array of other occupational pursuits. The ability of community mobility to serve as a conduit to engagement in other occupations has led to the recognition of community mobility as an *occupation enabler* (Stav & Lieberman, 2008). This additional purpose beyond transportation from location to location as an occupation enabler further strengthens the need to address community mobility in practice through the identification of needs and resolution of issues through interventions.

Importance of Addressing Community Mobility Needs

The importance of community mobility in an individual client's life is important from the time an infant is transported home from the hospital to the choices an aging client makes regarding travel to participate in community events. Clients that are organizations (e.g., transit companies, school systems) also view community mobility as important; they strive to transport riders of all ages and abilities while adhering to regulatory guidelines and laws. Even populations recognize the value of community mobility as governing bodies build and revise communities that support safe travel using several modes of transportation, including walking, bicycling, driving, bus, train, boat, and plane travel. Because community mobility is so widely used and regarded as a vital aspect of daily life among individuals, organizations, and populations, it is incumbent upon occupational therapists and occupational therapy assistants to address the community mobility needs of clients in support of occupational engagement, healthy clients, and healthy communities.

The range of potential issues in the area of community mobility is vast and can span the entire spectrum of age, affect function in clients with almost any type of disability, and be of concern in most practice settings. Fortunately, all occupational therapists possess the knowledge and skills to address this important IADL on some level, depending on the therapist's role as a generalist or specialist in community mobility (AOTA, 2010a). Although some therapists possess the skills to actively evaluate and address clients' community mobility needs, all therapists possess the knowledge and ability to refer clients to the most appropriate local, state, or national resources to meet the client's needs. It is the individual therapist's judgment that determines when it is appropriate to approach this critical area, to what depth various issues are explored, what type of interventions are indicated, and at what point a client should be referred to a specialist in the field. Because no "cookbook" protocol exists to manage the complex issues associated with community mobility concerns, the needs of each client, whether a person, organization, or population, are determined and addressed on a case-by-case basis.

> **All occupational therapists possess the knowledge and skills to address this important IADL on some level, depending on the therapist's role as a generalist or specialist in community mobility.**

Addressing Community Mobility Across Practice Areas

Occupational therapy practice can be categorized in several ways, such as by age of client, by placement on the continuum of care, by specific populations served, or by practice areas. The following section incorporates practice areas as they are represented in AOTA's Special Interest Sections and forums, as each uniquely presents special considerations in relation to community mobility practice.

Administration and Management

Occupational therapists with a role or interest in administration and management should not forego their attention to community mobility simply because they are not providing direct services. Rather, these therapists need to attend to community mobility issues from a managerial perspective in terms of program development or establishment of referral pathways. Addressing community mobility needs from an administrative perspective can be difficult because of an array of barriers that hinder development and sustainment of community mobility programs (Stav, Snider Weidley, & Love, 2011). Once programs are developed, there are numerous tasks and expectations associated with operating these programs, such as marketing, training, and documentation (Stav, 2012), which are important for administrators to understand so they can provide the necessary support.

In addition to the daily operations associated with providing the services, managers and administrators must keep abreast of the regulatory guidelines—such as billable services, paratransit laws, medical reporting guidelines, child passenger safety best practices and laws, graduated licensing, and bike helmet laws—to support their staff in abiding by those policies in the provision of interventions related to community mobility. Finally, resources are available to managers and administrators who wish to provide more stable, comprehensive programming to meet the community mobility needs of their clients. Many of these resources are available through Web sites and can be found through AOTA:

- **Toolkit for Professionals:** www.aota.org/Older-Driver/Professionals/Toolkit/Professional.aspx
- **Driving Rehabilitation Program Development Toolkit:** www.aota.org/Older-Driver/Professionals/Toolkit/Programs.aspx.

Developmental Disabilities

Occupational therapists who work with children and adults with developmental disabilities must address safety and independence issues related to community mobility, including, but not limited to,

- Safety or stability while being transported in vehicles;
- Use of a tricycle, bicycle, or wheeled device;
- The amount of freedom an individual safely can be allowed related to walking in the neighborhood (or using a tricycle, bicycle, or other piece of equipment);
- Determining eligibility and application for paratransit services;
- Use of public or private alternative modes of transportation (e.g., buses, paratransit, cabs);
- Use of power equipment (e.g., electric scooter, power wheelchair); and
- Driving a vehicle.

Although clients with developmental disabilities may have impairments, occupational therapists capitalize on the strengths and resources of the client to support community mobility.

Serving this population may necessitate the advocacy of an occupational therapist to address all areas of community mobility from an occupational justice perspective. Chapter 13 addresses the important issues that surround working with young drivers who have special needs.

Early Intervention

Occupational therapists explore the safety issues related to community mobility as part of early intervention programming. Therapists assess

- How a child is transported in a vehicle,
- Whether there are any special positioning needs in using a stroller or other wheeled device, and
- Whether the medical needs of a child (e.g., oxygen tanks, other equipment) necessitate special adaptations during community mobility.

To best meet the child passenger safety needs of the client and provide up-to-date education to parents and caregivers, therapists may choose to become certified in child passenger safety through **Safe Kids USA.** This credential allows therapists to facilitate educated decisions about which child safety seat is the best for the child's age, height, and positioning needs while also considering the best fit with the caregiver's vehicle (Safe Kids USA, 2007a, 2009b). Safety needs of child passengers vary and progress from infancy through 12 years of age and remains highly dependent on the child's age, height, and weight. Detailed guidelines and child-specific recommendations are addressed thoroughly in the child passenger safety technician training and through the National Highway Traffic Safety Administration (http://www.nhtsa.gov/Safety/CPS).

Following are the primary questions to be asked of parents in serving the early intervention population:

- When do you take your child out of the home?
- Where do you take your child?
- What mode of transportation do you use?

Therapists also instruct and facilitate the development of cognitive and motor skills for functional and community mobility so that all forms of travel can be executed safely, including walking (Safe Kids USA, 2007b), bicycling, and skating (Safe Kids USA, 2009a). Occupational therapists use narrative reasoning to collaborate with families and develop a "future story" related to the upcoming needs of the child and the hope for adaptation, growth, and participation in the community as the child develops.

School System

Many of the same child passenger safety issues that exist in the school system are present in early intervention, although some interventions may be organization-wide. School bus safety is a paramount concern for school systems and gives occupational therapists a role in ensuring that children, particularly those with special needs, are transported safely. In addition, there are national programs, some with funding, that school-based therapists can implement, such as **International Walk to School Day** (National Center for Safe Routes to School, 2011) and **Safe Routes to School** (Federal Highway Administration, 2010).

International Walk to School Day is a worldwide event in October encouraging pedestrian travel as a safe and healthy alternate mode of transportation to school. Safe Routes to School is a nationally funded initiative aimed at building collaborative partnerships among school administrators, teachers, parents, students, law enforcement, community planners, community leaders, and others to foster safe travel to school.

Sensory Integration

Therapists working in the area of sensory integration should be aware of community mobility concerns that may present themselves related to how well children tolerate or seek sensory input. Clients who are sensitive to vestibular input may perceive car movements as noxious or demonstrate fear when learning to ride unstable devices such as bicycles or scooters. Conversely, clients who crave vestibular input may exhibit high-risk behaviors on mobile equipment and require additional supervision. Auditory sensitivity in clients may raise issues with noises generated from bike horns or bells and should be addressed according to the client's needs.

Physical Disabilities

Clients with a broad array of physical disabilities—including neurological conditions with paresis, paralysis, or abnormal muscle tone; orthopedic injuries with decreased range of motion, decreased strength, or loss of a limb; cognitive deficits; visual changes; or any combination of the above—may present with community mobility needs specific to the operation of a motor vehicle or ability to travel within the community. The needs of these clients are met in different settings, depending on where the client is receiving treatment in the continuum of care.

Acute Care Hospitals and Sub-Acute Care

Clinicians in acute and sub-acute settings often serve clients who are focused on survival issues. In the United States, the time a patient stays in the acute care setting has become increasingly shorter because of changes in reimbursement and health care delivery patterns (Ottenbacher et al., 2004). Nevertheless, the role of the occupational therapist in these settings is critical for guiding the client, family, and subsequent health care providers in issues related to driving and community mobility.

Historically, occupational therapists in the inpatient settings have focused on self-care activities; these are, after all, the activities of daily living (ADLs) that a hospitalized client often is struggling to resume. The larger role of the occupational therapist, however, includes helping a client and family see the entire picture of what meaningful activities may be affected by the new loss, impairment, or disease process. Certainly, this is not a time for final judgments to be made regarding the ability to return to the role of driver, but rather a time to set the stage for further exploration and discussion of the important IADLs related to community mobility, including driving.

Evaluation forms used in these settings can include questions related to driving and community mobility, such as the following:

- Does the client currently hold a driver's license?
- Does the client use a bicycle or drive any power-operated vehicles?
- What form of transportation does the client use to access community services?
- How often does the client leave the home? Where does he or she go?
- How does the client get there?

Client answers to these questions can guide therapists in the next level of health care to further address these issues. Therapists in rehabilitation centers, skilled nursing facilities, and home health care settings often receive documentation from the acute care therapist; simple questions asked and documented in a nonthreatening manner in the acute care setting can provide therapists in these subsequent settings an opportunity to explore an area of the person's life.

It is critical to begin the discussion about driving safety as early as possible to establish realistic expectations about timelines and potential long-term outcomes, especially if a client has a disease process at work that will result in progressive cognitive decline. The role of driving is too important to ignore; the questions related to how a client will be able to participate in meaningful activities may take time to explore and problem solve. Family members are often hopeful that someone else will bring the subject up; it is critical that occupational therapists recognize their responsibility to do so. Clinicians in the acute care setting must be sensitive to the importance of community mobility needs in a person's life, "call the questions" to begin important discussions, prepare clients for the role of occupational therapy in the next level of care, and refer clients to appropriate sources for further intervention post-discharge.

Family members are often hopeful that someone else will bring the subject up; it is critical that occupational therapists recognize their responsibility to do so.

Rehabilitation Centers and Skilled Nursing Facilities

Whether serving children, adolescents, or adults, therapists in rehabilitation centers and skilled nursing facilities have a responsibility to explore the needs of clients related to community mobility, including, if appropriate, a person's history and future goals related to driving a vehicle. Although the focus of therapy in these settings is on the remediation of dysfunction, occupational therapy is always, ultimately, about a return to meaningful *occupations*.

The occupational profile of clients receiving inpatient rehabilitation should include a clear picture of the client's routines and habits related to community mobility. Occupational therapy cannot be so short-sighted as to focus simply on the current self-care needs, or issues related to the home (e.g., home safety issues, meals, laundry), without considering issues related to the client's patterns of living outside of the home. How will the client purchase groceries? What activities (e.g., social, civic, faith based, family oriented) did the client enjoy outside of the home before the hospitalization? Will the client be able to return to these community-based activities? How did the client access these activities before the hospitalization?

Many rehabilitation centers have driving rehabilitation specialists or senior clinicians who have developed competencies related to the use of simulators or specialized screenings to provide information to clients regarding driving skills. All occupational therapists in these settings, however, should have the skills necessary to assess driving-related skills and to carefully assess the client's psychosocial skills related to driving and community mobility. Moreover, all clinicians should be able to provide input to clients regarding how specific skills (e.g., head and neck rotation, visual fields, visual attention skills, memory) relate to driving and community mobility.

Outpatient Clinics

For a client even to be able to receive outpatient therapy services, transportation related to getting the client to the clinic must be arranged. Nevertheless, occupational therapists in outpatient settings are in an excellent position to further address community mobility needs and to establish community mobility goals. The client's occupational profile should be very specific regarding driving and community mobility issues. Clients' attitudes, preferences, and goals regarding driving and community mobility and participation in community-based activities should be a standard part of every outpatient occupational therapy program.

Home Health Care (Medicare Part A)

Occupational therapists who provide services under Medicare Part A are aware that clients must be considered homebound to receive Part A benefits. Occupational therapists working in this health care delivery model, however, should develop an occupational profile that explores the client's prior level of function regarding driving and community mobility as well as lead the client and his or her family in the process of establishing realistic goals in these IADLs. The difficulty is that as a client progresses and develops the motivation and skills to leave the home, he or she becomes ineligible for Part A services to support the development of these skills. This situation should not, however, stop the occupational therapist from supporting a client in establishing community-based goals; once a client is no longer homebound, he or she can be directed to an outpatient clinic or a private practice therapist who can continue the intervention plan.

Home- and Community-Based Occupational Therapy (Medicare Part B)

Medicare recognizes the occupational therapist in private practice (OTPP) as an important part of the continuum of care; the OTPP provides therapy to clients in the home and community and supports a return to full participation in meaningful activities. The OTPP is in an excellent position to address driving and community mobility needs; the occupational therapy evaluation should apply information about the client's impairments to all occupations, including driving and community mobility–related concerns. Not only can the OTPP provide evaluation and training for driving-related skills, but if a client is unable to drive (whether on a temporary or a permanent basis), the OTPP can provide instruction and training regarding alternative modes of transportation. The OTPP is in a perfect position to advance the role of the occupational therapist in the area of driving and community mobility. Whether the OTPP obtains the credentials to do the actual on-road evaluation or partners with other professionals in the locality regarding the behind-the-wheel evaluation, the OTPP can serve clients by increasing awareness of how impairments affect driving and by supporting the client and family in obtaining further evaluation by the appropriate assessor.

Low Vision

Occupational therapists have a particular interest in driving and community mobility because their clients often wish to continue driving, are experiencing difficulties with driving cessation, or need to transition to transportation alternatives. Therapists serving clients with low vision need to pay particular attention to the vision requirements for driving as dictated by the laws in the states in which their clients drive. Each state has a unique set of requirements that may include minimum standards for visual acuity, visual fields, binocular vision, or permission for the use of bioptic equipment for driving.

For clients who are no longer driving, therapists will likely develop goals and interventions related to community mobility so that clients can continue to be mobile and access their necessary and preferred occupations in the community. Knowledge of transportation resources in the region for visually impaired clients is an essential aspect of practice therapists serving clients with low vision.

Mental Health

Community mobility is often an area of top priority for clients receiving mental health services, particularly because for many individuals with chronic conditions, their symptoms and medications make it impossible to drive an automobile (Ménard & Korner-Bitensky, 2008; Rouleau, Mazer, & Ménard, 2010). Without the ability to drive, these clients experience substantial difficulty accessing the community. In fact, in a study of long-term care needs among adults with mental illness, the most commonly identified area of IADL impairment was "getting to places out of walking distance" (Kellet, Shurgrue, Gruman, & Robison, 2010).

This area of concern for clients was identified by more participants than other IADLs that occupational therapists tend to concentrate a lot of time and effort on, including meal preparation, grocery shopping, money management, and household chores (Kellet et al., 2010). Directing individuals with mental illness to the nearest transit service likely will not resolve the community mobility issues among this population, because they are often "transportation handicapped" in that they cannot negotiate a transit system without special resources and assistance to develop way-finding skills (Taylor & Taylor, 1996). The inability to drive combined with the continued need to access the community, along with difficulties navigating transit systems, creates a substantial role for occupational therapists to address community mobility related to travel training with individuals and organizations.

Gerontology

Occupational therapists working with older adults likely are familiar with driving, community mobility, and driving cessation issues. During the past decade there has been considerable attention to older driver issues, with associated funding awarded to occupational therapists and to several other disciplines. There is a clear need for attention to community mobility on the basis of the effects of aging and age-related illnesses on one's ability to safely operate a motor vehicle. Unfortunately, with so much of the focus on driving, there is little evidence of programming dedicated to community mobility, despite the fact that older adults continue to need access to their communities. The undeniable role for occupational therapy with this population involves education to drivers, education to health care providers, client evaluation and determination of fitness-to-drive, intervention to prolong driving, development of transportation alternatives with travel training, assistance with transitions to driving cessation, and support for community design to promote multimodal community mobility.

Technology

Occupational therapists with an interest in technology typically do not consider community mobility as an area of focus, but there are abundant opportunities to develop, adapt, and train individuals and organizations in technology. Many of the adaptations used on vehicles are technology based to allow drivers with limited physical capacity to enter, exit, and operate a motor vehicle. Other technologies are growing in use to compensate for both cognitive and visual deficits; they include global positioning systems, sonar technology to aid in following distance and parking, and cameras to increase visual access.

Eventually, intelligent transportation systems may replace our need to operate a motor vehicle altogether as vehicles will communicate with the roadway and with each other, completely eliminating human errors (Intelligent Transportation Systems Joint Program Office, 2012). Technology use is growing in the transit industry as well to assist with scheduling and to adapt buses. As the role of technology grows in the community mobility arena, so too will the role for occupational therapists with an interest in technology to address the growing needs related to the person–technology interface.

Work and Industry

Although a relatively small portion of the occupational therapy workforce is employed in the area of work and industry, such therapists have an important role in driving and community mobility. Some clients in the work and industry practice area may present with issues because they drive or operate transit as a major part of their work responsibilities. In these cases, the issues should be addressed as they would be for any other client with the same physical, cognitive, or visual impairment. That said, the duration of the engagement in driving presents a unique element to address from the work rehabilitation perspective because many professional drivers are on the road for several hours straight. Most other clients undergoing rehabilitation to return to work ultimately will need to drive, use transit, bicycle, or walk to get to their place of employment, and thus community mobility becomes a relevant concern for occupational therapists practicing in the area of work and industry.

Education

Academic occupational therapists working in higher education have a vested interest in driving and community mobility for teaching and scholarship. The Accreditation Council for Occupational Therapy Education (ACOTE) specifically identifies driving and community mobility in one of the standards related to intervention that reads, "Provide recommendations and training in techniques to enhance mobility, including physical transfers, wheelchair management, and community mobility, and address issues related to *driver* rehabilitation" (ACOTE, 2007; B.5.11). In addition to the required curriculum content per the accreditation standards, ACOTE also explores the inclusion of "emerging niche" practice areas, one of which is *community mobility and older drivers*, during the accreditation process.

Teaching content is not the only mechanism to address community mobility in higher education settings—service, service learning, and scholarship opportunities exist for students. The **CarFit** program, which is a community-based educational program aimed at optimizing driver–vehicle fit among older adults, has been a growing presence in academic programs since 2006. Participation in CarFit gives faculty and students the opportunity to engage in community practice, provide service to the community, demonstrate wellness and injury prevention programming, develop relationships with community partners and stakeholders, and even conduct research. Some academic programs have explored similar opportunities through involvement in other areas of community mobility, including child passenger safety and bicycle helmet fittings.

Finally, most faculty members have to engage in some level of scholarship activity, which might include grant writing, research, evidence-based literature reviews, or generating publications. There are ample opportunities in the driving and community practice area regardless of the population of specialization, as noted by the previous sections in this chapter. Although grant funding is diminishing in many areas, funding for community mobility projects continues to be stable in the areas of transportation alternatives for older adults, individuals with disabilities, and veterans with disabilities, as well as pedestrian safety for children. In addition, the body of evidence in the area of driving and community mobility is still quite small relative to other practice areas, leaving an abundant field of scholarship opportunities for conducting research supporting evidence-based practice.

Clinical Fieldwork

Driving rehabilitation and community mobility are generally considered a specialty practice area and not suitable for newly graduated occupational therapists. With that in mind, it is unlikely that an entry-level student will complete a Level II fieldwork in a setting solely devoted to this practice area. However, this does not preclude students from completing specialty fieldwork or post-professional fieldwork or residency experiences in driving rehabilitation and community mobility. Both clinicians and fieldwork coordinators should keep these alternate clinical experiences in mind, as participation in such a specialized fieldwork will expand the professional development of the students and help alleviate the workforce shortage in this practice area. Therapists wishing to develop a fieldwork experience at their site should collaborate with fieldwork coordinators in academic programs nearby to establish expectations, curricula, assignments, and opportunities for students.

How Occupational Therapists Address Community Mobility

Therapists addressing community mobility in practice should follow procedures that are consistent with the process outlined in the *Framework–II* (AOTA, 2008) and *Standards of Practice for Occupational Therapy* (AOTA, 2010b). The *Framework–II* outlines three major categories in the occupational therapy process:

1. Evaluation that includes an occupational profile and analysis of occupational performance;
2. Intervention that includes an intervention plan, intervention implementation, and intervention review; and
3. Outcomes to determine success (AOTA, 2008).

Evaluation

Occupational therapists typically begin addressing community mobility by recognizing the possibility for occupational performance issues based on the client's diagnosis and community mobility needs for a client of a particular age and circumstance. Oftentimes, an occupational therapist will conduct a screening of the client, which involves "obtaining and reviewing data relevant to a potential client to determine the need for further evaluation and intervention" (AOTA, 2010b, p. S107). These screenings may be for clients who are already on the therapy caseload to determine whether they specifically need community mobility services, or they may be for clients who are not receiving services, such as children with special needs who will need to use transit services, older adults transitioning to driving retirement, or participants in CarFit who may need further performance evaluations or adjustments to their vehicles.

If it is determined that a client does need further evaluation or intervention and the therapist is not sufficiently skilled to provide those services, the therapist is ethically obligated to refer the client to another provider. That other provider may be an occupational therapist who specializes in driving rehabilitation or community mobility but also could be a psychologist, social worker, eye care specialist, physician, or transit agency. It is advisable to set up referral pathways and network with professionals and agencies that provide specialized services so that clients can have choices and make educated decisions. Tips and resources for establishing referral pathways can be found on AOTA's Web site, on the older-driver page (AOTA, n.d.).

Clients who need additional services as noted by a referral or on the basis of screening results will undergo an *evaluation*, which is the "process of obtaining and interpreting data necessary to intervention. This includes planning for and documenting the evaluation process and results" (AOTA, 2010b, p. S107). Occupational therapists conducting a community mobility evaluation should incorporate an occupational profile into the evaluation process (AOTA, 2008) to capture the presence, need, and desire of the client to be mobile in the community as well as to identify the occupational performance patterns of the client requiring community mobility to access the locations of participation.

The evaluation process continues with measures of client factors, performance skills, and contexts in which the client engages in community mobility to identify strengths and areas of need. Therapists are responsible for selecting the "specific tool or instruments that are used during the evaluation process" (AOTA, 2010b, p. S107). Some assessments used in the area of driving and community mobility are drawn from other practice areas and disciplines, while other assessments have been developed specifically for use in the practice area. Detailed information about these assessments is provided in Chapter 9.

Intervention

Ultimately, the intention of an evaluation is to develop an intervention plan and make appropriate recommendations to the client for safe participation in community mobility. Interventions in driving and community mobility involve "the process and skilled actions taken by occupational therapy practitioners in collaboration with the client to facilitate engagement in occupation related to health and participation" (AOTA, 2010b, p. S107). These interventions are specialized (AOTA, 2010a) and are focused on the community mobility needs of the client, depending on the age, health condition, mode or modes of travel, and context in which travel takes place.

The range of intervention services is broad, encompassing clients at the individual, organization, and population levels; the full spectrum of ages across the lifespan; and any mode of transportation. Examples of these services are identified in further detail in later chapters, as well as in the AOTA (2010a) official document on driving and community mobility (pp. S119–S123).

At the conclusion of a community mobility evaluation or during the intervention process, recommendations may be made related to the client's continued or future participation in community mobility or the provision of community mobility services. As with interventions, these recommendations are individualized to the client based on performance, community mobility needs or desires, and the community mobility context. Table 1.1 illustrates the categories of recommendations

Table 1.1. Recommendations in Community Mobility Services

Category of Recommendation	Role of Occupational Therapist
Appropriate modes of transportation	• Identification of paratransit services • Identification of type of child safety seat
Adaptation needs	• Prescription of adaptive equipment in a motor vehicle • Modification of buses and bus stops for accessibility
Modified performance suggestions	• Alternate contexts of travel (e.g., routes, time of day) • Use of supportive technology such as GPS
Driving cessation	• Transition to driving retirement
Future planning	• Reevaluation intervals to track performance for clients with progressive illnesses • Strategic planning for transit systems to enhance equipment, train staff, and build infrastructure

Note. GPS = global positioning system.

and examples of the role the occupational therapist plays in making those recommendations.

Consultation

Some of the occupational therapy services provided in the area of driving and community mobility are traditional in that they are administered directly to clients and follow the occupational therapy process (AOTA, 2008) using typical approaches as defined in the *Standards of Practice* (AOTA, 2010b). These services are described in further detail in later chapters. Other services are provided using consultation in a format that is oftentimes less direct, in an "interactive process of helping others, identifying and analyzing issues, and developing problem solving strategies to prevent current and future problems" (Jaffe & Epstein, 1992, p. 724).

Occupational therapists with more experience or recognized expertise in a topic area often seek to provide community mobility services through a consultation model. Consultation services are approached in very different ways, depending on the model of consultation being used and the needs of the client. Table 1.2 outlines the different models of consultation, definitions of each model, and examples of consultation in the area of community mobility.

Conclusion

Community mobility is an occupation enabler; it is within the scope of occupational therapy practice as an IADL and therefore should be attended to or addressed in all areas of practice. The beginning of the occupational therapy process includes an analysis of all aspects of a client's occupational performance; occupational therapists should explore community mobility as part of the evaluation process. It is critical, at this point in our profession's development, that all occupational therapists recognize the vital role of community mobility in a person's life and that therapists in all practice settings consider the community mobility needs of their clients. Driving, albeit an important and highly valued occupation in American society, is only one form of community mobility.

Table 1.2. Models of Consultation

Model	Definition	Examples in Community Mobility
Clinical	Client-focused, "case-specific consultation model based on the unique circumstances, with an emphasis on remediation and treatment" (Jaffe & Epstein, 1992, p. 723)	• Administering a behind-the-wheel assessment on a physically impaired client in an adapted van per referral from a driving rehabilitation practice that only owns a sedan • Performing a child safety seat check and adaptation for a parent with a physical impairment
Professional	Provision of expert advice based on specialized knowledge for the purpose of formulating a decision or plan	• Serving as an expert witness in a court case determining fitness-to-drive for a driver involved in a crash • Participating with a municipal planning board during the design phase of a community to advise about sidewalks, bicycle paths, and avoiding interaction of high-risk road users
Educational	"Information-centered ... focusing on enhancement of client knowledge and skills; utilizing in-service training, staff development, and dissemination of information" (Jaffe & Epstein, 1992, p. 725)	• Delivering an in-service to a pediatric clinic about bicycle helmet fittings for its clientele • Offering an educational program and sensitivity training for schedulers and transit operators about riders with cognitive deficits • Participating in a CarFit educational event
Organizational development	"Organization-centered, management-focused model ... emphasizing organizational structure, interrelationships, conflict resolution, and planned change" (Jaffe & Epstein, 1992, p. 728)	• Offering problem-solving strategies to alleviate conflicts between a paratransit provider and riders in the transportation disadvantaged community • Coordinating the transportation needs of students with special needs in a school system undergoing redistricting
Process management	"Group-based model ... focusing on specific management-oriented organizational processes and dynamics; intervention strategies emphasizing interpersonal and intergroup process, communication patterns, group roles and functions" (Jaffe & Epstein, 1992, p. 729)	• Coordinating a referral pathway system between a multi-unit hospital system and community providers to manage client community mobility needs • Collaborating with the state licensing agency about the revision of medical reporting processes and guidelines
Program development	"Service-centered model ... based on development of new programs or modification of existing programs to improve a service delivery system" (Jaffe & Epstein, 1992, p. 730)	• Collaborating with school personnel, parents, and community leaders to initiate a Safe Routes to School program • Consulting with a hospital to assist in the development of a new driving rehabilitation program

Table 1.2. Models of Consultation (*cont.*)

Model	Definition	Examples in Community Mobility
Social action	"Social-reform based model … focusing on social values and policies; action-oriented intervention strategies utilizing advocacy, and occasional confrontational approaches to effect change" (Jaffe & Epstein, 1992, p. 730)	• Working with lawmakers to implement regulations and a revenue stream to fund transportation resources for individuals with disabilities • Performing advocacy activities related to bicycle helmet use or the inclusion of bike paths on roadways
Systems	"Model … based on general systems theory focusing on the mission, goals, values, and culture of a system … or organization; utilizing planned change strategies to effect long range changes in the system" (Jaffe & Epstein, 1992, p. 731)	• Working with a transit agency to assist in meeting its organizational goals of access and inclusion • Providing support for strategic planning activities with safety organizations such as AAA or Safe Kids USA

Occupational therapists play a vital role in our society by addressing not only community mobility skills (including the role of driver) but also the underlying skills (visual, motor, cognitive) and the environmental and other contextual factors that enable and empower a person to participate in the community. Moreover, occupational therapists actively promote a healthy, overarching perspective of the importance of *occupation* in a person's life. Meaningful occupation is the core of a healthy lifestyle and the objective of valuable occupational therapy programs.

References

Accreditation Council for Occupational Therapy Education. (2007). Accreditation standards for a master's-degree-level educational program of the occupational therapist. *American Journal of Occupational Therapy, 61,* 652–661. doi:10.5014/ajot.61.6.652

American Occupational Therapy Association. (2008). Occupational therapy practice framework: Domain and process (2nd ed.). *American Journal of Occupational Therapy, 62,* 625–683. doi:10.5014/ajot.62.6.625

American Occupational Therapy Association. (2010a). Driving and community mobility. *American Journal of Occupational Therapy, 64,* S112–S124. doi:10.5014/ajot.2010.64S112

American Occupational Therapy Association. (2010b). Standards of practice for occupational therapy. *American Journal of Occupational Therapy, 64,* S106–S111. doi:10.5014/ajot.2010.64S106

American Occupational Therapy Association. (n.d.). *Setting up referral pathways.* Retrieved July 27, 2011, from http://www.aota.org/Older-Driver/Professionals/Toolkit/Professional/Referral-Pathways.aspx

Centers for Disease Control and Prevention. (2011). *Motor vehicle safety.* Retrieved March 10, 2011, from http://www.cdc.gov/motorvehiclesafety/index.html

Federal Highway Administration. (2010). *Safe routes to school.* Retrieved March 8, 2010, from http://safety.fhwa.dot.gov/saferoutes/

Healthy People. (2010). *Healthy People 2020 topics and objectives: Injury and violence prevention.* Retrieved March 10, 2011, from http://www.healthypeople.gov/2020/topics objectives2020/objectiveslist.aspx?topicid=24

Intelligent Transportation Systems Joint Program Office. (2012). *About ITS*. Retrieved January 22, 2012, from http://www.its.dot.gov/about.htm

Jaffe, E. G., & Epstein, C. F. (1992). *Occupational therapy consultation: Theory principles and practice*. St. Louis: Mosby.

Kellet, K., Shurgrue, N., Gruman, C., & Robison, J. (2010). Mental illness and long-term-care needs: Identifying the long-term-care needs of older and middle-aged adults with mental illness. *International Review of Modern Sociology, 36*(2), 143–168.

Ménard, I., & Korner-Bitensky, N. (2008). Fitness-to-drive in persons with psychiatric disorders and those using psychotropic medications. *Occupational Therapy in Mental Health, 24*(1), 47–64.

National Center for Safe Routes to School. (2011). *International walk to school in the USA*. Retrieved July 27, 2011, from http://www.walktoschool.org/index.cfm

Ottenbacher, K. J., Smith, P. M., Illig, S. B., Linn, R. T., Ostir, G. V., & Granger, C. V. (2004). Trends in length of stay, living setting, functional outcome, and mortality following medical rehabilitation. *JAMA, 292*, 1687–1695.

Rouleau, S., Mazer, B., & Ménard, I. (2010). A survey on driving in clients with mental health disorders. *Occupational Therapy in Mental Health, 26*(1), 85–95.

Safe Kids USA. (2007a). *Safe kids buckle up*. Retrieved October 3, 2007, from http://www.usa.safekids.org/tier2_rl.cfm?folder_id=3120

Safe Kids USA. (2007b). *Safe kids walk this way*. Retrieved October 3, 2007, from http://www.usa.safekids.org/tier2_rl.cfm?folder_id=3124

Safe Kids USA. (2009a). *Bicycling and skating safety*. Retrieved July 27, 2011, from http://www.safekids.org/safety-basics/safety-resources-by-risk-area/bicycling-and-skating/

Safe Kids USA. (2009b). *Car seats, booster, and seat belt safety: Fact sheet*. Retrieved March 11, 2011, from http://www.safekids.org/our-work/research/fact-sheets/car-seats-booster-and-belt-safety-fact-sheet.html

Stav, W. B. (2012). Developing and implementing driving rehabilitation programs: A phenomenological approach. *American Journal of Occupational Therapy, 66*(1), e11–e16. doi:10.5014/ajot.2012.000950

Stav, W. B., & Lieberman, D. (2008). From the Desk of the Editor. *American Journal of Occupational Therapy, 62*, 127–129. doi:10.5014/ajot.62.2.127

Stav, W. B., Snider Weidley, L., & Love, A. (2011). Barriers to developing and sustaining driving and community mobility programs. *American Journal of Occupational Therapy, 65*(4), e38–e45. doi:10.5014/ajot.2011.002097

Taylor, B., & Taylor, A. (1996). A way-finding perspective in mental health: Generating a sense of community among people with multiple handicapping conditions. *Psychiatric Rehabilitation Journal, 20*(2), 77–81.

World Health Organization. (2001). *International classification of functioning, disability and health (ICF)*. Geneva, Switzerland: World Health Organization.

Appendix 1.A. Community Mobility and Driving–Related Resources

- **Toolkit for Professionals:** http://www.aota.org/Older-Driver/Professionals/ CE/Toolkit/Professional.aspx
  The Toolkit for Professionals was developed as part of a cooperative agreement between AOTA and NHTSA. The toolkit contains numerous resources and templates for expanding programs and services that address driving and community mobility. Each resource (e.g., how to develop a brochure, conducting an educational seminar for varied audiences, how to estimate costs when proposing the development of a driving rehabilitation program) was developed by the recipients of the mini-grant funding.

- **Driving Rehabilitation Program Development Toolkit:** http://www.aota. org/Older-Driver/Professionals/CE/Toolkit/Programs.aspx
  The Driving Rehabilitation Program Toolkit housed on the AOTA Web site lists an ever-expanding array of resources and links. This portion of the Web site is available to both AOTA members and nonmembers. The term "toolkit" is used to reflect the varied resources that may be of interest to practitioners, physicians, families, and clients.

- **Safe Kids USA:** www.safekids.org
  Safe Kids USA is a nonprofit organization solely dedicated to eliminating preventable childhood injuries, the leading cause of death and disability to children. The Web site offers a range of resources and information including Safe Kids research and statistics, unintentional injury fact sheets, and position statements on critical injury risks.

- **International Walk to School Day:** http://www.iwalktoschool.org/
  If you are looking for a way to get involved in community mobility, consider Walk to School. The goal of the walk varies from community to community. Some walks rally for safer and improved streets, some promote healthier habits, and some advocate conserving the environment.

- **Safe Routes to School:** http://safety.fhwa.dot.gov/saferoutes/
  Safe Routes to Schools proactively supports walking to school with community-centered initiatives. Occupational therapy involvement may reach out to children with disabilities and special needs.

- **CarFit:** http://www.car-fit.org
  CarFit is a community education program that offers older adults the opportunity to see how well their personal vehicles "fit" them. The CarFit program also provides information and materials on community-specific resources that could enhance safety for drivers or increase their community mobility options.

- **Lifelong Driver:** www.lifelongdriver.com
  Lifelong Driver is a preventative intervention designed to extend the driving longevity of the well elderly. The program addresses visual and cognitive skills through video driving simulations that target the top 5 causes of older driver crashes.

- **Distracted Driving Information:** http://www.distraction.gov
  NHTSA's Web site on distracted driving includes many videos for instructing and educating occupational therapists, clients, or families.

- **Roadwise Review:** http://www.roadwisereview.com
  Roadwise Review is a free online screening tool developed by AAA to help
  seniors measure certain mental and physical abilities important for safe
  driving. The self-screen suggests that a second person act as an assistant.
  It can be completed within 30 minutes. Results are interpreted in relationship to driving and a summary results page can be printed.

CHAPTER 2

The Big Picture: Comprehensive Community Mobility Options

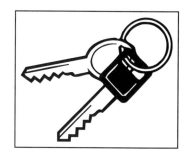

Jennifer L. Womack, MA, MS, OTR/L, SCDCM, and Nina M. Silverstein, PhD

Learning Objectives

At the completion of this chapter, readers will be able to

- Identify multiple forms of community mobility options used within the United States;
- Recognize ways to assess transportation options in local communities;
- Recognize specific legislation and policy relevant to community mobility;
- Describe the relationship between community mobility and life participation;
- Identify community mobility challenges specific to people with disabilities and age-related limitations;
- Determine specific strategies available to occupational therapists to address community mobility with clients;
- Determine local, regional, and national transportation and community mobility resources beneficial to occupational therapy clients;
- Identify opportunities for collaborative work with agencies, providers, and consumers to maximize community mobility options; and
- Select evaluation and intervention tools and methods to address comprehensive community mobility issues.

Key Words

- **commercial transportation**
- **community mobility**
- **eligibility**
- **liveability**
- **personal transportation**
- **public transportation**
- **supplemental transportation**
- **transportation culture**
- **travel instruction**
- **travel training**

Introduction

Although the majority of content in this publication addresses driving evaluation and rehabilitation, driving is only one element of the more comprehensive construct of community mobility that encompasses all the ways in which people move about their communities and the world. Driving rehabilitation has become a focus for occupational therapists as client needs and reimbursement mechanisms have provided fertile ground for the growth and financial viability of this practice area.

The bigger picture that must be considered, however, is how people move about their communities in multiple ways—the private automobile being only one of a number of transportation options for connecting with goods, services, vocations, and occupations outside the home.

Given the changing demographics of the United States, coupled with current environmental concerns and economic uncertainty, we assert that broadening the focus from driving rehabilitation toward a more comprehensive consideration of community mobility at the individual, community, and societal levels is necessary to fully serve occupational therapy clients and their family members. More importantly, this shift is essential to ensure that older adults with functional limitations; people with disabilities; and indeed all of us have safe, accessible, and viable options for moving about the communities in which we live, work, and play.

The *Occupational Therapy Practice Framework: Domain and Process, 2nd Edition* (*Framework–II;* American Occupational Therapy Association [AOTA], 2008a) categorizes *community mobility* as an instrumental activity of daily living (IADL) and provides the following definition: "moving around in the community and using public or private transportation, such as driving, walking, bicycling, or accessing and riding in buses, taxi cabs, or other transportation systems" (p. 631). Addressing the varied means of moving about the world and the fit between these means and clients' abilities not only will serve individual clients and their families but also will provide opportunities for occupational therapists to be engaged in a broader dialogue with transportation providers, health and human services agencies, and policy makers.

Community mobility represents connectedness to others, to goods and services, and to the occupations of everyday life (Marottoli et al., 2000; Vanderbur & Silverstein, 2006; Vine & Hamilton, 2005). For these reasons alone, holistically addressing community mobility and the relevant abilities of clients is not only an opportunity but a mandate for occupational therapists. Beyond the individual level of impact, however, the existence of safe, reliable means of community mobility also carries economic implications based on access to goods and services and affects social opportunities for civic engagement and participation in community life.

Furthermore, the urgency to reduce traffic congestion and, subsequently, negative effects on the environment is a particularly critical issue for those most in need of alternate transportation resources (Rosenbloom, 1993). In other words, populations that use public transportation with greater frequency also are disproportionately exposed to the ill effects of traffic congestion. Before exploring the specifics of these relationships, however, it is helpful to understand the context for community mobility in the United States.

Community Mobility in the United States: A Historical Perspective

People living in the United States use the passenger automobile as their primary means of transportation to an extent far greater than any other nation in the world (NationMaster.com, 2011). Although there are many advantages to travelers who either drive or ride in private automobiles, there are also environmental consequences and social and financial considerations. Those who do not drive, whether by choice or inability to do so, must be willing and able to pay for mobility options or rely on family and friends to transport them, particularly in situations in which there is poor access to public transportation. Limited financial resources or limited social connections may result in reduced mobility outside the home.

Reliance on the Passenger Automobile

How did this dominance of the passenger automobile take hold in the United States? At the end of the 19th century, several industrialized nations were involved in small-scale manufacturing of automobiles primarily based on the development of steam engine and electric technology (Hyde, 2006). Early on, the gasoline-powered engine emerged as the dominant form of production due in part to the discovery of large domestic oil deposits in the United States in the early 20th century (Flink, 1970). During the first three decades of the 20th century, ownership of automobiles, almost all of them gasoline powered, increased 50-fold (Flink, 1970).

Despite these rapid advancements in the automobile industry, private ownership of automobiles was still restricted to slightly more than half of U.S. citizens as late as 1950 (Hyde, 2006). The use of mass transit, particularly for transportation to and from work, was common in urban areas even into the 1950s, and multiple non-automotive transportation options (e.g., horses, walking) remained in use in rural areas during the same time period (Berger, 1979). Between 1950 and 1970, however, that scenario would drastically shift.

Transportation historians (Foster, 1981, 2003; St. Clair, 1986) have noted the alliance between automobile manufacturers and the oil industry in creating an increased desire for and reliance on the passenger car, effectively reducing the availability and efficiency of mass transit systems. Transportation funding priorities also shifted with passage of the Federal-Aid Highway Act of 1956 (P. L. 84-627; Federal Highway Administration, n.d.), which focused on building the interstate highway system. Subsequently, between 1950 and 1970, private automobile registrations more than doubled. The dominance of the private passenger car as the primary means of transportation within the United States was firmly entrenched at this point.

Decline of Mass Transit

Mass transit options—buses, trains, and subways—declined dramatically within the same time period and continued to decline until 1995, when the combination of an economic boom, stable transit fares, rising gasoline prices, and expansions in light rail transportation systems, particularly in dense urban areas, fueled a rebirth of public transportation (Pucher, 2002). The infrastructure for mass transit lags far behind that in place for automobile traffic, however, because of the earlier funding priorities. As of 2009, the American Public Transportation Association (APTA) reported modest increases in the use of public transportation each year since 2000, yet the private automobile remains the preferred mode of transportation for most Americans. For adults ages 65 or older in particular, the travel mode of the majority (89%) continues to be either as the driver or passenger in a private automobile (Coughlin & Cobb, 2000; ICF Consulting, 2006).

Sociocultural Considerations

The scientific and technological advances that led to the dominance of the private automobile are much easier to outline than are the sociocultural factors that allowed them to take root and flourish within U.S culture.

Consumerism and Success

Pellerito and Lysack (2006) noted the intertwined relationship of the automobile and consumerism in the United States, the former a hallmark of the development of technological ingenuity and the latter a celebration of the triumph of capitalism. The private automobile, initially a luxury afforded only by a wealthy minority, eventually came to be seen as a necessity for the average U.S. household and in that role symbolized economic success; not owning an automobile carries the cultural connotation of economic and, therefore, social inferiority (Pellerito & Lysack, 2006).

There is no doubt that the automobile symbolizes much that is revered as success and achievement in U.S. culture. Consider, for example, how often the automobile is associated with milestones in life: obtaining a driver's license, buying or receiving a first car to go to college or to work, buying the house with the two-car garage, fixing up classic cars, and—particularly pertinent to our discussion—driving retirement, which rather than an achievement often is considered the most poignant marker of decline in aging (Marottoli et al., 1997). Freund (2003) noted that the automobile is "the most popular form of transportation in history" (p. 68), so much so that using it for personal mobility comes to define our ability to be independent.

Individualism and Independence

Individualism and fierce independence have been touted as characteristics of U.S. culture, and the way in which people travel in the United States seems to affirm those concepts. According to the 2009 National Household Travel Survey, the majority of trips made across all persons in the United States occur in single-occupancy passenger cars, followed by high-occupancy passenger cars (2 or more passengers) as the second most common form of personal mobility, and public transit as a distant third (U.S. Department of Transportation, 2011). This is particularly true for older drivers, who conduct 45% of trips in single-occupancy vehicles (Pucher & Renne, 2003).

It is important to grasp the dominance of driving an automobile as the most accepted form of community mobility in the United States, because those who do not drive—whether due to disability, finances, functional losses related to aging, or choice—encounter consequences that affect their ability to easily and spontaneously participate in some aspects of life. Equally important, research is emerging that suggests that populations with a greater dependence on driving have greater rates of obesity and ill health effects related to more sedentary lifestyles (McCann & Ewing, 2003; Samimi, Mohammadian, & Madanizadeh, 2009).

Rural–Urban Divide and Poverty

One environmental characteristic that greatly defines transportation use not only in the United States but around the world is the rural–urban divide. In both developing and developed nations, those who reside in cities have more access to transportation options, both public and private, beyond the realm of the passenger car. In the United States, however, this divide is embedded in a cultural context in which wide-open spaces and the ability to privately own land is highly valued and associated with independence and freedom (Rome, 1998). As we entered the new millennium, 49% of Americans lacked access to public transportation, and 41% of rural counties did not have public transportation at all (Bailey, 2004).

The migration away from urban living to suburban fringes and rural spaces has continued for most of the past half-century. For older Americans in particular, the move away from city centers—referred to as the "graying" of the suburbs (Leslie, 2011)—creates a potential conflict between the desire to age in place and more limited access to transportation options (Rosenbloom, 2005). One cannot assume, however, that access to public transit equates to use of public transit; on the contrary, although multiple researchers have indicated that public transportation is not a common, or at times appropriate, choice for older adults who do not drive (Bailey, 2004; Crabtree, Troyer, & Justiss, 2009; U.S. Department of Transportation, 2011), there appear to be two specific populations that do use public transportation with a greater frequency: (1) persons with disabilities and (2) older minority adults who have lower incomes. Latino and African-American older adults are more than twice as likely to use public transportation than White, non-Hispanic older adults (Bailey, 2004), and the typical profile of a public transportation user as presented by Rosenbloom (2005) is older, female, a city-center dweller, and poor.

Why public transportation in the United States has been relegated to a status of being only for the poor is socially complex and beyond the scope of this chapter, but this assumption is reflected in the transportation choices of more well-to-do older adults as they transition through driving retirement. Sources have stated that only 1%–2.5% of trips taken by older adults are based on public transportation use (Collia, Sharp, & Giesbrecht, 2003; Rosenbloom, 2005), and those trips are heavily skewed toward poorer inner-city residents. Without transportation policy that recognizes this disparity, Rosenbloom (2005) argued that women in particular—and poor women of color specifically—will bear an inordinate burden of transportation dependence as they age (p. 3).

The rural context is not alone in affecting access to and feasibility of safe and sustainable transportation options beyond the private automobile. Urban areas, while traditionally offering more public transportation options and pedestrian-friendly contexts, can present challenges for travelers with functional limitations in terms of unsafe or inaccessible walking areas, congested streets and transit systems, and built environments that sometimes preference high-density commercial development over traveler-friendly design (Clarke, Ailshire, & Lantz, 2009). In recent decades, urban planning has extended to regional planning, and the concepts of *livability, walkability,* and *smart growth* have interwoven aspects of health promotion with the built environment and landscape design (Florida Department of Transportation, 1995; Sandt et al., 2008; U.S. Department of Transportation, 2010). These concepts related to land use and the built environment are important for occupational therapists to understand and will be revisited in a later section.

Disability Legislation and Policies

Within the past two decades, legislation and policies have been enacted in the United States that affect the design, accessibility, and affordability of transportation for people with disabilities, those who earn lower incomes, and older adults. Historical legislation has contributed to the recognition that older adults and persons with disabilities should have alternatives to institutional care.

The Supreme Court decision from the case of *Olmstead v. L.C.* (1999) was influential in enforcing that older adults and persons with disabilities should be served in the most integrated and least restrictive settings possible that comply with the Americans with Disabilities Act of 1990 (ADA, P. L. 101-336; Kaiser Commission on Medicaid and the Uninsured, 2004; Keigher, 2006). ADA is a comprehensive civil rights law that protects Americans with disabilities, and states are required to comply with ADA by providing services in community-based settings when possible (Keigher, 2006).

Access to appropriate and affordable transportation is a key factor in enabling individuals to be maintained in "the most integrated and least restrictive" settings. Specific transportation-related mandates set in motion by ADA will be examined in more detail in a later section.

Transportation Culture

Several realities pertinent to community mobility become evident for travelers in the United States:

- Reliance on transportation via any means other than a private automobile is uncommon in all but the most urban environments;
- Public transit options, despite legislation such as ADA, are primarily geared toward fixed-route systems that are less accommodating to people with functional limitations; and
- The breadth of geographic space creates challenges for operational efficiency and financial solvency of transportation systems.

The opportunity is ripe for a *transportation culture* to emerge that situates options other than the private automobile as equally desirable and accessible forms of community mobility.

Given current economic and environmental circumstances, the opportunity is ripe, however, for a *transportation culture* to emerge that situates options other than the private automobile as equally desirable and accessible forms of community mobility.

Economics of Community Mobility

Economic issues associated with community mobility are of interest for three reasons:

1. The potential economic stimulus provided by the availability of comprehensive public transportation options to consumers,
2. The financial challenges encountered in managing and expanding accessible transportation options, and
3. The economic disparities evident in public transportation–user demographics.

The economic impact of investment in public transportation occurs through expenditures of funds on the creation, maintenance, and operation of public transportation infrastructure and services as well as through contributions to overall economic growth by providing access for consumers to goods and services (APTA, 2009). Using a formula in which current expenditures on public transportation and the resultant economic activity are projected a decade into the future, researchers working on behalf of APTA noted a potential cost savings to taxpayers if funding for transportation were to shift from private investment in automobiles to increased public funding for mass transit options. Presenting two economic scenarios—one in which the investment in, and use of, public transportation continues at the same rate of growth as in the past decade (2.4%; APTA, 2009, p. 56), and a second in which ridership and public investment are doubled—the authors estimated that the latter scenario would result in greater household savings, an increase in the gross domestic product that outpaces tax increases needed to build infrastructure, and hundreds of thousands of jobs added in the public transportation sector.

While the authors of the APTA study specifically cautioned that they were not attempting to address broader, non-economic impacts, they did propose that more widespread societal benefits such as equitable access to health care and services, improved air quality, and reduced dependence on fossil fuels may parallel the economic benefits (APTA, 2009, p. 60). Despite this compelling evidence regarding the potential economic benefits of an expanded public transportation system, the current situation of public transportation provision is one of tough economic realities. APTA (2010) noted that nationwide, public transportation providers are consolidating routes, cutting staff hours, and trying to determine how to continue providing effective paratransit services while contending with rising fuel and vehicle maintenance costs. Many systems are facing the need to increase fares, a situation that will disproportionately affect those most in need of affordable transportation options.

Social Impact of Community Mobility

Occupational therapists typically are most aware of the challenges of community mobility for individuals and their families experiencing disabling conditions or functional losses because of aging. The rates of social isolation and depression experienced by seniors who transition through driving cessation are well documented (Fonda, Wallace, & Herzog, 2001; Marottoli et al., 1997; Ragland, Satariano, & MacLeod, 2005; Taubman-Ben-Ari, Mikulincer, & Gillath, 2004) and widely discussed in professional materials and clinical practice settings serving older adults.

Studies addressing the use of public transportation by younger persons with disabilities tend to focus on models or programs designed around paratransit use, travel training, or individualized approaches to promote community reintegration (Denson, 2000; Shaw, 2000; Sohlberg, Fickas, Lemoncello, & Hung, 2009) rather than on social aspects of transportation use, such as achieving desired destinations or social connectedness. Although there is anecdotal evidence to suggest that community mobility is addressed with younger clients, particularly as they transition to community living or work roles, literature within occupational therapy related to comprehensive community mobility is relatively scarce (Stav, 2008). Understanding the social impact of transportation availability for all potential clients necessitates that we go beyond thinking about the functional logistics of access to considering ways in which public policy, personal choice, and civic engagement are intertwined with the ability to travel.

Personal Choice and Transportation

Many clinicians who work with clients facing driving cessation can recount stories of individuals who report that despite the availability of transportation options, the ability to travel when they choose and with the means they choose is less than optimal. Personal choice is a highly valued commodity in U.S. society, and the independence and spontaneity of travel offered by the personal automobile are unparalleled. It is plausible that one major reason why public transportation is not heavily used in this country is because of its inability to replicate these characteristics. To conduct publicly funded transportation options in a cost-effective manner, some form of moving multiple people simultaneously is necessary. Even in paratransit systems designed to serve riders with functional limitations, the need to combine destinations and passengers results in advanced scheduling, shared rides, and potentially long waits for pickup.

Experts working in transportation research and development acknowledge the need to address community mobility shortcomings. Joseph Coughlin, director of the Massachusetts Institute of Technlology AgeLab, often refers to "the ice cream cone test" as a true test of a good transportation system (Coughlin, 2007). Simply stated, if it is a hot summer's night and someone decides she would like a chocolate ice cream cone at 7:00 p.m., can she get to the ice cream shop and back? Coughlin's point is that we don't typically call 2 days in advance for that ice cream cone, we would rarely find a bus that runs late enough for a round trip to the ice cream store, and we can't be assured that there would be a pedestrian path with sufficient lighting and places to rest to encourage walking.

Helen Kerschner, president of the Beverly Foundation, has her own version of the ice cream cone test. For Kerschner, a true test of a good transportation program is one that will get you to the hairdresser (Kerschner, 2003). Kerschner believes that quality-of-life trips, such as going to the hairdresser, deserve as much consideration in maintaining a healthy lifestyle as do trips to medical appointments, grocery stores, and faith communities.

Individuals who can access fixed-route public transportation may carry out quality-of-life trips successfully during the hours that the system operates, but those who need to travel outside those times or those who cannot access fixed-route systems often benefit more from other types of transportation programs, such as those staffed by volunteer drivers. These programs provide the supportive assistance that many paid driver programs do not, and as such, they fill important roles in supplemental transportation programs for seniors. Characteristics of these types of programs will be covered in the "Terminology, Concepts, and Resources in Community Mobility" section of this chapter.

Employment, Civic Engagement, and Transportation

In 1996, Congress enacted the Personal Responsibility and Work Opportunity Reconciliation Act (P. L. 104-93) that created a system of time-limited benefits and work requirements. This led to an urgency of finding work within quickly approaching deadlines and raised the consciousness of many to the institutional barriers and emotional challenges that unemployed people face, with transportation as one of those major challenges. The U.S. Department of Transportation's

Joblinks program underscored the importance of transportation to successful welfare-to-work initiatives. When Congress enacted the 1998 Transportation Equity Act for the 21st Century (P. L. 105-178)—a $217 billion transportation bill—it included up to $750 million over 5 years for the Job Access and Reverse Commute competitive grant program (Community Transportation Association of America, 2010).

The Safe, Accountable, Flexible, Efficient Transportation Equity Act (P. L. 109-59) was signed into law in 2005 and includes acknowledgment of the role of state and local transportation decision makers in bringing attention to safety concerns related to individual users of different transportation modes. Specific areas of safety concerns (relevant to occupational therapists) include older drivers, pedestrians, children walking to school, bicycle safety, and motorcycle safety. Metropolitan and statewide planning processes must include safety and security and represent tribal, bicycle, pedestrian, and disabled interests (Federal Highway Administration, n.d.).

Although travel for employment or carrying out daily routines is considered a necessity, and travel for reasons that enhance quality of life is advocated by transportation experts, travel for the purpose of engaging in community life warrants equal attention. Civic engagement connotes ways in which individuals contribute to their communities, and it includes a variety of activities such as political activity, religious activity, social activism, and volunteerism. Beyond the ability to travel for means of personal necessity or benefit, the ability to travel for civic engagement ensures that individuals can contribute to the maintenance and well-being of others through organizational, systemic, or personal outreach.

Occupational therapists often consider how a specific individual with specific functional limitations can interface with personal or public transportation vehicles and services to reach destinations relevant to the maintenance of that client's life. What might be equally important is the opportunity to connect with, and give back to, one's broader community that is inherent in the ability to access transportation.

Hammel (2007) and Boschen, Tonack, and Gargaro (2003) have offered examples from research with individuals with spinal cord injury (SCI) who report a strong desire to live productive and connected lives, not only within the context of employment but also in the context of multiple community roles. Hammel's (2007) meta-synthesis of research related to quality of life after SCI concludes with the statement that people with SCI want "to be busy . . . to give back . . . to participate and be involved in meaningful roles" (p. 131); this, coupled with the finding by Lysack, Komanecky, Kabel, Cross, and Neufeld (2007) that transportation is one of the top three barriers to community reintegration for people with SCI, serves as examples reinforcing the need for health and human services providers to address the importance of access to transportation for purposes of community engagement.

Building on this foundation that outlines a broad scope of community mobility and the relationships between access to transportation and personal, economic, and social well-being, the next section of this chapter offers a comprehensive overview of various forms of community mobility and related resources. The occupational therapist is encouraged to develop familiarity with current concepts related to public transportation and personal mobility options before moving to the final section of the chapter addressing clinical assessment and intervention.

Terminology, Concepts, and Resources in Community Mobility

So what are we referring to when discussing various forms of community mobility? What options do our clients have when considering how to travel beyond their own home? What dictates the availability, cost, and accessibility of transportation options? The *Framework–II* (AOTA, 2008a) definition of community mobility encompasses private and commercial automobiles, walking, and using public transit, but it also mentions "other transportation systems." This section addresses public, volunteer, and private transportation options; personal mobility; and related resources.

Public Transportation

Public transportation, according to APTA (2010), consists of at least a dozen forms of travel that move more than one person at a time between locations and represents those services operated at least, in part, through taxpayer funding and available to all citizens of a specified geographic area. APTA members include organizations and businesses involved in the planning, design, construction, and operation of public transportation systems classified in the following categories: bus, paratransit, light rail, high-speed rail, commuter rail, subways, and waterborne passenger services (APTA, 2010). Within these categories, only those systems operated in whole or part with public funding constitute *public* transportation; transportation services that operate as private businesses do not fall into this category. This distinction is important for understanding which types of transportation systems are mandated by law to provide accessible options for persons with functional limitations.

Title II–Part B of ADA mandates that public transit providers offering fixed-route services also must offer parallel services (paratransit) for those individuals who live within the service provision area but have functional limitations preventing use of the fixed-route system (U.S. Department of Transportation, 1991). The paratransit system must be accessible to wheelchair users, and new vehicles purchased within the fixed-route system following passage of ADA also must have the capability to transport wheelchairs. The cost of each paratransit trip cannot exceed twice the cost of a standard fixed-route trip for the user.

Since passage of ADA (1990), transit providers have implemented various methods for complying with the law, launching smaller bus systems, using existing taxi services, managing fleets of vans and shuttles, and developing eligibility determination procedures to ensure that limited financial resources are allocated to those most in need of paratransit services (Denson, 2000; Griffin & Priddy, 2005; Rosenbloom, 2005). Implementation of aspects of ADA relative to transportation falls under the mandate of the U.S. Department of Transportation, which also manages formula grants and capital investments (Vanderbur & Silverstein, 2006).

The U.S. Department of Health and Human Services is responsible for allocating and overseeing funding for a different aspect of subsidized transportation: Medicaid benefits for those who need transportation for health care and life maintenance but cannot afford to pay for it (Vanderbur & Silverstein, 2006). Although eligibility for these benefits is based on socioeconomic status, persons with disabilities are disproportionately represented among Medicaid beneficiaries and in that circumstance may qualify for transportation assistance under related guidelines.

Public transportation systems, then, are designed to be available to all members of a community within a specified service area, and they are mandated to provide paratransit for those who are functionally unable to access usual fixed-route services. These paratransit options typically offer somewhat more flexible travel times, use vehicles that are equipped to more readily accommodate mobility limitations, and have operators specifically trained to assist passengers with disabilities.

However, paratransit services have some limitations. Most transit systems require advance reservations—often 24 hours or more—and restrictions on the amount of assistance vehicle operators can provide are common. For example, operators cannot routinely assist a rider from the door of his or her residence to the vehicle (door-to-door), but they can provide assistance to the rider using a mobility device to board and disembark from the vehicle. These services operate on a curb-to-curb basis; that is, the individual must be able to meet the transit at the curb without assistance. In addition, transit systems may prioritize uses of paratransit based on funding for the system; many paratransit systems offer unlimited rides for medical appointments and grocery shopping but do not prioritize travel for other reasons.

Other Transportation Options

Supplemental Transportation Providers

The term *supplemental transportation* typically refers to services accessed by clients who are eligible for Medicaid or Medicare waivers for transportation, and it most often relates to non-emergency medical transportation or other transportation deemed necessary for health and well-being (Council on Aging of Southwestern Ohio, 2009). These programs are administered by departments of health and human services at the city or county levels throughout the country, and the actual transportation providers, which may include commercial taxi or van companies, are determined by contractual agreements with those entities.

Used in a more specific way, the term *Supplemental Transportation Programs (STPs)* for seniors is used to connote transportation systems designed to serve older adults and people with disabilities who cannot access other existing transportation options. The term refers to community-based options set up as complements to or in the absence of existing transportation systems (Beverly Foundation, 2004). The Beverly Foundation (2004), working in conjunction with the AAA Foundation for Traffic Safety to understand the scope and purpose of STPs, identified characteristics of programs across the United States that shared the goal of serving the transportation needs of older adults (see Exhibit 2.1).

The Beverly Foundation has been instrumental in advancing the cause of dignified and accessible transportation for older Americans. Originally a foundation focused on health policy and research, it has for more than a decade addressed transportation issues relative to older adults, and it is considered the pioneer in researching and documenting supplemental transportation programs for seniors (Beverly Foundation, 2009). Because of its extensive work in this area, concepts initiated by the Beverly Foundation have set the tone for other entities working on community mobility issues. Among these concepts is a set of principles—"Five A's of Senior-Friendly Transportation" (Exhibit 2.2)—outlining characteristics of transportation programs that are essential for them to be considered adequate providers of transportation for seniors (Beverly Foundation, 2002).

Exhibit 2.1. Characteristics of Supplemental Transportation Programs

- Sponsored by a variety of agencies or organizations for a variety of reasons
- Tend to have low or no cost to the rider
- Do not limit rides based on trip destination; quality-of-life trips are considered equal to life-essentials trips
- Most offer door-to-door or door-through-door service, meaning that riders can receive assistance to exit their home and access the vehicle
- Most rely on some grant funding but also have revenue from other sources, including governmental sources, civic organizations, and private donations
- Some rely on volunteer drivers, while others have a paid staff or mix of personnel relative to other transportation providers
- Serve more adults over the age of 85
- Many use personal automobiles as their vehicle fleet, but others have mixed fleets including larger vehicles.

Note. Beverly Foundation (2004).

Many agencies and researchers are concerned with senior transportation issues because of the compelling evidence indicating changes in health and quality of life following driving retirement. A lifespan perspective on community mobility also necessitates attention, however, to other aspects of community mobility relevant to other age groups: (1) to children, who are dependent on others for motorized transportation, and (2) to adults with disabilities, who may require adaptations to typical forms of mobility.

One type of transportation common to most children in the United States is the school bus, which is a hybrid between public transportation and a supplemental transportation program. Like the former, it is taxpayer funded and available to all riders in a specific area; more like the latter, it is operated free of charge to the rider and uses different vehicles to meet different needs. The National Highway Transportation Safety Administration administers the regulations for school-based transportation, which are then carried out at the state level. Although a complete overview of school bus mobility issues is beyond the scope of this chapter, various occupational therapy authors have advocated for the involvement of practitioners in school bus safety at both individual and policy levels (Loveland, 2009; Shutrump, Manary, & Buning, 2008; Stav, 2009).

 As a national coalition of organizations working to prevent unintentional childhood injury, **Safe Kids USA** is a nonprofit entity with chapters in all 50 states that addresses, among other things, community mobility. Safe Kids maintains

---

Exhibit 2.2. Five A's of Senior-Friendly Transportation

1. *Availability*—transportation exists and is available when needed (including evenings or weekends)
2. *Accessibility*—transportation can be reached and used (e.g., bus stairs can be negotiated, bus seats are high enough, vans come to door, bus stops are reachable)
3. *Acceptability*—refers to conditions such as cleanliness (the bus is not dirty), safety (bus stops are in safe areas), and user-friendliness (operators are courteous and helpful)
4. *Affordability*—refers to cost of transportation (e.g., fees are less than or comparable to driving a car, vouchers or coupons help offset costs)
5. *Adaptability*—transportation can be modified or adapted to meet special needs (e.g., trip chaining is possible, wheelchairs can be accommodated).

Note. Beverly Foundation (2002).

information on research, policy, and safety statistics relevant to childhood mobility, and it also provides car seats to needy families, monitors product safety, and conducts initiatives focused on pedestrian and bicycle safety (see **Appendix 2.A** for a list of community mobility resources). These community mobility options will be revisited in a later section on personal mobility options.

Commercial Transportation Providers

Commercial transportation, unlike public or supplemental transportation systems, is operated under a business model for profit making. *Commercial transportation* refers to services, for which people pay privately, that provide ways to move about in the world. These may be private transportation systems (e.g., bus line, airline company) or transportation systems for hire that operate on either a common carrier or contractual basis (e.g., taxis; Garber & Hoel, 2009). What is typical of commercial transportation systems is that the safety and integrity (and in some instances, the accessibility) of the vehicles they operate are subject to regulation by the U.S. Department of Transportation, but the service provision is typically not regulated by any outside agency (Garber & Hoel, 2009, p. 48).

The manner in which commercial transportation is operated may or may not be conducive to use by customers with special needs; commercial operators sometimes orient their business, however, toward service to customers who cannot easily use public transportation. Larger entities that are more heavily regulated by subsidiaries of the U.S. Department of Transportation (e.g., airlines regulated by the Federal Aviation Administration) must follow federal guidelines for accessibility, while smaller providers (e.g., taxi companies, private livery services) do not have the same mandate but may choose to use accessible vehicles for various reasons.

In many public transit systems, existing private companies are contracted to provide all or part of the paratransit services because of the relative savings realized in using an existing fleet of vehicles (Burkhardt, 2010). In these cases, the taxis must be accessible for use as stipulated by ADA. In other instances, disability rights groups have successfully advocated for accessible vehicles to be included in taxi fleets (Perez, 2008) or argued that taxi companies and similar private transportation should be mandated under Title III of ADA (public accommodations) to meet the standards described for other transportation providers. In both situations, advocates argue that private transportation options offer independence and spontaneity in travel for persons with disabilities and older adults that have not yet been realized by public transportation entities (Perez, 2008).

Personal Transportation Options

Personal transportation refers to ways in which individuals move about in the world, using either their own bodily capacity or nonvehicular transportation technology. Within this category fit walking, biking, skiing, running, skating, and use of a wheelchair, Segway,™ scooter, skateboard, golf cart, or other personal device. Note that in clinical situations, a distinction is typically drawn between using these devices for leisure versus using them for transportation purposes.

In the realm of transportation devices, manufacturers must meet safety standards and provide user instructions, but users are at liberty to use the devices as they see fit. Although adapting personal mobility devices for specific needs might invalidate product warranties, many personal transportation users with disabilities are finding individuals or companies willing to customize products to fit their needs. Several national organizations engage in advocacy or provide resource information relative to this topic. The **National Complete Streets Coalition, National AMBUCS™ Inc.,** and **AmericaWalks** are examples of nonprofit entities that provide information useful to occupational therapy clients and are included in the list of resources in Appendix 2.A.

The National Complete Streets Coalition is a network of organizations interested in safe mobility that seeks to transform the way streets and roads are designed in the United States to incorporate universal access. The coalition maintains federal policy updates, publishes a periodic newsletter, and advocates for changes in design practices that benefit all users. In the realm of personal mobility, it addresses not only pedestrian issues but also bicycling, the use of scooters and wheelchairs, and the intersection of these users with vehicular traffic.

National AMBUCS Inc. is a nonprofit organization dedicated to creating mobility and independence for persons with disabilities. AMBUCS has been integrally involved with occupational therapists for many years through an adapted cycling program called AmTrykes.™ AmTrykes are therapeutic tricycles, typically provided free to the user, that can be operated with either hands or feet and are designed for persons of all sizes and ages. Beyond this specific project, AMBUCS also is involved in ramp-building and playground accessibility projects nationwide as part of the overall emphasis on mobility and inclusion.

An organization with a focus on pedestrian rights, AmericaWalks is a nonprofit coalition of local advocacy groups promoting walkability (a concept that will be more fully discussed in the next section). In its declaration of pedestrian rights, AmericaWalks states that the definition of *pedestrian* includes wheelchair users and anyone who uses a mobility aid. In conjunction with the National Safe Routes to School organization, AmericaWalks sponsors Webinars designed to educate parents, professionals, and other interested parties in ways to advocate for safe and accessible pedestrian pathways for users of all ages and abilities. A specific concern regarding safe walking routes for school-age children is that pedestrian injury is the second leading cause of accidental death for children ages 5 to 14 years in the United States (Safe Kids Worldwide, 2009).

The above-mentioned organizations can help occupational therapists understand and develop the skills to address personal transportation safety with clients. As with all other areas considered in this chapter, *client* may refer to an individual, an organization, or a system. In the case of personal mobility, for example, the occupational therapist may work with an older adult who wishes to address walking safety, a parent group concerned with cycling accessibility for their children with special needs, or a community designing a new walking route throughout the area.

Matching the Abilities of the User to Transportation Options

It is not enough to assume that if someone is a nondriver, he or she will be able to access public transportation; it is also inaccurate to assume that if someone cannot walk, he or she will be able to use wheeled transportation. Each person's capabilities will intersect in different ways with various mobility options, and being involved in assessing and helping to create a fit that maximizes participation falls within the expertise of the occupational therapist. Three examples of user–transportation fit will be outlined in this section: determining eligibility for paratransit use, carrying out travel training or travel instruction, and assessing environmental factors.

Paratransit Eligibility

Implementation of ADA by public transportation providers included provisions for granting conditional, or trip-by-trip, eligibility to paratransit users (U.S. Department of Transportation, 1991). This type of eligibility indicates that the user may at times require the use of a paratransit vehicle but at other times can use the fixed-route system. For example, a user with multiple sclerosis whose mobility is affected by extreme heat may be deemed eligible to use paratransit only when the outside temperature exceeds a specified level. Because the use of paratransit services is more expensive for the transit provider, the eligibility determination process necessitates a fair and standard means of determining when paratransit—rather than fixed-route service—should be used.

Conditional eligibility refers to people who have inconsistent functional capacities because of a disabling condition or for whom environmental conditions may present barriers at certain times or in certain locations but not others. For example, a person with a disability affecting higher-level cognitive functions may be able to use fixed-route transportation for familiar routes but be eligible for paratransit when traveling novel routes. The eligibility determination process as outlined by ADA may consist of any or all of the following: an interview, certification by a professional, and a performance assessment of those functions relevant to using public transportation (Transit Access Project, n.d.). Functional performance assessments typically include physical, visual, and cognitive aspects of using transportation and also may include consideration of other functional limitations as presented by the applicant.

ADA stipulates that a transit system must have an eligibility determination and appeals procedures. These documents must be available to users in accessible formats. Within those parameters, however, transit systems can establish their own methods of eligibility determination, and the practices have historically varied widely (Transportation Research Board, 1998). The partner concept to trip-by-trip eligibility is that transit systems also are encouraged to provide training to transition riders from paratransit to fixed-route use, particularly for frequently traveled routes.

Travel Training and Travel Instruction

The terms *travel training* and *travel instruction* have both specific and general uses within the lexicon of language related to community mobility. In specific use, they refer to the process of educating people with disabilities to used fixed-route public transportation (Easter Seals Project Action, n.d.). The two terms often are used interchangeably, but Project Action, an Easter Seals initiative funded by the U.S. Department of Transportation to promote cooperation between the transportation and disability communities, specifies *travel instruction* as serving people with disabilities other than blindness or visual impairment, while *travel training* is the more inclusive

Being involved in assessing and helping to create a fit that maximizes participation falls within the expertise of the occupational therapist.

term. Used generally, these terms also apply to initiatives to introduce a broad array of travel options to all citizens, not just those with disabilities or functional limitations because of aging.

Travel training and instruction offered by public transportation providers must be specific to the user's needs and cannot be mandated. For example, if a rider has been determined to be eligible for paratransit and is offered but refuses travel training, he or she cannot be coerced to accept the training or denied paratransit services because of the refusal. Although professionals providing travel training to those with blindness or visual impairment often receive highly specialized education in teaching orientation and mobility skills, the basic academic competencies outlined by Easter Seals Project Action (n.d.) for travel training and instruction relative to users are more than met in occupational therapy educational programs. What occupational therapists more often lack is the knowledge of transportation systems and the legal and ethical issues surrounding mobility instruction. To provide education regarding these issues, Easter Seals Project Action offers numerous online and on-site courses (see Appendix 2.A).

Environmental Considerations

Most theoretical foundations of occupational therapy include a consideration of environment or context. It is well understood within the profession that disability does not exist within a person but lies in the transaction among person, action, and context (Brown, 2009; Dickie, Cutchin, & Humphry, 2006). Application of this theoretical orientation is easily achieved in regards to community mobility: Any consideration of the ability for people to move about in the world necessitates attention to not only the person's capacity for movement but also the desired destination and the context in which the mobility is enacted. The natural and built environments in which people travel are at the forefront of contextual considerations, yet equally important are mobility technologies and social support. The preceding sections have focused on capabilities of the traveler and systems or technologies by which travel occurs. Two additional concepts related specifically to the built environment warrant attention here: walkability and livability.

Walkability is a concept emerging from the disciplines of urban planning and environmental engineering (Muraleetharan, Takeo, Toru, Seiichi, & Ken'etsu, 2004), and although it has been defined in various ways, it is most simply described by Abley (2005) as "the extent to which the built environment is walking friendly" (p. 2). Technical audits of community walkability are common within urban planning and landscape design (Abley, 2005), but there are also tools in the public domain that are listed in Appendix 2.A under "Environmental Audits."

A broader concept, but one inclusive of walkability, is *livability*, or the extent to which a community fulfills 6 core principles (National Council on Disability, 2006):

1. Provides affordable, appropriate, accessible housing
2. Ensures accessible, affordable, reliable, safe transportation
3. Adjusts the physical environment for inclusiveness and accessibility
4. Provides work, volunteer, and education opportunities
5. Ensures access to key health and support services
6. Encourages participation in civic, cultural, social, and recreational activities.

In other words, a livable community strives to enable maximal participation of all dwellers regardless of age or abilities. Livability audits seek to understand how fully a community fulfills that mission by assessing the six characteristics listed.

The Public Policy Institute of the AARP has been a leader in operationalizing livability relative to older adults through the publication and free distribution of two editions of livability evaluation guides (AARP, 2004; see the link to ***Livable Communities: An Evaluation Guide*** in Appendix 2.A). These comprehensive community surveys encompass checklists about transportation options, walkability, drivability, safety and security, recreation opportunities, and shopping. The checklists provide a helpful exercise for occupational therapy students and professionals to observe their communities from the perspectives of their clients (Silverstein, Johns, & Griffin, 2008).

Community Mobility and Occupational Therapy

Role of the Occupational Therapist

The role of a driving rehabilitation specialist has achieved recognition as a practice area with specifically identified skills and credentials within occupational therapy, but specialization in comprehensive community mobility has not been circumscribed in quite the same way. Despite the inclusion of community mobility in the *Framework–II* (AOTA, 2008a), it is rare to find occupational therapy assessment tools that address community mobility in a comprehensive way. Inquiries related to community mobility are often limited to driving and walking status, and they fail to address the availability of transportation resources and the congruence of those resources with the financial, social, and personal factors of the client.

Acknowledging the challenge of a shift in emphasis in our clinical settings from personal mobility and driving to approaches that are more inclusive of a broad array of community mobility options, we propose 10 priorities for occupational therapists to embark upon (Exhibit 2.3). These priorities range from actions that can be taken within individual clinical practice settings to awareness of local, state, and national policies and resources.

Priority 1: Understand the official position of your professional association regarding community mobility and the resources available about this topic.

As stated at the beginning of this chapter, AOTA (2008a) firmly situates community mobility as an area of occupational performance to be addressed by occupational therapists. The occupation of driving and the practice of driving rehabilitation have, in particular, benefited from the resources of our professional organization over the past decade in the form of a dedicated staff person, Web and print resources, and professional advocacy relevant to this arena. There have been several national conference institutes and multiple continuing education offerings sponsored on this topic.

Although driving rehabilitation continues to be the realm of personal transportation most associated with clinical practice options, AOTA gradually has expanded activities and resources relevant to other forms of community mobility as well. Between 2000 and 2010, 23 articles or official documents that included content about a breadth of community mobility issues have appeared in the *American*

Exhibit 2.3. Top 10 Priorities for Addressing Community Mobility as an Occupational Therapist

Role of the occupational therapist

- *Priority 1:* Understand the official position of your professional association regarding community mobility and the resources available about this topic.

Broadening the concept of community mobility within clinical practice

- *Priority 2:* Include community mobility in initial evaluations and documentation of treatment planning.
- *Priority 3:* Include either actual or simulated practice in using community mobility options within intervention plans for all clients.
- *Priority 4:* Maintain a resource library about community mobility options relative to the area in which your client population lives and travels, and keep information updated.
- *Priority 5:* Work with clients to develop a broad array of travel options, regardless of their current driving status.

Becoming a community mobility advocate: action at the local to state level

- *Priority 6:* Join or establish a network of health and human services and transit providers in your geographic area to share concerns and knowledge about community mobility.
- *Priority 7:* Develop awareness of local human services agencies and state-level or governmental organizations that may provide funding or actual mechanisms for travel.
- *Priority 8:* Volunteer or consult professionally with transportation providers to understand the fit between the abilities of individuals and the transportation context.

Developing awareness of national-level transportation advocacy efforts

- *Priority 9:* Bolster your knowledge of national-level organizations that provide training and resources and lead advocacy and policy efforts related to community mobility.
- *Priority 10:* Stay abreast of legislation, policy, and broader concepts that encompass and influence community mobility options.

Journal of Occupational Therapy, indicating an increase of professional expertise in this domain.

Collaborative efforts with other national associations advocating for the successful use of multiple mobility options have resulted in an increase in professional resources relevant to transportation. The AOTA (2008b) fact sheet titled ***The Occupational Therapy Role in Driving and Community Mobility Across the Lifespan,*** about the role of occupational therapy in addressing community mobility across the lifespan, clearly situates transportation as a means of enabling participation in occupation. The fact sheet emphasizes occupational therapists' role in addressing community mobility at the individual, organizational, and societal levels to ensure safety and promote participation and inclusion in all spheres of life.

Priority 2: Include community mobility in initial evaluations and documentation of treatment planning.

The length and the content of documentation have been abbreviated within many health care settings in the past several decades, with transitions to electronic documentation increasing efficiency but resulting in the recording of functional abilities as numerical scores, with little space allocated for narrative commentary (Siegler, 2010). Widespread assessment tools used by occupational therapists within inpatient rehabilitation and long-term care settings address only the status of basic activities of daily living (BADLs; James, 2009), without the opportunity to officially document an IADL such as community mobility. There are instruments that prompt the collection of information related to community mobility, but these require supplemental use of tools outside the scope of most initial evaluation processes to gain complete information regarding community mobility. We assert that every evaluation process should include a single question (at minimum) regarding how the client moves about in the community to engage in his or her occupational routines—not simply whether or not that person drives.

The *Framework–II* (AOTA, 2008a) advocates for occupational therapy evaluations to begin with an occupational profile. Several instruments (e.g., the Canadian Occupational Performance Measure [Law, Baptiste, Carswell, Polatajko, & Pollock, 2005], the Occupational Performance History Interview–II [Kielhofner et al., 2004]) prompt the clinician to ask questions regarding transportation use as part of an initial profile. In addition, the combination of different forms of mobility for engagement in different occupations should be explored. That is, occupational therapists have the opportunity to gain more valuable information about community mobility by asking not only about types of transportation used by clients but also about how they travel to what destinations and for which occupations. This type of information gathering provides greater opportunities for intervention that targets client capacities through an occupational means.

Community mobility has relevance for occupational therapy clients in every practice setting across the lifespan. AOTA (2008b) suggested that the developmental lessons learned through engagement in community mobility tasks—from being seated in a car seat to learning to ride a bike to obtaining a driver's license—affect identity, independence, and participation in occupations. Assessment of community mobility issues relies on the same skills as other occupational therapy performance areas: analyzing needs, capacities, strengths, resources, and the fit between the client and the context.

For school-age clients with special needs, the assessment process may consist of determining the adequacy of a school system's bus fleet, while for the teen, readiness to drive takes priority. For the adult with onset of chronic progressive illness, assessing family mobility options may be in order, and for the older adult who is facing driving retirement, pedestrian safety and capacity may take precedence. As in other realms of clinical practice, the needs of the client and the context drive the evaluation process.

Another concept useful to an initial evaluation in many practice settings is the issue of *readiness* for mobility transitions. Understanding how a client perceives impending transitions in community mobility allows the practitioner to use the most appropriate approach in addressing these changes in the course of evaluation and intervention. King and colleagues (2011) have offered the **Assessment of Readiness for Mobility Transitions (ARMT)**, which measures readiness for mobility transitions among older adults through the collection of subjective responses to statements regarding mobility options and status.

Priority 3: Include either actual or simulated practice in using community mobility options within intervention plans for all clients.

Just as many practice settings engage clients in practicing household transfers or IADL tasks in spaces that approximate their natural contexts, community mobility skills also can be practiced in whole or in part in most clinical environments. Even in settings focused on specific aspects of function, opportunities exist to include

---

Exhibit 2.4. Addressing Community Mobility in a Hand and Upper-Extremity Rehabilitation Setting

- While teaching protection of the injured extremity, include concepts regarding positioning and protecting structures when driving, riding, or accessing public transportation.
- Include in sensory retraining the manipulation of materials related to community mobility such as money, tickets, passes, hand grips (steering wheel or handlebars), and handrails.
- Analyze upper-extremity motion demands related to the client's preferred modes of community mobility and include in sessions facilitating motor recovery (e.g., reaching and gripping steering wheel or bike handlebars, handling doors and keys, donning clothing related to walking or biking).

---

awareness of community mobility skills and safety into intervention sessions. Exhibit 2.4 and Exhibit 2.5 provide examples of practice settings that emphasize rehabilitation of impaired performance and ways in which community mobility issues might be integrated into relevant intervention protocols.

Priority 4: Maintain a resource library about community mobility options relative to the area in which your client population lives and travels, and keep information updated.

When working with a client on community mobility transitions, it is crucial to have information already in place to supplement conversations about options for travel. Particularly for clients facing a transition from driving to driving cessation, it is helpful to be able to put printed information into their hands regarding community mobility options at the time that discussion takes place. Consider building this resource electronically so that it may be updated easily and also easily accessible by others. Even if the clients are grieving the transition and not ready to engage in future planning, providing information to which they can later refer has been shown to assist clients in revisiting options when they are ready (Oxley & Charlton, 2009). Local Area Agency on Aging organizations may have compiled this information for older adults in their region; efforts by occupational therapists to distribute this information in the community would be appreciated. Exhibit 2.6 illustrates materials pertinent to a community mobility resource library.

Priority 5: Work with clients to develop a broad array of travel options, regardless of their current driving status.

Begin conversations and practice with mobility options early, particularly in clinical settings when working with people who have a higher incidence of mobility dependence (older adults, people with newly acquired disabilities, those living in poverty). Introducing the idea of using transportation options at a time when the client is not adjusting to a difficult personal transition often makes the conversation

---

Exhibit 2.5. Suggestions for Including Community Mobility in Psychosocial Rehabilitation

- Use actual materials related to community mobility (e.g., bus schedules, transportation brochures) to provide opportunities for practice with transportation use.
- Role-play transportation-related scenarios (e.g., asking for directions, requesting a specific destination on public transit, handling travel emergencies).
- Educate and ask for return demonstration of personal safety strategies during travel (e.g., protecting belongings, handling difficult interpersonal exchanges, protecting money).

Exhibit 2.6. Materials for a Community Mobility Library in a Clinical Setting

- Applications for local or regional paratransit services
- Bus, subway, train, or ferry schedules
- Information on how to obtain fare passes, including eligibility criteria for discounted passes
- Information about transportation provided by human services agencies in the community (see "Terminology, Concepts, and Resources in Community Mobility" section for possibilities)
- Information regarding city or county pedestrian walkways and bikeways
- Phone numbers for supplemental transportation providers (public and private) in the vicinity
- Information about personal safety during travel
- Information on travel training and mobility management assistance
- Information about accessibility and safety tips for long-distance travel by air or sea.

---

less threatening (Stern et al., 2008). Beyond conversation, providing therapeutic intervention relative to the use of community mobility alternatives is also critical. Having the support of a care provider in using public transportation improves the likelihood that someone will continue use of that same mode of travel independently in the future (Sterns, Antenucci, Nelson, & Glasgow, 2003).

Priority 6: Join or establish a network of health and human services and transit providers in your geographic area to share concerns and knowledge about community mobility.

There are many health and human services providers who have an interest in community mobility options for persons with functional limitations. Among these are social workers, case managers, public health representatives, primary health care providers, and transit providers. If you practice in an area with established municipal transit systems, check first with those systems or with the city or county government in your area to determine existing interest groups formed around this topic. Many city and county government structures have transportation advisory boards with rotating membership who seek residents of the area to serve on those committees. In rural areas, check with county government agencies such as the department on aging. In addition, invite transit providers to join in addressing the challenges. If there are no apparent existing groups meeting about these issues, consider hosting a networking session of local health and human services and transit providers and local occupational therapists to determine interest in forming an action coalition.

Priority 7: Develop awareness of local human services agencies and state-level or governmental organizations that may provide funding or actual mechanisms for travel.

Knowledge of health and human services agencies that provide transportation will likely become apparent as you develop a library of resources for your workplace. Occasionally, however, entities that provide some funding for community mobility may differ slightly from those that actually provide transportation services. City and county social services departments, for example, often assist with funding for travel relevant to life necessities through the allotment of Medicaid funds, although they rarely operate transit services. Relative to older adults and people with limited incomes, resident services departments with urban housing units also may have available funds for travel; in this case, being familiar with where your clients live may provide new travel alternatives.

Faith communities offer another possibility for transportation in terms of either funding or services. Many churches, synagogues, and temples organize transportation for their members who are nondrivers; likewise, many carry out a social mission of assisting those with lower incomes to access transportation resources. Some of these faith communities limit their resources to those who belong to their particular congregation, while others offer supplemental funding for transportation through local social services agencies.

Social workers are invaluable in understanding these resources, and many occupational therapists may defer to these professionals when determining available resources. What is crucial, however, is that occupational therapists also develop a working knowledge of the types of transportation resources available in the area to determine appropriate referrals as well as the fit between the available transportation or funding option and a particular client's abilities and situation.

Priority 8: Volunteer or consult professionally with transportation providers to understand the fit between the abilities of individuals and the transportation context.

An exciting and emerging opportunity for the occupational therapist in the realm of community mobility is that of serving in a consultative role for transit service providers and supplemental transportation programs. The emphasis in occupational therapy on conducting an analysis of person–environment–task fit and modifying one or more of those factors to maximize performance offers great promise for evaluating the match between the skills of a transportation user and the system he or she is trying to access.

Griffin and Priddy (2005) provided evidence that rehabilitation professionals acting to design and carry out paratransit eligibility determination processes can ensure that riders have needed access while also helping transit systems to allocate scarce resources where they are most needed. The first author (Womack) collaborated in 2000–2001 with a midsize city in the design of its paratransit eligibility system, resulting in an effective cost savings of several thousand dollars in the first few months of implementation.

Travel training as an intervention fits well within the scope of occupational therapy services.

For those transportation users who may not be eligible for paratransit, travel training relative to the use of fixed-route services may be indicated and is another area in which occupational therapists may offer expertise. Crabtree and colleagues (2009) suggested travel training as an intervention that fits well within the scope of occupational therapy services. These authors suggested that travel instruction be included in every rehabilitation discharge plan for adults with newly acquired disabilities and older adults facing driving retirement. While the provision of occupational therapy services for repeated travel instruction may be cost-prohibitive, the involvement of an occupational therapist to design individualized instruction from the outset of training may effectively use resources in the long run (Crabtree et al., 2009).

Supplemental transportation programs, which typically serve older adults (Beverly Foundation, 2001), frequently rely on volunteer drivers to provide door-through-door service to riders. A third consultative role for the occupational therapist consists of service to these transportation providers through the training of volunteers who provide added assistance. Issues of liability in helping someone with compromised mobility in and out of a vehicle are cited as a common concern for volunteer drivers with supplemental transportation programs (Beverly Foundation, 2007). The occupational therapist can teach effective mobility assistance skills to maximize the confidence and capability of the volunteers and can document the intent of the transportation provider to provide adequate training for risk management purposes.

The need for accurate determination of fit between the capabilities of the traveler and the mode of community mobility cannot be overemphasized. Rosenbloom (2005) noted that one of the myths influencing transportation policies is a belief that when older adults cease driving, they transition to the use of public transportation and, when that fails, to walking. Not only do transportation data indicate that this is untrue (U.S. Department of Transportation, 2001), but Rosenbloom (2005) has contended that driving is, in regards to physical access, the easiest form of transportation for older adults (p. 52), and the need to retire from driving is most often due to factors that also will affect the successful use of public transportation. Impairments in vision and cognition, two factors heavily implicated in driving cessation, also present challenges in terms of using public transportation and exercising safe pedestrian skills. Impairments in mobility and endurance, which can often be accommodated in driving with vehicle modifications, are inordinately challenging in relationship to using mass transit and functioning in a pedestrian environment. The occupational therapist can assess and intervene in regards to each of these performance capacities.

Sohlberg and colleagues (2009) also provided an example relative to individuals with cognitive disabilities resulting from brain injury, identifying common characteristics of the types of interventions carried out by occupational therapists in facilitating transportation for these clients. Trip planning, destination navigation, management of personal possessions, and pedestrian safety are frequently practiced skills in the context of cognitive impairment from head injury, leading these authors to propose a community transportation model for intervention with these clients.

Priority 9: Bolster your knowledge of national-level organizations that provide training and resources and lead advocacy and policy efforts related to community mobility.

In the "Terminology, Concepts, and Resources in Community Mobility" section of this chapter, we offered an introduction to national organizations that are focused on transportation issues, primarily those in the realm of increasing or ensuring access to community mobility options for persons with disabilities or income status preventing the use of standard public transportation modes. Choose one or two of these organizations to follow on a routine basis by bookmarking their Web sites and visiting them periodically for updates. A more comprehensive list of community mobility resources categorized by subject area is provided in Appendix 2.A, and others can be found on the AOTA Older Driver Web site.

Priority 10: Stay abreast of legislation, policy, and broader concepts that encompass and influence community mobility options.

For busy practitioners, it is often tempting to deal with immediate client needs relative to community mobility and to assume that broader transportation policy is not within our realm of concern. It is helpful, however, to know what influences transportation policy and where opinions about policies under consideration can be shared. Both governmental and nonprofit organizations that provide policy briefing and advocacy related to community mobility are categorized according to interest area in Appendix 2.A. Several specific Web sites may be useful in gaining a broader understanding of legislative, political, and financial implications related to community mobility.

Summary

Community mobility represents all the ways in which people move themselves about in the world, and the ability to successfully engage with community mobility options facilitates participation in valued occupations. Although driving rehabilitation has been at the forefront of the professional conscience for several decades, expanding occupational therapists' knowledge of and capacity to address all forms of community mobility clients will ensure that access to transportation and preparation for mobility transitions are not an afterthought but rather part of a comprehensive consideration of well-being. Multiple local, state, and national resources exist to facilitate this outcome, and the goal of this chapter has been to increase awareness of these resources and how occupational therapists might use them in conjunction with professional training to better serve individuals, organizations, and society relative to community mobility needs.

References

AARP. (2004). *Enhancing mobility options for older Americans: A five-year national action agenda.* Washington, DC: Author, Public Policy Institute.

Abley, S. (2005*). Walkability scoping paper.* Retrieved February 17, 2011, from http://www.levelofservice.com/walkability-research.pdf

American Occupational Therapy Association. (2008a). Occupational therapy practice framework: Domain and process (2nd ed.). *American Journal of Occupational Therapy, 62,* 625–683. doi:10.5014/ajot.62.6.625

American Occupational Therapy Association. (2008b). *The occupational therapy role in driving and community mobility across the lifespan.* Retrieved December 2, 2010, from http://www.aota.org/Older-Driver/Professionals/Toolkit/Professional/Brochures-and-Fact-Sheets/41773.aspx?FT=.pdf

American Public Transportation Association. (2009). *Economic impact of public transportation investment.* Retrieved March 3, 2011, from http://www.apta.com/resources/reportsand publications/Documents/economic_impact_of_public_transportation_investment.pdf

American Public Transportation Association. (2010). *Facts at a glance.* Retrieved October 28, 2010, from http://publictransportation.org/takesusthere/docs/facts_at_a_glance.pdf

Americans with Disabilities Act of 1990, P. L. 101-336, 42 U.S.C. 126.

Bailey, L. (2004, April). *Aging Americans: Stranded without options.* Surface Transportation Policy Project. Retrieved August 5, 2010, from http://www.transact.org/library/reports_html/seniors/aging.pdf

Berger, M. M. (1979). *The devil wagon in God's country: The automobile and social change in rural America, 1893–1929.* Hamden, CT: Archon Books.

Beverly Foundation. (2001). *Supplemental transportation programs for seniors.* Washington, DC: AAA Foundation for Traffic Safety.

Beverly Foundation. (2002). *The 5 A's of senior-friendly transportation.* Retrieved December 4, 2010, from http://www.beverlyfoundation.org/wp-content/uploads/Fact-Sheet-5-the-5-as.pdf

Beverly Foundation. (2004). *Supplemental transportation programs for seniors: A report on STPs in America.* Pasadena, CA: Author & AAA Foundation for Traffic Safety.

Beverly Foundation. (2007). *Risk and risk management strategies: Important considerations for volunteer driver programs and volunteer drivers.* Pasadena, CA: Author & Partnership to Preserve Independent Living.

Beverly Foundation. (2009). *The history of the Beverly Foundation.* Retrieved November 20, 2010, from http://www.beverlyfoundation.org/aboutus/history.html

Boschen, K., Tonack, M., & Gargaro, J. (2003). Long-term adjustment and community reintegration following spinal cord injury. *International Journal of Rehabilitation Research, 26,* 157–162.

Brown, C. E. (2009). Ecological models in occupational therapy. In E. B. Crepeau, E. S. Cohn, & B. A. B. Schell (Eds.), *Willard and Spackman's occupational therapy* (11th ed., pp. 435–445). Baltimore: Lippincott Williams & Wilkins.

Burkhardt, J. E. (2010, June). *Potential cost savings from taxi paratransit programs.* Paper presented at the 12th International Conference on Mobility and Transport for Elderly and Disabled Persons, Hong Kong.

Clarke, P., Ailshire, J. A., & Lantz, P. (2009). Urban built environments and trajectories of mobility disability: Findings from a national sample of community-dwelling American adults. *Social Science and Medicine, 69,* 964–970.

Collia, D. V., Sharp, J., & Giesbrecht, L. (2003). The 2001 National Household Travel Survey: A look into the travel patterns of older Americans. *Journal of Safety Research, 34,* 461–470.

Community Transportation Association of America. (2010). *A brief history of the Job Access and Reverse Commute Program.* Retrieved December 4, 2010, from http://web1.ctaa.org/webmodules/webarticles/anmviewer.asp?a=108&z=5

Coughlin, J. (2007). Disruptive demographics, design, and the future of everyday environments. *Design Management Review, 18,* 53–59.

Coughlin, J. F., & Cobb, R. W. (2000). How will we get there from here? *Journal of Aging and Social Policy, 11,* 201–210.

Council on Aging of Southwest Ohio. (2009). *Medicaid waiver programs and transportation.* Retrieved February 12, 2012, from http://www.help4seniors.org/page.asp?ref=77

Crabtree, J., Troyer, J. D., & Justiss, M. D. (2009). The intersection of driving with a disability and being a public transportation passenger with a disability. *Topics in Geriatric Rehabilitation, 25,* 163–172.

Denson, C. R. (2000). Public sector transportation for people with disabilities: A satisfaction survey. *Journal of Rehabilitation, 66*(3), 29–37.

Dickie, V., Cutchin, M. P., & Humphry, R. (2006). Occupation as transactional experience: A critique of individualism in occupational science. *Journal of Occupational Science, 13,* 83–93.

Easter Seals Project Action. (n.d.). *Competencies for the practice of travel training and travel instruction.* Retrieved November 10, 2010, from http://projectaction.easterseals.com/site/DocServer/04COMP.pdf?docID=6363

Federal-Aid Highway Act of 1956, P. L. 84-627, 70 Stat. 374.

Federal Highway Administration. (n.d.). *Dwight D. Eisenhower National System of Interstate and Defense Highways.* Retrieved December 29, 2010, from http://www.fhwa.dot.gov/programadmin/interstate.cfm

Flink, J. J. (1970). *America adopts the automobile, 1895–1910.* Cambridge, MA: MIT Press.

Florida Department of Transportation, State Safety Office Pedestrian and Bicycle Program. (1995). *Walkable communities: Twelve steps for an effective program.* Tallahassee: Author.

Fonda, S. J., Wallace, R. B., & Herzog, A. R. (2001). Changes in driving patterns and worsening depressive symptoms among older adults. *Journal of Gerontology: B. Psychological and Social Sciences, 56,* S343–S351.

Foster, M. S. (1981). *From streetcar to superhighway: American city planners and urban transportation, 1900–1940.* Philadelphia: Temple University Press.

Foster, M. S. (2003). *A nation on wheels.* Belmont, CA: Thomson-Wadsworth.

Freund, K. (2003). Mobility and older people: Independent transportation network—The next best thing to driving. Replicating the travel characteristics of the private auto. *Generations, 27,* 68–71.

Garber, N. J., & Hoel, L. A. (2009). *Traffic and highway engineering* (4th ed.). Toronto: Cengage Learning.

Griffin, J., & Priddy, D. A. (2005). Assessing paratransit eligibility under the Americans with Disabilities Act in the rehabilitation setting. *Archives of Physical Medicine and Rehabilitation, 86,* 1267–1269.

Hammel, K. (2007). Quality of life after spinal cord injury: A metasynthesis of qualitative findings. *Spinal Cord, 45*, 124–139.

Hyde, C. K. (2006). Driving and community mobility: An historical perspective. Section I: History of the automobile. In J. Pellerito (Ed.), *Driver rehabilitation and community mobility* (pp. 23–31). St. Louis: Mosby.

ICF Consulting. (2006). *Estimating the impacts of the aging population on transit ridership* (NCHRP Project 20-65[4]). Transportation Research Board of the National Academies. Retrieved December 4, 2010, from http://drcog.org/documents/Estimating%20 impacts%20of%20aging.pdf

James, A. B. (2009). Activities of daily living and instrumental activities of daily living. In E. B. Crepeau, E. S. Cohn, & B. A. B. Schell (Eds.), *Willard and Spackman's occupational therapy* (11th ed., pp. 538–578). Baltimore: Lippincott Williams & Wilkins.

Kaiser Commission on Medicaid and the Uninsured. (2004, June). *Olmstead v. L.C.: The interaction of the Americans with Disabilities Act and Medicaid.* Retrieved December 4, 2010, from http://www.kff.org/medicaid/7096a.cfm

Keigher, S. (2006). Policies affecting community-based social services, housing, and transportation. In B. Berkman (Ed.), *Handbook of social work in health and aging* (pp. 877–891). New York: Oxford University Press.

Kerschner, H. (2003). Rural transportation and aging: Problems and solutions. In R. J. Ham, R. T. Goins, & D. K. Brown (Eds.), *Best practices in service delivery to the rural elderly* (pp. 133–147). Retrieved March 16, 2011, from http://www.red-elaia.com/ adjuntos/176.1-Best_Practices-Rural_Elderly.pdf#page=150

Kielhofner, G., Mallinson, T., Crawford, C., Nowak, M., Rigby, M., Henry, A., et al. (2004). *Occupational Performance History Interview II (OPHI–II), Version 2.1.* Chicago: University of Illinois–Chicago, Model of Human Occupation Clearinghouse.

King, M. D., Meuser, T. M., Berg-Weger, M., Chibnall, J. C., Harmon, A., & Yakimo, R. (2011). Decoding the Miss Daisy Syndrome: An examination of subjective responses to mobility change. *Journal of Gerontological Social Work, 54*, 29–52.

Law, M., Baptiste, S., Carswell, A., Polatajko, H., & Pollock, N. (2005). *Canadian Occupational Performance Measure* (4th ed.). Ottawa: Canadian Association of Occupational Therapists.

Leslie, L. (2011). *Staying on in a sprawling space: Getting involved and speaking out.* Retrieved February 7, 2012, from http://search.proquest.com/docview/919905195?account id=14244

Loveland, J. (2009). School buses + safety belts = good idea. *OT Practice, 11*(11), 17–18.

Lysack, C., Komanecky, M., Kabel, A., Cross, K., & Neufeld, S. (2007). Environmental factors and their role in community integration after spinal cord injury. *Canadian Journal of Occupational Therapy, 74*(ICF Special Issue), 243–254.

Marottoli, R. S., Mendes de Leon, C. F., Glass, T. A., Williams, C. S., Cooney, L. M., Jr., & Berkman, L. F. (2000). Consequence of driving cessation: Decreased out-of-home activity levels. *Journal of Gerontology, B: Social Sciences, 55*, S334–S340.

Marottoli, R. A., Mendes de Leon, C. F., Glass, T. A., Williams, C. S., Cooney, L. M., Jr., Berkman, L. F., et al. (1997). Driving cessation and increased depressive symptoms: Prospective evidence from the New Haven EPESE. Established Populations for Epidemiologic Studies of the Elderly. *Journal of the American Geriatrics Society, 45*, 202–206.

McCann, B., & Ewing, R. (2003). *Measuring the health effects of sprawl.* Washington, DC: Smart Growth America and Surface Transportation Policy Project.

Muraleetharan, T., Takeo, A., Toru, H., Seiichi, K., & Ken'etsu, U. (2004). *Evaluation of pedestrian level of service on sidewalks and crosswalks using conjoint analysis.* Presented at the 83rd Annual Meeting of the Transportation Research Board, Washington, DC.

National Council on Disability. (2006). *Creating livable communities.* Retrieved February 12, 2011, from http://www.ncd.gov/publications/2006/Oct312006#executive

NationMaster.com. (2011). *Transportation statistics—Motor vehicles by country.* Retrieved February 24, 2011, from http://www.nationmaster.com/graph/tra_mot_veh-transportation-motor-vehicles

Olmstead v. L. C. (1999), (98-536) 527 U.S. 581.

Oxley, J., & Charlton, J. (2009). Attitudes toward and mobility impacts of driving cessation: Differences between current and former drivers. *Topics in Geriatric Rehabilitation 25*(1), 43–54.

Pellerito, J. M., Jr., & Lysack, C. L. (2006). The role of the automobile in American culture. In J. M. Pellerito, Jr. (Ed.), *Driver rehabilitation and community mobility* (pp. 35–52). St. Louis: Elsevier.

Perez, C. (2008). *Justification for wheelchair accessible private transportation in the United States of America.* National Council for Independent Living. Retrieved February 2, 2011, from http://www.ncil.org/news/AccessibleTaxis2.html

Personal Responsibility and Work Opportunity Reconciliation Act of 1996, P. L. 104-93, 110 Stat. 2105.

Pucher, J. (2002). Renaissance of public transport in the U.S.? *Transportation Quarterly, 56*(1), 33–49.

Pucher, J., & Renne, J. L. (2003). Socioeconomics of urban travel: Evidence from the 2001 NHTS. *Transportation Quarterly, 57*(3), 49–77.

Ragland, D. R., Satariano, W. A., & MacLeod, K. E. (2005). Driving cessation and increased depressive symptoms. *Journal of Gerontology: Medical Sciences, 60A*, 399–403.

Rome, A. W. (1998). William Whyte, open space, and environmental activism. *Geographical Review, 88*(2), 259–275.

Rosenbloom, S. (1993). Women's travel patterns at various stages of their lives. In C. Katz & J. Monk (Eds.), *Full circles: Geographies of women over the life course* (pp. 208–242). London: Routledge.

Rosenbloom, S. (2005). The mobility needs of older Americans. In B. Katz & R. Puentes (Eds.), *Taking the high road: A metropolitan agenda for transportation reform* (pp. 227–254). Washington, DC: Brookings Institution Press. Retrieved December 15, 2011, from http://www.brookings.edu/reports/2003/07transportation_rosenbloom.aspx

Safe, Accountable, Flexible, Efficient Transportation Equity Act of 2005, P. L. 109-59, 119 Stat. 1144.

Safe Kids Worldwide. (2009). *Pedestrian safety.* Retrieved January 6, 2011, from http://www.safekids.org/safety-basics/safety-resources-by-risk-area/pedestrian/

Samimi, A., Mohammadian, A. K., & Madanizadeh, S. (2009). Effects of transportation and the built environment on general health and obesity. *Transportation Research Part D: Transport and Environment, 14*, 67–71.

Sandt, L., Schneider, R., Nabors, D., Thomas, L., Mitchell, C., & Eldridge, R. J. (2008). *A resident's guide for creating safe and walkable communities.* Retrieved August 1, 2010, from http://safety.fhwa.dot.gov/ped_bike/ped_cmnity/ped_walkguide/index.cfm

Siegler, E. L. (2010). The evolving medical record. *Annals of Internal Medicine, 153*, 671–677.

Shaw, G. (2000). Wheelchair rider risk in motor vehicles: A technical note. *Journal of Rehabilitation Research and Development, 37*, 89–100.

Shutrump, S. E., Manary, M., & Buning, M. E. (2008). Safe transportation for students who use wheelchairs on the school bus. *OT Practice, 13*(15), 8–12.

Silverstein, N. M., Johns, E., & Griffin, J. (2008). Students explore livable communities. *Gerontology and Geriatrics Education, 29*, 19–37.

Sohlberg, M. M., Fickas, S., Lemoncello, R., & Hung, P. (2009). Validation of the activities of community transportation model for individuals with cognitive impairments. *Disability and Rehabilitation, 31*, 887–897.

Stav, W. B. (2008). Review of the evidence related to older adult community mobility and driver licensure policies. *American Journal of Occupational Therapy, 62*, 149–158. doi:10.5014/ajot.62.2.149

Stav, W. (2009, August 31). Seats belts on school buses: Not a good idea. *OT Practice, 15*, 18–20.

St. Clair, D. J. (1986). *The motorization of American cities.* Westport, CT: Praeger.

Stern, R. A., D'Ambrosio, L. A., Mohyde, M., Carruth, A., Tracton-Bishop, B., Hunter, J. C., et al. (2008). At the crossroads: Development and evaluation of a dementia caregiver group intervention to assist in driving cessation. *Gerontology and Geriatrics Education, 29*, 363–382.

Sterns, R., Antenucci, V., Nelson, C., & Glasgow, N. (2003). Public transportation: Options to maintain mobility for life. *Generations, 27*(2), 14–19.

Taubman-Ben-Ari, O., Mikulincer, M., & Gillath, O. (2004). The multidimensional driving style inventory–scale construct and validation. *Accident Analysis and Prevention, 36*, 323–332.

Transit Access Project. (n.d.). *ADA paratransit eligibility standards.* Retrieved March 26, 2011, from http://www.transitaccessproject.org/paratransit

Transportation Equity Act for the 21st Century of 1998, P. L. 105-178, 112 Stat. 107.

Transportation Research Board. (1998). *Synthesis of transit practice 3: Paratransit eligibility certification practices.* Washington, DC: Author.

U.S. Department of Transportation, Federal Highway Administration. (2011). *Summary of travel trends: 2009 national household travel survey.* Retrieved December 11, 2010, from http://nhts.ornl.gov/2009/pub/stt.pdf

U.S. Department of Transportation, Federal Transit Administration. (1991*). Preamble: Transportation for individuals with disabilities [September 6, 1991].* Retrieved December 1, 2010, from http://www.fta.dot.gov/civilrights/ada/civil_rights_4058.html

U.S. Department of Transportation, National Highway Traffic Safety Administration. (2010). *Pedestrian safety workshop: A focus on older adults.* Prepared by the University of North Carolina Highway Safety Research Center. Retrieved January 11, 2011, from http://www.nhtsa.gov/staticfiles/nti/older_drivers/pdf/PedSafetyWorkshop-02.pdf

Vanderbur, M., & Silverstein, N. M. (2006). *Community mobility and dementia: A review of the literature.* Washington, DC: NHTSA & Alzheimer's Association.

Vine, X. K. L., & Hamilton, D. I. (2005). Individual characteristics associated with community integration of adults with intellectual disability. *Journal of Intellectual and Developmental Disabilities, 30,* 171–175.

Appendix 2.A. Comprehensive Community Mobility Resources

Children's Community Mobility

- **National AMBUCS AmTryke program:** www.ambucs.org/amtryke/
- **National Center for Safe Routes to School:** www.saferoutesinfo.org
- **SafeKids USA:** http://safekids.org

Disability and Community Mobility

- **Easter Seals Project Action:** www.projectaction.org
- **National Council on Disability Transportation Policy:** www.ncd.gov/policy/transportation

Livability

- **National Complete Streets Coalition:** www.completestreets.org
- **Partners for Livable Communities:** www.livable.org
- **U.S. Department of Transportation Livability Web site:** www.dot.gov/livability/101.html

Public Transportation

- **American Public Transportation Association:** www.apta.com and www.publictransportation.org

Senior Community Mobility

- **AARP transportation information:** www.aarp.org/home-garden/transportation/
- **American Occupational Therapy Association Older Driver microsite:** www.aota.org/Older-Driver
- **The Beverly Foundation:** www.beverlyfoundation.org
- **National Center for Senior Transportation:** www.seniortransportation.easterseals.com

Walkability

- **AmericaWalks:** www.americawalks.org
- **WalkScore:** www.walkscore.com

Environmental Audits

- **AARP Livable Communities Evaluation Guide:** http://assets.aarp.org/rgcenter/il/d18311_communities.pdf
- **Robert Wood Johnson Foundation Walkability app:** www.rwjf.org/files/newsroom/interactives/walkability/walk_app.html
- **Walkability checklist:** www.walkinginfo.org

CHAPTER 3

Welcome to the Team! Who Are the Stakeholders?

Anne Dickerson, PhD, OTR/L, FAOTA, and
Elin Schold Davis, OTR/L, CDRS

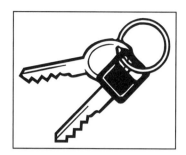

Learning Objectives

At the completion of this chapter, readers will be able to

- Identify the roles, motivations, and background of stakeholders invested in driving and community mobility across the lifespan;
- Delineate the relationships between stakeholders when considering community mobility; and
- Recognize the methods, strategies, and opportunities for interactions and partnerships between team members or stakeholders that facilitate an effective and efficient system to address driving and community mobility across the lifespan.

Key Words

- **certified driver rehabilitation specialist**
- **collaboration**
- **driver rehabilitation specialist**
- **stakeholders**

Introduction

Addressing driving and community mobility as a routine part of occupational therapy practice cannot be accomplished working in isolation. Therefore, the goal of this chapter is to introduce readers to the range of stakeholders who may play a role in this important practice area. These stakeholders include the levels of the individual consumer, the occupational therapist, and the larger social community. To build a network of services with other stakeholders, occupational therapists need to understand the options and resources, available via Web sites or located within their own community, that range from traditional partners (e.g., physicians) to unique partnerships with entities such as the state and local law enforcement.

Driving and community mobility services in occupational therapy practice settings should not be restricted to screening and evaluation but must ensure access to the wide spectrum of services, including training, rehabilitation, and the identification of and training in alternative transportation options. Currently, few occupational therapy programs have the size and scope to directly offer this extensive range of services. In some cases, the network of services that address driving and community mobility may involve a group of practice settings or stakeholder resources that are critical to access and affordability. As resources tighten, we have an obligation to our programs and clients to bridge gaps, incorporating the services and expertise of partners and stakeholders.

This chapter will highlight a sampling of stakeholders who share the vision of ensuring safe mobility and access to driving and community mobility services. Thus, stakeholders include not only providers of services but also those influencing policy and licensure. This chapter will describe the role of the occupational therapy generalist and the driver rehabilitation specialist as members of an interdisciplinary team of individuals or agencies concerned with driving and community mobility.

Within the Health Care System

This section highlights the roles and responsibilities of the team members of the medical model or the broader health care system, as the most familiar model of practice. In addition to the obvious members (e.g., physicians, social workers) associated with occupational therapy, there are other partners in driving and community mobility who are unique to this area of practice.

Occupational Therapist (Generalist)

In the hospital, rehabilitation center, subacute/long-term care, or home health care setting, it is critical that occupational therapists consider all aspects of the occupational therapy domain when evaluating and planning interventions for clients (American Occupational Therapy Association [AOTA], 2008). The essential activities of daily living (e.g., dressing, bathing, eating) are usually at the forefront of treatment priorities, while instrumental activities of daily living (IADLs) elevate in priority as the client progresses. Community mobility as a driver, pedestrian, or passenger, as discussed throughout this publication, needs to be an essential component of the occupational therapist's intervention plan, whether directly, through education, or by referral. It is the ethical responsibility of the occupational therapist to not miss, avoid, or skip over this crucial IADL with the expectation or assumption that others will address it.

The ethical responsibility of addressing driving and community mobility extends to recognizing when there is simply a concern about mobility. When addressing the implications of impairment, the occupational therapist must make the client and family aware of the client's risk and vulnerability with all complex tasks, including driving. One should not assume that the client or family members will automatically know if and when it is time to either stop (for a recovery interval or long term) or return to driving. Among many confounding factors is the recognition that the family member or client is potentially conflicted and may understandably avoid the potential struggle surrounding the discussion of such a highly valued activity. Family members or clients may not ask the question to avoid an unwanted outcome.

Through the occupational therapist's intervention, the discussion of the IADL of driving and community mobility is relevant to the client's goals and the discharge plan. Including driving and community mobility in the evaluation and discharge criteria appropriately positions the discussion as intervention on the basis of evaluation results and client performance interpreted through evidence and data, not one of emotion, opinion, or (age) bias. The occupational therapy evaluation and person-centered plan offer information that is clear and factual, allowing clients and their families to know what is expected and to be open to alternative options. Accordingly, there may be an assumption that because the client is not presently able to drive, non-driving will remain a permanent recommendation. Over-restriction may occur when a client abandons hope to resume driving and is unaware that when recovery occurs, driving may again become an option. In addition, dependence on Americans with Disabilities Act Amendments (P. L. 110-325, 2008) paratransit services is costly to individuals and communities. As recovery progresses, occupational therapists need to ensure that clients have access to the least restrictive form of transportation options available.

Even occupational therapists who do not specialize in driving and community mobility must address the IADL of driving appropriately within their scope of practice. By including driving and community mobility, occupational therapy intervention will ensure that the client has the means of mobility to get to where he or she needs and wants to go to fulfill the IADL. This may or may not include self-driving at any point, but if the client has identified the goal to resume or learn to drive, the occupational therapist should help with resources and access to services to optimize the client's opportunity to meet his or her goal. The occupational therapy general practitioner should determine which partners need to be informed or involved in goal setting or decision making.

There is always the issue of early discharge (e.g., short stays, with discharge long before it is appropriate to address IADLs) and the dilemma of determining priority interventions while the client is involved in therapy. In reference to driving and community mobility, the occupational therapist should consider the provision of information and referrals as an *intervention*. With driving primarily under the domain of occupational therapy, the interaction with the occupational therapist may be the client's only opportunity to discuss his or her concerns and questions about driving and community mobility. Thus, with the exception of the most infirm, mobility (transportation) *must* be considered an IADL critical for clients' transportation needs from home to destinations including medical appointments and social engagement. Engagement and participation are also critical parts of the occupational therapy domain of practice (AOTA, 2008), and occupational therapists have the responsibility to help clients and their families appreciate risk, the potential options, and the avenues to explore when the time is right to consider driving again.

Driver Rehabilitation Specialist

The driver rehabilitation specialist (DRS) plans, develops, coordinates, or implements driving rehabilitation services for individuals with disabilities. *Driver rehabilitation specialist* is a general term that encompasses a diverse group of providers who may include engineers, driving instructors, and health care professionals. Currently, the mandated requirements for certification and education are vague and inconsistent from state to state, contributing to the variability in the training of the provider who uses the title DRS. Ideally, the DRS who is also an occupational therapist understands his or her ethical responsibility (which may or may not be mandated) to acquire the specialized education and training, beyond professional education, to

The driver rehabilitation specialist plans, develops, coordinates, or implements driving rehabilitation services for individuals with disabilities.

Exhibit 3.1. Baby Boomers

The *baby boomers* are individuals born post–World War II, between 1946 and 1964. In addition to the population bulge that this generation brings, these individuals grew up in the 1960s, 1970s, and 1980s, known for redefining traditional values. In terms of driving, the baby boomers grew up with the automobile and value driving as a "right" rather than a privilege. In 2010, approximately 13% of the population in the United States was over 65, and in 2030, it is projected to be 19%, with more than 40 million aging baby boomers on the road (National Highway Traffic Safety Administration [NHTSA], 2009).

---

be prepared to offer needed driving rehabilitation evaluation and intervention for novice and experienced drivers.

It is important to realize that the historical development of the DRS is from a physical and developmental disabilities perspective. The profession has a long history of evaluating individuals with disabilities to appropriately adapt motor vehicles and to teach these individuals how to drive the adapted vehicles. It has been the extension of the lifespan and the increased numbers of individuals living with chronic conditions that has significantly expanded and altered the DRS's service populations. Moreover, the "gray tsunami" of the baby boomers (see Exhibit 3.1) will continue to increase the numbers of older adults and medically at-risk drivers (see Exhibit 3.2).

It is important for occupational therapy generalists and their clients to recognize and understand that individuals who describe their credential as DRS and practice driving rehabilitation can be as different as the practice areas of occupational therapy (e.g., school-based therapists vs. long-term-care therapists).

Program Administrator

As a manager of an occupational therapy program, it is important to ensure that the program incorporate the IADL of driving and community mobility within its menu of services. This critical IADL can be addressed by identifying the network of services as well as by developing clear criteria for referral that meet the needs of clients in the program's service area. Some clients will require screening to determine whether driving is

---

Exhibit 3.2. Medically At-Risk Driver

The Medically at-Risk Driving Centre of the University of Alberta (2011) defines a *medically at-risk driver* as the following:

> A person who, regardless of age, has a medical condition or conditions that could affect driving performance, but further assessment or testing is needed to determine whether their medical condition(s) have made them unsafe to drive (e.g., some drivers with diabetes are safe to drive, others are not).

The term *medically at risk* is being used with greater frequency by the transportation research community (e.g., NHTSA, Transportation Research Board), consistently and internationally in place of the previous term *older driver*, because it defines the issue more clearly (Dobbs, 2005). Specifically, just because an individual is older does not mean that he or she is an unsafe driver. In fact, there is no reason a driver who is healthy and 90 years old should be judged as unsafe based on birth date alone.

However, as one ages, the potential for medical conditions that may affect driving risk significantly increases. It is the older adults with health conditions that may affect driving who are the individuals of interest. The question is whether their medical condition puts them at risk for being able to continue driving, manage as a pedestrian, or safely use transit. Therefore, *medically at-risk driver* is a more appropriate term for occupational therapy practice.

---

at risk or is an option. Others will require the therapist to determine whether there are public transportation services available or whether the family will manage transportation without undue burden.

It is the responsibility of program administrators to require, educate, and encourage their occupational therapists to address this essential IADL that falls solidly within our scope of practice. Recent evidence demonstrates that even experienced occupational therapists are not adequately addressing this IADL and would benefit from education specifically addressing community mobility and driving (Dickerson, Schold Davis, & Chew, 2011).

Physician

As the traditional leader of the medical team, the physician is and will remain one of the significant decision makers in the intervention and discharge planning for the client. Clients, especially older adults, tend to look to the physician to make the decision in terms of driving (Carr, Schwartzberg, Manning, & Sempek, 2010), and many hospital-based occupational therapy driving rehabilitation programs require a physician's order before completing a comprehensive evaluation, regardless of the payer of services. However, physicians' decisions and recommendations for referrals are dependent on the critical and comprehensive input of team members. Although there are resources specifically designed for the physician, such as the *Physician's Guide to Assessing and Counseling Older Drivers* (Carr et al., 2010), physicians traditionally are not trained in the tools and resources for making the decision or referring their clients if they believe them to be at risk (Brooks, Venhovens, Healy, & McKee, 2011).

Occupational therapists are in an ideal position to be the "go-to" profession. Thus, as an important stakeholder, a physician needs to be educated as to what the occupational therapy generalist can provide in terms of information about community mobility and what the driving specialist can provide for the appropriate referrals. Dr. David Carr of Washington University, St. Louis, and editor of the recent *Physician's Guide,* offers specific suggestions or strategies encouraging occupational therapists to inform physicians about driving services by attending physician conferences and contacting the office managers when seeking to send information or meet with a physician (as cited in Dickerson, Schold Davis, & Carr, 2010). He encourages therapists to offer useful information to physicians about their clients that will facilitate a collaborative relationship between therapist and physician to assist clients in their community mobility needs, including historical information on driving behavior; results of vision, cognitive, and motor domain assessments; opportunities to improve any functional impairment; a summary of the road test; recommendations; and alternative transportation options.

Client or Patient

Occupational therapists are sensitive to client needs and work diligently to be client centered. This sensitivity should carry through the whole process, ensuring that the client has the ability to get to where he or she needs to go regardless of driving status. In some programs, a social worker or similar professional is the referral source for alternative mobility needs, but if not, the occupational therapist should follow up with the client so that he or she continues to have mobility options.

Clients may not view driving evaluations as client centered. If the outcome is a recommendation to cease driving, the therapist may be seen as the adversary. The program model should include a method of providing the appropriate counseling or intervention at the *appropriate* times so that the client can benefit. For example, speaking to the client about alternative methods of transportation immediately after hearing a non-driving recommendation may be counterproductive. Furthermore, counseling about the results of an assessment may involve more than a quick summary. It may take the therapist time to integrate the information to give a succinct report that allows the client, family, and therapist to prepare for the give-and-take of this communication.

Just as reading an MRI or neurological test is not done immediately after the testing, driving evaluation conclusions might be integrated into a subsequent occupational therapy intervention session, strategically conveying the interpretation of driving evaluation results and integrating the results' implications to develop a person-centered plan. It may be the time to involve the generalist occupational therapist to focus on the support of the IADL of community mobility for successful transitions and access to alternative methods of transportation.

Family Member or Caregiver

As with the client, family members should be involved in the evaluation and discussion of community mobility. Although family members may not be surprised by a "cease driving" recommendation, they may be overwhelmed by the implications of this recommendation or resist it because of the impact their loved one's transportation dependence places on their personal lives. For example, the adult child may now need to be responsible for all transportation of both elderly parents who live in a rural area with limited services. Similarly, the parents of a child may be overwhelmed to hear that their child might not be able to drive at 16 years of age along with his or her friends and to think how that distinction will affect future plans for the child, parents, and family as a whole.

The entire family is a major stakeholder, as any outcome will affect the circumstances of the family structure. Information gathered from family members before a driving evaluation is critical, as is information when preparing the final report or referral plan. It is important for the clients, family members, and therapists to knowledgably exchange information about available resources. Communities likely have some transportation resources, but it may take work on the part of the therapist, social worker, or health care team to identify them. If it is difficult for professionals to understand public and private service systems, it's no wonder families become so overwhelmed and discouraged, concluding that no options exist. Therapists need to be familiar with the resources, add any needed or local information, or appropriately refer the family and client.

Therapists address the IADL of mobility around the home, bathroom, and stairs with their clients and their families. These needs extend to the motor vehicle and include getting in and out of vehicles as drivers or passengers and addressing the storage and management of adaptive or mobility devices, ensuring that clients and their families can get them in and out of their automobiles. This educational process is an opportunity for occupational therapists to be proactive and to allow clients and family members to begin to appreciate the impact of disability on community mobility while still within the therapeutic environment.

Early awareness by family members is important. Consider the decisions that many clients or families face with changes in medical status, living situations, and transportation. Awareness of options is of critical importance when making informed decisions. Without appropriate guidance, clients might replace a vehicle damaged in a crash with a vehicle that cannot effectively accommodate the most cost-effective or beneficial mobility devices or will be more costly to modify for hand controls. With ready Internet access, family members may purchase an adapted vehicle or adaptive equipment before having all the facts to understand the safety risks or range of options that fit the vehicle purchased. It is essential to inform the family about the various levels of complexity and the diversity of equipment options. What clients, families, and some professionals do not know or understand is that the DRS is an *expert* in this process and can evaluate and prescribe the specific equipment, devices, or vehicles that will work best for an individual and his or her family circumstances.

Social Worker or Case Manager

Generally, medical practice settings have a designated individual managing the overall treatment plan for each individual patient. It is usually a social worker or case manager with roles and responsibilities unique to the setting. It is advisable for the occupational therapist to understand the role and scope of the social worker or case manager when addressing community mobility options as the client and family prepare for discharge. It may be in the purview of the social worker to make arrangements if alternative transportation is needed. Regardless, the occupational therapist's driving and community mobility plan should incorporate the social worker or case manager's role in determining current and future transportation needs. This collaboration between disciplines is particularly important for clients facing progressive disorders. The social worker or case manager may understand the progression of a particular disease process but will not necessarily understand the impact of the disease process on functional performance and the client's current and future ability to drive or travel within the community.

It is important not to assume that others have the knowledge or awareness of the mobility needs and future potential. The social worker or case manager commonly is responsible for initiating the exploration of transportation alternatives to determine eligibility and funding resources. In some cases, as an advocate for the client's mobility, the occupational therapist may need to work collaboratively with the social services department to build awareness of and access to transportation alternatives and driver rehabilitation services.

Ophthalmologist or Optometrist

Vision is often the first screen to driving. The occupational therapist completing a visual screening or evaluation might be the first health care professional to suspect a vision problem. For example, if an issue with an older adult's performance on paper-and-pencil tests is detected, impaired vision must be considered and appropriate referrals made. Cataracts are probably the best example of a possible intervention. Older adults lose their eyesight with cataracts very gradually and often do not realize the extent of their visual deficit and that it can be corrected. Thus, the referral to the ophthalmologist or optometrist is the appropriate next step.

It is also important for the occupational therapist to realize that each state has visual guidelines for driver licensing and to know these guidelines (see the *Physician's Guide* or the individual state licensing agency). It is the ethical responsibility of the therapist to inform the client, family, and team members if there is a visual deficit that may have implications for driver licensing. It becomes the responsibility of the team, and particularly the ophthalmologist or optometrist, to evaluate the possibility of corrective measures.

When the client has a complex visual issue (e.g., nystagmus, field cut, depth perception), there may be referral options for intervention. The neuro-optometrist or neuro-ophthalmologist can evaluate an individual and may be able to intervene with a vision rehabilitation program. Again, it's important to be aware of the network of services available and, if the client does not meet minimum state guidelines for vision, to consider those options.

Just as with the physician, the DRS would be wise to build relationships with optometrists in his or her service area. Older adults may see an optometrist every year to check their status of glaucoma or to get another pair of eyeglasses. An optometrist evaluates an individual's vision, and it is very reasonable for the optometrist to become aware of cognitive change during the eye exam. For example, consider the demands of the eye exam. The client is asked to read lines of numbers or letters and compare them from one view to the other. Although a senior may "pass" the vision test, the optometrist may be able to offer some information about a change in cognitive status and should be encouraged to convey this concern to the medical doctor or DRS.

Psychologist or Neuropsychologist

Occupational therapists familiar with driving evaluations recognize that some of the assessments used in the clinical component of the comprehensive driving evaluation may be the same assessments completed by neuropsychologists, particularly assessments of cognitive and processing speed components. As part of the network of services, it is important to clarify what testing is done by the neuropsychologist, what is done by the occupational therapist in the normal course of practice, and what is uniquely included in the comprehensive driving evaluation, because it is contraindicated to subject a client to repetition of the same test when results could be shared.

Furthermore, the expertise of the neuropsychologist interpretations could contribute to the overall picture of the client. Accordingly, while assessing a client for driving and community mobility, it is possible to find evidence of impairments that have not yet been brought to the attention of the client, family, or other team members. As with all occupational therapy evaluations, referrals to the psychologist or neuropsychologist for signs of depression, medication imbalances, cognitive impairment, behavioral problems, and so forth are appropriate.

Other Health Professionals

The occupational therapist recognizes that problems identified within the driving screening or evaluation should be referred to other health professionals as appropriate.

The occupational therapist recognizes that problems identified within the driving screening or evaluation should be referred to other health professionals as appropriate. For example, a referral to a physical therapist would be warranted if gait problems are obvious and not addressed in the client's history. A good review of medications is always warranted if the evaluation reveals multiple physicians prescribing multiple medications. Both the types of medications and the interactions of medications can cause a change in consciousness and performance. There are resources available that offer guidelines regarding medications and driving, and therapists should be familiar with the most common types of medications that will affect driving (see the *Physician's Guide*). A pharmacist is a good partner and can be of assistance to therapists, other team members, family members, and clients in exploring medications and identifying potential problems.

Community Partners

Because driving and community mobility occur outside the physical environment of the medical care system, the DRS requires partners who are part of the environment not directly related to the medical care system. These partners include driving educators or instructors, mobility dealers and equipment vendors, state licensing agencies, transit authority, law enforcement, and judicial and public health systems, and they are critical to clients or consumers achieving successful mobility within their communities.

Driving Educator or Driving Instructor

There is a difference between a driving educator and a driving instructor. The *driving educator* has a degree in education with a specialized degree in driver education (Stav, Hunt, & Arbesman, 2006). The *driving instructor* is an individual who has gone through an educational program that prepares him or her to teach individuals how to drive within the state. Driving instructors' state-specific education typically consists of "rules of the road" content and an on-road component designed to prepare them to teach driving to teenagers and novice drivers.

Some driving instructors have extended their service model to offer driver training to individuals returning to the road, older drivers, or individuals using a new adaptive device in their vehicle. Additionally, some driving educators and driving instructors have fulfilled the criteria and passed the examination offered through the **Association of Driving Rehabilitation Specialists (ADED)** to use the designation of *certified driver rehabilitation specialist (CDRS)*. Although there are differences in the training and job responsibilities, no national protocols or labels consistently distinguish the services provided by a driving instructor, a driving educator (with or without CDRS), and a DRS (a multidisciplinary field) in a manner free of misinterpretation by the health care professional or consumer. All of these providers offer a service called a *driving evaluation*.

Obviously the skills and scope of services differ between the various providers and all offer a genuine valued contribution, but the services are indistinguishable by titles alone. This ambiguity creates confusion for consumers, family members, and health professionals. The occupational therapist, as the facilitator of driving and community mobility for clients, needs to be prepared to describe the differences and refer the client to the appropriate service that benefits him or her. Ideally, the individual professionals will work together to address the unique needs of individual clients.

For example, how might roles be delineated in a program for a client with a lower-extremity amputation? The occupational therapist DRS would evaluate the client to assess the ability to learn hand controls, recommend the specific model, and initially instruct the client in the use of hand controls. The driving instructor, however, may be the individual who offers the on-road training sessions to actually practice with the controls, once installed, in the client's neighborhood and community.

Another example of driving evaluations is the model used in Australia and commonly in California. The occupational therapist sits in the back seat of the vehicle while a driving instructor sits in the front seat. The driving instructor monitors both the client and other drivers in order to intervene with the vehicle controls or the instructor brake while the occupational therapist evaluates the *driving performance* of the client (Kay, Bundy, & Clemson, 2009). Driving instructors and educators are in every community, and they can provide a unique service and valuable resource to the overall driving evaluation program. Once the initial evaluation or vehicle fit is determined by the DRS, a skilled driving instructor has the skill set to train a driver in the context of a motor vehicle.

Mobility Dealer or Equipment Vendor

Mobility dealers (vehicles) and (driving adaptive) equipment vendors are significant stakeholders in the driver rehabilitation network (see Chapter 10 for a full description). DRSs with comprehensive driving rehabilitation programs have developed relationships with equipment vendors and mobility dealers. The equipment vendors work directly with occupational therapy DRSs and clients to modify vehicles or adapt a vehicle for modifications based on the client's individual needs (e.g., wheelchair lift, hand controls), and mobility dealers market fully equipped vehicles for adapted driving. Because some adaptations to a motor vehicle are particularly expensive, possibly amounting to thousands of dollars, it is important for clients and family members to understand all the considerations before adapting a vehicle or purchasing a vehicle for adaptation. Furthermore, it is critical that any equipment selected be installed by a mechanic correctly, with safety as the ultimate priority. The DRS needs to have an honest and collaborative relationship with vendors so that the client receives the best model adaptation with a vehicle that is appropriate for his or her disability.

Most occupational therapists are not engineers. Thus, the therapist must recognize that mobility and equipment dealers have the expertise needed to offer the best advice for vehicle modification. This is particularly true when high-tech modifications are required, such as minimum-effort steering or computerized controls. Many DRSs are trained in basic options. Few specialists study and attain expertise required to prescribe the range of choices required by drivers with, for example, extremely limited mobility. When seeking expertise in high-tech adaptations, it is important for the specialist to seek education and mentorship, be it another occupational therapist, a DRS, or a rehabilitation engineer. In Chapter 10, the process and components of the technology of vehicle modification are explained in detail.

State Licensing Agency

Each state in the United States has a licensing agency that has developed its own licensing regulations and renewal systems for drivers of private motor vehicles. Although the department title may vary depending on where it is located in the state government structure, this agency is often called the *Department of Motor Vehicles (DMV)*. This department is tasked with the business of determining who has the privilege of driving. To appropriately address the driving needs of clients, occupational therapists should be knowledgeable about the minimum requirements for licensure and the process for reporting the at-risk driver. Two resources that are helpful are the **Physician's Guide to Assessing and Counseling Older Drivers** (Carr et al., 2010) and a Web site sponsored by the **AAA Foundation for Traffic Safety** (www.AAAfoundation.org).

Many, but not all, states have a group charged with collecting adequate data to make licensing determinations for the medically at-risk driver. The name of this group varies by state, but the most common title is the *Medical Review Board*. This board is commonly made up of physicians and nurses. In some states these are volunteer appointments; in a few, the positions are paid.

Increasingly, DRSs are appropriately becoming more involved. The Medical Review Board is usually responsible for reviewing individual cases of at-risk drivers submitted through its state dependent process (which may include reports from law enforcement, physicians, clinicians, or the public). This may generate a referral to DRSs. The driving evaluation offers data contributing to an informed determination of a client's driving potential or risk. It is critical for occupational therapists to know about the Medical Review Board process in their state, understand its function, and ensure that the board is aware of the evaluation information their program can contribute.

Because licensing falls under the jurisdiction of the state, there is no national between-state consistency in the process or criteria. The state-specific structure, rules, and implementation of restrictions give occupational therapists a challenge and an opportunity. Occupational therapists need to recognize the value of networking with their state licensing agency, becoming an advocate, and building awareness of their clients' need for services and local resources. As licensing agencies better understand how occupational therapy services may address the needs of the at-risk driver, referral links are established or strengthened. Access to appropriate and skilled individualized assessment and interventions protects the rights of citizens in need of rehabilitation services that allow them to continue to drive as a legally licensed driver or to secure appropriate transportation support services.

Transit Authority

State transportation authorities are as diverse as the states' driver licensing agencies, if not more so. Typically, public transportation is governed broadly from the individual state's Department of Transportation, but individual cities, regions, and even companies have services unique to their region of the country. For example, medium to large cities have some type of fixed bus systems for their citizens; large metropolitan or regional areas have huge integrated systems (e.g., Washington, DC, or New York City); and universities provide free transit for students from parking areas, dorms, or apartment complexes to campus.

The American Public Transportation Association (APTA) is an organization for all transportation groups at the state, city, regional, and private levels. APTA's mission includes strengthening and improving public transportation. It also advocates for public transportation to be available and accessible for all citizens across the

United States. **APTA's Web site** (www.apta.com) includes links to every state's public transportation groups.

For the occupational therapist, it is important to be familiar with the options for public transportation in a client's home community. If the client is expected to take a transit bus, the therapist may need to work on functional skills such as reading the timetables, address issues of accessibility within the system, or recommend that a family member or travel trainer be enlisted to support the learning process.

Law Enforcement

As public servants, law enforcement officers must keep the public safe, including ensuring safe driving on roads, in cities, and on highways. A law enforcement officer might be the first person to identify an at-risk driver if the driver is observed performing a moving violation. The role of the violation ticket has been recognized as a valuable indicator for identifying potential at-risk drivers (Carr et al., 2010)

NHTSA developed an educational initiative on the topic of ticketing and the potential actions an officer may take when coming upon an at-risk driver. This sponsored law enforcement training encourages officers to ticket the senior driver committing an infraction as the ticket represents an error, and a pattern of tickets may serve as a meaningful "red flag" for drivers and particularly for their families. The NHTSA-sponsored law enforcement education module is rich with content developed for law enforcement, describing changes associated with aging and medical conditions and the important role of law enforcement.

Occupational therapists should consider reaching out to local law enforcement agencies, such as offering information to educate the officers on the services their programs offer and building their awareness of resources available to citizens they may feel are at risk. Law enforcement officers are highly trained, but generally not on medical conditions or the aging process. The occupational therapist might volunteer to work with the local precinct's law enforcement education coordinator to offer the NHTSA law enforcement education module (developed by NHTSA and available to law enforcement educators as an educational resource) or contact the safety officer in the community. In many communities, *safety officers* are specially designated officers who are tasked with doing community presentations to groups, creating an opportunity for a partnered presentation.

Judicial System

In 2008, AOTA entered a cooperative agreement with NHTSA entitled the Judicial Project. The goal was to address the potential for occupational therapy programs to contribute expertise when courts are asked to make decisions on driving competence. As a result of the project, AOTA has a better understanding of the role of the judge as a stakeholder in driving and community mobility. AOTA found that there was active interest on the part of judges to understand and potentially access DRSs to identify drivers medically at risk who may benefit from corrective intervention and to assist with determining driver competence. AOTA developed two fact sheets to be used by occupational therapists and judges: *Facilitating Judgments About Driving: A Guide for Judges* (AOTA, n.d.-a) and *Occupational Therapy's Role in Judicial Decisions About Older Drivers: A Guide for Occupational Therapists* (AOTA, n.d.-b).

Occupational therapists should consider reaching out to judges in their area and informing them about the potential benefit of the comprehensive driving evaluation report as guidance for determining driver competence. Generally, judges can require additional information before making a final decision when faced with a complex dynamic. When faced with a senior driver or a driver who is medically compromised, the informed judge might require an additional evaluation or expert information before making a decision. In many areas, judges are elected, so it is in the judge's best interest to understand the dynamics of the community to make fair and objective decisions on a factual foundation, such as a comprehensive driving evaluation.

By understanding that judges or others in the judicial system are a potential stakeholder group, occupational therapists have an opportunity for advocacy and outreach. An occupational therapy program could work with the court system to better understand the needs within that community and how the evaluation program could fill a gap in service.

Public Health

The U.S. public health system is charged with considering the health and quality of life from a population perspective in terms of prevention of disease and illness. The system focuses on broad issues such as vaccinations, serving impoverished groups, and infant health. Many states have recognized the growing numbers of older adults, and their public health systems are working on fall prevention and the needs of at-risk drivers.

The local public health structures vary considerably but usually consist of social workers and public health nurses charged with advising families and seniors. Reaching out to the public health sector as a stakeholder group is another opportunity for occupational therapists to

- Advocate for the medically at-risk driver;
- Advise by matching seniors and medically at-risk drivers with appropriate transportation options; and
- Respond to consumers, including families seeking assistance with complying with mandates from physicians or licensing agencies requiring an individual to stop driving.

Occupational therapists reaching out to the public health sector can identify gaps in service, work with local providers to understand services for education and direct intervention that may address these needs, and build a pathway for service.

An example of this successful outreach can be found in California. Since 2005, San Diego State University's School of Public Health research division, the **Center for Injury Prevention Policy and Practice (CIPPP)**, has facilitated a collabora-tive public health systems approach to increase the number of seniors who remain safely in their communities and successfully age in place. Together with the Epidemiology and Prevention for Injury Control Branch of the California Department of Public Health and the Occupational Therapy Association of California, CIPPP developed a strategic action plan to increase the number of occupational therapists who can address the driving and community mobility needs of the senior population. The project focused on the needs of the at-risk seniors, and occupational therapists were identified as an integral member of this stakeholder group. This project was funded through the California Office of Traffic Safety and resulted in the creation of a comprehensive Web site of services, including a database of occupational therapy driving rehabilitation services. The **final report** (CIPPP, 2005) and other useful documents can be downloaded from the **Elder Safety Web site** (www.eldersafety.org).

The California example illustrates the value of a group of diverse stakeholders addressing the needs in their community together. Efforts such as these can take months or years. Occupational therapists should understand that the broader stakeholder initiatives are ongoing as they build understanding of the array of services essential to addressing the driving and community mobility needs of seniors. The California Web site serves as an example of a place to start and of what a stakeholder group might achieve.

Professional Organizations

This section describes professional organizations whose mission includes either addressing the transportation needs of their constituents or assisting their constituents in meeting the mobility and transportation needs for client groups. Each of these professional organizations has significant value for its membership as a resource for information; networking with other professionals; and searching for evidence about driving, community mobility, and transportation options. For the occupational therapist concerned with driving, membership in these associations is beneficial. **Appendix 3.A** lists each organization's Web site.

AOTA: Driver Safety Initiative

The AOTA Older Driver Initiative (ODI) was formalized in 2003. It began by bringing together key stakeholders. AOTA conducted this meeting with funding from NHTSA. The priorities identified by this stakeholder group became the initial goals of ODI, which included building a microsite, developing educational resources for occupational students and therapists, and reaching out to the broader stakeholder community through conference presence and presentations (Peterson & Somers, 2003; **see Older Drivers Opportunities**).

AOTA's **Driver Safety Web site** (www.aota.org/older-driver) provides essential information to occupational therapists, consumers and caregivers, DRSs, and other health care professionals. For occupational therapists, there are resources to start programs and enhance skill sets and knowledge. Consumers can access sources of information about driving and community mobility and the role of occupational therapy and search for specialists in their geographic area. AOTA's Older Driver Safety Awareness Week won a national award for advocacy and will continue to promote the profession in this growing practice area.

Association of Driving Rehabilitation Specialists

ADED is a professional organization "devoted primarily to the support of professionals working in the field of driver education and transportation equipment modification for persons with disabilities" (ADED, 2012). ADED provides (1) key components of education for DRSs, (2) the structure for certification testing of DRSs, and (3) information for consumers. Although most of the professionals using the designation of DRS are licensed occupational therapists, the ADED membership represents a multidisciplinary group of individuals who address driving through screening, assessment, training, the engineering and development of adaptive driving equipment, and intervention.

Specifically for consumers, ADED has a Web site that allows individuals to locate DRS members in their immediate area. For occupational therapists, ADED provides unique educational opportunities that specifically address driving rehabilitation on the practical level. The annual conference facilitates the networking of specialists and mentor options that provide the opportunity to expand skills, abilities, and knowledge. The exhibit hall has many of the vehicle modifications and dealers can demonstrate the latest adaptive equipment available. ADED does not have a professional journal but publishes a newsletter called *Newsbrake* that includes upcoming events, short articles about driving rehabilitation, membership news, and advertisements.

National Mobility Equipment Dealers Association

The **National Mobility Equipment Dealers Association (NMEDA)** is an organization whose mission is to provide a quality and safe vehicle modification. It is a nonprofit trade association whose membership includes primarily equipment dealers and manufacturers of adaptive equipment for vehicles. In conjunction with DRSs who are members, NMEDA's members "work together to improve transportation options for people with disabilities" (www.NMEDA.org). To be an equipment dealer or manufacturer member, NMEDA requires adherence to the safety standards of NHSTA and the guidelines set forth by NMEDA. Thus, for the consumer, NMEDA serves as a quality assurance network that strives to assist with the selection of quality equipment that adheres to quality standardization. For the driving specialist, it offers a professional dealer network that can be used to compare and contrast the variety of options for vehicle modifications.

Transportation Research Board

The **Transportation Research Board (TRB)** is one of five major divisions of the National Research Council (NRC). NRC is a private nonprofit that is the principal operating agency of the National Academies in providing services to the government, the public, and the scientific and engineering communities. The National Academies (National Academy of Science, National Academy of Engineering, and Institute of Medicine) are institutions that provide expert advice on science, engineering, and medical challenges and produce reports that help shape policies, inform public opinion, and advance science.

The mission of TRB is to "provide leadership in transportation innovation and progress through research and information exchange, conducted within a setting that is objective, interdisciplinary, and multimodal" (TRB, 2011, p. 2). TRB covers every aspect of transportation, including aviation, highways, marine, motor carriers, pedestrians and bicyclists, public transportation, pipelines, and rail. It has five major divisions: (1) design and construction; (2) operations and preservation; (3) planning and environment; (4) policy and organization; and (5) safety, system components, and users. Under this last section are the TRB committees related to safety and human factors, with more than 30 committees. Although there are several committees of interest to occupational therapists, the most relevant committee is ANB60, Safe Mobility for Older Persons, which was established to stimulate high-quality research and allow interested researchers and practitioners to disseminate research and related information to those interested in improving the safety and mobility of older drivers.

It is critical that occupational therapists who understand the importance of transportation research represent the profession on this committee to ensure that researchers and key stakeholders clearly appreciate the value of occupational therapy and driving rehabilitation, especially in terms of research on evaluation and assessment. There are other committees and subcommittees to which occupational therapists can contribute (e.g., Medical Review, Women and Driving, Novice Drivers), but overall TRB is a significant source of the latest research and policy development in the area of transportation. The TRB Web site (www.TRB.org) is available to consumers but may be difficult for them to negotiate because of the massive amount of materials in all areas of transportation and documents geared for the researcher. However, in this respect, TRB is an excellent organization for therapists who are doing transportation research to join and become an active contributing member.

Gerontological Society of America

The Gerontological Society of America (GSA) is a multi- and interdisciplinary organization dedicated to research, practice, and education in the area of aging. The society's purpose is to "advance the study of aging and disseminate information among scientists, decision makers, and the general public" (GSA, 2008). The members of this large association (more than 5,000) select to be associated with one of four sections: (1) Biological Sciences; (2) Health Sciences; (3) Behavioral and Social Sciences; or (4) Social Research, Policy and Practice. GSA publishes several peer-reviewed journals (*The Gerontologist, The Journals of Gerontology Series A: Biological and Medical Sciences*, and *The Journals of Gerontology Series B: Psychological and Social Sciences*), and there is an annual scientific conference that offers research sessions and educational programming in each of the four sections. The association also has special interest groups that meet about common topics and are offered special sponsoring of programs and presentation platforms.

The Transportation and Aging Interest Group is a sanctioned group that meets annually offering a networking meeting for researchers interested in transportation issues. This interest group was effective in developing a white paper (Dickerson et al., 2007) that is considered a landmark paper summarizing research in this area. For researchers, membership and participation in this association are important, and occupational therapy is a well-recognized profession with leading occupational therapy researchers participating as active members. For the therapist, membership links practice to research, and the association is a strong advocate for increasing aging education and practice. For the consumer, membership or information is less pertinent, as it is more a professional organization.

American Society of Aging

The **American Society on Aging** (ASA) is also a professional association whose mission is "to support the commitment and enhance the knowledge and skills of those who seek to improve the quality of life of older adults and their families" (http://

www.asaging.org). Rather than focus primarily on research, ASA's publications, Web site, and annual conference emphasize practice and continuing education for professionals on issues of aging. ASA offers webinars and publications centered on aging and diversity, environments, technology, multiculturalism, mental health, and leadership. There are several constituent groups but only an informal transportation group. For therapists, ASA is an influential link to best practices in the area of aging and offers multiple opportunities for expanding professional education beyond occupational therapy. For consumers, ASA, like GSA, is a professional association and will not have practical information for the client level.

Southern Gerontological Society

The **Southern Gerontological Society (SGS)** is a network of gerontological professionals in the South. Although smaller and in a focused area of the United States, this association provides a bridge between research and practice. SGS has an annual conference and publishes a peer-reviewed and respected *Journal of Applied Gerontology*. Members include researchers, aging network personnel, educators, health professionals, and policy makers. For therapists in the Southern region of the country, this association can offer meaningful support, an annual scientific conference for best practice and research, and assistance in "translating and applying knowledge in the field of aging" (SGS, 2011).

National Stakeholder Groups and Their Resources

In addition to associations of which occupational therapists may choose to become members, there are other stakeholder groups that are critical in terms of finding resources both professionally and for our clients. Each of the organizations described in this next section contributes to the goal of mobility for all citizens and may be used by the therapist or passed on as a resource to the consumer.

National Highway Traffic Safety Administration

NHTSA (http://www.nhtsa.gov) is a federal agency established by the Highway Safety Act of 1970 (P. L. 91-605) to develop and disseminate programs that increase safety on U.S. roads and highways. It is responsible for reducing deaths, injuries, and economic losses resulting from motor vehicle crashes. This includes investigating safety on motor vehicles, conducting research on driver behavior and traffic safety, and providing grants to state and local governments to provide highway safety programs. For consumers, NHTSA offers current news or issues on a comprehensive amount of information on driving safety, vehicle safety, laws and regulation, research information, and data. For the occupational therapist, the NHTSA Web site is a rich source of reports, presentations, and resources that are invaluable. For example, there are summaries as well as full reports that include polypharmacy and older drivers; intersection crashes among drivers in their 60s, 70s, and 80s; multiple medications and vehicle crashes; traffic safety facts for children, pedestrians, and the older population; and many sources of materials for the education of clients, community members, and professionals.

NHTSA has been a longtime supporter of occupational therapy through the Driving Safety Initiative at AOTA. AOTA has managed several grant-funded programs from NHSTA that assisted in the creation of many of the materials currently

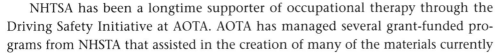

available on the AOTA Web site, such as ***Guidelines for Creating a Transportation Resource Guide,*** which outlines the steps for creating a usable list of transportation options for clients (www.aota.org/documentvault.driving/guidelines.aspx). Anything funded by NHTSA is readily available for therapists, clients, and consumers, and is free of charge.

American Association of Motor Vehicle Administrators

The American Association of Motor Vehicle Administrators (AAMVA) is a nonprofit organization that represents the state and provincial public officials, including driver licensing, in North America who administer and enforce motor vehicle laws. The association serves as a liaison between government and the private sector to facilitate uniformity and reciprocity in motor vehicle laws and guidelines. Its membership includes associations, organizations, and businesses that share the goal of developing model programs for motor vehicle administration, law enforcement, and highway safety.

Clinicians may look to this organization for information on driver licensing laws (vehicles and motorcycles), vehicle standards, guidelines for licenses, and initiatives related to safety and security. **AAMVA also maintains a Web site** (www.aamva.org) rich with resources and initiatives of interest to occupational therapy programs. For example, ***Driver Fitness Medical Guidelines*** (NHTSA & AAMVA, 2009) was a joint collaborative effort between NHTSA and AAMVA. The GrandDriver project is another example of an AAMVA project addressing safe mobility for seniors. This project offers a toolkit of resources available for replication, including a Web-site framework, ideas for community outreach, and a format for listing community resources.

National Center for Senior Transportation

The National Center for Senior Transportation (NCST) was established as part of the reauthorization of the Older Americans Act Amendments of 2006 (P. L. 109-365). It is administered by Easter Seals, in partnership with the National Association of Area Agencies on Aging. The mission of NCST is to increase the transportation options for older adults so they can live more independently within their communities. NCST

develops, collects, and distributes information and resources for communities, transportation providers, government entities, human services providers, and older adults and their caregivers. Its **Web site** (www.seniortransportation.easterseals.com) contains a rich source of publications, resources, and training, particularly for the occupational therapist who is invested in providing information to clients about options for transportation alternatives.

NCST also offers instructions and a template for professionals to use in creating a brochure regarding transportation options (NCST, n.d.). Additionally, NCST has offered free webinars about transportation for health professionals and in the past few years has offered small scholarship programs for graduate students who pursue a project on transportation. For example, the *Transportation Resource Guide* (Dickerson, Evans, Webster, & Faircloth, 2008) was developed by five occupational therapy graduate students with a small grant to Dr. Anne Dickerson. This guide was developed as an occupational therapy intervention tool to guide the discussion of community mobility with clients and was found to be effective by the therapists who piloted it. The resource guide is available free for use (http://www.roadi.org/Resource_Guide/Transportation_OT_RG/trans_rg_home.html). For the consumer, NCST provides

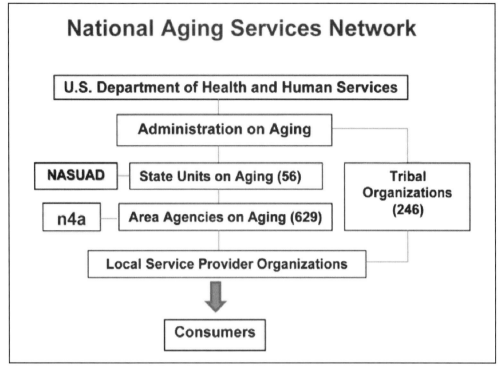

Figure 3.1. Organizational chart for aging services in the United States.

Source. From "Aging Services Network," available at http://n4a.org/about-n4a. Copyright © 2012, by the National Association of Areas on Aging. Used with permission.

information about accessible transportation and guidance in using transportation systems.

National Association of Area Agencies on Aging

The **National Association of Area Agencies on Aging (N4A)** is the national advocacy organization for the members of the Area Agencies on Aging (www.n4a.org). The federal agency of the Administration on Aging (AoA) is responsible for the concerns of older adults and their caregivers. Through the U.S. Department of Health and Human Services, AoA administers funds to the Area Agencies on Aging and tribal service groups. (*Note.* The confusion between the Area Agencies on Aging and the Auto Club is well known. In the aging community, this is commonly referred to as "the other AAA".)

Most states are divided into service and planning areas so that each specific Area Agencies on Aging office can serve the needs of its consumers at a local level. N4A provides training and technical assistance and frequently offers small grants to Area Agencies on Aging member offices (see Figure 3.1).

For the occupational therapist, N4A is an important advocacy group. There is an annual joint conference of N4A and the American Society of Aging. Both of these organizations are important for therapists because both provide critical resources about the political and social changes in the changing demographics of the United States.

At the local and state levels where occupational therapists work within a community, the Area Agencies on Aging offices in the therapists' area are a crucial resource for clients. Although services may differ from area to area, generally Area

Agencies on Aging services include transportation options or at least information for that service area at the consumer level.

State Highway Safety Offices

All states and territories have highway safety offices, most located within the U.S. Department of Transportation, although some are located in the public safety department or other state agency. Each of these entities submits highway safety plans to NHTSA to assist its state's department of transportation and receive funding to implement the plans. Occupational therapists in nonprofit organizations may be eligible to submit proposals for programs that will affect safety on the state's highways through their individual state's highway safety program.

The **Governors Highway Safety Association (GHSA)** is a national organization that represents the highway safety offices, providing leadership and advocacy to improve traffic safety, influence national policy, promote best practices, and manage programs. Although GHSA's Web site (www.ghsa.org) is geared for safety officers of state agencies, therapists can find useful information about safety programs, crash statistics, and model programs that can be used to advocate change in one's own state.

AAA

AAA, formerly the American Association of Automobiles, is well known for its on-road services, insurance, and travel advice. However, this national organization has expanded to offer additional services and products, including a focus on senior drivers. There are two components of AAA in terms of driver safety: (1) the membership organization for individual members of AAA and (2) the AAA Foundation for Traffic Safety.

The membership organization is the larger of these two components, with AAA clubs existing in almost every community in the country. Although there are corporate office programs such as CarFit, the community clubs manage different programs based on individual community needs. The AAA corporate Web site (www.aaa.com) links to a driver safety page that assists individuals in finding driving schools and traffic safety courses in the local club area. Additionally, there are tools and information on separate links for teenagers and their parents and seniors and their caregivers. Specifically, **SeniorDriving.AAA.com** concerns how to help the senior driver with early planning, communication, and skills assessment information. For the consumer, this is a resource geared for caregivers of clients needing supportive information, resources, or safe driving tips.

The second component of the AAA organization is the AAA Foundation for Traffic Safety. As a not-for-profit charitable organization, it is separate from the AAA insurance companies and club members but funded from voluntary contributions from the clubs and other groups. The foundation's mission is to "identify problems, foster research that seeks solutions, and disseminate information and educational materials that promote good traffic safety practices" (AAA Foundation for Traffic Safety, 2007, p. 2). For the clinician, the foundation offers a wealth of research reports on diverse driver safety projects, many of them directly related to occupational therapy practice in the area of driving and community mobility. One rich source of information is a link (www.seniordrivers.org/lpp) with all driver-licensing policies and practices in the United States, including noteworthy initiatives. For driving specialists, this is a useful resource when in need of DMV information from a specific state.

For the consumer, the foundation has a Web site for senior drivers (www.seniordrivers.org). Unlike the AAA motor club site, this Web site is designed for senior drivers, family members, researchers, and providers of alternative transportation. It includes general safe-driving information, self-assessment or "measuring your driving skills/needs," education and training, and planning for continued mobility. For seniors without medical impairments, this can be a rich source of information on self-assessment tools, tips on how to maintain or improve safe driving habits, and planning for alternatives in the future.

The Hartford

To meet the needs of the 50-plus age market, **The Hartford** has employed gerontologists for the past 25 years to advance the development of research and educational materials covering diverse topics, including motor vehicles and driving, home safety and disaster planning, healthy aging, and brain fitness. Being a partner with the MIT Aging Lab, AARP, and AOTA, the Hartford has produced a Web site (www.safedrivingforalifetime.com) that contains quality information that is useful for consumers and therapists. Particularly useful are the series of guidebooks that the Hartford has produced either to be downloaded or ordered free of charge. Although all the guidebooks are useful, for driving specialists, three are especially important to have available to show physicians, consumers, family members, and other health care professionals.

First, *We Need to Talk: Family Conversations with Older Drivers* (The Hartford, 2010b) offers suggestions and worksheets for starting the conversation about driving retirement. It is useful for the senior and the adult child who wonder when the right time is to turn in the keys. Second, *At the Crossroads: Family Conversations about Alzheimer's Disease, Dementia, and Driving* (The Hartford, 2010a) is helpful for family members when their loved one has developed dementia and offers strategies to manage the changes. Finally, a Guidebook that was designed in collaboration with AOTA, *Your Road Ahead: A Guide to Comprehensive Driving Evaluations* (The Hartford & AOTA, 2010) is a critical resource for occupational therapy, as it describes the benefits of having a comprehensive driving evaluation from an occupational therapist. Describing the usefulness of the comprehensive driving evaluation from a professional in easy, friendly terms extends the understanding of the benefits of a comprehensive driving evaluation far greater than what driving specialists can do individually.

AARP

AARP (www.aarp.org), once the American Association of Retired Persons, is a non-profit member organization for individuals 50 years or older. Dedicated to "enhancing quality of life for all as we age," AARP is one of the largest contingency groups advocating for social change and meeting the needs of older citizens. Through its national and regional offices and Web sites, AARP provides extensive and diverse services, products, and information on health, money, work, retirement, politics, food, travel, entertainment, technology, and other topics. AARP has made significant contributions in driver safety, especially for the consumer. For many years, AARP has offered driver safety classes for a low fee in the local community. These courses, which review the rules of the road and newer regulations, are popular and advertised as a possibility for a discount on insurance rates. More recently, an online driver safety class has been added.

For therapists, the contributions of AARP have been significant. AARP partnered with The Hartford (www.theHartford.com/lifetime) to provide the guidebook *We Need to Talk* (The Hartford, 2010b). In collaboration with the MIT Aging Lab and The Hartford–developed tools, AARP has taken a step further with structured online seminars and training volunteers to offer a *We Need to Talk* educational seminar to clients or any public groups. In addition, AARP has developed other mobility resources that provide great tools for therapists working with older adults in enhancing their community mobility.

Beverly Foundation

The Beverly Foundation is recognized in the transportation community as offering the model of the *5 A's of Senior-Friendly Transportation* (Beverly Foundation, n.d.), specifically, *availability, acceptability, accessibility, adaptability,* and *affordability*).

> The Beverly Foundation's mission is to foster new ideas and options to enhance mobility and transportation for today's and tomorrow's older population. The foundation pursues this mission through research activities, community outreach, and technical assistance products. The Foundation emphasizes transportation options for older adults which are essential to their ability to get where they need to go when they have limited their driving or have outlived their driving expectancy. (Beverly Foundation, 2011)

The **Beverly Foundation's Web site** (http://beverlyfoundation.org) offers a vast array of reports and resources specifically addressing the need for transportation options in every community. Tools offered on the Web site include a *Transportation and Dementia* factsheet recognizing the unique needs and vulnerability of the passenger with impaired cognition (Beverly Foundation, 2008). This factsheet offers a checklist of considerations when selecting services for the person with dementia. In recognition of the need to identify transportation options in a local community, the Beverly Foundation joined with Easter Seals to produce and make available a **Transportation Options Template** (http://seniortransportation.easterseals.com/site/PageServer?pagename=NCST2_tsc_options_download). This template (a workbook of sorts offering guidance through headings and boilerplate content) is formatted to simplify the development of a local resource guide. Once completed, the guide easily can be printed and updated.

The Transportation Options Template developed by the Beverly Foundation was in direct response to an occupational therapist speaking up at a national conference and asking the president of the Beverly Foundation for assistance finding local resources. From that exchange, this widely used tool was developed, and occupational therapists became more involved in the activities of the Beverly Foundation.

National Advocacy Groups

Many national advocacy groups address transportation on their Web sites or in their materials. One of the best examples of groups advocating for community mobility is the National Alzheimer's Association (www.alz.org) because of the needs of its caregivers and clients. In 2011, the Alzheimer's Association launched a microsite called the **Driving Resource Center** that specifically addresses the driving needs of persons with dementia (www.alz.org/safetycenter/we_can_help_safety_driving.asp). The launching of this Web site represents a significant step forward in the acknowledgment of the devastating effect dementia has on the ability to retain driving privileges over time. The Web site references occupational therapy as a significant resource and occupational therapy programs are encouraged to continue to build the services so desperately needed by persons with this progressive degenerative disease.

Partnerships Between Stakeholders

Although occupational therapists identify partnerships within the medical community to address driving, the need to build unique partnerships with other stakeholders is significant, especially as society attempts to meet the needs of the baby boomers. This section illustrates a few examples of these unique partnerships that define and enhance the experience of occupational therapists in the area of driver rehabilitation.

State Highway Patrol

North Carolina, with its Executive Committee for Older Drivers Safety Working Group, was one of seven states to participate in a project funded by NCST–NHTSA to promote older driver safety in their respective states. One of the requirements was to have representatives from specific government agencies, including the state highway patrol. As the team leader, Dr. Anne Dickerson contacted the leadership of the North Carolina State Highway Patrol (NCSHP), and eventually Sergeant Billy Overton was assigned, not because of his interest in older drivers, but because he happened to be in the state office when the decision was made to assign someone and his duty assignment in accident reconstruction was in the city of Greenville, where Dr. Dickerson is employed. Sgt. Overton dutifully contacted Dr. Dickerson, attended the meetings as assigned, and participated in the NCST workshops. However, through active engagement and collaboration, Sgt. Overton has become a champion for older driver safety. Significant contributions from his participation include the following:

- Sgt. Overton arranged for a visit with the commanding officer of the NCSHP training facility. Dr. Dickerson offered a brief lecture describing older drivers and driver rehabilitation. Understanding the need for education, the commanding officer asked for the PowerPoint presentation so she could present it to officers in their training.
- Sgt. Overton arranged a meeting with one of the developers of education of the training facility for law enforcement (for all law enforcement, not just State Highway Patrol). Through this link, Dr. Dickerson and other members of the older drivers working group had the opportunity to provide significant input to the educational module about older drivers for all North Carolina law enforcement.
- With input from Sgt. Overton and others, an older adult "cue card" for traffic stops was developed. Because of Sgt. Overton's support and participation, this cue card was distributed to more than 2,000 State Highway Patrol officers, and feedback was elicited via the Web to evaluate the effectiveness of the cards. With Sgt. Overton's influence, officers did respond, and the positive response will be reported at conferences.

> Although occupational therapists identify partnerships within the medical community to address driving, the need to build unique partnerships with other stakeholders is significant, especially as society attempts to meet the needs of the baby boomers.

White House Conference on Aging

The 2005 White House Conference on Aging (WHCoA) was held December 11–14, 2005, in Washington, DC, and was the fifth WHCoA in history. Like its predecessors, its purpose was to make recommendations to the president and Congress to help guide national aging policies for the next 10 years and beyond. The 2005 WHCoA, which had as its theme "The Booming Dynamics of Aging: From Awareness to Action," focused on the aging of today and tomorrow, including 78 million baby boomers who began to turn 60 in January 2006 (WHCoA, 2005). Seven occupational therapists participated as delegates from their respective states. As members of the 1,200 delegates, these occupational therapists had the unique opportunity to influence social policy, affect funding for aging issues, and interact with leaders of state and federal government and nationally known figures in the aging field. As delegates, all of the occupational therapists actively influenced workshops related to occupational therapy, including several on transportation issues. That transportation was ranked as the No. 3 issue (WHCoA, 2005) indicates how important older adults and their constituents view transportation issues.

It is now the time to begin preparation to become a delegate. To be a state delegate, an individual must be nominated by the governor of the state, a state senator, or a representative. It is critical for occupational therapists to make contact with their state leaders now to show an interest in this critical political process. If interested, therapists must be vigilant for any announcements for when the next White House Conference on Aging is planned.

Challenges and Opportunities

One of the most rewarding aspects of driver rehabilitation is the rich relationship that occupational therapists have with other stakeholders. Astute occupational therapists appreciate the unique skill set and contribution of key stakeholders, the resources (e.g., educational brochures, meeting space, speakers), and the providers of transportation. Collaboration is efficient in time and money, and this chapter has highlighted some inspiring examples where a phone call or site visit changed practice.

Researchers, state licensing officials, aging advocates, and others involved with transportation understand the critical role that occupational therapists have in driving, particularly within the aging and transportation community. Many national leaders in the field of aging specifically identify occupational therapy as a key component in meeting the needs of the aging population.

However, there are still significant stakeholders or subgroups of stakeholders who do not even know that DRSs exist or comprehend the complexity of the systems in which DRSs might operate. For example, most physiatrists might know to refer an individual with a spinal cord injury to the DRS; however, many gerontologists, internal medicine physicians, neurologists, or family practitioners do not know that such a service is even available. In presentations to physicians, most have welcomed the information and are interested to know they can refer their clients for driving assessments. Even the physicians who refer for comprehensive driving evaluations need education about driving rehabilitation—that is, there is more beyond the evaluation, that there is reason for referring for intervention. Further, physicians, although an important group of stakeholders, are only one group of many stakeholders.

Many developed programs across the United States have successfully addressed gaps in service through engagement of occupational therapy clinicians with the various stakeholders. However, within driving and community mobility, occupational therapy outreach is hindered by a lack of awareness and no common language to identify need and link with services already in place. Now is a time of challenge and opportunity for occupational therapy, and all therapists, specialists and generalists, must work toward defining and clarifying the roles, responsibilities, and partnerships of driver rehabilitation in their community. As communities strive to address safe mobility, occupational therapy professionals have the opportunity to participate in an essential role to ensure that members of the community have access to programs and services addressing the IADL of driving and community mobility—a fundamental task that will ensure our clients are living life to its fullest.

References

AAA Foundation for Traffic Safety. (2007). *2006–2007 annual report*. Washington, DC: Author.

American Medical Association, & National Highway Traffic Safety Administration. (2010). *Physician's guide to assessing and counseling older drivers*. Washington, DC: Author.

American Occupational Therapy Association. (2008). Occupational therapy practice framework: Domain and process, 2nd edition. *American Journal of Occupational Therapy, 62*, 625–683. doi:10.5014/ajot.62.6.625

American Occupational Therapy Association. (n.d.-a). *Facilitating judgments about driving: A guide for judges*. Bethesda, MD: Author.

American Occupational Therapy Association. (n.d.-b). *Occupational therapy's role in judicial decisions about older drivers: A guide for occupational therapists*. Bethesda, MD: Author.

Americans with Disabilities Act Amendments of 2008, P. L. 110-325, 122 Stat. 3553.

Association for Driver Rehabilitation Specialists. (2012). *Welcome to ADED*. Retrieved March 22, 2012, from http://www.driver-ed.org

Beverly Foundation. (2008). *Transportation and dementia*. Pasadena, CA: Author.

Beverly Foundation. (2011). *Senior transportation options*. Retrieved March 22, 2012, from http://beverlyfoundation.org

Beverly Foundation. (n.d.) *The five A's of senior-friendly transportation*. Pasadena, CA: Author.

Brooks, J., Venhovens, P., Healy, S., & McKee, J. (2011). *Seniors and physicians view of using driving simulators in clinical settings*. Poster session presented at the Gerontological Society of America, Boston.

Carr, D. B., Schwartzberg, J. G., Manning, L., & Sempek, J. (2010). *Physician's guide to assessing and counseling older drivers*. National Highway Traffic Safety Administration.

Center for Injury Prevention Policy and Practice. (2005, September). *Building a network of convenient, affordable, and trustworthy driving assessment and evaluation programs: Reflections of California occupational therapists*. Retrieved February 10, 2012, from http://www.eldersafety.org/images/stories/CA%20OT%20Driving%20Programs.pdf

Dickerson, A., Schold Davis, E., & Carr, D. (2010, August). *From data to decision: What physicians want in a driving rehabilitation report*. Paper presented at ADED: Association of Driving Rehabilitation Specialists Annual Conference, Kansas City, MO.

Dickerson, A. E., Schold Davis, E., & Chew, F. (2011, September). *Driving as an IADL in the medical setting: A model for intervention and referral*. Paper presented at the Transportation Research Board Conference: Emerging Issues in Safe and Sustainable Mobility for Older People, Washington, DC.

Dickerson, A. E., Molnar, L., Eby, D., Adler, G., Bedar, M., Berg-Weger, M., et al. (2007). Transportation and aging: A research agenda for advancing safe mobility. *The Gerontologist, 47*, 578–590.

Dickerson, A. E., Evans, L., Webster, L., & Faircloth, S. (2008). *Transportation resource guide*. [Unpublished document].

Dobbs, B. (2005). *Medical conditions and driving: A review of the literature (1960–2000)* (Report No. DOT HS 809 690). Retrieved February 3, 2012, from http://www.nhtsa.gov/people/injury/research/Medical_Condition_Driving/pages/TRD.html.

Gerontological Society of America. (2008). *About us*. Retrieved March 22, 2012, from http://www.geron.org/About%20us

The Hartford. (2010a). *At the crossroads: Family conversations about Alzheimer's disease, dementia, and driving*. Retrieved February 24, 2012, from http://hartfordauto.thehartford.com/UI/Downloads/Crossroads.pdf

The Hartford. (2010b). *We need to talk: Family conversations with older drivers*. Retrieved February 24, 2012, from http://hartfordauto.thehartford.com/UI/Downloads/FamCon Htd.pdf

The Hartford, & American Occupational Therapy Association. (2010). *Your road ahead: A guide to comprehensive driving evaluations*. Retrieved February 24, 2012, from http://hartfordauto.thehartford.com/UI/Downloads/Your_Road_Ahead.pdf

Highway Safety Act of 1970, P. L. 91-605, 84 Stat. 1739.

Kay, L. G., Bundy, A., & Clemson, L. (2009). Validity, reliability, and predictive accuracy of the Driving Awareness Questionnaire. *Disability and Rehabilitation, 31*, 1074–1082.

National Association of Areas on Aging. (2012). *Aging services network*. Retrieved March 23, 2012, from http://www.n4a.org/about-n4a

National Center on Senior Transportation. (n.d.). *Transportation solutions for caregivers: Senior transportation options template*. Retrieved March 22, 2012, from http://seniortransportation.easterseals.com/site/PageServer?pagename=NCST2_tsc_options_download

National Highway Traffic Safety Administration. (2009). *Traffic safety facts*. Retrieved February 24, 2012, from http://www-nrd.nhtsa.dot.gov/Pubs/811391.PDF

National Highway Traffic Safety Association, & American Association of Motor Vehicle Administrators. (2009, September). *Driver fitness medical guidelines*. Washington, DC, & Arlington, VA: Authors.

Older Americans Act Amendments of 2006, P. L. 109-365, 120 Stat. 2522.

Peterson, M. F., & Somers, F. (2003, November 19). Older driver opportunities. *OT Practice*, pp. 23–24.

Southern Gerontological Society. (2011). *Welcome to the Southern Gerontological Society*. Retrieved March 22, 2012, from http://www.southerngerontologicalsociety.org

Stav, W. B., Hunt, L. A., & Arbesman, M. (2006). *Occupational therapy practice guidelines for driving and community mobility for older adults*. Bethesda, MD: AOTA Press.

Transportation Research Board. (2011). *2011 annual report*. Washington, DC: Author.

University of Alberta, Faculty of Medicine & Dentistry. (2011). *The Medically At-Risk Driver Centre: Frequently asked questions*. Retrieved February 4, 2012, from http://www.mard.ualberta.ca/Home/FAQ/#What

White House Conference on Aging. (2005). *Report to the President and Congress: The booming dynamics of aging: From awareness to action*. Retrieved from http://www.whcoa.gov/

Appendix 3.A. Stakeholders-Related Resources

- **Association of Driving Rehabilitation Specialists (ADED):**
  http://www.driver-ed.org
  ADED aims to support professionals working in the field of driver education or training and transportation equipment modifications for persons
  with disabilities through education and information dissemination.

- **AAA Foundation for Traffic Safety:** http://www.aaafoundation.org
  A public education and research organization, the AAA Foundation for
  Traffic Safety funds projects designed to discover the causes of traffic
  crashes, prevent them, and minimize injuries when they do occur. Its Web
  site contains articles on studies and helpful links to increase driver safety.

- **American Public Transportation Association (APTA):** www.apta.com
  APTA is a trade association for organizations that are engaged in the areas
  of bus, paratransit, rail, subways, waterborne passenger services, and high-
  speed rail; large and small companies who plan, design, construct, finance,
  supply, and operate bus and rail services worldwide; and government agencies, metropolitan planning organizations, state departments of transportation, academic institutions, and trade publications.

- **Center for Injury Prevention Policy and Practice (CIPPP):** www.cippp.org
  CIPP offers resources aimed to reduce the frequency and severity of injuries
  by assisting government agencies, and community programs by compiling
  and posting a wealth of information and resources including publications,
  data as well as conferences and educational / training opportunities. They
  host two additional Web sites, including SafetyLit.org (safety literature)
  and ElderSafety.org (facilitating safe mobility for seniors).

- **Elder Safety Web site:** http://www.eldersafety.org
  ElderSafety.org is the product of collaboration and offers California wide
  resources for safe mobility for seniors including a database for locating
  occupational therapy driving rehabilitation programs in California. The
  site also offers a wonderful literature review of current research (http://
  www.eldersafety.org/images/stories/CA%20OT%20Driving%20Programs.
  pdf).

- **AOTA Driver Safety/Older Driver Web site:** http://www.aota.org/
  older-driver
  The AOTA Driver Safety-Older Driver Web site is a dedicated site offering
  practitioners, professionals, and consumers information and resource links
  on the topic of driver safety. It offers a database of driving rehabilitation
  specialists searchable by state.

- **National Mobility Equipment Dealers Association (NMEDA):**
  www.nmeda.com
  NMEDA is the not-for-profit trade association for mobility equipment
  manufacturers, dealers, driver rehabilitation specialists, and others.

- **Transportation Research Board:** www.trb.org/main/Home.aspx
  The Transportation Research Board, which is part of the National Academies, links transportation practitioners, researchers, public officials, and
  others with credible, high-quality information and research.

- **Gerontological Society of America (GSA):** www.geron.org
  GSA has a Transportation Interest Group, which offers an opportunity to network with researchers from a range of disciplines concerned with safety.
- **American Society on Aging (ASA):** www.asaging.org
  ASA is a multidisciplinary association seeking to improve the quality of life of older adults and their families. Members include professionals who are concerned with the physical, emotional, social, economic, and spiritual aspects of aging.
- **Southern Gerontological Society (SGS):** http://www.southerngerontologicalsociety.org
  SGS is a network of gerontology professionals in the South, including educators, aging network personnel, researchers, health professionals, and policy makers. SGS aims to bridge between research and practice, translating and applying knowledge in the field of aging.
- **National Highway Traffic Safety Administration (NHTSA):** http://www.nhtsa.gov/Senior-Drivers
  NHTSA is a federally funded agency that focuses on highway safety. The Web site offers a range of educational resources. The description leads to the senior driver section and lists search terms and where to go to order resources.
- **American Association of Motor Vehicle Administrators (AAMVA):** http://www.aamva.org
  AAMVA is a tax-exempt, nonprofit organization involved with motor vehicle administration, law enforcement, and highway safety. AAMVA represents the state and provincial officials in the United States and Canada who administer and enforce motor vehicle laws.
- **National Center for Senior Transportation (NCST):** http://seniortransportation.easterseals.com/site/PageServer?pagename=NCST2_about
  NCST is administered by Easter Seals, Inc., in partnership with the National Association of Area Agencies on Aging. The mission of NCST is to increase transportation options for older adults and enhance their ability to live more independently within their communities.
- **National Association of Area Agencies on Aging (N4A):** http://www.n4a.org
  N4A is the national association for the Area Agencies on Aging and a champion for Title VI Native American aging programs. Through advocacy, training, and technical assistance, n4a supports the national network of 629 area agencies on aging and 246 Title VI programs. Area agencies on aging were established to respond to the needs of Americans 60 and over in every local community. They make it possible for older adults to remain in their homes and communities as long as possible.
- **Governors Highway Safety Association (GHSA):** www.ghsa.org
  GHSA represents the state and territorial highway safety offices that implement programs to address behavioral highway safety issues, including occupant protection, impaired driving, and speeding.

Welcome to the Team! Who Are the Stakeholders?

77

- **AAA SeniorDriving.AAA.com:** http://seniordriving.aaa.com
  In 2012, AAA launched SeniorDriving.AAA.com, which is dedicated to helping seniors drive safer and longer. In addition to traditional resources offered by AAA, this site offers links that range from screening, to education, to selecting vehicles, to transiting from being driver to a nondriver.
- **The Hartford:** http://www.thehartford.com/lifetime
  The Hartford's Web site is sponsored by The Hartford Advance 50 Team, a division staffed by gerontologists with the mission of addressing driver safety. This Web site offers resources and educational materials; a series of brochures can be ordered free of charge. A 3-minute video is posted featuring Mary M. Johnson, MS, OTR/L, CDRS, McLean Driver Rehabilitation Program, explaining the comprehensive driving evaluation.
- **AARP:** http://www.aarp.org
  The AARP Web site offers programs, educational materials, and resources for senior drivers.
- **Beverly Foundation:** http://www.beverlyfoundation.org
  The Beverly Foundation Web site offers resources to enhance mobility and transportation for current and future older populations. The foundation pursues this mission through research activities, community outreach, and technical assistance products. The foundation emphasizes transportation options for older adults, which are essential to their ability to get where they need to go when they have limited their driving or have outlived their driving expectancy.
- **Transportation Options Template:** http://seniortransportation.easterseals.com/site/PageServer?pagename=NCST2_tsc_options_download
  Transportation Solutions for Caregivers offers instructions and a template for professionals to use in creating a brochure regarding transportation options.
- **Dementia and Driving Resource Center:** http://www.alz.org/care/alzheimers-dementia-and-driving.asp
  Launched by the Alzheimer's Association, this microsite specifically addresses the driving needs of persons with dementia and cites occupational therapy as a significant resource.
- **AARP's Online Driver Safety Course:** http://www.aarpdriversafety.org
  The AARP Driver Safety Course is designed as a refresher course for drivers ages 50 years and older to help drivers remain safe on today's roads. The course is offered both in person and online formats.

CHAPTER 4

Understanding Psychosocial Needs and Issues Related to Driving and Community Mobility and the Role of Occupational Therapy

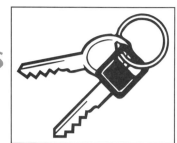

Christine Raber, PhD, OTR/L; Susan Martin Touchinsky, OTR/L; and Mary Jo McGuire, MS, OTR/L, FAOTA

Learning Objectives

At the completion of this chapter, readers will be able to

- Identify and describe the psychosocial needs and issues associated with driving, transitioning to driving retirement, and the use of community mobility;
- Identify the role of occupational therapists in addressing psychosocial needs and issues related to driving, driving retirement, community mobility, and transitions within this continuum; and
- Identify intervention strategies to address psychosocial needs of clients related to safe engagement in driving and community mobility.

Introduction

The freedom and ability to navigate through the world outside of one's personal living spaces is an essential occupation for most people. Engagement in productive leisure, self-care, and social occupations is often dependent upon the ability to access the community; one's sense of autonomy and self-determination often is associated with issues related to driving and community mobility. In Western society, transportation, in the form of driving and community mobility, has both utilitarian and symbolic meaning. This meaning is reflected in the following statement:

> For many individuals, obtaining a license to drive is a rite of passage. It represents freedom and a greater degree of mobility and independence. Driving becomes a regular part of an individual's routine, and not being able to drive is tantamount to being confined and dependent. (Bednarcik & Chew, 2009, p. 5)

To be effective in helping clients and families deal with questions related to driving and community mobility, therapists must recognize often-unspoken psychosocial issues, including attitudes and feelings related to independence, freedom,

Key Words

- awareness
- beliefs
- empathic breaks
- grief
- interpersonal reasoning
- loss
- metacognition
- psychosocial needs
- self-awareness
- therapeutic use of self

and self-determination. Analysis of the psychosocial skills necessary for safe community mobility skills reveals that emotional regulation skills, such as demonstrating patience, the ability to cope with stressors, and the ability to exhibit self-control, are important in all areas of community mobility. The ability to effectively regulate emotions intersects with the cognitive skills needed for a person to effectively drive, ride a bus, or move in the community as a pedestrian. Cognitive and emotional regulation skills, along with the underlying motivation to be mobile in the community, are intertwined with critical client factors of self-awareness, values, and beliefs (American Occupational Therapy Association [AOTA], 2008). Occupational therapy considers and addresses all of these areas.

Occupational Therapy and Psychosocial Needs: A Key Perspective

Central in the development of an occupational profile is consideration of psychosocial components, such as confidence, awareness, definitions of one's roles, and self-concept.

Occupational therapy offers a unique role and significant value when addressing psychosocial needs and issues related to driving and community mobility. Occupational therapists address the psychosocial skills essential for driving and community mobility by evaluating and intervening when impairments or issues affect the ability to successfully engage in these occupations. As team members, occupational therapists offer an integrated, holistic perspective in which psychosocial aspects are critical to occupational performance (AOTA, 2004). Occupational performance is seen as a dynamic interplay of underlying biomechanical, functional, and psychosocial components. Central in the development of an occupational profile is consideration of psychosocial components, such as confidence, awareness, definitions of one's roles, and self-concept. Christiansen and Baum (1991) identified this centrality in the following:

> Psychosocial aspects of human experience are essential determinants of competent occupational performance. These aspects of human function determine the nature of occupational behavior and the manner in which one perceives his/her functional abilities. (p. 306)

In the context of driving and community mobility, occupational therapists explore not only the purpose and mechanics of community mobility (e.g., where the clients want to go, how they can get there) but also the meaning of mobility to the individual. Therapists may pose the following questions:

- How does transportation define the client?
- What does it mean to be able to have a license or to own keys to a car?
- How important is it to be mobile at a moment's notice or at a time of one's choosing?
- What changes may happen to a client's life roles when driving and community mobility are challenged?
- What is the value of community mobility for this client?
- What is the client's view of driving and alternative modes of transportation?

Through exploration of these questions, occupational therapists demonstrate an empathetic understanding of the psychosocial considerations of a client, which may lead to increased understanding and stronger empowerment of the client. An example of this type of empathetic approach is illustrated in Exhibit 4.1, which shares a therapist's reflections on experiences and challenges in addressing driving as part of the rehabilitation process.

Exhibit 4.1. An Empathetic Approach

Most individuals can recognize the concrete impacts of a condition. For example, someone who has had a stroke affecting the right arm and leg immediately experiences difficulty with eating, dressing, or walking. These are tangible activities that the client engages in on a daily basis. The client recognizes these changes, understands their impact, and starts working. In many cases these areas improve. The routine daily frequency of these activities is experienced and addressed. As a result, these fundamental life skills are more acceptable.

Oddly enough, there tends to be little connection (on the client's part and often the treating clinician as well) between being able to walk and move and driving and community mobility. The lack of connections comes from both the distance from the activity and the lack of discussion. For many years, when I was faced with a patient who had just lost the use of his or her arm, my initial response was not one of, "This may affect your driving and your major life roles," but, "How can we start working on immediate small gains?" By addressing the client's immediate life roles—being able to bathe, dress, and feed self—instead of addressing *all* of his or her life roles, was I meeting all of the client's needs?

Certainly there is a time and place for a discussion on community mobility. But more often than not, the discussion is either forgotten or avoided, leaving the topic unaddressed. Consequently, this results in little discussion about driving and community mobility. What is holding occupational therapists back from addressing driving and community mobility with our clients? Is it the fear that we will damage our client–clinician rapport, or our own hesitations with either not knowing the answer or not wanting to take responsibility for such a valuable topic? Is this in response to the client's value of mobility? Or a response to comfort of this topic? I believe that both play a major role. Both relate back to psychosocial components of Who am I, Who is my client, and How do we each use community mobility to define ourselves?

—Reflections by Susan Martin Touchinsky, OTR/L

It is the responsibility of all occupational therapists, regardless of setting or population, to begin approaching the topic of driving and community mobility (Schold Davis, 2003). This topic is critical to most individuals. For example, driving and community mobility will be as important to a client who just experienced a midlife stroke and cannot move the right side of her body as it is to the 17-year-old with cerebral palsy who wants to reach life's milestones. A client facing the journey of early-onset dementia will have as many concerns as a 90-year-old, long-term-care resident with congestive heart failure whose family wants to take him out for Sunday meals.

For each individual, whether the person is a driver or not, the need to be mobile in the community remains a crucial part of that person's occupational profile. In considering these occupations, occupational therapists need to identify their perceived barriers to making driving and community mobility and its concomitant psychosocial aspects a priority in practice. The psychosocial aspects of occupational performance are central skills that occupational therapists possess and apply to the occupational therapy process (AOTA, 2004).

Community mobility includes a wide range of activities (e.g., driving a car, using public transportation, carpooling, walking, using a golf cart, riding a bicycle), and each means of transportation has unique activity demands, performance skills, and body functions. Occupational therapists possess unique skills for addressing community mobility skills by integrating knowledge of medical conditions with the requisite cognitive, sensory–perceptual, emotional, and motor and praxis performance skills (AOTA, 2008) associated with the preferred transportation form. This information is integrated further with knowledge of psychosocial components that affect driving and community mobility. This collection of critical information provides a holistic view of the client and his or her experience of driving and community mobility. This chapter explores specific psychosocial needs of clients and related occupational therapy intervention strategies to support positive outcomes in the important instrumental activities of daily living of driving and community mobility.

Driving and Community Mobility and the Psychosocial Needs of Clients

A Framework for Identifying Psychosocial Needs

Community mobility comprises a complex spectrum that progresses from possessing all of the skills needed for safe mobility in the community, to exhibiting some impairments that affect driving and community mobility skills, to demonstrating serious impairments, to being unfit to drive safely or being mobile in the community. Figure 4.1 illustrates the community mobility spectrum. This spectrum is intended to encompass a broad range of ages, health levels, and community mobility decisions across situations, including the stages of attainment, temporary interruptions, changing modes, and cessation. It is incumbent upon occupational therapists to fully understand how each of these stages along the continuum presents unique psychosocial needs and challenges for the person experiencing them. The Framework for Identifying Psychosocial Needs (Exhibit 4.2) provides suggested questions that may be useful during the evaluation process.

The Novice Driver

Occupational therapists work with clients across the lifespan who have medical problems that interfere with the acquisition of driving and community mobility skills, such as cerebral palsy, autism, Asperger's syndrome, congenital defects, developmental disabilities, attention deficit disorders, and learning disabilities. Chapter 13 addresses issues related to younger drivers in detail.

In working with young, novice drivers, occupational therapists serve clients whose skills are still developing; summative decisions about a person's ability to drive or be independent in using public transportation must be withheld until the individual's performance skills are fully developed. In some cases, occupational justice issues often need to be addressed, as society (including loving support systems) must be willing to permit a person to grow into the high-risk activity of community mobility. Often, the therapist's objective analysis of the underlying skills is needed to free a client from overprotective and fearful attitudes of society. For example,

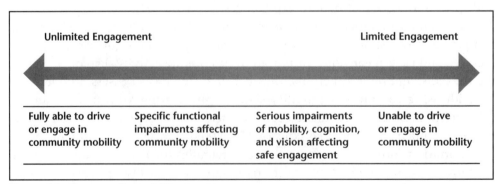

Figure 4.1. Community mobility spectrum.

Exhibit 4.2. Framework for Identifying Psychosocial Needs

- Who is the client?
- What are the life roles of the client?
- What is the history of the client in terms of driving and community mobility?
- Where does the client regularly go in the community?
- What will being able to drive mean to this client?
- What transportation options are available?
- How are these options different from the client's expectations?
- How does community mobility support the client's identified life roles?
- How will different transportation options expand this client's current life roles?
- What will not being able to participate in community mobility activities mean to this client?
- How will engagement in driving and community mobility change or restrict engagement in current life roles?
- How will this change or affect the client's definition of self?
- What support systems are in place?
- What is the involvement or impact of those individuals (such as a physician, parent, or other clinician)?
- What are the rights of this individual (occupational justice)?

---

community mobility for some younger clients might currently be limited to transportation by a parent or caregiver.

Various factors may interfere with the attainment of driving and community mobility skills; these factors include

- The individual's stage of development,
- The challenge of learning a new task,
- Mismatched expectations between the driver and significant others, and
- Self-awareness versus attitudes of others (see Table 4.1).

Consideration of these factors that impact a person's psychosocial status is vital, and the information can be gathered through conversations with the client, family, caregivers, physicians, and primary medical providers. It is important to work with the client and his or her support system to gather information and gain a full occupational profile.

An example of developing the occupational profile is found in Case Example 4.1. In Jennifer's case, these conversations provided insight to the occupational therapist assisting her in this journey. In addition to evaluating the performance skills associated with driving and community mobility, such as vision, cognition, and motor skills, the therapist took into consideration the impact of the social environment, in this case, Jennifer's relationship with her mother. Psychosocial components of this case included tension related to conflicting expectations as well as potential communication differences between Jennifer and her mother. Evaluation of all these components must be completed to determine the optimal recommendations and plan for engagement in successful community mobility options.

When Medical Conditions Trigger Temporary Changes in Driving and Community Mobility

Individuals experiencing a temporary restriction of mobility because of medical conditions may benefit from education, support for identification of options,

Table 4.1. Factors Affecting Attainment of Driving and Community Mobility

Stage of Development	New Task Attainment	Mismatched Expectations	Self-Awareness vs. Attitudes of Others
The clinician must assess the client's developmental level as well as manage the impact of any existing condition. Because of maturation issues, younger clients who may not have the full capacity for mature decision making may be affected further by deficits in cognition, attention, the ability to see a problem and anticipate what action will be needed, and the ability to notice environmental cues and respond accordingly.	Community mobility often may be a new task for the individual; with new tasks come a sense of uncertainty. When one is facing unknown situations, a common response may be anxiety, apprehension, and a sense of fear, as well as feelings of hope as one envisions the prospect of changing one's roles by being able to access the community independently. Clinicians should be prepared for a client experiencing "mixed emotions" and provide feedback to support coping with such inconsistent feelings.	There may be differences in expected outcomes between the person working toward driving and community mobility attainment and others in his or her environment. This mismatch often may occur as a result of limited discussions about driving and community mobility issues. Parents may harbor their own fears and apprehensions that they have not shared, and teens may be harboring thoughts and dreams that have not yet been communicated. Careful discussion, and the opportunity for all involved to reconsider the facts as well as the full implications of others' thoughts, should be facilitated.	It is critical to understand a client's awareness of his or her limitations, strengths, and aspirations and to compare it to the parent's or caregiver's level of awareness and attitude. Consider the situation in which the overprotective caregiver has already made the decision that the individual should not drive. Or, consider the overconfident caregiver or client who has not fully accepted the true impact of changes brought on by a condition. In both situations, the more a practitioner can know about the client, the clearer evidence can be when offered for specific recommendations. Therapists need to understand the beliefs and attitudes of both the client and his or her caregiver(s) when evaluating the client's potential to attain driving and community mobility.

preparation for driving retirement, or use of alternative modes of transportation. Temporary restrictions to community mobility often can be one of the most frustrating experiences for individuals. The medically imposed restriction is often a temporary change related to a major medical condition such as a joint replacement (e.g., 6-week restriction post-surgery) or related to immediate loss of license because of a variety of traffic violations.

For these clients, established life roles are supported by existing community mobility options, and the condition affects multiple areas of their lives and sense of self-worth. In these situations, psychosocial issues include

- Fears that the condition will never resolve,
- Stress in not being able to fulfill life roles,
- Financial concerns,
- Pressure to perform as they did before onset of the condition,
- Managing the responses of others,
- Denial of the condition,

> **Case Example 4.1. Facing New Challenges: Jennifer's Story**
>
> **Jennifer is an 18-year-old teenager** anxiously looking to obtain her driver's license. She is diagnosed with developmental delays and therefore the Department of Motor Vehicles for her state of residency needs her physician's review to consider her a candidate for licensure. Her doctor has reservations but refers Jennifer to occupational therapy for review of her driving skills. Her mother calls to schedule the visit and expresses that she is concerned about her daughter's ability to manage driving and is worried about Jennifer being alone. The mother reports that Jennifer has needed additional instruction for learning and needs supervision for "life decisions." The mother reports that she wants to give her daughter the chance to talk to someone about driving, but she does not want to be the person to tell her she cannot drive.
>
> Both Jennifer and her mother arrive for the driving appointment. During the evaluation, the occupational therapist identifies some deficits with divided attention and visual–spatial skills. A review of her school records shows that despite needing compensatory strategies, she has done quite well. During part of the evaluation, the occupational therapist excuses the mother so she can work individually with Jennifer. Once alone, Jennifer tells the occupational therapist that she feels like she would be a good driver and that her parents often hold her back because of her "different abilities."
>
> What psychosocial considerations must the occupational therapist consider for this situation? How should the occupational therapist work to address the psychosocial needs of Jennifer with the concerns of her mother?

- Driving and community mobility concerns,
- Anger and frustration with changes to established routines, and
- Feelings of dependency or guilt that stem from having to asking for help and rely on others.

Occupational therapists should be especially proactive with individuals in the temporary change category. It is critical to consider the psychosocial needs of these clients by identifying areas of concern, helping to clarify precautions or doctor recommendations, identifying problem-solving solutions, providing support to lessen fears, and offering information to clearly help with reattainment of previous levels of performance regarding driving and community mobility.

For clients whose driving privileges are temporarily suspended, the occupational therapist's unique perspective and consideration of the psychosocial demands plays a vital role in helping the traveler adjust to abrupt temporary changes and works with the individual to regain participation in life roles. As a whole, this group may be more open to alternative modes of transportation or change in general, as the impact on community mobility is temporary and the sense of loss may be less. These individuals may be "biding their time" until they can return to their preferred transportation. Alternately, this group may be less likely to seek out alternative modes of transportation. The occupational justice issues regarding return to driving are fraught with challenges to people's sense of dignity, their rights, and their overall occupational performance. Case Example 4.2 gives an example of a client whose community mobility privileges were placed on temporary hold.

When Medical Conditions Trigger Major Changes in Driving and Community Mobility

Clients experiencing a medical event might struggle with a wide range of questions: "How and when will I know if I may return to driving?" "Who may I turn to for help?" "What if I have no clear recommendations from my doctor?" Stress also can occur for this group when an individual is judged as incapable while capacity exists,

> **Case Example 4.2. Temporary Cessation of Driving: Louis's Story**
>
> **Louis is a 50-year-old professional man** who recently experienced a hold on driving. He was working in a full-time management position in the medical field and prided himself on being able to provide for others. He had a great balance of work, play, and family, fulfilling many life roles as a manager, employee, father, and runner.
>
> He was enjoying his summer weekend by participating in a 5K run when he suffered a medical event in which he lost sense of time and place. He was taken to the hospital, where his condition was coded as a seizure. While the exact nature of his event was reviewed, it became the responsibility of the physician to report his condition to the state's Department of Motor Vehicles (DMV). (Motor vehicle information on reportable conditions for each state may be obtained from the state's DMV or the *Physician's Guide to Assessing and Counseling Older Drivers* [Carr, Schwartzberg, Manning, & Sempek, 2010].) His license to drive was suspended, and this individual's world suddenly changed.
>
> Still a manager and father, without his license to drive, Louis now felt restricted, weak, and debilitated. He had to rely on others for transportation, needed to learn new ways to get around, had to face his perceived barriers with community transportation options—it takes too long, the bus does not run on time, public transportation may be dangerous—and then ultimately needed to work to regain his own confidence once he was released to drive again.
>
> He also needed coaching and support for working his way through the DMV system, which led to a lot of frustration because the DMV was not set up for the "proactive driver." Occupational therapy provided Louis with a stable sounding board where he could sort out his thoughts and emotions in reaction to a state system that offered vague direction regarding the resumption of his right to drive.
>
> Louis eventually returned to driving, resumed his management role, and carried away a deep appreciation for the role of occupational therapy in his life.

as well as the opposite scenario, when an individual is judged as capable but may have questionable skills because of his or her injury or the recovery process.

Driving and community mobility remains an uncomfortable discussion topic for many physicians and health care professionals, often because of a lack of knowledge, resources, time, confidence, and awareness. For these reasons, issues related to driving and community mobility frequently are underaddressed. Certain conditions, such as seizure disorders, have clear state guidelines regarding driving restrictions, but for many others, such as a stroke or transient ischemic attack, guidelines may be ambiguous or missing. Often the question "How should I be traveling?" is unspoken by the client and thus not addressed by health care providers. It is imperative that therapists consider the role of community mobility in the occupational profile and the impact of the current condition on safe participation in mobility.

When clients experience major changes that affect driving and community mobility, occupational therapists need to be prepared to respond to a wide range of emotions. Although some clients may accept feedback about transportation options, other clients may be angry or shocked. A range of client responses also may occur around anticipating limitations and the individual's level of emotional preparedness to handle changes to driving and community mobility. Other responses may include fear or a tendency to be overly restrictive or limiting of one's engagement, even when skills to safely resume mobility tasks exist. Clinical experience suggests that clients whose injuries were incurred from involvement in motor vehicle accidents are particularly vulnerable to psychosocial problems related to the return to driving. Consider the stories of Maria (Case Example 4.3) and Nancy (Case Example 4.4), and compare and contrast both the psychosocial issues and the approaches used to respond to these issues.

It is critical for all occupational therapists to be aware of the strategies and adaptations available for independence in driving and community mobility, particularly

Case Example 4.3. Dealing With Amputation and Setbacks: Maria's Story

Maria, a woman in her mid-40s, was referred to a driving program after losing her left arm in a driving crash. She was a wife, an employee, and, most importantly, a mother of 3 very active children. She had gone through several months of rehabilitation focused on the use and function of her remaining arm.

When Maria came to the program, she was knowledgeable and confident. In a very frank conversation, she shared how she had lost her left arm after suffering a motor vehicle crash involving her vehicle and a tractor trailer. She had been traveling home on the beltway when the tractor trailer changed lanes into her car. The result was a devastating crash resulting in several injuries. Her left arm was crushed and ultimately amputated. She had gone through months of therapy and was now "ready" to drive. She was referred by her doctor for adaptations to help her turn the steering wheel with her right arm (a spinner knob). Maria needed to return to driving to be able to fulfill her role as a mother—transporting her 3 children to various sports games, getting to the grocery store, getting to work, and so forth.

Maria's evaluation was completed, and she began to progress quickly with her training. Mastering control of the spinner knob came easily for this client, and she quickly progressed from the quiet, empty training lot to more advanced driving conditions. During her sessions her driving rehabilitation specialist (DRS) began reintroducing Maria to increasingly more difficult driving environments with more traffic and eventually more speed. The client was progressing and performing extremely well until she returned to driving on the highway, with tractor trailers. She began having a panicked, emotional response. She lost her confidence, decreased her speed, and worked to exit the highway. This initial response surprised the client.

The occupational therapist knew that if she was going to help Maria regain her independence, she would need to help her cope with her body's emotional response. The occupational therapist needed to dig deeper and find out more about her client.

Case Example 4.4. Integrating Psychosocial Interventions for Head Injury and Posttraumatic Stress Disorder: Nancy's Story

Nancy, a woman in her mid-40s, was referred for home- and community-based occupational therapy 4 years after surviving a traumatic brain injury as the result of a motor vehicle accident. She and 2 of her coworkers at a recycling center were walking along the side of the road on a work-related task, picking up recyclable materials that had blown off of trucks headed for their center. A motorist, blinded by the sun, veered off the road and "mowed over" all 3 women. Nancy was comatose for 3 weeks; as she became able, she participated in rehabilitation for 7 months. She went through many surgeries, including bilateral knee replacements, and "graduated" from outpatient speech, physical, and occupational therapies.

Four years later, Nancy was spending all of her time alone in her home, still with a long list of occupational performance problems, including her major goal, which was to return to riding as a passenger on her husband's large motorcycle; they used to spend many weekends doing long rides with groups of motorcyclists in town. Nancy was ambulating with a quad cane in her home, and she was afraid to walk outside because of the broken sidewalks.

Nancy had returned to driving about 3 years after the accident, but at the 4-year mark, she had stopped driving; she was under the impression that the man who hit her would come back to "finish off the job." She was always looking for him when she was on the road. Nancy's husband, Joe, was adamant that Nancy return to driving. He worked full-time; Nancy was at home on full disability, still recovering from the accident. If Nancy wouldn't drive, Joe was responsible for participating in grocery shopping and doing other family-oriented errands that Nancy used to do on her own. Joe saw how her ability to drive to medical appointments also would benefit her.

The occupational therapist contacted the neuropsychologist and the physician and requested an evaluation at a clinic that serves clients with posttraumatic stress disorder. Meanwhile, the occupational therapist developed a graded activity program for Nancy and her husband to follow, providing support and supervision to adjust the goals and encouraging Nancy as she slowly built her confidence in driving and overcame her paranoia. Her husband even told Nancy he would buy her a new car if she would return to driving. Slowly, Nancy developed the skills to drive in her neighborhood; at discharge, she had a long list of places she had driven independently.

The occupational therapist also worked on functional mobility skills and developed the lower-extremity flexibility skills that permitted Nancy to return to riding as a passenger on her husband's motorcycle (Figure 4.2).

The occupational therapy program also supported Nancy's return to walking around the neighborhood using a four-wheeled rollator to compensate for balance problems that made her a high risk for falls on the broken sidewalks that surrounded her home.

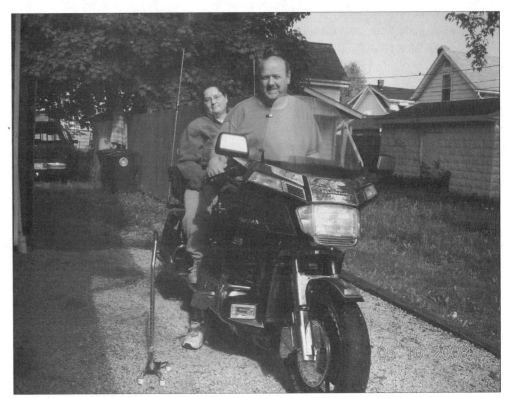

Figure 4.2. Returning to a meaningful community mobility activity after brain injury and posttraumatic stress disorder.

for clients experiencing major physical limitations. The role of the generalist is to provide the hope for independence and the guidance in locating and selecting professionals who can perform the evaluation and intervention necessary for driving and community mobility skills.

When Medical Conditions Cause Gradual Decline in Driving and Community Mobility

Many conditions produce a slow decline or deterioration in occupational performance that affects the safe ability to drive and use community mobility. During middle and older adulthood, individuals may face functional challenges associated with chronic conditions such as multiple sclerosis, Parkinson's disease, epilepsy, amyotrophic lateral sclerosis, and various forms of dementia, as well as the combined impact of multiple health issues. Clients with the physical ability to drive often may have to alter their habits as a result of medication regimes that cause drowsiness.

Individuals with these challenges often experience gradual decline and may have difficulty recognizing the overall impact of their limitations until they reach a critical point of challenge, or the multiple factors affecting performance coalesce to create a significant inability.

When medical conditions produce progressive decline, clients' awareness of their declining cognitive skills and acknowledgment of their psychosocial needs (e.g., anger, feelings of hopelessness, fear related to not being able to access services) is crucial. Offering limited conversations or imposing what may be perceived as arbitrary judgments, such as "Given your condition, you cannot drive," without therapeutically exploring the reasons behind the recommendation not to drive contributes to further negative emotions for clients. Occupational therapists can provide insight and support to these clients and their support system through information and resources. Occupational therapy intervention may offer clients therapeutic activities as well as computer-based assessments that provide a client with clear evidence of cognitive–perceptual problems that may result in unsafe driving. Upon receiving this information, the client should then be given time to process these deficiencies and be supported in discussions that facilitate the generalization of this information to driving and community mobility. Therapists play a key role in encouraging these essential discussions and promoting the development of coping mechanisms.

Preparing for Retirement From Driving

When a therapist recognizes that a client may be approaching a time when driving is no longer a safe option, it is critical to conduct a detailed analysis of where the client goes and what the client does in the community. Therapists need to promote a therapeutic milieu that focuses on providing the support to problem solve continued occupational participation in community activities.

Occupational therapy is most effective when the therapeutic work focuses on meeting the client's occupational and psychosocial needs and avoids a focused struggle over the right to hold onto the keys. Primary psychosocial responses associated with driving retirement include grief, withdrawal, isolation, depression, and loss of self-worth (Liddle & McKenna, 2003; Marottoli et al., 1997, 2000). Goals should relate to safety for the client, loved ones, and the community at large and to the client's community mobility needs. Therapists present driving a car as only one of many community mobility options; clients and families may need time to assimilate this point of view.

Therapists should not be surprised if this point of view is rejected when it is first presented, as it may be a view that clients and families "grow into" as awareness of impairments grows and as therapists help the client explore the benefits of using alternative modes of transportation. Strategies for addressing grief and loss are discussed later in this chapter.

When supporting a client's development of an awareness of the need to retire from driving, it is widely recognized that there is great value in having early conversations, before the time that driving must stop (The Hartford/AARP, 2007). Research addressing conversations about driving (The Hartford/AARP, 2007) revealed that older drivers have specific preferences regarding with whom they want to discuss issues related to driving retirement that are based on their own life experiences and varying psychosocial factors. These preferences are identified in the following:

- Men prefer to have discussions about driving with their spouse, although 15% of married men also identified that their spouse was the last person they wanted to have a conversation with regarding this topic.
- Twenty-seven percent of married drivers and 40% of single drivers would want to have the conversation with their doctor.
- Drivers ages 70 years or older tend to be more receptive to conversations with their adult children and also are more open to children who live geographically closer than those who live far away.

- Women are more receptive to conversations with their adult children than are men.

Occupational therapists may help the client identify who among the individuals in his or her support system is best for starting the conversation about driving retirement. There may be many individuals within the support system who are willing, but who is best for the driver? Who would the driver want to talk to about driving retirement? Once someone is identified, it helps to start several small conversations about driving. Topics of discussion may include recent related news events about older drivers, or changes in road conditions, traffic flow, or volume. Occupational therapists facilitate these conversations to build rapport with the driver and to facilitate understanding about the driver's perceptions and feelings.

When planning conversations, in addition to consideration of the person's driving record and driving pattern, current driving performance, occupations supported by driving and community mobility, and the availability of alternative modes of transportation, the therapist should give attention to the traveler's personality, support systems, acceptance of the impacting condition, and the meaning of driving for that individual. Therapists can use the *We Need to Talk: Family Conversations with Older Drivers* brochure (The Hartford/AARP, 2007) to facilitate discussion and provide support for change.

Time for Change

Occupational therapists must assess a client's readiness for change as well as recognize that people need time both to process information and to make a decision to change. Change takes time, and it is critical to acknowledge temporal factors necessary for a client to change routines and habits. If therapists rush the process of decision making and change and make premature recommendations, they may find that a client becomes resistive and angry. In fact, the client may be in an ambivalent state because of the continued processing of information and may not yet be able to make a choice for change. Miller and Cook (2008) have outlined behavioral theories and models of change that can be used to guide the occupational therapy process. Applying these models provides excellent guidance for effective therapy. One model, the Transtheoretical Model of Behavior Change (TTM; Prochaska & DiClemente, 2005), is useful to understanding the stages of change in the context of transitions that clients make related to community mobility. Table 4.2 applies TTM to occupational therapy intervention.

When information about driving and community mobility is initially provided, a client may not show any positive reaction. In the precontemplation or contemplation stage, the lack of a decision to change is to be expected; it is critical that therapists not perceive clients in this stage as "resistive" or "noncompliant." Therapists should remain hopeful that when provided with adequate evidence and information, clients will make a decision to change for their own good and for the good of others. Clients who resist change, despite evidence that their impairments impose dangerous risks to themselves or to others (whether driving a car, riding a bicycle, or engaging in any other form of community mobility), and who are provided with resources and therapeutic support to make appropriate transitions, are considered to have impaired judgment. Clients with impaired judgment need more intensive

Table 4.2. Applying the Transtheoretical Stages of Change to Driving and Community Mobility

Stages	Characteristics	Appropriate Intervention
1. Precontemplation	Client is not aware of need for change; client is not interested in discussion; family may be asking for intervention but has not discussed the topic with the client; client is not likely to make a change.	Occupational therapy evaluation to identify strengths and weaknesses; use of tools to "begin the discussion."
2. Contemplation	Client has some awareness that impairments are interfering with driving safety and is considering making a change; client is interested in discussing the topic; client is open to information.	Exploring benefits and consequences of various community mobility options; discussing appropriate restrictions in driving to reduce the risk of crash; exploring alternative modes of transportation in community; providing information on local resources.
3. Preparation	Client creates a plan; client may make small changes (permitting spouse to drive, expressing willingness to sign up for paratransit); client decides to restrict driving behavior.	Facilitating application to paratransit system or other community-based forms of transportation; discussion of self-restrictions on driving behavior.
4. Action	Client decides to sell car; client is willing to use forms of community mobility other than "driver of a car"; client uses paratransit system or develops a list of alternative modes of transportation for participation in community.	Facilitating development of skills and training for using paratransit system; identifying community mobility options for all meaningful occupations.
5. Maintenance	Client has established routines regarding safe community mobility options.	Intermittent evaluations to ensure that community mobility options are working.

Note. Adapted from Prochaska and DiClemente (2005).

therapy to recognize impairments and to cope with the imposition of limitations that they do not understand.

Self-Awareness

The World Health Organization (WHO; 2001) classifies *self-awareness* as a specific mental function category in the *International Classification of Functioning, Disability and Health (ICF)*. *ICF* also states that client factors, such as values and beliefs, contribute to awareness. The *Occupational Therapy Practice Framework: Domain and Process, 2nd Edition (Framework–II;* AOTA, 2008) defines *awareness* as body functions, categorized by *ICF* as *specific mental functions* (WHO, 2001). From this perspective, awareness is a key psychosocial function that supports safe community mobility skills. An individual's morals and beliefs affect ethical judgments, including the choice to follow transportation laws or to respect the rights of other drivers and travelers. A person's values influence attitudes about driving (e.g., considering driving a right vs. a privilege) and options regarding the use of public transportation (e.g., "Poor people ride the bus") or the services of family and friends (e.g., "I do not want to impose").

The psychosocial skill of awareness may be considered from both cognitive and psychological perspectives. Viewed from a cognitive perspective, the construct of *awareness* is defined as an integral part of executive function within metacognition (Katz & Hartman-Maeir, 2005). *Metacognition* has been defined as "thinking about one's thinking" and "knowing about knowing" (Katz & Hartman-Maeir, 2005, pp. 3–4) and encompasses the ability to examine one's thoughts, abilities, and beliefs.

In the context of driving and community mobility, awareness is the ability to accurately assess one's skills in relation to the requirements of the preferred form of transportation. In the psychosocial domain, awareness includes cognitive beliefs, which affect one's ability to recognize emotions, behaviors, and the impact of beliefs on daily activities and relationships. The *Framework–II* categorizes *beliefs* as a client factor, defined as "cognitive content held as true" (Moyers & Dale, 2007, p. 28). As such, layers of beliefs exist, which include automatic thoughts, rules for living, and core beliefs or schema (McCraith, 2011). Awareness of beliefs may allow a client to understand how emotions might affect his or her behaviors, and it assists the person in making choices that are congruent with his or her values, beliefs, and sense of abilities. Beliefs about one's capacity and efficacy are part of a person's *volition,* or motivation for occupation, and are dynamic and highly influenced by the environment (Kielhofner, 2008).

> When the construct of psychological awareness is applied to driving, it allows a person to understand his or her behaviors in context.

When the construct of psychological awareness is applied to driving, it allows a person to understand his or her behaviors in context, including concomitant emotions stemming from personal experiences. Awareness includes the ability to reflect upon experiences, such as why an error was upsetting or how feelings of anxiety may interfere with effective functioning.

The construct of awareness has been examined from neurological, psychological, and learning perspectives (Katz & Hartman-Maeir, 2005) as well as from occupational performance perspectives (Katz, 2005). For example, the Dynamic Interactional Approach (Toglia, 2005) proposes that self-awareness involves two distinct concepts: (1) self-knowledge and (2) online awareness. (Readers are referred to Toglia [2005] for further discussion of self-awareness.) Problems with self-awareness, regardless of etiology, may result in distorted judgments that affect both the effectiveness and the efficiency of occupational performance. A dynamic relationship exists between experiences and self-efficacy (Kielhofner, 2008; Toglia, 2005), as illustrated when driving errors such as the inability to find a location cause a person to hold the belief that he or she gets lost easily. Regardless of theoretical definitions and approaches to understanding awareness and metacognition, these constructs are essential psychosocial components of all occupational performance and clearly apply to driving and community mobility.

Medical conditions that affect awareness deficits contribute to safety issues, as declines in this critical skill lead to faulty decisions about whether and how to engage in safe driving or the use of alternative modes of transportation. Awareness is a multidimensional skill that comes to bear on all aspects of community mobility, such as whether one is accurately matching one's abilities to the task demands, recognizing possible deficits to be willing to make changes or adaptations, and understanding the consequences of one's choices. For example, older drivers who have minimal cognitive impairment may not be aware of how their slowed information processing and decreased memory skills affect driving safety, but occupational therapists can provide objective feedback through testing, facilitate increased awareness, and provide opportunities for clients to "change their minds" regarding the risks they take when they get behind the wheel.

Awareness is of particular concern for clients with acquired brain injury or diseases that cause cognitive decline. Clients who are not aware of their impairments (e.g., visual field cuts, impulsivity in decision making, distractibility, disinhibition, problems with divided attention, decreased speed of information processing) will often base their judgments about safety in driving and community mobility on their former, well-established self-image and sense of self-efficacy (Patomella, Johansson, & Tham, 2009). Therapists work with these clients to develop an awareness of their impairments, including how they will affect safety in community mobility.

It is critical for therapists to monitor clients' psychosocial response to this new level of awareness. For example, if a client becomes aware of deficits that indicate a need to retire from driving, there is a need for therapeutic support that provides a vision for independent community mobility using alternative modes of transportation.

Intervention Strategies for Psychosocial Needs

The case examples presented in this chapter demonstrate a range of psychosocial issues that may need to be addressed in occupational therapy related to the areas of driving and community mobility. Community mobility is a significant enabler for major occupations, and loss of access to the community as a result of impairments that affect this occupation threatens a person's sense of identity as a competent adult. Occupational therapists must approach driving and community mobility with the attitude and skills necessary to empower the client to maintain his or her identity, capable of self-determination and independence.

Occupational therapists use the occupational therapy process, knowledge of models of change and the grief process, and careful communication and counseling skills as part of therapeutic use of self to facilitate healthy changes in a person's life regarding issues related to driving and community mobility. *Therapeutic use of self* is "an occupational therapy practitioner's planned use of his or her personality, insights, perceptions, and judgments as part of the therapeutic process" (AOTA, 2008, p. 653). The initial evaluation, including the selection of assessment tools to create an occupational profile, begins the therapeutic process. Developing an empathetic understanding of the client and his or her story (Taylor, 2008) is also a central aspect of therapeutic use of self. The therapist's attitudes and approach toward driving and community mobility issues are a critical part of the therapeutic process. Is the client safe? Is the community safe? How can the client continue to participate in community activities if community mobility is challenged?

Although therapeutic use of self has been identified as a critical skill in all areas of occupational therapy practice (Taylor, Lee, Kielhofner, & Ketkar, 2009), specific guidance identifying the requisite skills and the strategies for using therapeutic use of self is missing from most literature in the profession. The Intentional Relationship Model (IRM; Taylor, 2008) provides a basis for understanding therapeutic use of self as well as a practice model with specific strategies. Taylor (2008) has contended that therapeutic relationships are always composed of an interaction among the client, the therapist, the desired occupation at hand, and interpersonal events that occur during the interaction.

Although all elements of the model are critical, its focus on the importance of interpersonal events of therapy is particularly relevant in responding to psychosocial issues related to driving and community mobility in the therapeutic relationship. It is incumbent upon therapists to develop the interpersonal skills that help build a therapeutic alliance and to use communication styles that best support the client's occupational needs at that moment in time. Otherwise, *"empathic breaks"* (Taylor, 2008, pp. 123–124), defined as instances in which communication from a client is misunderstood, are likely to occur. IRM asserts that "the client defines a successful relationship" (Taylor, 2008, p. 57) and charges therapists with the responsibility of responding with "mindful empathy" to support client needs.

IRM (Taylor, 2008) highlights the importance of *interpersonal reasoning*, defined as "the process by which a therapist monitors the interpersonal events of therapy, the client's unique personal characteristics, and his or her own behavior in a reflective way" (p. 138). Taylor advocated use of this information to determine appropriate interactive styles, or modes, which are collaborating, instructing, advocating, encouraging, empathizing, and problem solving. Although therapists' mode selection is typically first influenced by their personalities, Taylor has recommended intentional use of modes with clients, because the clients' experience of the therapist's mode is paramount. IRM also asserts that therapists must consider clients' unique interpersonal characteristics and preferred ways of interacting when choosing among the six therapeutic modes. (Readers are referred to Taylor [2008] for further explicit guidance in using this model to both develop and guide therapeutic use of self.)

Establishing a Therapeutic Approach in the Initial Evaluation

The approach that an occupational therapist takes during an initial evaluation, and the therapeutic relationship that he or she establishes with a client, is an important part of the intervention plan. This is true in all cases, but it is particularly important in cases in which driving and community mobility are involved. Driving and community mobility are an emotionally sensitive area, which can become more intense if a client is facing driving retirement. However, the occupational therapist does not know the client, nor does he or she have a comprehensive picture of all of the factors in the case, until after the evaluation is completed. The therapist must skillfully adjust questions and select tools according to the client's and family members' responses. This skillful adjustment of the process creates a safe environment for the client and family to share their concerns, fears, and hopes with the therapist regarding driving and community mobility.

The therapist's attitude toward driving and community mobility establishes a therapeutic milieu for the plan of care; the atmosphere and tone create a "safe and caring" place for discussion of sensitive issues related to driving and community mobility. A careful, matter-of-fact approach with questions related to driving and community mobility supports an objective discussion of the issues. It is important for clinicians to ask basic questions early in the health care delivery system (acute care); if simple questions are asked in a nonthreatening manner and documented in the medical record, therapists in subsequent delivery models can follow up on the information in the record. Therapists should use exploratory questions during the initial evaluation to establish an attitude toward driving that can open the client's mind to accepting alternative modes of transportation as viable options.

Using assessment tools that clarify where a client drives and the frequency of those outings can help identify the extent of his or her particular deficits in community mobility. Tools that examine the client's attitudes can be useful in establishing an effective intervention plan. The **Assessment of Readiness for Mobility Transition** (ARMT; Meuser, Berg-Weger, Chibnall, Harmon, & Stowe, 2011) was developed by researchers at the St. Louis Consortium for Older Driver Education and Research with funding from the National Center on Senior Transportation. The ARMT is a 24-item self-rating scale that assesses emotional and attitudinal readiness to cope with the transitions related to driving and community mobility. The client's responses are analyzed according to how they cluster in four categories: (1) anticipatory anxiety, (2) perceived burden, (3) avoidance, and (4) adverse situation.

This tool is designed to increase the client's awareness, as it provides an opportunity for discussion of sensitive issues and a look at the client's real concerns related to mobility transition. The authors of the ARMT consider the tool to be part of the public domain for educational, supportive, and clinical care purposes; it is available for free on the ARMT's authors' Web site and is an appendix to this text.

Many stakeholders have developed tools to support the interview process regarding driving and community mobility. Selecting the appropriate tools begins the intervention process by increasing the client's (and family's) awareness of the importance of driving and community mobility. Chapter 11 provides a variety of resources the therapist could use as part of the evaluation process, and Chapter 9 provides a list of standardized tools that could be administered. The selection of appropriate tools not only will guide the evaluation process but also will increase a client's awareness of his or her strengths, weaknesses, and needs related to driving and community mobility. The awareness of problems and the need for intervention is the foundation for further intervention.

Therapeutic Approaches to Support and Motivate

Understanding reactions to changes in driving and community mobility can help support transitions. The stages of grief described by Elisabeth Kübler-Ross (2005) often can be observed as an individual develops an awareness of limitations that may affect his or her ability to drive or use other forms of transportation safely. Table 4.3 provides examples of behaviors related to stages of loss that may be

Table 4.3. Experiences of Loss and Grief Associated With Driving and Community Mobility

Stage of Grief	Client Response to Occupational Therapy Evaluation and Intervention
Denial	Refusal to be evaluated in the clinic; denial that the problems identified interfere with safe driving; refusal to follow through with recommendation for on-road evaluation.
Anger	Anger often directed at family members who express concerns; it may be directed at clinician or DRS regarding the choices of tools or methods used that revealed impairments; accusations that the therapist did not perform the assessment properly.
Bargaining	Although it is a healthy and normal response for older adults to limit driving behavior (avoiding night driving, driving in bad weather, or expressway driving), self-limiting behavior is an indicator that the individual is aware of impairments; self-limiting behavior is a healthy "bargaining" regarding driving, and it often precedes an individual's choice to retire from driving.
Depression	Withdrawal from communicating with others about this issue; refusal to request or accept offers to be transported; refusal to register to use alternative modes of transportation; withdrawal from community activities that require transportation.
Acceptance	Self-limiting behavior regarding driving; active problem solving regarding alternative modes of transportation; registering for public or faith-based systems of transportation.

Exhibit 4.3. Rosenfeld's Sequence of Strategies to Motivate Clients

1. Build a relationship of respect, concern, and partnership.
2. Restore the client's identity by discussing occupational history in depth.
3. Listen to the client's story or recent events and normalize the emotions caused by illness, injury, surgery, admission, and displacement.
4. Challenge unrealistically negative assumptions about recovery and rehabilitation intervention.
5. Define the challenge of intervention: Seek and clarify goals by imagining a realistic future, and tie goals to specific intervention activities and expected outcomes.
6. Select meaningful tasks and occupations for intervention that are relevant to the occupational history of the client and, therefore, can restore a sense of life continuity.
7. Strongly support and reward the client's efforts, and advocate and monitor reasonable self-assessments of performance.

Note. From *Motivational Strategies in Geriatric Rehabilitation*, by M. Rosenfeld, 1997, p. 27. Bethesda, MD: American Occupational Therapy Association. Copyright © 1997, by the American Occupational Therapy Association. Used with permission.

observed as a client becomes aware of impairments affecting community mobility. Rosenfeld (1997) has provided clear guidelines for therapists working with older clients who are depressed. These guidelines are listed in Exhibit 4.3, providing a "sequence of strategies" that clarify therapeutic approaches for therapists to use to motivate clients.

A healthy therapeutic relationship provides the client with a safe environment for exploring strengths and weaknesses related to driving. It is critical that the client sense a therapist's sincere commitment to supporting him or her in examining the facts, to fostering self-determination, and to providing guidance and resources to support any decision to self-limit or retire from driving. The Model of Human Occupation offers useful conceptualization of motivation. Motivation for occupation, or volition, has three aspects: (1) interests, (2) values, and (3) personal causation, which includes self-efficacy and sense of capacity (Kielhofner, 2008). Understanding a client's perspective about his or her personal causation in particular is essential to determining interventions that may support motivation for change in occupations of community mobility. Personal causation relates to a client's view of effectiveness, capability, and sense of capacity, which are all key components to safe engagement in any community mobility occupation.

Exploring the client's occupational history, including information related to driving and community mobility, provides a basis for meaningful communication and reinforces and affirms the client's identity as a competent adult. Using a narrative approach, the therapist facilitates a clarification of the significant events that have caused the client or family to wonder about driving safety. The narrative approach is facilitated with the use of a structured interview assessment, such as the Occupational Performance History Interview (Kielhofner et al., 2004), which is designed to capture a client's narrative and assess the subjective experience of his or her performance capacity.

Therapists provide a sounding board for clients who express fears and anxieties regarding community mobility. Clients often will need support in reframing negative assumptions about loss of driving or other modes of transportation. Therapeutic responses that can create opportunities for adapting to changes in community mobility include helping clients recognize the places, experiences, and values that are important to them and exploring options that resonate with clients' values and interests. For instance, a client may be encouraged to recognize that life may be enjoyed just as fully without driving as long as the individual can participate in self-identified events such as attending church on Sundays, eating at favorite restaurants, enjoying scenic rides in the country, shopping at a favorite grocery store, and shopping weekly at the farmers' market. Motivation for change is further enhanced when therapists provide positive feedback to clients regarding any attitude or effort that embraces healthy transitions and reflects movement toward behavior modification or lifestyle redesign.

Addressing Psychosocial Issues Related to Motor Impairments

When a person has physical impairments that interfere with the normal development of driving skills, or when motor impairments are acquired through disease or injury, it is relatively easy for the client and therapist to address the issue of driving and community mobility because the ability to perform a specific task related to driving and community mobility can be evaluated objectively, and the client is typically able to see for oneself whether he or she is capable of safe, independent performance. Clients who are unable to develop adequate skills for driving may experience feelings of inadequacy as well as the range of emotions related to grieving a significant loss, but therapists often do not find it difficult to bring up driving in these situations. The physical limitations are evident, and the need for intervention is typically welcomed by the client. It is the therapist's responsibility to be responsive to the feelings expressed from these changes in ability and mobility.

Addressing Psychosocial Issues Related to Cognitive Skill Impairments

Cognitive impairments that cause awareness, safety, and competence issues related to driving and community mobility are more sensitive to address than motor skills.

Clients who have cognitive impairments that cause parents, caregivers, and health care workers to wonder about their safety alone in the community will typically have protective restrictions placed upon them by these significant others; in some instances, these restrictions may be overprotective. For example, Kara is 47 years old and living in her own rented room in a residence run by an order of religious women. Although many of the residents have the freedom to come and go as they please, Kara has intellectual disabilities and has been told she cannot leave the building alone. An occupational therapy evaluation has determined that Kara could walk safely from her residence to the public library. She is very excited about the potential freedom of walking to the library on her own, as she is tired of being disabled by the fears of others regarding her safety. This situation highlights the need to consider the appropriateness of restrictions and whether they pose an occupational justice issue.

Clients who are becoming aware that their cognitive impairments may affect their competence in driving may be hesitant to broach the topic, fearing that they may cause a therapist to impose limitations. Clients who lack the judgment to realize that their impairments may interfere with safety in driving or in the community certainly will not raise the conversation, as they are not aware that safety is a problem. In these latter cases, it is common for family members to share their concerns with the clients as well as with professionals, with the hope that the professionals will intervene. In either case, it is the therapist's responsibility to explore these areas.

Informing Clients of Options and Promoting Self-Determination

Occupational therapy not only helps a client relate his or her strengths and weaknesses to driving and community mobility, but it also informs and works with clients to remediate any dysfunction that can be overcome, provides adaptations to compensate for impairments, and addresses the environment and resources in the community to help a client participate in life to its fullest. Once impairments are identified, it is the therapist's responsibility to instruct the client and family on the evidence that exists related to remediation or adaptation, as described in the earlier chapters. It is unfortunate and bad practice for any therapist to inform a client that he or she "shouldn't be driving" without addressing the psychosocial impact and the occupational ramifications of this professional recommendation.

If it is determined that a client's impairments render the person an unsafe driver, then the therapist should design an intervention plan that addresses both the psychosocial and occupational issues related to this recommended transition. A therapeutic plan should be put in place to facilitate the client's awareness of the deficits that are related to the determination to stop driving as well as to develop the coping and problem-solving skills that will be required to function without the privileges of driving. Other forms of community mobility should be explored, and the client should receive training to empower him or her to continue to participate in community-based activities.

Conclusion

The psychosocial issues related to delayed development of driving and independent community mobility skills, as well as the responses related to losing driving privileges and the need to develop skills using alternative modes of transportation, are critical areas for occupational therapists to recognize and address. Occupational therapists possess the skills necessary to respond to the complex psychosocial issues associated with the essential occupations of community mobility (AOTA, 2010; Classen, Winter, & Lopez, 2009). Through continued professional development, these skills are further enhanced and strengthened and serve to make occupational therapy services truly holistic and responsive to clients' community mobility needs.

References

American Occupational Therapy Association. (2004). Psychosocial aspects in occupational therapy. *American Journal of Occupational Therapy, 58,* 669–672.

American Occupational Therapy Association. (2008). Occupational therapy practice framework: Domain and process (2nd ed.) *American Journal of Occupational Therapy, 62,* 625–683. doi:10.5014/ajot.62.6.625

American Occupational Therapy Association. (2010). Specialized knowledge and skills in mental health promotion, prevention, and intervention in occupational therapy practice. *American Journal of Occupational Therapy, 64,* 530–543. doi:10.5014/ajot.2010.64530

Bednarcik, K., & Chew, F. (2009). *Active aging: Transportation and community mobility.* Kennett Square, PA: Genesis Rehab Services.

Carr, D. B., Schwartzberg, J. G., Manning, L., & Sempek, J. (2010). *Physician's guide to assessing and counseling older drivers.* Washington, DC: National Highway Traffic Safety Administration.

Christiansen, C., & Baum, C. (1991). Psychological performance factors. In C. H. Christensen & C. Baum (Eds.), *Occupational therapy: Overcoming human performance deficits* (p. 304–332). Thorofare, NJ: Slack.

Classen, S., Winter, S., & Lopez, E. D. S. (2009). Meta-synthesis of qualitative studies on older driver safety and mobility. *Occupational Therapy Journal of Research, 29,* 24–31.

Katz, N. (2005). *Cognition and occupation across the life span: Models for intervention in occupational therapy* (2nd ed.). Bethesda, MD: AOTA Press.

Katz, N., & Hartman-Maeir, A. (2005). Higher-level cognitive functions: Awareness and executive functions enabling engagement in occupations. In N. Katz (Ed.), *Cognition and occupation across the life span: Models for intervention in occupational therapy* (2nd ed., pp. 3–25). Bethesda, MD: AOTA Press.

Kielhofner, G. (2008). *A model of human occupation: Theory and application* (4th ed.). Baltimore: Lippincott Williams & Wilkins.

Kielhofner, G., Mallinson, T., Crawford, C., Nowak, M., Rigby, M., Henry, A., et al. (2004). *Occupational Performance History Interview–II (OPHI–II; version 2.1).* Chicago: Model of Human Occupation Clearinghouse, Department of Occupational Therapy, College of Applied Health Sciences, University of Illinois.

Kübler-Ross, E. (2005). *On grief and grieving: Finding the meaning of grief through the five stages of loss.* New York: Simon & Schuster.

Liddle, J., & McKenna, K. T. (2003) Older drivers and driving cessation. *British Journal of Occupational Therapy, 66*(3), 125–132.

Marottoli, R. A., Mendes de Leon, C. F., Glass, T. A., Williams, C. S., Cooney, L. M., Berkman, L. F., et al. (1997). Driving cessation and increased depressive symptoms: Prospective evidence from the New Haven Established Populations for Epidemiologic Studies of the Elderly. *Journal of American Geriatrics Society, 45,* 202–206.

Marottoli, R. A., Mendes de Leon, C. F., Glass, T. A., Williams, C. S., Cooney, L. M., & Berkman, L. F. (2000). Consequences of driving cessation: Decreased out-of-home activities. *Journal of Gerontology, 55,* S334–S340.

McCraith, D. B. (2011). Cognitive beliefs. In C. Brown & V. C. Stoffel (Eds.), *Occupational therapy in mental health: A vision for participation* (pp. 262–279). Philadelphia: F. A. Davis.

Meuser, T. M., Berg-Weger, M., Chibnall, J. T., Harmon, A., & Stowe, J. (2011). Assessment of Readiness for Mobility Transition (ARMT): A tool for mobility transition counseling with older adults. *Journal of Applied Gerontology.* doi:10.1177/0733464811425914

Miller, P. A., & Cook, A. (2008). Interventions along the care continuum. In S. Coppola, S. Elliott, & P. Toto (Eds.), *Strategies to advance gerontology excellence: Promoting best practice in occupational therapy* (pp. 391–394). Bethesda, MD: AOTA Press.

Moyers, P. A., & Dale, L. M. (2007). *The guide to occupational therapy practice* (2nd ed.). Bethesda, MD: AOTA Press.

Patomella, A., Johansson, K., & Tham, K. (2009). Lived experience of driving ability following stroke. *Disability and Rehabilitation, 31,* 726–733.

Prochaska, J. O., & DiClemente, C. C. (2005). The transtheoretical approach. In J. C. Norcross & M. R. Goldfried (Eds.), *Handbook of psychotherapy integration* (2nd ed., pp. 147–171). New York: Oxford University Press.

Rosenfeld, M. (1997). *Motivational strategies in geriatric rehabilitation.* Bethesda, MD: American Occupational Therapy Association.

Schold Davis E. (2003). Defining OT roles in driving. *OT Practice, 8,* 15–18.

Taylor, R. R. (2008). *The intentional relationship: Occupational therapy and use of self.* Philadelphia: F. A. Davis.

Taylor, R. R., Lee, S. W., Kielhofner, G., & Ketkar, M. (2009). Therapeutic use of self: A nationwide survey of practitioners' attitudes and experiences. *American Journal of Occupational Therapy, 63,* 198–207.

The Hartford, & AARP. (2007). *We need to talk: Family conversations with older drivers* (Brochure). Hartford, CT: The Hartford.

Toglia, J. P. (2005). A dynamic interactional approach to cognitive rehabilitation. In N. Katz (Ed.), *Cognition and occupation across the life span: Models for intervention in occupational therapy* (2nd ed., pp. 29–72). Bethesda, MD: AOTA Press.

World Health Organization. (2001). *International classification of functioning, disability and health (ICF).* Geneva, Switzerland: Author.

Occupational Therapy's Ethical Obligation to Address Driving and Community Mobility

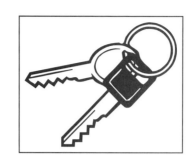

Linda A. Hunt, PhD, OTR/L, FAOTA, and Deborah Yarett Slater, MS, OT/L, FAOTA

Learning Objectives

After completion of this chapter, readers will be able to

- Identify the ethical and professional responsibility of occupational therapists to address clients' occupational performance in driving and community mobility through evaluation, contextual assessment, and clinical reasoning;
- Delineate the ethical and clinical importance of fully explaining components of the occupational therapy evaluation or the comprehensive driving evaluation process and recommendations that derive from it;
- Recognize the ethical obligation for occupational therapists to collaborate with clients in carrying out a safe driving or mobility plan, including alternative transportation strategies and referral for additional services as needed; and
- Identify a framework for ethical decision making and demonstrate the ability to analyze ethical dilemmas related to client safety and driving on the basis of type and severity of impairment.

Key Words

- *Code of Ethics and Ethics Standards*
- **competence**
- **confidentiality**
- **ethical reasoning**
- **scope of practice**

Introduction

Occupational therapy evaluation and intervention is philosophically based on addressing the client's occupational performance abilities and deficits to maximize participation in daily activities that are necessary and important. Activities of daily living (ADLs) and instrumental activities of daily living (IADLs) are perhaps the most important skills for individuals to acquire or relearn following injury or disease to best resume the routines of their lives.

Just as occupational therapists typically evaluate and provide training in self-care and home management skills, to meet the professional standards of care they also have an ethical responsibility to consider the client's mobility needs to truly participate in his or her daily routines. Mobility needs can include the need or desire not only to drive but also to use alternate community mobility strategies to achieve the client's goals.

The ethical responsibility to address driving and community mobility is not limited to older adults. This responsibility is relevant across the lifespan and might include adolescents with attention deficit hyperactivity disorder, traumatic brain injury, or other conditions that may result in an impaired ability to drive safely (or use alternate mobility options such as bicycles or public transportation). These individuals, as well as young or middle-aged adults who have had strokes or various neurological diagnoses, can have perceptual, visual, attention, or cognitive deficits that may increase the likelihood of harm to themselves or the public while driving, using alternative community mobility options, or even moving around as a pedestrian.

Occupational therapists need to be alert to ethical considerations such as client autonomy, competency, appropriate levels of personnel and supervision issues, documentation, and reporting. The extent of interventions and recommendations should be based on the client's needs as well as the therapist's competency and level of expertise to meet those specific needs. This may involve, in certain cases, referral to an occupational therapist driver rehabilitation specialist (DRS) who has more advanced knowledge and skills in this area. However, *all* occupational therapists have an ethical obligation to consider driving and community mobility in their initial evaluation and as part of comprehensive occupational therapy services.

> **Occupational therapists need to be alert to ethical considerations such as client autonomy, competency, appropriate levels of personnel and supervision issues, documentation, and reporting.**

Ethical Considerations Related to Driving and Community Mobility: Evaluation and Recommendations

Ethical Reasoning

Ethical reasoning, defined as "reasoning directed to analyzing an ethical dilemma, generating alternative solutions, and determining actions to be taken" (Schell & Schell, 2008, p. 7), is a critical skill to appropriately address many of the sensitive issues in clinical practice related to driving and community mobility. One particularly challenging issue is balancing the needs or desires of clients (autonomy and the right to self-determination) with those of the general public. Safety is of paramount concern, and all practitioners have an obligation to not inflict and to prevent foreseeable harm to their clients while also providing benefit through their interventions. However, the public also has a right to be safe. So, which priority is more compelling—individual autonomy or the greater good?

Weighing these priorities is complex, and the most appropriate decision can depend on the context and the individuals involved. A framework for ethical decision making can provide a systematic method for evaluating these questions and assist in making the best decision based on the specific circumstances (see Exhibit 5.1).

U.S. society generally supports individual rights and values, but there may be a point at which limitations should be placed on the expression of those values and desires to create benefit (or to prevent harm) for the larger public. Although occupational therapists must acknowledge the difficulty of these decisions and the need for help with resolution, they nevertheless have an ethical obligation to not remain

---

Exhibit 5.1. Framework for Ethical Decision Making

- What is the nature of the perceived problem (e.g., ethical distress, ethical dilemma), and what is the specific problem (i.e., "name and frame" the problem)?
- Who are the players—not just those immediately involved, but others who may be influenced by the situation or any decision that is made?
- What information is known, and what additional information is needed to thoroughly evaluate the situation and formulate options?
- What resources are available to assist?
- What are the options and likely consequences of each option?
- How are values prioritized (e.g., prioritize moral values, despite potential negative personal repercussions, to act on best decision)? Good intentions do not always bring about good deeds (Kanny & Slater, 2008).
- What action is being taken, and is it defensible?
- Was the outcome expected? Would one make a different decision if confronted with a similiar situation in the future?

Note. From "Ethical Dimensions of Occupational Therapy," by L. C. Brandt and D. Y. Slater, in K. Jacobs and G. L. McCormack (Eds.), *The Occupational Therapy Manager* (5th ed., p. 478), Bethesda, MD: AOTA Press. Copyright © 2010 by the American Occupational Therapy Association. Used with permission.

silent if they have the knowledge and skills to make a reasonable clinical judgment on the ability of a client to safely resume driving or access community mobility options. Objective data and clinical and ethical reasoning guide the recommendation process in this area, just as they do when making judgments about safety and ability related to other ADL or IADL tasks.

Ethical Responsibilities Related to Evaluation

Occupational therapists have an ethical responsibility, through the evaluation process, to identify impairments in occupational performance that may correlate with driving risks and to inform clients (and caregivers or significant others, if applicable), even if they do not have a legal responsibility to report them to the state. Principle 1 (Beneficence) of the ***Occupational Therapy Code of Ethics and Ethics Standards*** (American Occupational Therapy Association [AOTA], 2010) is central to guiding ethical conduct in these and other situations. This principle states that "occupational therapy personnel shall demonstrate a concern for the well-being and safety of the recipients of their services" (AOTA, 2010, p. S18).

The corollary to this is Principle 2, Nonmaleficence, which mandates that "occupational therapy personnel shall intentionally refrain from actions that cause harm" (AOTA, 2010, p. S19). This can include not only protecting the safety of clients but also, by extension, protecting the public from actions that have a high likelihood of causing harm (e.g., an impaired driver). Clients are not deriving benefit when occupational therapists do not share objective clinical findings and recommendations that have an impact on their well-being and that of others.

Competence

An occupational therapist's evaluation of his or her own skill is important, as is knowledge about the competency of the individuals to whom one is considering making a referral. This precludes any referrals that may be influenced by friendship, financial gain, and so forth, as noted in Principle 2J of the *Code and Ethics Standards:* "Occupational therapy personnel shall avoid exploiting any relationship established as an occupational therapist or occupational therapy assistant to further one's own physical, emotional, financial, political, or business interests at the expense of the best interests of recipients of services, students, research, participants, employees or colleagues" (AOTA, 2010, p. S20). Occupational therapists can and should evaluate and provide driving-related services at their level of competence. Competence to provide any occupational therapy service is an ethical imperative; Principle 1E states that "occupational therapy personnel shall provide occupational therapy services that are within each therapist's level of competence and scope of practice (qualifications, experience, and the law)" (AOTA, 2010, p. S19).

Therapists who are generalists may use standard occupational therapy evaluation components such as range of motion, muscle strength, and perceptual and cognitive testing, the results of which may definitively rule out driving as a safe occupation for clients who have identified driving as a necessary or important activity. Recommendations then should focus on community mobility alternatives.

Other occupational therapists may have more specialized training and can use in-clinic simulation or other equipment, potentially including an on-road evaluation to provide more precise information in cases where the recommendations are not as clear-cut. When generalists find themselves in an uncertain situation, they are ethically required to "refer to other health care specialists based solely on the needs of the client" (Principle 1I, Beneficence; AOTA, 2010, p. S19). However, because all occupational therapists have a responsibility to advocate for clients to receive necessary services (Principle 4E, Social Justice; AOTA, 2010), therapists need accurate information about all potential resources to make appropriate referrals and to ensure that clients' needs are met without a gap between providers.

On-Road Evaluation

Some occupational therapists believe they cannot even discuss the important occupation of driving because they lack knowledge about adaptive equipment, may not know how to weigh evaluation components to arrive at a valid and safe conclusion, or may believe that a road test is essential in all cases. Therapists tend to place emphasis on an in-car road assessment without understanding that it is only one piece of information in the evaluation process.

As in many areas of medicine, comprehensive driving evaluation is made up of a series of components. Occupational therapists need to understand that the in-car evaluation is essential for some (e.g., when vehicle adaptation is required) but not all (e.g., in cases of severe dementia) clients. (*Note.* Subsequent chapters will address the individual components.)

It is important to consider that the following limitations are inherent with an in-car road test:

- The high cost of testing, which may bring additional emotional stress to clients while being tested
- The subjectivity of scoring by the evaluator
- The inability to control variables such as traffic flow, road conditions, and other drivers' behaviors.

These limitations may decrease the strength of a correlation with neuropsychological tests or provide a false conclusion that someone is safe because the evaluator "saw" him or her drive. Therefore, occupational therapists also have an ethical responsibility to carefully consider whether their assessment tools, and the evidence guiding the application of results to driving, will provide valid data to aid in making realistic and appropriate intervention decisions and recommendations.

In addition, therapists sometimes allow reimbursement issues to influence their clinical decision making. Even when driving evaluations are not covered by payers, this is not a defendable reason to withhold information from clients that they need an evaluation or that their driving ability may be in question.

Ethical Responsibilities Related to Recommendations and Reporting

Occupational therapists have the ability and obligation, based on their knowledge and skills, to accurately and objectively assess potential risk and benefit. When assessing risk, identification should lead to warning, the scope of which can be determined by the context and degree of risk. However, while most individuals recognize potential ethical issues, moral courage is required to take action, even when the positive outcome is protection of both client and society. Change will not occur without action.

When risk is identified, there are legal and ethical considerations that influence taking action such as reporting. Although many people consider the terms *legal* and *ethical* to be synonymous, they are not always so. An action can be legal but still unethical. An occupational therapist may not be legally required to make recommendations that driving cease based on clinical evaluation data, but he or she still has an ethical obligation to document safety concerns and inform the client as well as the referring physician.

> **An occupational therapist may not be legally required to make recommendations that driving cease based on clinical evaluation data.**

From an ethical perspective, Principle 1M of the *Code and Ethics Standards* states that "occupational therapy personnel shall report to appropriate authorities any acts in practice, education, and research that appear unethical or illegal" (AOTA, 2010, p. S19). Equally important, occupational therapists need to know and understand state law with regard to their legal obligation or ability to report.

Concerns may exist about breaching confidentiality, which is a core ethical principle and expectation in the therapeutic relationship between client and therapist. Although Principle 3G states that personnel must "ensure that confidentiality and the right to privacy are respected and maintained regarding all information obtained about recipients of service," it continues, "The only exceptions are when a practitioner or staff member believes that an individual is in serious foreseeable or imminent harm. Laws and regulations may require disclosure to appropriate authorities without consent" (AOTA, 2010, p. S21). Serious consideration must be given to the multiple potential risks of not warning or not reporting when appropriate.

Consider Case Example 5.1, which discusses an 80-year-old client and her daughter. There are a number of potential issues in this case, such as judgment about performing the evaluation, client autonomy and rights, client versus society's well-being and prevention of harm, accuracy in communicating clinical information, compliance with applicable laws and regulations, and resource allocation. One issue is whether the occupational therapist should take the time and resources to

Case Example 5.1. Client With a Neurological Disorder

A daughter wants her 80-year-old mother evaluated for driving ability prior to discharge from the occupational therapy program because she has a neurological disorder (now under control) and has had numerous accidents. The daughter believes that her mother is cognitively impaired and states that her mother will not come in for an evaluation if she knows it has to do with driving. Therefore, the daughter requests that the occupational therapist not discuss driving issues but instead just perform the evaluation and make the recommendation to the physician and herself.

perform what may be an unnecessary evaluation, as he or she already has (or has access to) considerable relevant data to make recommendations about driving ability. For example, state guidelines for driving (which are unique to each state) inform decisions for generalists and specialists alike. If a client is legally blind or has a field cut, the generalist has the duty to warn the client that his or her vision no longer meets state guidelines and driving must stop until addressed and licensing requirements are met. Some states license low vision, and this generalist would inform and refer for specialized service.

Case Example 5.1 supports the value of an occupational therapist making a judgment on the basis of multiple factors, including making reasonable assumptions based on what is known about the effect of cognitive or neurological deficits and their relationship to future performance, particularly in a high-risk area such as driving. In addition, this case illustrates the potential for conflicts between client rights and wishes; the responsibilities of the daughter, physician, and therapist; and the societal "greater good."

Case Example 5.1 also raises issues related to transparency and autonomy, as the evaluation is being requested under deceptive circumstances. Why is an evaluation even being requested, as there is already significant probability that driving will be a concern? In this case, a generalist occupational therapist could use history and evidence, test results, and his or her clinical judgment to make an appropriate recommendation that driving is not a safe option or that additional information is required and make the referral to a comprehensive driving evaluation.

The goal of a driving evaluation is to identify whether an individual is likely to be safe to resume driving and whether any interventions (e.g., education, access to adaptive equipment through a DRS, training, intervention to address cessation and associated strategies) are necessary to achieve that outcome. By requesting to have evaluation results shared only with the physician and herself, the daughter is adopting a paternalistic attitude and is not respectful of her mother's right to make a decision by being fully informed before giving consent to an evaluation. The concept of autonomy, discussed in Principle 3 of the *Code and Ethics Standards,* supports the individual as his or her own agent and acknowledges a "person's right to hold views, to make choices and to take actions based on personal values and beliefs" (Beauchamp & Childress, 2009, p. 103). If the mother cannot comprehend relevant information to make thoughtful decisions about the need for and purpose of an evaluation, then she is not likely to have adequate cognitive ability to drive.

Further, more specialized evaluation may be an unnecessary use of resources to confirm what is already known. In this scenario of moderate to severe cognitive impairment, a collaborative discussion of the risks of driving and alternative community mobility strategies among the daughter, mother, physician, and occupational therapist would be more productive and ethically appropriate than undermining the mother's autonomy.

Transparency in communicating concerns, risks, and options is necessary, as is ensuring that clients and families comprehend the information that is being conveyed. Not allowing the mother the opportunity to understand the full purpose of the evaluation, nor receive the results, would not demonstrate transparency or respect for the dignity of the individual. The AOTA Specialty Certification in Driving and Community Mobility includes an Ethical Reasoning Standard, Competency A.9, which further reinforces this concept, as the occupational therapist is required to "communicate evaluation results to the client or necessary authorities as required to ensure safety of the client and the community" (AOTA, 2009).

The occupational therapist in this case also needs to be aware of any applicable laws, regulations, or requirements that can guide decision making and may even supersede ethical preferences. Principle 5 (Procedural Justice) of the *Code and Ethics Standards* requires compliance with "institutional rules, local, state, federal and international laws and Association documents applicable to the profession of occupational therapy" (AOTA, 2010, p. S22). If driving cessation is recommended and the client or family refuses, both legal and ethical actions may be needed.

Laws may require reporting or warning, but if the laws are silent, the occupational therapist can have an ethical obligation to warn not only the client and his and her family but also the physician and the state. Some states (e.g., Massachusetts) have passed legislation that protects health care providers, including occupational therapists, who report in good faith. The details of the reporting laws differ broadly by state, and advocacy efforts requesting change demand that therapists seek the most up-to-date information. The ***Physician's Guide to Assessing and Counseling Older Drivers*** (Carr, Schwartzberg, Manning, & Sempek, 2010) lists each individual state and its reporting laws at the time of printing. The department to contact also is listed and therapists are encouraged to check for the most current information.

When reporting information in compliance with applicable regulations, Principle 6 (Veracity) of the *Code and Ethics Standards* (AOTA, 2010) mandates that reported information be accurate. In this case, if the documentation for the occupational therapist's evaluation is accurate, it would need to include the reason for the evaluation and the client's cognitive status. Because the medical record is a legal document, misinformation can have serious consequences for treatment by other providers or if subpoenaed in litigation. Failing to include a recommendation to cease driving if the assessment data warranted it is misleading and incomplete.

Finally, the *Code and Ethics Standards* asks occupational therapists to "be diligent stewards of human, financial, and material resources of their employer" (Principle 7H; AOTA, 2010, p. S25). Given limited health care resources, a comprehensive evaluation may be unnecessary when the evidence points to a likely outcome. However, this does not negate the importance of a valid recommendation and action related to the client's ability to continue to drive on the basis of data that are already available.

Occupational Therapy's Domain and Scope of Practice

Occupational therapists are positioned and qualified to provide information on one's capacity that includes determination of driver fitness and transportation options that are an appropriate fit for the individual client. Determining capacity is a complicated process of evaluation along with professional and ethical reasoning based on multiple sources of information.

Ensuring Safety

Occupational therapists are involved with and experienced in the evaluation, decision-making process, and recommendations regarding safe transportation options across the spectrum of ages and diagnoses. Occupational therapists must consider the context in which a client will perform an activity. In the area of driving and community mobility, occupational therapists recognize that some environments and situations may not be safe, and restrictions and clarifying factors need to be discussed with clients and their families.

For example, clients with dementia require door-through-door transportation services to avoid confusion and the possibility of getting lost. It is the responsibility of the therapist to explain to caregivers what type of transportation options will and will not work for populations with memory loss, disorientation, and other cognitive impairments. From an ethical perspective, this is supported by Principle 1 of the *Code and Ethics Standards*, which states that "occupational therapy personnel shall demonstrate a concern for the well-being and safety of the recipients of their services" (AOTA, 2010, p. S18).

Decision-Making Process

Because driving assessment and training are in the domain of occupational therapy practice, the general public expects that occupational therapists are qualified to make recommendations that protect individuals as well as public safety in this area. The decision-making process therefore needs to be broad-based and comprehensive to ensure that all relevant factors are considered. The Multifactor Older Dementia/Driver Evaluation model (MODEM; Hunt, 2010) is one such tool to meet this goal and can be applied to decisions about driving in other age groups (Figure 5.1; Exhibit 5.2). One area should not necessarily be weighed more than other sources of information.

Driver evaluations must include comprehensive data collected from many sources, filtered through a system of professional reasoning to determine an ultimate decision regarding fitness-to-drive. Assessing an individual's fitness-to-drive must be carefully designed according to the individual's unique clinical picture. This design is consistent with Principle 1B of the *Code and Ethics Standards*, which states that "occupational therapy personnel shall provide appropriate evaluation and a plan of intervention for all recipients of occupational therapy services *specific* to their needs" [italics added] (AOTA, 2010, p. S19). See Schell and Schell (2008) for a complete review of the definitions of professional reasoning that occupational therapists should use to positively influence client outcomes. Accurate professional reasoning leads to an informed decision that requires action based on evidence and should occur in all practice settings.

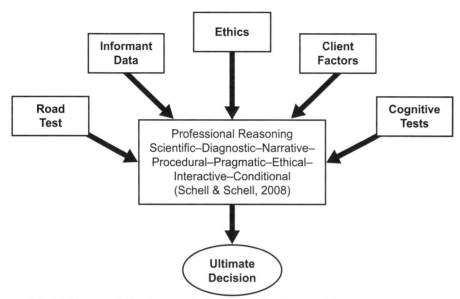

Figure 5.1. Multifactor Older Dementia/Driver Evaluation Model.
Note: From Hunt (2010). Copyright © 2010 by Linda A. Hunt, PhD, OTR, FAOTA. Used with permission.

Although the effect of cognitive impairment on driving ability may be most frequently studied in conditions such as Alzheimer's disease, it also can be an important factor in the ability to drive for those with other diagnoses. Case Example 5.2 describes a generalist occupational therapist who works at an outpatient community facility. She is well versed in evidence-based practice and the

---

Exhibit 5.2. Clinical Application of MODEM

MODEM (Hunt, 2010) is a tool to ensure that the decision-making process considers all relevant factors. Therefore, this tool individualizes the approach to assessing fitness-to-drive. In addition, the model does not rely on only one method of professional reasoning. Rather, it includes comprehensive data collection from many sources, filtered through a system of professional reasoning to determine an ultimate decision regarding fitness-to-drive.

The various components of the model guide therapists through the decision-making process. The Road Test data come from an actual in-car road test. However, a therapist may decide that the other components, such as a moderate diagnosis of dementia, may preclude using this assessment. The Informant Data section is defined as information collected from the client, caregiver, physician, or other individuals who provide information that may lead to a better understanding of the client's fitness-to-drive. The Ethics section of the model refers to the occupational therapist considering all evaluation information and coming up with the best recommendations that keep in mind benefiting the client and doing no harm. It is an ethical responsibility to choose and correctly administer the appropriate evidence-based assessments and to use them, along with therapists' expertise to guide and communicate to all stakeholders throughout the evaluation process. The Client Factors section reflects the client's roles, values, needs, and bodily functions, including visual, sensory, perceptual, and biomechanical. If the Cognitive Tests section is used, the tests should be evidence-based with regard to driving and consistent with the diagnosis.

An example of both client factors and ethical reasoning is explaining to a client and his family that the client's untreated depression may be creating some impairment in the client's thinking. The potential benefits of anti-depressive medications and the relationship of depression to impairment can be explained. The client is therefore informed of all the options and consequences; ethical reasoning may result in the postponement of driving until anti-depressive medications are tried. As part of ethical reasoning, all relevant information is disclosed to facilitate client and family autonomy in making a decision that is safe, is beneficial, and prevents harm to all parties. Using ethical reasoning is an important component in protecting all stakeholders. The use of MODEM turns the driver evaluation into a multistep and comprehensive process. Therapists must consider that decisions may proceed in steps as information is received and reviewed.

—Linda Hunt, PhD, OTR/L, FAOTA

importance of using the *Occupational Therapy Practice Framework: Domain and Process, 2nd Edition* (AOTA, 2008). In addition, she recently attended a workshop on assessing drivers with dementia.

Ethical Discussion

In considering the most appropriate venue and personnel to deliver services, important factors are competence, cost, convenience, and client preference. Depending on the situation, there may be additional factors as well. In Case Example 5.2, the therapist knew the skill set of the driving school and understood that they could work together to meet the client's needs in a cost-efficient manner so that all criteria were met. However, in a different situation, ethical challenges may include how these factors weigh in the decision-making process and who ultimately makes the final determination. Clients need to understand the implications of alternatives to reach outcomes so they are autonomous and can make a fully informed decision. They need to understand how the interventions and skills of potential providers may differ and, as a result, how outcomes may be affected.

In Case Example 5.2, the occupational therapist synthesizes all the data, including feedback from the driving school, and integrates it into the final discharge recommendations. The clinician must ensure that the client understands all options and their consequences but is offered appropriate choices where feasible. The process in this case example was collaborative and a plan was outlined that met the client's needs and to which he agreed. In other situations, careful consideration and perhaps intensive education from other team members involved with the client may be necessary to arrive at an appropriate plan that is acceptable to all parties.

In the case of driving rehabilitation, where reimbursement can be challenging, the clinician's recommendations should nevertheless be based on client abilities and needs; alternative strategies to achieve goals are a separate discussion and should not be unduly influenced by payment. Even if a recommended service is not paid, clinicians need to talk about it and offer the client options with open disclosure to meet their ethical obligation to deliver appropriate services. As previously stated in Principle 4E, therapists should make "efforts to advocate for recipients of occupational therapy services to obtain needed services through available means" (AOTA, 2010, p. S22).

Because occupational therapists have an obligation to provide (or recommend) services for which there is an expectation that a benefit will result (Principle 1, Beneficence) and also to prevent foreseeable harm (Principle 2, Nonmaleficence), the clinician in Case Example 5.2 ensured that the client's deficits that could negatively impact the ability to resume driving were addressed not only in occupational therapy, but also in the "real-world" training of the driving school. Communication was essential to provide critical information to the driving school personnel so that their intervention was appropriately focused and achieved the client's goals.

Even if a recommended service is not paid, clinicians need to talk about it and offer the client options with open disclosure to meet their ethical obligation to deliver appropriate services.

Communication

This chapter seeks to reinforce the ethical obligation of occupational therapists to discuss driving and community mobility needs and desires across various practice settings with their diverse clients. One way to address this obligation is to establish

Case Example 5.2. Client With Asperger's Syndrome

A young man 26 years of age with a diagnosis of Asperger's syndrome and mild residual left hemiparesis (from birth) contacted the local driving school about his desire to resume driving. He described having driven between the ages of 20 and 22 until his license was revoked for 1 year following a DUI. Because of family opinion and financial restrictions, he has not attempted to reinstate his license until now. The driving school had a close working relationship with occupational therapy at the local hospital. The initial interview at the driving school identified concerns related to medical diagnoses; therefore, the driving school asked him to begin his exploration with occupational therapy, and he was given the forms and contact information.

The occupational therapist's evaluation began with developing his occupational profile. His goals included returning to community college, driving, and meeting new friends. He described living in an apartment in town and using public transportation to get to work and to the store. He would like to expand his evening activities and build social relationships with friends, but he is uncomfortable using the bus system in the evening and recognizes that the limited bus routes and schedule of operation restrict his activity options. He has successfully completed treatment for alcohol abuse and is committed to remaining chemical free. His family is supportive, offering to sell him their vehicle in relatively good repair.

On the basis of the data gathered, the occupational therapist designed the clinical evaluation to build on the basic measures for vision, physical ability, and cognition with the addition of an evaluation tool that would measure strengths and limitations in bilateral dexterity, speed of response, and planning and problem solving (executive deficits associated with Asperger's syndrome) to comprehensively address all of the relevant skills for safe driving. The occupational therapist then scheduled an on-road evaluation to be done by the driving school.

Following the clinical and on-road evaluations, the occupational therapist then got permission from the client to set up a meeting with the driving school personnel, the therapist, the client, and his family to review the results and recommendations. It was determined that physical adaptations were not necessary but that intervention should focus on compensatory skills training with an emphasis on anticipatory planning for problem solving and vigilant attention.

Potential Ethical Considerations (for this case or similar ones)

1. Where and to whom should a referral go (if a referral is necessary)? What factors should be considered in making that decision?

    - If the occupational therapy program and the driving school both are highly skilled to offer this training but the occupational therapy program is more costly, how should factors be weighted in making a decision?

    - Should a client go to a driving school for compensatory skills training? In this case, a relationship had been developed with the driving school. The local driving school had excellent experience and skill and had developed a strong relationship with the occupational therapy program. The therapist was confident that the training would include addressing the subtle executive deficits the client exhibited. The driving school charged a much lower hourly fee for training. The therapist working closely with a driving school would have the opportunity to recognize the strengths each discipline brings to the evaluation and training.

2. How does a therapist evaluate the equality of skills and services from different potential providers?

3. What if the local driving school lacked the experience and training to deliver the recommended treatment? But the driving school was far less costly and the client had limited funds—how does that influence the decision, if at all?

4. What if the occupational therapist's program or employer discouraged or did not allow referrals to outside agencies, mandating that the therapist must keep the intervention revenue in-house, but the occupational therapy staff did not have appropriate competency to best serve the needs of the client?

5. Is it the responsibility of the occupational therapist to advocate for the client to receive needed services (regardless of reimbursement)?

6. What, if any, is the role or responsibility of the client in deciding what type of services he will receive and where he will obtain them?

7. What if the client's self-assessment and wishes are not in agreement with therapist or driving school recommendations? What options exist to support the safety of the client and the public, and whose safety is most important?

Case Example 5.2. Client With Asperger's Syndrome *(cont.)*

Because of the close working relationship developed between the occupational therapy driving rehabilitation program and the driving school in this case, it was determined jointly in the meeting (of therapist, client, and driving school personnel) that the client's needs would best be served by seeking training at the driving school, supporting the principle of collaborative goal setting and client autonomy. The driving school plan was to integrate the occupational therapist's recommendations by including demands on attention and concentration, problem solving, and speed of response into the skills training. The therapist suggested a phone conference following the first week of lessons, and the client agreed (permissions and releases were signed). A reevaluation with the occupational therapist was planned to occur before the final decision if there was a recommendation to return to driving. That reassessment would include subtle high-level executive function deficits and the ability to be self-aware: Can the client describe a realistic plan for returning to driving and avoiding alcohol and safety considerations related to driving?

---

driving or community mobility as a line item on the occupational therapy evaluation to ensure that it is covered. Another way to keep addressing driving and community mobility as part of standard occupational therapy services is to initiate and maintain contact with DRSs for potential referral of clients whose needs exceed the individual therapist's competency in this area. Finally, it is within the scope of occupational therapy practice to facilitate the client's communication with community agencies regarding the use of alternative modes of transportation.

As stated in Chapter 1, occupational therapists should consider addressing driving and community mobility at some level in all settings of occupational practice. For example, if a client is in the intensive care unit after heart surgery, an occupational therapist may be focused on very basic upper-body ADLs. Just sitting up on the side of the bed unsupported might be a goal. However, the occupational therapist can introduce the topic of driving and community mobility to identify whether it is an activity that is desired or needed and of interest to the client. Clients can be encouraged to discuss this further with the occupational therapist after transitioning to a future program, such as outpatient cardiac rehabilitation.

Handouts on resources for assessment and community mobility options should be available and offered. In rehabilitation settings, occupational therapists need to determine whether clients are at risk, whether driving and community mobility are client goals, and whether more specialized driving evaluation is warranted. When driving competence is in question, therapists have an obligation to optimize the potential for client success through addressing clinical sub-skills and considering the timing of referral for a comprehensive driving evaluation.

Finally, in home care and outpatient settings, therapists should discuss options and referrals and possibly provide the driver evaluation, if appropriate. If there is demand but few referral options to address more specialized driving evaluation, occupational therapists should consider expanding their expertise and services to meet the need.

Conclusion

Determining capacity to drive is an evolving and complex functional–psycho–legal construct with clinical, ethical, and legal dimensions. Each state maintains the primary responsibility, from a legal point of view, for determining whether a citizen is safe to drive; the state has the power to give and to remove a driving license.

Professional and ethical reasoning should guide the occupational therapist's reflection and actions in evaluation, planning, intervention, and outcomes in regard to driving and community mobility.

If occupational therapists are going to maintain a key role in determining driver capacity, they need to better use all the types of professional reasoning along with a clear understanding of their ethical obligations to determine a level of risk for both the client and society. Further, because driving and community mobility are solidly within the scope of occupational therapy practice, therapists must have the confidence to provide information in all applicable settings and with all relevant populations. Effective occupational therapists need to know what community resources are available for driver rehabilitation, alternate transportation options, and appropriate referrals to other services when they do not offer driver evaluations at their own facility. Such knowledge is necessary to meet both ethical and practice standards.

References

American Occupational Therapy Association. (2008). Occupational therapy practice framework: Domain and process (2nd ed.). *American Journal of Occupational Therapy, 62,* 625–683. doi:10.5014/ajot.62.6.625

American Occupational Therapy Association. (2009). *Competencies, criteria, and client outcomes: Specialty certification in driving and community mobility: Occupational therapist.* Retrieved February 24, 2011, from http://www.aota.org/Practitioners/ProfDev/Certification/Info.aspx

American Occupational Therapy Association. (2010). Occupational therapy code of ethics and ethics standards (2010). *American Journal of Occupational Therapy, 64*(Suppl.), S17–S26. doi:10.5014/ajot.2010.64S17

Beauchamp, T. L., & Childress, J. F. (2009). *Principles of biomedical ethics* (6th ed.). New York: Oxford University Press.

Brandt, L. C., & Slater, D. Y. (2010). Ethical dimensions of occupational therapy. In K. Jacobs & G. L. McCormack (Eds.), *The occupational therapy manager* (5th ed., pp. 469–482). Bethesda, MD: AOTA Press.

Carr, D. B., Schwartzberg, J. G., Manning, L., & Sempek, J. (2010). *Physician's guide to assessing and counseling older drivers.* Washington, DC: National Highway Traffic Safety Administration.

Hunt, L. A. (2010). *Determining capacity to drive for drivers with dementia using research, ethics, and professional reasoning: The responsibility of all occupational therapists* [CEonCD]. Bethesda, MD: American Occupational Therapy Association.

Kanny, E. M., & Slater, D. Y. (2008). Ethical reasoning. In B. A. B. Schell & J. W. Schell (Eds.), *Clinical and professional reasoning in occupational therapy* (pp. 188–208). Baltimore: Lippincott Williams & Wilkins.

Schell, B. A. B., & Schell, J. W. (2008). *Clinical and professional reasoning in occupational therapy.* Baltimore: Lippincott Williams & Wilkins.

CHAPTER 6

Analyzing the Complex Instrumental Activities of Daily Living of Driving and Community Mobility

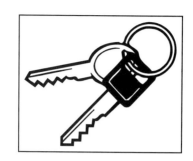

Anne Dickerson, PhD, OTR/L, FAOTA,
With Pat Niewoehner, OTR/L, CDRS

Learning Objectives

At the completion of this chapter, readers will be able to
- Delineate the process of an activity analysis for one component of driving a motor vehicle,
- Identify the complexity of driving a motor vehicle,
- Identify the multiple components and factors that influence the performance of driving, and
- Recognize the variety of issues affecting safe driving as illustrated through an occupation-based activity analysis.

Introduction

The overall goal of this chapter is to discuss the instrumental activity of daily living (IADL) of community mobility from the perspective of activity analysis, with the objective of illustrating the complexities of community mobility and, in particular, driving a motor vehicle. Occupational therapists' unique contribution as health care professionals is our ability to take everyday tasks and analyze their components. In being able to break tasks into steps or smaller components, therapists are able to grade the task to be simpler or more complex depending on the needs of the client. Thus, this chapter is a critical review of the process of analysis and its application to driving. Although community mobility comprises many activities, such as riding a bus or bicycle, this chapter will specifically address the task of *driving an automatic motor-vehicle sedan.*

The profession of occupational therapy has actively moved from using the term *activity* in defining our domain to the now common use of *occupation,* with a clear distinction occurring with the first edition of *Occupational Therapy Practice Framework* (American Occupational Therapy Association [AOTA], 2002) replacing *Uniform*

Key Words
- activity analyses
- body functions
- body structures
- client factors
- community mobility
- contexts
- driving
- environments
- occupational analysis
- performance patterns
- performance skills

Terminology for Occupational Therapy—Third Edition (AOTA, 1994). However, *activity* is still an important term in occupational therapy vocabulary, as the expertise of activity analysis should be considered one of our profession's unique contributions to the health care collaboration. In fact, we make a distinction between *activity analysis* and *occupation-based activity analysis*. *Activity analysis* is the generic, broader term that incorporates the demands of an activity—the skills involved in the performance as typically performed in a culture (AOTA, 2008). *Occupation-based activity analysis* addresses the performance of the activity by a specific individual within his or her actual environmental context. This chapter will address both the activity analysis of driving and the occupation-based activity analysis of driving.

When clients receive occupational therapy, the IADL of community mobility may not be addressed. Reasons include the acute nature of the disability or the limits imposed by the time frame of intervention. However, frequently the occupational therapy generalist may not view driving as within his or her scope of practice and consequently may not consider it in intervention plans or goals. As noted in previous chapters, it is imperative that occupational therapists deal with the issue of community mobility as a critical IADL.

Experienced occupational therapists complete an activity analysis automatically using clinical reasoning and observation skills.

With common therapeutic interventions, experienced occupational therapists complete an activity analysis automatically using clinical reasoning and observation skills. They intuitively break the activities into steps to provide an accurate amount of challenge for the client to succeed in the desired occupation. If initially too easy or too difficult, the therapist will adjust the steps or tasks accordingly. Although most occupational therapists freely travel their community as experienced drivers, they probably have not specifically considered the process of driving using the components of an activity analysis.

Just as a student needs to write out his or her *first* activity analysis through a detailed examination of a specific task, this chapter will detail an analysis to demonstrate the multifaceted task of driving a car. This analysis will help readers appreciate driving as one of the most complex and dynamic IADLs and to appreciate the need to address driving and community mobility with clients who want to resume driving regardless or in spite of their disability. The *Occupational Therapy Practice Framework: Domain and Process, 2nd Edition* (*Framework–II;* AOTA, 2008) will be used as the framework for illustrating the activity analysis and occupation-based activity analysis related to driving.

Community Mobility and the Domain of Occupational Therapy

The domain of occupational therapy is the established knowledge and expertise that occupational therapists should address in their practice, service, and research (AOTA, 2008). The domain covers areas of occupation, client factors, performance skills, performance patterns, contexts and environments, and activity demands. We will address each of these aspects individually as they relate to the task of driving an automatic sedan automobile.

Community mobility is one of the 12 IADLs (AOTA, 2008); driving is one method of community mobility. By definition, IADLs support daily life in the home and community. Typically, they require more complex interactions than basic activities of daily living (BADLs) (AOTA, 2008). It is not surprising that after the valued ADLs are met, adult clients, particularly those in rural areas, often identify driving as one of their most meaningful and valued activities (Dickerson, Reistetter, & Gaudy, in press). In fact, the reality is that participating in other IADLs (e.g., shopping, social participation) is often dependent on the ability to drive independently or access transportation in rural and suburban communities.

Occupational Analysis

Client Factors

There are three elements of *client factors*: (1) body structures; (2) body functions; and (3) values, beliefs, and spirituality that affect the performance in occupation (AOTA, 2008).

Body Structures

When driving is a desired outcome for a specific client, the client's *body structures* must be considered. There will be some body structures that will be essential to the task of driving, such as eyes, the nervous system, and structures related to movement. However, for some body structures, vehicles may be modified to fit the needs of the driver. An example may be hand controls, so that arms can steer and control acceleration and braking if an individual's legs are not functional.

Body Functions

Accordingly, some body functions will be more essential for driving than others. These include the mental functions, sensory functions, and neuromusculoskeletal functions. It is the task of the occupational therapist to evaluate each client and consider which of the body functions and structures affect the occupation of driving and how they relate to performance skills associated with driving. How has the client's injury, illness, or process of aging affected his or her body structures and functions? Does the client have congenital or acquired body structure differences? Is there a disease process that is progressive that will affect the manner in which his or her body structures or functions will change over time? Does the client take medication for treatment of some disease or illness that will affect the manner of the body functions? If so, does the medication have side effects that affect any body function or speed of processing?

Values

The question to consider with the task of driving is what *value* does driving have for the client? Is the occupation of driving important to the person, and to what degree? Does the ability to drive affect others in the client's social world, such as a mother who picks up her children from school? How meaningful is driving to the client?

Beliefs

What *beliefs* are inherent in the occupation of driving? With many older adults, there is a strong belief that independence is dependent on driving, and young adults may consider getting a license as a major step to independence and adulthood.

Spirituality

Spirituality refers to the source of meaning in one's life. For most people, it is important to gather together to encourage one another and to participate in rituals and ceremonies that sustain one another's spirituality. Driving is often the preferred mode of transportation that permits a person the freedom and ability to participate in groups related to one's faith-based community (e.g., church, synagogue, Alcoholics Anonymous meetings). Therefore, it is critical to explore alternative modes of transportation when a person is no longer able to drive safely.

Performance Skills

Performance skills are the abilities that clients demonstrate in the actions performed during a step of an activity (AOTA, 2008).

Motor and Praxis Skills

Motor and praxis skills include the physical actions of moving body or body parts as well as the skilled, purposeful movements that are sequenced, organized, and part of an overall plan to carry out a learned or novel motor activity rather than an individual act (AOTA, 2008). Although driving a sedan does not require significant strength or agility, sequencing and skilled planning of the motor tasks are essential. Moving between brake and acceleration pedals must be automatic, with sufficient dexterity and adequate speed. The motor actions of using the steering wheel and pedals rely on procedural memory that must be integrated with the ability to scan the environment to execute instant action judgments. Can the client manipulate the key to unlock the door and start the vehicle, or reach and apply the safety belt, or open the gas cap, or apply the parking brake? Can he or she reach the pedals and other driving controls adequately? Can the client pace and coordinate his or her movements to complete the driving task? Can the client anticipate and adjust his or her body position in response to environmental clues?

Sensory–Perceptual Skills

When considering driving, the sensory–perceptual skill most essential to the task is *visual–perceptual*. At this time, no technical substitution exists for the ability to visually locate, identify, interpret, organize, remember, and respond to the environment to drive a vehicle. The critical question to consider is, What are the minimum requirements for visual–perceptual deficits? For example, How much of a field cut can be compensated by substitution strategies before a driver is unsafe? How much does a client's glaucoma or cataract affect his or her ability to visually scan the environment and drive safely?

The sensory inputs of auditory, vestibular, proprioception, and tactile also need to be considered with each client, although usually the threshold of disability can be greater in these areas in most cases. For example, sensory input from the feet and legs is important for control of foot pedals, but compensation is possible with adaptive equipment.

Emotional Regulation Skills

Learning to drive a motor vehicle takes persistence and patience, especially if a client needs to learn how to compensate for deficits. The *regulation of emotions* needs to be considered with each client. Can the client respond appropriately when driving a powerful machine in heavy traffic if the individual is simultaneously experiencing feelings of frustration, anger, or grief? Can the client tolerate hours of practice to ensure an automatic response when encountering a red light, other drivers driving too slowly, being cut off by other drivers, a pedestrian in the street, or a dog running out between parked cars?

Cognitive Skills

Cognitive skills, the actions or behaviors a client uses to plan and manage the performance of an activity (AOTA, 2008, p. 640), are sometimes the most difficult skills to evaluate when considering driving. Driving for most adults is an overlearned, automatic activity that can be fairly simple when traveling on a mostly empty, rural, two-lane road in a client's familiar environment. However, the complexity multiplies when another vehicle, person, animal, or object appears on the road ahead. The cognitive skills needed for safe driving include simultaneously multitasking the ability to judge the importance of an upcoming object in the road, selecting the appropriate action quickly, sequencing the order of the motor response, and responding if another vehicle appears from behind as well as in front on the roadway.

The abilities to identify, remember, and organize the steps to get to a destination safely in the motor vehicle are vitally important. Visual–perceptual and cognitive skills are the two most essential performance skills that require the most attention when addressing a client's occupational analysis.

Communication and Social Skills

Perhaps not an essential skill compared to visual–perceptual and cognitive skills, *communication* while driving a motor vehicle is still important. Maintaining acceptable physical space between vehicles and making eye contact to take turns at a four-way intersection with stop signs require an individual to communicate his or her intentions and maintain appropriate *social skills*. Using the horn when a driver pulls out from a parking space and does not see an oncoming driver, using the turn signal, and gesturing to indicate the driver's intention are important communications needed to keep all drivers aware of each other's actions in a dynamic environment. Communication can be affected when a person has decreased vision and he or she is unable to identify a hand wave or has difficulty distinguishing between a hand wave to go ahead and one of anger.

Performance Patterns

Considering performance patterns, we know that individual drivers (1) have specific driving *habits*, (2) follow *routines* of driving, (3) may have *rituals* associated with their personal motor vehicles, and (4) fulfill *roles* during their performance.

Habits

Most drivers have specific driving habits such as using the seat belt, using turn signals, locking the vehicle when leaving, playing music, and so on. Wearing seat belts and using turn signals are positive habits that increase the safety of the driver. Unfortunately, drivers often have negative habits such as speeding, slowing down rather than stopping for stop signs, or using a cell phone or other electronic device while driving. It is important for the occupational therapist to observe and ask about habits to reinforce the positive habits and initiate strategies to change the negative habits.

Routines

Routines in driving are very strong. Drivers have specific routines of starting the car, parking the car, and taking steps in cleaning the car. As driving becomes more automatic, routes become so familiar that drivers follow the route without consciously thinking of what they are doing. For example, it is not uncommon for the driver to intend to stop on an errand on the way to work and then pass by the extra stop because it was not part of the usual routine. Tragic examples include parents who forget to drop off the sleeping baby at day care on the way to work, leaving the baby in the back seat of a car, because going to day care is not part of their usual routine in the morning.

In most cases, however, routines assist in managing time and energy in the process of driving. Driving routines help the individual with beginning dementia to continue to find his or her way back and forth from home and familiar destinations. The main question is, When a disruption of the routine occurs, can the driver with cognitive impairment respond to novel situations and environments to drive safely *outside of the driving routine?*

Older drivers frequently make changes to their routines to increase safety—such as driving only during daylight hours, avoiding rush hour, limiting left turns, and selecting to stay off highways (Dellinger, Sehgal, Sleet, & Barrett-Connor, 2001). Some of these proactive changes establish safer routines that can help individuals to safely postpone driving retirement.

Rituals

Driving can have a ritualistic or sacred value. With some people, the actual act of driving is revered; for others, the actual possession of the motor vehicle has great meaning. This is particularly true for baby boomers (see also Chapter 2). Owners of classic or high-end sports cars will have rituals of cleaning their vehicle; preparing for a particular drive; or displaying their vehicle in their home, garage, or showcase car show. For many individuals, their truck is a part of their extended self, similar to the wheelchair for a person with quadriplegia. Consider also the aging baby boomers purchasing increasing numbers of motorcycles. These are not vehicles for merely transportation but are part of a sacred return to some former young lifestyle, for enjoying the fruits of one's labors, or part of one's life review (e.g., movies such as *Wild Hogs* [Becker, 2007]). Recognizing these rituals or symbolic meanings can promote a more sensitive approach when the therapeutic intervention requires a therapist to interfere with an individual's transportation choices.

Roles

As with all occupations, individuals have specific roles depending on their family structure, gender, or age. For example, with adults 80 years or older, it is not unusual for the male of the family structure to be the primary or only driver. However, for baby boomers, the role of driving is coupled with independence. Driving cessation is often a traumatic event regardless of whether an individual chooses this role change or is forced to stop driving by family members, licensing authorities, or even the economics of owning a car. In addition, driving cessation often affects a person's ability to participate in other significant roles, such as worker, volunteer, grandparent, or friendly chauffeur.

Contexts and Environments

The external *physical* and *social environments* refer to surroundings within which the individual drives. The *context* of driving includes cultural, personal, temporal, and virtual factors.

Physical

The physical environment significantly affects the occupation of driving. Whether an individual drives in a rural, suburban, or urban area, or a combination of these, will determine his or her level of skills, knowledge, and amount of experience. The physical environment of living on primarily flat land, hills, or mountains affects the speed of driving and the type of vehicle. Weather conditions of the Northern U.S. states with snow versus the South with intense heat and the states in between will influence the methods of teaching driving, adapting vehicles, and accommodating to changing and potentially dangerous driving circumstances. For example, the heat of the South will determine how one might adapt or modify a vehicle, do training, and protect a vehicle (e.g., window screens).

Physical structures of roadways should be considered with driving. City streets are different from rural scenic byways and major expressways; negotiating one-way streets, interpreting traffic signals, using shared left-turn lanes, and reading roadway signs are all part of the complex physical environment of city driving. To add to the complexity, other motor vehicles, pedestrians, motorcycles, trucks, and animals interact within this environment. The physical environment of even a familiar route is different during various times of the day because of lighting changes, traffic changes, and weather conditions. Rush hour traffic can be extreme, while the same roadway may be deserted during midday or on a weekend.

In addition to the physical environment of the land and roadways, the motor vehicle also has a physical environment. What type of motor vehicle does the client drive? Driving a four-wheel-drive truck is vastly different from driving a compact vehicle, four-door sedan, or minivan. Considering the various types and models of motor vehicles, the therapist needs to examine and consider the client's specific motor vehicle to get an accurate sense of this element of the physical environment. Does the client have a door that opens wide enough for entry and exit? Does the seat adjust for appropriate seating? Does the client have appropriate reach for the pedals?

> In addition to the physical environment of the land and roadways, the motor vehicle also has a physical environment.

Social

The social environment of the driving task can be considered in terms of two aspects: (1) public or societal rules and interactions and (2) personal or familial relationships. The *rules of society* dictate that drivers obey traffic control signals, keep in their lane of traffic, signal intentions to change positions, and follow an appropriate distance behind other vehicles, to name a few. However, there are *informal rules* of the social environment, such as allowing others to merge when there is a crowded exit or waving hello to a neighbor when passing by his or her home. When analyzing driving, the therapist needs to consider whether the client understands the social environment and the formal and informal rules and so can appropriately respond to the normal expectations of the roadways in his or her community or in other environments, if the driver ventures outside familiar communities.

The other aspect of the social environment is the relationships of individuals and organizations around the client. A significant other who can or cannot drive will affect the client's social environment. Does the client have a spouse, caregiver, family member, or friend who can transport the client if he or she cannot drive at night or at all? How will the transition from driver to passenger for the older adult, or from passenger to driver for the young novice driver, affect relationships? What relationships will be affected for the male client who cannot drive his child to school or his wife to the physician? What relationships are critical to ensuring the community mobility of the newly disabled young person?

Cultural

As with other tasks, the cultural aspect of driving is often not visible, but it is still powerful in terms of personal impact. The acquisition of the driver's license is often seen as a rite of passage, particularly to the baby boomers who grew up with the automobile (Trilling, 2001). Although the privilege of holding a driver's license is governed by the state's licensing agency, some adults who depend on their "wheels" to participate in life often consider driving a *right* (Trilling, 2001). The loss of the ability to drive is difficult in many ways. Driving, freedom, and independence are interwoven in the North American culture. Unlike retirement from work, which can be viewed as a positive life progression, for many individuals the loss of the driver's license represents a catastrophic loss in status and mobility. Although being a licensed driver is not a right, therapists should advocate for their clients and help society embrace the concept that mobility—the access to transportation—is a right.

U.S. driving culture is typically orderly and structured, with drivers generally obeying the rules of the road. However, there are common customs that are actually illegal but are tolerated and passively endorsed by those who would otherwise be considered law-abiding citizens, such as driving 5 to 10 miles over the speed limit. Other driving customs may be more regionally based, such as pulling to the side of the road for funeral processions.

Personal

The personal context includes age, gender, socioeconomic status, and educational status (AOTA, 2008). Certainly, an individual's age affects if and why the individual drives a vehicle (e.g., school, work, leisure). Gender or socioeconomic status might influence what type of vehicle a person may drive, while educational status may affect driving as a vocation (e.g., high school degree needed for a commercial license). Conversely, the ability to drive can have a tremendous impact on both educational and socioeconomic status. If one can freely move within the community, that individual can pursue educational opportunities that affect his or her socioeconomic status. With the exception of living in major cities with extensive public transit systems, the inability to drive limits employment and training opportunities, which are sure to affect socioeconomic status.

Temporal

The environmental element of time is important for the activity of driving. Getting from place to place requires patterns of driving as well as time. Thus, a driver has to estimate the distance, environment, and speed to determine how long it will take to get to or from a destination. The time of day also contributes to the context. Many drivers make a point of avoiding rush hour traffic or traveling on the interstate during the holiday weekends. Older adults might begin self-restriction of driving by avoiding nighttime driving because of age-related visual changes, while parents might monitor a teenager's driving during the weekend or evening hours as a precaution against risky behaviors.

Virtual

In some ways, the use of computer mapping and GPS (global positioning system) has revolutionized the ways we give and receive directions. Traveling "virtually" (e.g., through Google mapping) to a place to even determine whether one wants to drive to the destination is becoming routine. Using GPS to find a particular type of restaurant, lodging, or point of interest provides immediate information that allows more options for all individuals, but especially for those who might have special mobility, physical, or dietary needs. Individuals with spatial challenges can use GPS to guide them to their destinations with programs that eliminate highways, back roads, or other parameters.

However, GPS is not without its issues. For example, an individual with cognitive challenges may depend too greatly on GPS and allow the system to lead him or her into danger, such as a road that is under construction, not plowed, or diverted because of natural events such as flooding.

The virtual environment includes the driving simulator. Much research has yet to be done on how occupational therapists can use driving simulators effectively, but as with all technology, it is likely their use for training, rehabilitation, and assessment will eventually become part of the occupational therapists' repertoire of therapeutic tools.

Occupational Profile: Don Weathers

To apply the occupational analysis information in this chapter, we introduce Case Example 6.1 with an *occupational profile* (AOTA, 2008), which is a summary of information describing a client's occupational history, experiences, patterns of daily living, interests, values, and needs to get an understanding of the client's perspective and background. (Chapter 12 will discuss the driving evaluation and intervention.) The occupational profile illustrates how driving and community mobility is usually critical to clients and part of the complex interweaving of their lives.

Activity Analysis

The process of analyzing a particular individual's performance, culture, and patterns associated with driving, as illustrated above, is an *occupational analysis,* as each individual client's attitudes, skills, and knowledge are unique. Conversely, an *activity analysis* is a description of the generic tasks; with the task of driving, it involves specifically describing the *activity demands*. In this case, the example will be driving an automatic motor vehicle sedan. The activity demands (AOTA, 2008) are the aspects of an activity that are needed to carry out the activity (see Table 6.1).

Case Example 6.1. Occupational Profile of Don Weathers: Dementia

Note. Information directly linked to driving is italicized.

Referral

Don Weathers was referred to occupational therapy by his primary physician, with the diagnosis of cognitive impairment. The family practice physician referred Mr. Weathers *when his daughter mentioned that her father had gotten lost while driving* and was demonstrating other difficulties with managing his finances and the household tasks. Mr. Weathers's daughter accompanied him to the occupational therapist's evaluation.

Occupational History

Mr. Weathers is a 75-year-old man who lives alone in the same town as his married daughter. He is a Korean War veteran and achieved a college degree in business. He was a supervisor at a grocery chain store until his retirement 10 years ago. He was married for 40 years with 2 children, including the daughter with no children living in the same city. A married son has 2 children and lives in an adjoining state. The son has regular contact through phone calls and visits 2–3 times a year. Mr. Weathers has several surviving older siblings, but they live out of state and only have contact through phone calls.

Areas of Occupation

Mr. Weathers has lived alone since his wife's death 7 years ago. He has been independent in his ADLs and IADLs, but his daughter took over his finances recently when there was a problem with his phone service being terminated because of nonpayment. More recently, she has noticed that his home is more cluttered and the stove was on when she arrived for a late morning visit, apparently left on after he prepared breakfast 2 hours earlier. The daughter recently purchased a pill dispenser that holds his medication for each day, and she noticed that some days he forgets to take his medication.

Client Factors

Values and beliefs. Mr. Weathers verbalizes *a high value on living independently, including driving to where he needs and wants to go.* Although he expresses trust in his daughter, he believes that she was premature in perceiving the need to take over his finances. However, he has been able to rationalize that with the electronic conversion of banks and billings, he is not prepared to deal with computerized banking, and he has relented to her taking over. *Mr. Weathers insists that he is a safe driver because he drives slowly and has not gotten any tickets. He feels that he should be able to drive, because he has a valid license and says no one should be able to infringe on his right to drive. When asked about driving retirement, he stated that if he had to give up driving, "I might as well be dead."*

Spirituality. Mr. Weathers was raised Catholic and attends services at least twice a week. He has participated in church activities throughout his life and verbalizes a strong sense of right and wrong.

Performance Skills

Note. Sensory–perceptual skills, motor and praxis skills, and cognitive skills will be addressed in Chapter 12, as they are directly related to driver rehabilitation intervention.

Emotional regulation. Mr. Weathers's daughter reports her father is generally quiet and even-tempered. *However, since beginning to discuss issues of giving up his finances and particularly driving, he easily becomes angry and expresses frustration when such topics are initiated.*

Communication and social skills. Mr. Weathers's speech seems slow and deliberate. He answers questions with a "yes" or "no" and needs encouragement to expand upon an answer. His daughter reported that he was always a quiet man, but his initiation of conversation has decreased over the past year.

Performance Patterns

Roles. Mr. Weathers's roles have decreased significantly in the past 10 years. He had a strong work ethic before retiring and had few hobbies. He was an attentive husband and had difficulty assuming the home management roles after his wife's death. However, he gradually assumed the necessary roles to live independently. Until recently, he had been an active religious participant by attending and volunteering in services and church activities. Although not an avid gardener, he does work outside to maintain his yard.

Case Example 6.1. Occupational Profile of Don Weathers: Dementia *(cont.)*

Habits and routines. Mr. Weathers's habit and routines are regular and vary little from day to day. Mr. Weathers eats simple meals at home, although he joins his daughter and her husband regularly on Sunday afternoon after church. He reads the newspaper every day, works in the yard or garage in the morning, shops at his former store every Thursday, attends church services on Sunday and Wednesday, and watches TV in the afternoon and evening. In the evenings, he often takes a walk in his neighborhood, circling several blocks. He does have a regular routine of browsing yard sales on Saturday mornings. This was an activity he and his wife did together and he has continued to enjoy, although he rarely purchases any items. When he has a doctor's appointment or special event, his daughter must remind him about it several times, as he is prone to forget. *Although he follows the same routes to the store and church, he proudly reported he drives on the highway, even during rush hour, and has never had an issue. In the past, it was his routine to use the Friday paper to plan a route for the next day's yard sales. However, he says now he "enjoys just driving around to find the good sales." Recently, he drove during a rain storm to check on yard sales and does not understand why it would be upsetting to his daughter.*

Rituals. One of Mr. Weathers's rituals is his faithful washing of his Crown Victoria every Saturday afternoon.

Contexts and Environments

Cultural. Mr. Weathers was born in the United States and was from a large Catholic family. His family was middle class, with his father an attorney, but as one of the younger children he had to go to work because the family's finances were stretched. Mr. Weathers was proud that he worked his way through college and valued hard work over hobbies or entertainment. *As a military veteran, he believes strongly in the country and particularly individual rights, such as making decisions about when to stop working, where to spend money, or driving a car. He states he would rather die than lose his driver's license.*

Personal. Mr. Weathers has enjoyed fairly good physical health, with the exception of high blood pressure that is currently controlled by medication. His daughter has reported he is much more forgetful lately, but Mr. Weathers insists that he is fine. He has a good income from his savings before retirement. *Although the daughter acknowledges her father appears more forgetful, she is adamant that there is nothing wrong with his driving. In fact, she had just rode with him and relates "he is a good driver." Both Mr. Weathers and his daughter denied any traffic citations (tickets), accidents, or near misses. However, with questioning, Mr. Weathers revealed he had been pulled over by the police recently for a problem at an intersection, but he was not ticketed and therefore insisted he had not done anything wrong—the police officer had made a mistake.*

Physical. Mr. Weathers lives in a one-story home that he has owned for 40 years in a middle-class neighborhood. He is content with the current furnishings, although he did purchase a new television after his wife's death. *His daughter reported that the garage door did have some damage, as did Mr. Weather's car, but again Mr. Weathers claimed someone else must have hit his car and garage. Two times per year, Mr. Weathers must drive from his home in the suburbs to the city (a more complex environment) to see his podiatrist. He does not allow his daughter to drive him for his podiatry appointments: "I do just fine down there. Why would it be a problem?"*

Social. Mr. Weathers's daughter reported that her father seemed to be well liked by his employees and enjoyed socializing with his wife in community, family, and church activities. After retirement and the death of his wife, he socialized less but still was active in the church. However, over the past year, Mr. Weathers's social skills have decreased significantly as he spends time only with a few longtime friends at the church. He is quiet during shared meals and does not initiate conversation easily.

Temporal. Mr. Weathers measures his days by mealtimes and regular routines in his life. He continues to set an alarm for 7 a.m. and goes to bed at 10 p.m. after watching the news. Except for his activities on the weekend, he rarely varies his activities.

Virtual. Mr. Weathers is proud of not owning a computer and reluctantly accepted a cell phone and service from his son, although he tends to forget to charge it or even turn it on.

Summary

Mr. Weathers appears to be independent in the BADLs *but is having difficulty with complex IADLs, including driving. The occupational therapist's plan would be to do a performance evaluation of several IADLs, including screening tools designed to address driving.*

Table 6.1. Activity Demands

Objects and Their Properties	Tools, Materials, and Equipment
Space demands (relates to physical context)	Size, arrangement, surface, lighting, temperature, noise, humidity, ventilation
Social demands (relates to social environment and cultural contexts)	Rules, expectations
Sequence and timing	Steps, sequences, timing
Required actions and performance skills	Sensory, perceptual, motor, praxis, emotional, cognitive, communication, social
Required body functions	Physiological functions, mobility of joints, level of consciousness
Required body structures	Anatomical parts, organs, limbs, and components

Objects Used and Their Properties

Objects used in driving a motor vehicle are typically the key (tool), fuel (materials), and motor vehicle (equipment), although the type of motor vehicle can vary greatly. The properties of the key are small, hard, and portable, although newer models are electronic keypunch that open the door and push buttons to start the vehicle rather than a key. The materials needed to drive include the various fluids needed for the motor vehicle, with the most obvious being gasoline to run the engine, although various other fluids (e.g., oil, brake, windshield washer) need to be added periodically. The properties of gasoline include liquid, flammable, strong odor, and limited access through controlled gas pumps. Motor vehicles, as equipment, all have the primary controls for turning a steering wheel and for operating the brake and acceleration pedals, although there is a wide range of variability.

Although not considered primary controls, nearly all vehicles have to be entered by opening a hinged door; drivers must be seated in a chair that may have various heights, and the driver must attach a seat belt. Secondary controls are those used while the vehicle is in motion, including headlights, turn signals, dimmer switch, horn, cruise control, and wipers. Tertiary controls should be used when the vehicle is stationary; these include shifting gears, airflow vents, heating and cooling systems, radio or stereo, GPS, and telephone options. The types of secondary or tertiary controls vary across vehicles, but actions to move the controls consist of turning, pushing, pulling, and adjusting knobs, buttons, or levers with fingers, hand, or foot actions.

Space Demands

The physical environmental requirements for driving range from the minimum of a large space for parking the vehicle to the infinite roadways of the immediate community and beyond. The roadway system usually controls where a vehicle can move, although some vehicles have the capacity to go off-road. Weather, temperature, and lighting (e.g., night driving) can affect the physical environment, but ultimately the public highway transportation system offers unlimited options for a driver to operate the motor vehicle as an occupation.

The space within a vehicle varies, but the driver seat usually has the flexibility of moving the seat back and forth from the seating wheel as well as up and down from the base seat. Primary and secondary controls should be within comfortable arm's reach with tertiary also within easy reach, although not necessarily without fuller extension of the arm.

Social Demands

The social demands of driving a motor vehicle are a critical component of the activity analysis. Most rules of the road are learned from an early age and do not change. However, in other cases, there are changes in laws that vary across states and even county lines. The driver must know, understand, and respond appropriately to traffic signals, signs, roadway markings, human gestures, other vehicles' signals, and unanticipated events.

Theoretically, one could consider two levels of social demands for driving. The critical level is the expectation that the driver will follow the rules regardless of his or her physical locale—for example, maintaining a safe speed on a roadway, making a full stop at a red traffic signal, or stopping for a school bus picking up children. The less critical may be the more socially acceptable or unacceptable demands such as allowing another vehicle into your lane of traffic, honking the horn at a slower driver, or waving someone on at a four-way stop sign. The activity analysis of driving could be considered to have an overwhelming list of cultural, legal, and social demands in which the participant must have appropriate command.

Sequencing and Timing

The process of driving a motor vehicle is composed of multiple-step processes of several concurrent tasks that are integrated together through precise sequence and timing to achieve a successful and safe driving performance.

Required Actions and Performance Skills

Required actions are the usual skills needed by a person to be able to do an activity. Each step of an activity can be described in terms of the detailed actions that a person will have to perform. For each required action, the performance skills needed to complete the action should be identified in an activity analysis. The performance skills (i.e., sensory–perceptual, motor and praxis, emotional regulation, cognitive, communication and social skills) are related to the demands of the activity. That is, as the activity increases in complexity, the demand of the performance skills increases.

In the included example (Exhibit 6.1), under each step of the maneuver, the performance skills needed for making a right-hand turn are listed in order. Note that this *right turn* is a relatively simple turn at a stop sign, but it still involves most performance skills. The addition of motor vehicle traffic, high pedestrian traffic, foul weather, or a broken or tilted mirror will further complicate the process of making a right-hand turn and will require a higher level of performance skills. The concept of evaluating the *activity demands* for an activity analysis is to determine how a client who has performance skill issues can manage the steps of the tasks necessary to perform the activity (see Figure 6.1).

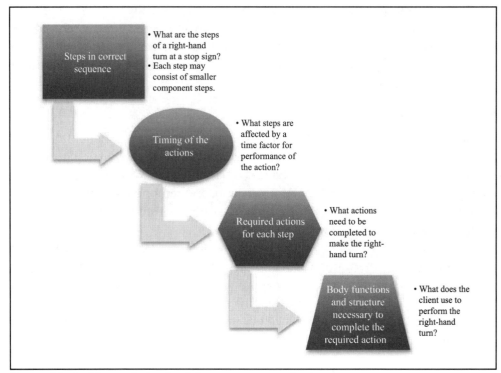

Figure 6.1. Activity analysis of a right turn at a stop sign.

Required Body Functions and Structures

Eight categories of body structures and six categories of body functions are identified in the *Framework–II* (AOTA, 2008). Although it is essential for all body structures and functions to be performing for one to be able to drive a motor vehicle (e.g., the respiratory system needs to be functioning to breathe, the cardiovascular system needs to function so that blood can flow to the blood and extremities), this chapter addresses the three key components that affect the act of driving: (1) visual–perceptual, (2) cognitive, and (3) motor abilities.

In the activity analysis of making a right turn, the anatomical parts and physiological functions of the human body for each of the *required actions* that make up each step of the activity process (i.e., a right-hand turn in a motor vehicle) should be identified. Thus, on the basis of the required actions identified, each required body function (e.g., visual acuity, motor proprioception functions, muscle power) and body structure (e.g., leg, arm, hands) needed to perform the actions should be listed for the completed activity analysis.

The example of the right turn here is not intended to be comprehensive, because the example is focusing on visual–perceptual, cognitive, and motor abilities, but it illustrates the complexity of all body functions and structures needed to perform driving. Even with the simplest of actions related to driving, such as a right turn, the need to be able to multitask and make quick and effective decisions is obvious. For example, the needed actions to determine that *a gap in traffic is great enough to merge or cross the road* require many aspects of body structures and functions as one determines what to do and executes the selected action within

Exhibit 6.1. Activity Analysis of a Right Turn

Steps in Correct Sequence

Step 1: Driver approaches the intersection, observing the stop sign.

    a. Activate turn signal.

    b. Slow vehicle down.

    c. Search to the left, front, and right as moving forward to the stop sign.

    d. Check the rear-view mirror to observe behind the motor vehicle.

Step 2: Search for pedestrians or other vehicles moving into the path of travel while approaching the stop sign.

Step 3: Stop behind the white line or line car bumper even with the curb.

Step 4: Search to the left and right.

    a. Look a full 90-degree angle to the left and right.

    b. If the view is blocked, pull up so there is a clear visual point.

    c. Look to the left and right again.

Step 5: Make the turn.

    a. Turn to head to the right.

    b. Begin to accelerate.

    c. Turn the steering wheel so the vehicle is 3 or 4 feet away from the curve.

Step 6: Complete the turn and accelerate into the lane of traffic.

    a. Complete the turn and straighten the wheels.

    b. Speed up to adjust to traffic.

Timing of the Steps

Step 1: Driver approaches the intersection, observing the stop sign.

Timing: See sign, slow vehicle as search areas around vehicle, then activate turn signal.

Step 2: Search for pedestrians or other vehicles moving into the path of travel while approaching the stop sign.

Timing: Continue slowing and searching the area for potential targets.

Step 3: Stop behind the white line or line car bumper even with the curb.

Timing: Stop the vehicle.

Step 4: Search to the left and right.

Timing: Look to the left, the right, move up if blocked, and search left and right.

Step 5: Make the turn.

Timing: Begin the turn and accelerate.

Step 6: Complete the turn and accelerate into the lane of traffic.

Timing: Accelerate and check mirrors.

"Required Actions" Necessary for Each Step of the Task

Step 1: Driver approaches the intersection, observing the stop sign.

    a. Observe and recognize the stop sign.

    b. Grip the steering wheel.

    c. Move left hand and push the turn signal up to activate.

    d. Move right foot from the accelerator to the brake pedal.

    e. Push on the brake smoothly to adjust the speed of the vehicle.

    f. Judge the speed of the vehicle and the distance to the stop sign.

    g. Move head to the left and right.

    h. Scan the environment.

    i. Perceive objects both near and far, determining any movement.

    j. Move eyes from forward to mirror back to forward.

    k. Process information to make decisions.

    l. Judge for any possible objects moving into the path of travel.

(continued)

Exhibit 6.1. Activity Analysis of a Right Turn (*cont.*)

Step 2: Search for pedestrians or other vehicles moving into the path of travel while approaching the stop sign.

    a. Continue slow compression on the brake with right foot.

    b. Judge the speed of the vehicle and the distance to the stop sign.

    c. Move head to left and right.

    d. Scan the environment.

    e. Perceive near and far, moving and nonmoving objects.

    f. Continue to judge for any possible objects moving into the path of travel.

Step 3: Stop behind the white line or line car bumper even with the curb.

    a. Complete and hold compression on the brake to stop.

    b. Perceive the curve for projecting the position of the vehicle to be in line.

    c. Judge the appropriate stopping position.

Step 4: Search to the left and right.

    a. Continue to hold the brake.

    b. Turn head completely side to side.

    c. Scan the environment.

    d. Decide if full visual field is visible to make decision.

    e. Move foot to accelerate to slowly move up, if needed.

    f. Make judgment about the gap in traffic.

Step 5: Make the turn.

    a. Turn head to right.

    b. Scan and search the environment.

    c. Process information quickly to make decision.

    d. Continue to hold the brake, until clear, then move right foot to the accelerator and slowly compress accelerator in a controlled movement.

    e. Grip the steering wheel and move hand over hand to turn.

    f. Turn head to left for a final scan.

    g. Turn the steering wheel, adjusting for the curve.

    h. Judge the distance from the curve and through the curve.

    i. Judge the speed of the vehicle.

Step 6: Complete the turn and accelerate into the lane of traffic.

    a. Adjust pressure of right foot on the accelerator pedal.

    b. Hands move steering wheel back into the straight position.

    c. Judge other vehicles' speed and match accordingly.

    d. Judge the posted speed limit and compare appropriately.

    e. Focus on the rear-view mirror and scan the environment.

Body Functions and Body Structures

Each step of the task (i.e., the right turn) has specific actions that need to be performed, described above as required actions. Each required action necessitates the use of specific body functions and structures. Thus, this section lists the structures and functions for completing the all the individual required actions for each of the 6 steps of the right hand turn.

Note. * indicates that the function or structure is necessary for *all* the required actions and is listed only once.

1. Observe and recognize the stop sign.

- *Global mental functions:* Conscious, oriented, awake, and maintaining energy.*
- *Mental functions (including):*
  - Attention to observe
  - Memory and recognition to know the sign
  - Thought process to understand and know what to do in response.
- *Sensory functions:* See the sign with adequate visual acuity, visual stability, and visual field.

Exhibit 6.1. Activity Analysis of a Right Turn (*cont.*)

2. Grip the steering wheel.

- *Neuromusculoskeletal and movement (including):*
  - Joint stability and mobility of head, trunk, arms, hands, and fingers*
  - Muscle power; muscle tone; muscle endurance; and no involuntary motions of head, trunk, arms, hands, and fingers.*
- *Sensory functions:* Touch to grip, proprioception to keep hands in place.

3. Move left hand and push the turn signal up to activate.

- *Mental functions:* Memory and thought process to know what to do and sequence the action.
- *Mental functions:* Attention
  - Divided attention among maintaining adequate grip on the steering wheel, pushing the turn signal, and keeping vision attention on the road
  - Selected attention to continue to watch for critical events in the environment.
- *Neuromusculoskeletal and movement:* Movement of hand and fingers to move the turn signal.
- *Sensory functions (including):*
  - Touch to grip
  - Proprioception to move hand without looking at the turn signal
  - Hearing signal functioning
  - Visually watching the environment.

4. Move right foot from the accelerator to the brake pedal.

- *Mental functions:* Attention
  - Divided attention among maintaining a grip on the steering wheel, moving the right foot to the brake pedal, and keeping vision attention on the road
  - Selected attention to continue to watch for critical events in the environment.
- *Sensory functions (including):*
  - Proprioception to move right foot to the brake pedal with visual cues
  - Touch and feel the brake pedal.
- *Neuromusculoskeletal and movement:* Movement of right foot and leg to reach from the accelerator to the brake pedal.

5. Push on the brake smoothly to adjust the speed of the vehicle.

- *Mental functions:* Attention
  - Divided attention among maintaining a grip on the steering wheel, putting pressure on the brake pedal, and keeping vision attention on the road
  - Selected attention to continue to watch for critical events in the environment
  - Sustained attention to the task.
- *Sensory functions (including):*
  - Touch and feel pressure of the brake pedal to apply smoothly
  - Proprioception of the right foot to use the brake pedal.
- *Neuromusculoskeletal and movement (including):*
  - Plantar flexion of the foot
  - Stability of the right leg and foot.

6. Judge the speed of the vehicle and the distance to the stop sign.

- *Mental functions (including):*
  - Attention
    - Divided attention among maintaining a grip on the steering wheel, putting pressure on the brake pedal, and keeping vision attention on the road
    - Selected attention to continue to watch for critical events in the environment
    - Sustained attention to the task of stopping.

(*continued*)

Exhibit 6.1. Activity Analysis of a Right Turn (*cont.*)

    ◦ Perception
       ▪ Discriminate the speed of the car
       ▪ Discriminate the distance to the stop sign.
    ◦ Thought
       ▪ Logically compare the speed of the car to the distance to determine needed pressure of the brake pedal.
    ◦ Sequencing of complex movement
       ▪ Make a decision of needed actions to make the motor vehicle stop at the stop sign.

7. Move head to the left and right.
- *Neuromusculoskeletal and movement:* Movement of head from side to side.

8. Scan the environment.
- *Mental functions:* Attention
    ◦ Divided attention among maintaining a grip on the steering wheel, putting pressure on the brake pedal, and vision attention for the task
    ◦ Selected attention to scan the environment for critical features
    ◦ Sustained attention to the task of scanning.
- *Sensory functions (including):*
    ◦ Visually scanning the environment.

9. Perceive objects both near and far, determining any movement.
- *Mental functions (including):*
    ◦ Perception
       ▪ Discrimination of visual input.
    ◦ Higher-level cognition
       ▪ Awareness of movement of objects and the meaning.

10. Move eyes from forward to mirror and back to forward.
- *Mental functions:* Attention
    ◦ Divided attention among maintaining a grip on the steering wheel, putting pressure on the brake pedal, and vision attention to scan the environment both forward and in the mirror
    ◦ Selected attention to scan the environment for critical features
    ◦ Sustained attention to the task of scanning.
- *Sensory functions (including):*
    ◦ Visual acuity, visual stability, and visual field.
- *Neuromusculoskeletal and movement:* Purposeful movement of the eye muscles.

11. Process information to make decisions.
- *Mental functions (including):*
    ◦ Higher-level cognition
       ▪ Judge the situation accurately
       ▪ Use all sensory information to make a decision.
    ◦ Emotional
       ▪ Keep strong emotions in check to make a logical decision.

12. Judge for any possible objects moving into the path of travel.
- *Mental functions:* Attention
    ◦ Divided attention among maintaining a grip on the steering wheel, putting pressure on the brake pedal, and vision attention to scan the environment
    ◦ Selected attention to scan the environment for critical features
    ◦ Sustained attention to the task for making a decision.
- *Sensory functions (including):*
    ◦ Visual acuity, visual stability, and visual field.

Exhibit 6.1. Activity Analysis of a Right Turn (*cont.*)

- *Mental functions:* Higher-level cognition
  - Judge the situation accurately
  - Use all sensory information to make a decision.

13. Continue slow compression on the brake with right foot.

- *Neuromusculoskeletal and movement (including):*
  - Plantarflexion of the foot
  - Stability of the right leg and foot.

14. Judge the speed of the vehicle and the distance to the stop sign.

- *Mental functions (including):*
  - Attention
    - Divided attention among maintaining a grip on the steering wheel, putting pressure on the brake pedal, and keeping vision attention on the road
    - Selected attention to continue to watch for critical events in the environment
    - Sustained attention to the task of stopping.
  - Perception
    - Discriminate the speed of the car
    - Discriminate the distance to the stop sign.
  - Thought
    - Logically compare the speed of the car to the distance to determine needed pressure of the brake pedal.
  - Sequencing of complex movement
    - Make a final decision for action to stop the motor vehicle at the stop sign.

15. Move head to the left and right (same as #7).

16. Scan the environment (same as #8).

17. Perceive near and far, moving and nonmoving objects.

- *Sensory functions (including):*
  - Visual acuity, visual stability, and visual field.
- *Mental functions:* Higher-level cognition
  - Judge the situation accurately
  - Use all sensory information to make a decision.

18. Continue to judge for any possible objects moving into the path of travel.

- *Mental functions (including):*
  - Attention
    - Divided attention among maintaining a grip on the steering wheel, putting pressure on the brake pedal, and vision attention to scan the environment
    - Selected attention to scan the environment for critical features
    - Sustained attention to the task for making a decision.
  - Higher-level cognition
    - Judge the situation accurately
    - Use all sensory information to make a decision.
- *Sensory functions (including):*
  - Visual acuity, visual stability, and visual field.

Note. Required body structures and functions for the rest of the required actions for Steps 3 through 6 of the right-hand turn are essentially already covered and not repeated because of space.

19. Make judgment about the gap in traffic.

- *Sensory functions (including):*
  - Visual acuity, visual stability, and visual field.

(continued)

Exhibit 6.1. Activity Analysis of a Right Turn (*cont.*)

- *Mental functions (including):*
  - Attention
    - Divided attention among maintaining a grip on the steering wheel, holding pressure on the brake pedal, and vision attention to scan the environment
    - Selected attention to scan the environment for critical features
    - Sustained attention to the task for making a decision.
  - Perception
    - Discriminate all other vehicles, their speed, and their path of travel
    - Discriminate other objects including pedestrians in the crosswalks.
  - Thought
    - Recognition of the rules of stopping and starting at a stop sign.
  - Higher-level cognition
    - Judge the relationship of the vehicle to the stop sign and the intended path of travel
    - Form a concept of where other vehicles will travel in relation to own vehicle
    - Judge the accurate amount of space to move safely into the turn.
  - Sequencing of complex movement
    - Execute the learned movement patterns to move.

Did you know?

On the flash drive, there is a QuickTime movie of two driving processes: (1) the steps for a right-hand turn; and (2) the steps to pass another vehicle on a rural, two-lane road. It is an animation from the perspective of being inside the motor vehicle and then from a "bird's-eye view" of the maneuver. It is an activity analysis of the task of passing another motor vehicle on a rural road— in 2D, using animation to demonstrate the complexity of a task.

seconds. The key for the occupational therapist to recognize is that if the client has a significant deficit in any of the required body functions or structures, one must consider how it will affect the complex IADL of driving.

Driving consists of many maneuvers using motor, cognitive, visual, and perceptual performance skills. Completing an activity analysis on the complete driving process is a daunting task, comparable to building the Great Wall of China! However, we illustrate the process with an example of a right-hand turn at a stop sign. This example demonstrates the complex dynamics of driving for a relatively simple driving maneuver. The occupational therapist must understand the details of the driving process to articulate the strengths, areas of need, and potential goals of clients.

Conclusion

The purpose of this chapter was to illustrate the complexity of the driving task. Based on *Framework–II* (AOTA, 2008), each of its domain areas is identified directly for driving and community mobility. When driving is a valued occupation of the client, almost all performance skills, client factors, performance patterns, and environments and contexts are linked to mobility.

In examining the actual task of the right-hand turn at a stop sign through an activity analysis, readers should use the example to further extend the analysis for more complex maneuvers. Most importantly, consider this driving activity analysis while assessing or observing clients performing other IADLs. An occupational therapist who documents that a client is unsafe in the performance of cooking activities can report the client is likely unsafe driving independently and can recommend a comprehensive driving evaluation.

Accordingly, when documenting that the client is able to be independent in most tasks to live by himself or herself, the therapist may want to scrutinize highly complex tasks, especially considering processing speed and reaction time. Performing budgeting and cooking a meal with slower processing is acceptable and even preferable for independence, but in the driving environment, slower performance may put the client (or community) at risk.

Most people, including older adults, want the independence of being able to go where they wish in the community. However, this independence may not always be possible for the safety of the client or the community. Thus, because driving is an IADL within occupational therapy's domain, occupational therapists must consider and address this occupation directly as a part of their regular scope of practice.

References

American Occupational Therapy Association. (1994). Uniform terminology for occupational therapy (3rd ed.). *American Journal of Occupational Therapy, 48,* 1047–1054. doi:10.5014/ajot.48.11.1047

American Occupational Therapy Association. (2002). Occupational therapy practice framework: Domain and process. *American Journal of Occupational Therapy, 56,* 609–639. doi:10.5014/ajot.56.6.609

American Occupational Therapy Association. (2008). Occupational therapy practice framework: Domain and process (2nd ed.). *American Journal of Occupational Therapy, 62,* 625–683. doi:10.5014/ajot.62.6.625

Becker, W. (Director). (2007). *Wild hogs* [Motion picture]. United States: Touchstone Pictures.

Dellinger, A. M., Sehgal, M., Sleet, D. A., & Barrett-Connor, E. (2001). Driving cessation: What older former drivers tell us. *Journal of the American Geriatrics Society, 49,* 431–435.

Dickerson, A. E., Reistetter, T., & Gaudy, J. (in press). The perception of meaningfulness and performance of instrumental activities of daily living from the perspectives of the medically-at-risk older adult and their caregiver. *Journal of Applied Gerontology.*

Trilling, J. S. (2001). Selections from current literature: Assessment of older drivers. *Family Practice, 18,* 339–342.

CHAPTER 7

Cognition: A Vital Component to Driving and Community Mobility

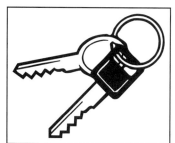

Peggy P. Barco, MS, BSW, OTR/L; Wendy B. Stav, PhD, OTR/L, SCDCM, FAOTA; Rosanna Arnold, MS, OTR/L; and David B. Carr, MD

Learning Objectives

At the completion of this chapter, readers will be able to

- Identify how cognitive deficits from a variety of medical conditions affect the complex instrumental activity of daily living of driving and community mobility;
- Recognize how the activity of driving and community mobility is affected by various components of cognition, including memory, attention, executive function, and visual perception; and
- Delineate the roles of cognition, insight, and functional level in clinician decision-making processes relating to driving recommendations and community mobility.

Introduction

Illnesses and diseases that occur in mid- to late life may cause functional decline and include impairment in cognitive abilities. Lidz (1987) defined *cognition* as the capacity to acquire and use information to learn and generalize. Cognition involves organizing, assimilating, and integrating new information with prior experiences and being able to apply this information to plan and structure behavior for goal attainment under conditions that may change (Baum & Katz, 2010).

Components of cognition commonly referred to in practice and in the literature are *attention, memory,* and *executive functioning.* Equally important and related to cognitive functioning are *processing speed* and *visual–perceptual abilities.* These domains of cognition and perception have been studied in relationship to driving ability, and impairments of varying levels in individuals have been shown to be related to driving safety concerns (Carr & Ott, 2010; Owsley & McGwin, 2010).

Key Words

- **alertness**
- **arousal**
- **attention**
- **awareness**
- **cognition**
- **executive function**
- **fatigue**
- **insight**
- **memory**
- **speed of processing**
- **visual perception**
- **visual processing**

The literature concerning cognition and driving has focused on various neuro-psychological, cognitive-based assessments, attempting to determine their relation to driving performance. Efforts also have been made to determine whether a single test or combination of cognitively based tests can predict driving safety. Several cognitive screening batteries have been explored to determine their relation to driving (De Raedt & Ponjaert-Kristofferson, 2001; Marottoli & Richardson, 1998; Staplin, Gish, & Wagner, 2003; Szlyk, Myers, Zhang, Wetzel, & Shapiro, 2002). Currently, cognitive tests appear to be most effective in identifying individuals *at risk* for unsafe driving and may be beneficial in establishing a need for additional evaluation in certain clinical situations (Anstey, Wood, Lord, & Walker, 2005; McKenna, Jefferies, Dobson, & Frude, 2004; Withaar, Brouwer, & Van Zomeran, 2000). However, there does not appear to be agreement about which areas of cognition should be tapped and what specific tests to adopt (Mathias & Lucas, 2009).

Further, a variability in findings is reported for the tests listed in this chapter when they are used in driving research. The myriad findings probably are related to studying different samples, deciding on different cutoff points or scoring methodology on tests, and having different outcome measures of driving safety. A recent meta-analysis (Mathias & Lucas, 2009) reviewed which standardized neuropsychological tests were able to best predict driving performance in community-dwelling older adults without dementia. The authors of this review concluded that a wide variety of cognitive tests was used to evaluate driving performance, and there was considerable variability in test prediction. That being said, the ability of clinicians to understand the role of cognitive skills in driving, and how cognition can change as the result of specific illnesses or diseases, is very important.

Medical Conditions Commonly Associated With Cognitive Deficits

When considering different medical conditions that can have symptoms of cognitive deficits, it is important to understand that each medical condition can affect individuals differently. Some medical conditions have an acute onset (e.g., traumatic brain injury [TBI]), while others are more slowly progressive (e.g., Parkinson's disease). Different patterns or types of cognitive deficits can show a different prevalence depending on the time course of the medical condition and the presence of comorbidities. Therefore, it is important to be familiar with myriad medical conditions and how cognition can be differentially affected. The following lists brief examples of the more common conditions that are associated with cognitive deficits.

It is important to be familiar with myriad medical conditions and how cognition can be differentially affected.

Traumatic Brain Injury

A *TBI* is an insult to the brain that is not the result of a degenerative or congenital nature and is caused by external force (Hsu, 2009). A TBI can result in a diminished state of consciousness, impaired motor skills, impaired cognitive functioning, and difficulties with emotional regulation. Different patterns of cognitive functioning can be observed in individuals, depending on the areas of the brain that are affected. The damage can be because of the primary mechanism, such as the point of contact of damage, as well as the diffuse axonal damage throughout the brain tissue due to acceleration–deceleration forces and rotational forces that affected the brain. Secondary mechanisms such as intracranial hemorrhages, brain swelling, and hypoxia can further reduce capacity (Boake, Francisco, Ivanhoe, & Kothart, 2000).

Cognitive impairment is the most common and disabling problem among survivors of head injury (Mayer & Badjatia, 2010). In a pilot study on visual exploration while driving following TBI, participants with TBI showed a reduction in visual exploration and difficulties in divided attention, anticipation, and planning (Milleville-Pennel, Pothier, Hoc, & Mathé, 2010).

Stroke

A *stroke* is a nontraumatic brain injury caused by occlusion or rupture of cerebral blood vessels that results in sudden neurological deficits characterized by loss of motor control, altered sensation, cognitive or language impairment, disequilibrium, or coma (Roth & Harvey, 2000). The location of the lesion, the extent of the injury, and the mechanism by which the vascular injury occurred play a role in recovery (Knesek, 2009). Symptoms include, but are not limited to, hemiplegia/paresis, aphasia, apraxia, dysarthria, visual–perceptual deficits, homonymous hemianopsia, sensory problems, cognitive deficits (impaired insight, judgment), psychosocial deficits, and incontinence (Knesek, 2009).

Legh-Smith, Wade, and Hewer (1986) noted that a significant number of community-dwelling stroke survivors continue driving (~42%). Yet in one study, the majority of stroke survivors (87%) did not receive any type of formal comprehensive driving evaluation but simply resumed the operation of a motor vehicle (Fisk, Owsley, & Pulley, 1997). The greater longevity after stroke suggests that health professionals will be faced with increasing numbers of survivors who continue to drive.

Preliminary studies on fitness-to-drive in stroke survivors note that those patients who fail on-road evaluations have scores that reflect impairment on measures of perception, cognition, and complex visual–perception or attention information (Engrum, Lambert, & Scott, 1990). Lundzvist, Gerdle, and Ronnberg (2000) found that evaluations requiring high-order cognitive functions such as mental control, working memory, and attention provided the best differentiation of driving skills in stroke survivors. Recently, a systematic review and meta-analysis in the literature noted that traffic sign recognition and the Compass Test from the Stroke Drivers Screening Assessment (Lincoln, Radford, & Nouri, 2004) and Trails B (Reitan, 1958) were predictive of impaired driving performance on an on-road evaluation (Devos et al., 2010).

Brain Tumor

Brain tumors can be malignant (progressive) or nonmalignant, and they can affect all age groups. The location of the tumor or lesion determines the resulting neurological deficits. For example, tumors in the frontal lobe can cause seizures, behavioral changes, dementia, gait disorders, hemiparesis, and expressive aphasia from the dominant hemisphere. Occipital lobe tumors are associated with hemianopsia and visual disturbances. Temporal lobe tumors can cause behavioral changes, language disturbance (dominant hemisphere), seizures, and visual-field deficits. Cerebellar tumors cause headache, ataxia, nystagmus, and neck pain (Deangelis & Rosenfeld, 2010).

Multiple Sclerosis

Multiple sclerosis (MS) is a progressive neurological condition characterized by patches of demyelination of nerves in areas of the brain and spinal cord (Beers & Berkow, 1999). The relapsing course of the disease varies with individuals. Symptoms can include the following (but all are not present in everyone with MS): muscle stiffness, tremulousness, paresthesias, numbness, partial or complete paralysis of extremities, visual deficits, fatigue, memory deficits, concentration difficulties, information-processing deficits, problem-solving deficits, visual–spatial deficits, articulation difficulties, emotional lability, and mood disturbance (Keller & Stone, 2009).

Recent findings (Schultheis et al., 2010) reveal an association with information processing and visuospatial skills and driving performance among patients with MS. Interestingly, a recent study (Marcotte et al., 2008) indicated that spasticity in addition to cognition appeared to negatively affect driving performance in patients with MS during a driving simulation study.

Parkinson's Disease

Parkinson's disease (PD) is a progressive neurodegenerative disease that affects motor function and sometimes cognitive function, which could potentially impair driving performance, thereby limiting mobility and independence (Wood, Worringham, Kerr, Mallon, & Silburn, 2005). PD presents with cardinal symptoms of bradykinesia, tremor, and rigidity, as well as difficulties with movement planning, subtle visual deficits, and impairments in shifting attention (Lieb et al., 1999; Wood et al., 2005).

Uc and colleagues (2009) demonstrated the presence of considerable variability among drivers with PD, with some performing normally, while Wood and colleagues (2005) found drivers with PD as a group to be less safe to drive than age-matched controls. Impairments in cognition—including attention (Uc et al., 2007, 2009), executive function, visual attention and visual perception (Stolwyk, Charlton, Triggs, Iansek, & Bradshaw, 2006; Uc et al., 2007), and visual-processing speed (Uc et al., 2009)—have been shown to be related to driving safety in PD.

Mental Illness

Cognitive impairment is recognized as a major symptom in schizophrenia (Penades et al., 2006). Cognitive impairments also are described in other mental health conditions, including depression (Kiosses, Klimstra, Murphy, & Alexopoulos, 2001), bipolar disorder (Martınez-Aran et al., 2004), obsessive–compulsive disorder (Boldrini et al., 2005), and substance abuse (Davies et al., 2005).

Dementia

According to the National Institute of Neurological Disorders and Stroke (NINDS; 2011), *dementia* is not a specific disease but a descriptive term for a collection of symptoms that can be caused by several disorders that affect the brain. Common symptoms of dementia include impairments in episodic memory (e.g., forgetting conversations, repetition, missing appointments, forgetting recent events or details), executive function (e.g., impaired function, attention, organizing, planning), language (e.g., dysnomia, aphasia), and visuospatial skills (e.g., staying in the lane, trouble getting in and out of a car). Physicians may use the Clinical Dementia Rating (CDR) for individuals with dementia to evaluate the presence or absence of dementia, rate the severity, and evaluate function; other health care professionals also may administer the CDR to document a client's status. (See Chapter 9 for more information on receiving free online training to administer the CDR.) A brief screen, the AD8 (Galvin, Roe, Xiong, & Morris, 2006), also can be used to determine the presence or absence of dementia.

Some individuals with mild dementia are able to continue to drive in the early course of the disease (Dobbs, 1997; Geldmacher & Whitehouse, 1996), with the recommendation that they be reevaluated as their condition progresses. Pooled data from two longitudinal studies indicated that 88% of drivers with very mild dementia and 69% of drivers with mild dementia were still able to pass a formal on-road evaluation. The median time to cessation of driving in very mild dementia was 2 years from the time of the evaluation; in mild dementia, it was 1 year (Duchek et al., 2003; Ott et al., 2008).

A meta-analysis of neuropsychological tests and driving performance–indicated tests of visuospatial skills were most relevant predictors of driving ability in older adults with dementia (Reger et al., 2004). Recent studies have indicated that tests of executive function and visual attention predict driving abilities in adults with early cognitive decline (Dawson, Anderson, Uc, Dastrup, & Rizzo, 2009; Ott et al., 2008; Whelihan, DiCarlo, & Paul, 2005). Carr and Ott (2010) reviewed predictive values for neuropsychological tests and found that they ranged from 66% to 81% accuracy in being able to correctly classify road test performance in individuals with Alzheimer's disease.

Medications

Many common medication classes have been studied and are associated with impaired driving skills. These include, but are not limited to, narcotics, benzodiazepines, antihistamines, antidepressants, antipsychotics, hypnotics, alcohol, antiepileptic agents, anti-emetic agents, and muscle relaxants (Carr, Schwartzberg, Manning, & Sempek, 2010). Wang and Carr (2004) noted that any drug that can depress the central nervous system (CNS) is associated with impairment in operating a motor vehicle. CNS side effects from drugs are myriad and may include sleepiness, fatigue, or sedation; lightheadedness, dizziness, or low blood pressure; blackouts or syncope; or impaired coordination.

However, it should be noted that many medication and driving studies are simply correlational in nature, and results may suggest an increased crash risk or impaired driving by a road test but not necessarily prove causation. Other factors may contribute to impaired driving, such as the disease that the medication is being used to treat or other comorbidities.

Cognition and Driving

Attention

Attention in its various forms is one of the most important and basic functions of the human brain and constitutes the basis for other cognitive processes (Gillen, 2009).

Attention is an essential part of information processing. Attention is related to many other cognitive functions. For instance, when a person attends to competing stimuli or any aspect of the environment, he or she is using judgment to determine which specific stimulus is most important. By attending only to specific inputs, the brain can decide which information is important and should be rehearsed and stored in long-term memory (Lou & Lane, 2005). Obviously, if stimuli are never attended to, then they are likely not to be remembered.

There are several classifications of types of attention, many of which are considered highly important in the driving literature:

- *Selective attention:* The process of deciding which aspects of the environment to attend to is known as *selectivity*. Selectivity allows people to focus on only the important aspects and ignore the rest. *Distractibility* is therefore a breakdown in selective attention and results in an inability to select key stimuli over other less-relevant information in order to concentrate on a task.
- *Sustained attention:* The ability to have the capacity to maintain attention for an extended period of time is known as *sustained attention*.
- *Alternating attention:* The ability to have flexibility by transitioning effectively between different stimuli is known as *alternating attention*.
- *Divided attention:* The ability to attend to two or more tasks (or stimuli) simultaneously is known as *divided attention*.
- *Neglect:* A *neglect* is the failure of an individual to report, respond, or orient to novel or meaningful stimuli on the side opposite a brain lesion—when the failure cannot be because of sensory or motor deficits (Heilman, Watson, & Valenstein, 2003). It has been conceptualized as a *lateralized attention deficit* (Gillen, 2009).

Understanding the role of attention in driving and community mobility is vital to being able to make safe recommendations. While driving, a person must use most, if not all, of the types of attention described earlier. The abundance of tasks necessary to concentrate on while driving is extensive. A very dangerous situation can occur when an individual is driving who has difficulty switching attention sets as he or she tries to make one decision at a time instead of "multitasking." This can result in the individual literally stopping the car unsafely in mid-traffic while trying to make a decision (e.g., where to turn) and impeding the flow of traffic. Consistently, researchers found that low scores on measures of attention were correlated with crash risk (Anstey et al., 2005).

A visual inattention or neglect (of either the right or left side; most often on the left) can be very detrimental in a driving situation. Visual inattention or neglect is distinguished from a visual field defect. A visual neglect usually coexists with significantly impaired insight, resulting in the individual being less able and less willing to compensate for it through typical strategies addressed in therapy.

For an individual with a significant visual neglect, driving usually is contraindicated (Akinwuntan, Feys, Baten, Arno, & Kiekens, 2006) because the individual is at a very high risk of not attending to the neglected side. This can result in inadequate lane positioning; not attending to pedestrians, signs, or vehicles on the affected side; or having a slower response time because of the lack of visual attention on the affected side (Coeckelbergh, Cornelissen, Brouwer, & Kooijman, 2002). Individuals with only peripheral visual field defects usually have a more preserved sense of awareness of the deficit and, thus, have more potential to compensate.

Attention impairments are common in many neurological illnesses (both traumatic and nontraumatic) and include, but are not limited to, TBI, MS, and stroke (Dujardin, Donze, & Hautecoeur, 1998; Robertson, Ridgeway, Greenfield, & Parr, 1997). People who experience a stroke or TBI often complain that they cannot finish a task that they have started or cannot fully focus on a task or situation (Zoltan, 2007). Fisk, Owsley, and Mennemeier (2002) found that those patients who had had a stroke demonstrated a higher attentional impairment than those who had not. They also found that stroke survivors scored higher on the Useful Field of View test, which indicates poorer performance. Some medications can cause CNS depression and impaired attention, including but not limited to narcotics, anxiolytics, antidepressants, antihistamines, and muscle relaxants (Lococo & Tyree, 2010).

The National Highway Traffic Safety Administration (NHTSA) databases have analyzed and researched the role of "driver distraction" in crashes for many years, with an increased focus on the dangers of cell phone use and texting while driving (Neale, 2005; NHTSA, 2009a; Ranney, 2008; Wang, Knipling, & Goodman, 1996). Many states have passed or are in the midst of legislating against the use of handheld cell phones and texting while driving. The term *distracted driving* is used by NHTSA and other stakeholders to describe the state of the driver when his or her attention is not focused on driving; NHTSA has investigated specific causes of crashes related to the visual and mental distractions that often precede crashes.

Table 7.1 provides a list of common causes of crashes and distracted behaviors often seen while driving. It is critical that clients with cognitive impairments fully understand the important role of visual and mental attention when driving. Therapists should instruct them in avoiding all these behaviors to attend to driving.

The results of this NHTSA research provide occupational therapists with a wealth of details to incorporate into patient education and programming regarding the need to attend to driving, to avoid distractions, and to develop skills to avoid distracted driving. For instance, a client with memory impairments who cannot freely recall where the windshield wiper controls are located will be placed in a dangerous situation behind the wheel if he or she must visually search for the controls while driving. Although a client may have the motor ability to control a vehicle, the importance of compensating for even mild cognitive impairments must not be overlooked. Table 7.2 offers examples of driving and community mobility activities adversely affected by cognitive impairment.

Memory

Memory is known to support independence and participation in daily life activities, including driving. There are varying types of memory and memory loss that result from disease or injury; different diseases or injuries are more susceptible to one type of memory loss over another. By understanding some of the more common types of

Table 7.1. Factors Related to Driver Distraction

Factor	Examples or Definitions
Emotional (e.g., depressed, angry, disturbed)	Fighting, disagreements, depression, emotional upset
Looking but not seeing	Paying attention but not seeing relevant vehicle or object (blind spot, intersection)
Distracted by other occupant	Includes conversing with or looking at other occupant
Talking or listening to cell phone	Multitasking by driving and using phone
Using cell phone or PDA	Reaching for phone or PDA, accessing voicemail, inputting data for dialing, texting
Adjusting climate controls	Air conditioning or heating controls
Adjusting or controlling equipment; inserting or retrieving equipment	Adjusting equipment such as radio, CD, or mp3 player
Using other devices or controls in vehicle	Adjusting window, door locks, rearview mirror, seat, steering wheel, seat belt, etc.
Using or reaching for other equipment brought into vehicle	Radar detector, razor, CD or portable CD player, headphones, cigarette lighter, etc.
Distracted by outside person, object, or event	Animals on roadside or previous crash
Eating or drinking	Food or drink related
Smoking	Any activity related to smoking
Inattentive or lost in thought	Daydreaming, talking to self, or singing
Taking care of personal hygiene	Combing or fixing hair, applying makeup, shaving, or performing any other personal hygiene activity
Reading	Book, magazine, computer, or other
Insect in vehicle	Startled by or swatting at insect

Note. Adapted from NHTSA (2009a).

memory, one can discern which ones have a more active role in affecting the ability to drive safely and independently. The more common terms when referring to memory impairments are as follows:

- *Short-term memory:* Involves storage of a limited amount of verbal or nonverbal material for a limited time. Short-term memory should not be confused with long-term or working memory. The average capacity of short-term memory has been defined as the storage of 7 items (± 2) for a limited time (Miller, 1965) and can be thought of as immediately repeating a 7-digit phone number after being told it.
- *Working memory:* Related to short-term memory, but includes the active manipulation of the information that is currently in short-term storage (e.g., doing a calculation with stored numbers).
- *Long-term memory:* Memory that has been encoded into relatively permanent storage.

Table 7.2. Examples of Attention Deficits in Driving and Community Mobility

Type of Attention Difficulty	Example of Affected Driving Behaviors	Example of Influence on Alternative Forms of Community Mobility
Selective attention	*Visual:* Difficulty selectively attending to a road sign while ignoring other distracters in the environment	*Visual:* Difficulty selectively attending to the correct schedule on a complicated bus route and ignoring distracting information on the page
	Auditory: Difficulty selectively attending to a siren coming from behind while ignoring the music on the radio	
Sustained attention	Difficulty sustaining attention for a prolonged period of time while driving on the highway	Difficulty sustaining attention to wait for a bus or cab without becoming too fatigued or falling asleep; not alert to current location and upcoming stop with appropriate readiness and follow-through to get off
Alternating attention	Difficulty preparing for a lane change when alternating attention from glancing back and forth while looking in the side mirror and back to monitoring traffic conditions in the front of the car	Difficulty alternating attention while on a bus from looking at other people and then back to monitoring what bus stop is currently coming up next
Divided attention	Difficulty maintaining safe control of the car while holding a conversation with a passenger at the same time	Difficulty safely walking in a crosswalk while simultaneously attending to people, dogs, uneven terrain or curbs, and traffic
	Difficulty maintaining safe control of the car while simultaneously attending to weather, road, and traffic conditions	
Neglect	Inaccurate lane positioning by not attending to the (affected) side of the road completely	A left neglect might cause an individual to bump into things on his or her left side
	Lack of attending to a vehicle or pedestrian on the affected side while driving	A left neglect may result in missing the left side of a bus schedule while reading it

- *Episodic memory:* Form of long-term memory for personally experienced events or episodes.
- *Semantic memory:* Form of long-term memory that is considered our "knowledge base" and can include learned facts, vocabulary, and general knowledge accumulated throughout our lives.
- *Procedural memory:* Also known as *implicit memory,* procedural memory is expressed in the form of actual performance of an activity (without the conscious retrieval of this memory from being learned in the past).

- *Prospective memory:* Known as a critical aspect of memory to support everyday living (Gillen, 2009), prospective memory is remembering to remember—it is remembering to follow through with an intention at some planned time in the future.

All types of memory are used at some point during the driving task. Some types are more related to safety issues with driving and community mobility than others. Driving, by its own accord, is visually based and therefore relies heavily on visual memory. If drivers get lost and need to turn around or retrace a route, they must hold in their visual working memory the mental image of their previous route, and they may be able to manipulate this image to return to the original destination.

Driving is usually a well-learned skill for many adults, which taps into procedural memory. It can be compared to riding a bike. You get on the bike and immediately know where to put your feet, how to balance the bike, and how to pedal. Similarly in driving, you know how to put the key in the ignition, what pedal to put your foot on for acceleration and braking, and generally how to change gears. Again, in many injuries (e.g., TBIs, brain tumors, many types of strokes) this form of procedural memory is preserved. However, diseases with dementia (e.g., Alzheimer's disease) can result in a loss of common procedural memories, especially as the dementia progresses in severity. When this happens, the individual may struggle with how to turn the key to start the car, may become confused over the procedure of which pedal to apply pressure for the brake versus the gas, or may forget how to put the car in reverse.

Semantic memory loss and procedural memory loss related to driving can be some of the most worrisome concerns in regard to safety.

Diseases and injuries can result in vastly different types of memory impairments. Semantic memory loss and procedural memory loss related to driving can be some of the most worrisome concerns in regard to safety. These are more common in Alzheimer's disease, especially as the condition advances. Other neurological disorders (e.g., TBI, stroke, brain tumors) result in more short-term and immediate memory loss and can be compensated for in many ways, assuming the individual has the insight and level of functioning in other areas to do so. Examples of how memory impairment may interfere with driving behaviors and safe community mobility are described in Table 7.3.

Executive Function

Executive function is an umbrella term that refers to complex cognitive processing requiring the coordination of several subprocesses to achieve a particular goal (Elliot, 2003). Executive functions act as a supervisor of other cognitive processes (e.g., attention, memory). In the literature, it has not been consistently agreed upon as to which processes are considered "executive" in nature. However, initiative; problem solving and judgment; decision making; impulsivity; flexibility in thinking or generation of alternatives; and planning, organizing, and sequencing complex actions are commonly referred to when discussing executive functions.

Executive functions provide control over information processing and are a key determinant of driver strategies, tactics, and safety (Rizzo & Kellison, 2010). Many cognitive assessments that have been shown to have some value in predicting

Table 7.3. Examples of Memory Deficits in Driving and Community Mobility

Type of Memory Difficulty	Example of Affected Driving Behaviors	Example of Influence on Alternative Forms of Community Mobility
Short-term memory	Difficulty immediately remembering directions offered by a good Samaritan responding to the driver's question asking for directions to where he or she was going	Difficulty scheduling alternative transportation on the phone or at a transit station by forgetting what the schedule (series of stops or transfers) was that was just arranged Leaving possessions on a bus or in a cab
Working memory	Difficulty mentally altering directions in some manner (e.g., due to road construction, reversing directions to return home); to do this, the individual needs to hold the original directions in mind while imposing the alteration	Difficulty scheduling alternative transportation through a bus or cab (e.g., retaining the time and location of where he or she needs to go while mentally processing the various options available through bus schedules and cab arrangements)
Episodic memory	Difficulty remembering where he or she parked the car after going grocery shopping Difficulty remembering how to go to a familiar location (e.g., grocery store) Difficulty remembering what type or year of car the individual owns or if he or she has had any recent accidents	Difficulty remembering the directions to a familiar location to tell the cab or bus driver where he or she would like to go
Semantic memory	Difficulty remembering what common traffic signs mean (e.g., yield sign, stop sign, railroad crossing) Difficulty remembering "rules of the road" (e.g., what to do when a siren comes up from behind, whether one can make a right on a red light in his or her town)	Difficulty remembering how to use the yellow pages in a phone book to look up phone numbers to schedule transportation (e.g., with a cab company)
Procedural memory	Difficulty remembering how procedurally to turn the key to start a car, to put the car in gear, or to apply pressure to the correct pedal to stop or start the car	Difficulty remembering the procedure of how to pedal a bike
Prospective memory	Difficulty remembering to follow through with the "intention" of putting gas in the car or doing routine car maintenance	Difficulty remembering to follow through with the "intention" of scheduling transportation or bringing money to pay for a cab

driving abilities are geared toward executive function (Anstey et al., 2005). Executive function skills are most challenged in novel situations. When one is driving or using alternative transportation, certain situations involving executive function skills are more obvious than others (see Table 7.4).

Decision making is part of executive functioning. Impaired decision-making abilities have been suggested to be a main factor resulting in vehicular crashes (Van Zomeran, Brouwer, & Minderhoud, 1987). Both neurological and non-neurological conditions can affect executive functioning. Neurological conditions that affect executive functioning include TBIs, strokes, and neurodegenerative impairments that result in damage to the prefrontal areas of the brain. People who have these conditions may have changes in their abilities to logically problem solve through challenging, novel situations of daily life. They also may not be able to benefit from feedback to control their behaviors.

Deficits in executive functioning have been identified in people who have PD and dementia and have been related to driving safety (Dobbs, 2005). Frontal-lobe damage (e.g., due to trauma, stroke), antisocial personality disorder, effects of drugs and alcohol, and fatigue also have been shown to be correlated with impaired decision-making skills (Bechara, Tranel, Damasio, & Damasio, 1996; Jones & Harrison, 2001; Rolls, Hornak, Wade, & McGrath, 1994; Stuss, Gow, & Hetherington, 1992).

Visual Perception and Processing

Visual perception is the process of obtaining and interpreting the visual information of the surrounding environment (Kohlmeyer, 2003). Zoltan (2007) discussed three steps involved in visual processing. The first, *input or reception,* uses the ocular motor skills to input the various visual stimuli from the environment. Next, this input is organized during the *perception* or *integration* step to understand the environment, integrate the information, and prepare a response. Finally, during the motor *output* or *behavior* step, the individual uses functional mobility and hand–eye coordination to react to the visual stimuli.

Visual perception skills include, but are not limited to, the following:

- *Depth perception:* The processes of the visual system that interpret depth and create an accurate understanding of the perception. Accurate depth perception is based on having binocular vision. Because the eyes see an image from two slightly different angles, the visual system must "interpret" the information to make judgments regarding depth and distance.
- *Spatial relations:* The ability to process and accurately interpret information about the location of objects relative to each other and to the individual.
- *Right–left discrimination:* The ability to accurately understand and interpret the directions of right and left.
- *Topographical orientation:* The ability to accurately be oriented to space and be able to negotiate surroundings without becoming lost.
- *Figure–ground discrimination:* The ability to distinguish objects in the foreground from objects in the background.

Table 7.4. Examples of Executive Function Deficits in Driving and Community Mobility

Type of Executive Function Difficulty	Example of Affected Driving Behaviors	Example of Impact on Alternative Forms of Community Mobility
Initiation	Difficulty initiating moving the foot to the gas at the appropriate speed when a traffic light turns from red to green	Difficulty initiating a phone call to begin the scheduling process for alternative transportation or initiating a call for follow-up when there is a breakdown in plans
Problem solving and decision making	Difficulty problem solving how to get out of a parking lot or garage

Difficulty problem solving what to do when the route changes because of unexpected road construction

Difficulty problem solving what to do when sirens come from behind | Difficulty deciding what cab company to use

Difficulty problem solving which family member might be best to call

Difficulty deciding the time or schedule of when one wants to go somewhere so that he or she arrives at the appointment on time |
| **Planning, sequencing, and anticipating** | Difficulty anticipating that another vehicle may turn in front of him or her

Difficulty planning for a lane change and not waiting until the last minute

Difficulty anticipating the need to brake as other traffic ahead is slowing down or stopped

Difficulty problem solving car maintenance or breakdown issues | Difficulty planning and scheduling when alternative transportation is needed; time management issues overwhelm the planning efforts

Difficulty planning appointments in advance by anticipating future needs |
| **Flexibility in thinking and generation of alternatives** | Difficulty thinking of route options if a road is unexpectedly closed or a detour occurs

Difficulty considering options of what to do if the car breaks down in traffic or where to get gas if outside of the ordinary route | If one form of alternative transportation does not work, difficulty thinking of what other options might be available |
| **Impulsivity** | Impulsively turning out into traffic without looking

Impulsively making a lane change without checking for other vehicles | Impulsively leaving the house to go somewhere without logically thinking through safety issues (e.g., walking safety, knowing the bus schedule) or planning needs (e.g., having money) |

Visuospatial impairment has been associated with a significant increase in falls, decreased functional performance in activities of daily living (ADLs), and decreased mobility (Nys et al., 2007; Olsson, Wambold, Brock, Waugh, & Sprague, 2005). Equally important, visual perception and processing skills are extremely important to safe driving and community mobility practices (see Table 7.5). Researchers have found that visual–perceptual tests showed moderate to high associations with driving outcome measures (De Raedt & Ponjaert-Kristofferson [2001] as cited in Anstey et al., 2005). Baker (2006) discusses the need for visual perception and processing skills to read road signs and recognize pedestrians and other vehicles. Visual–perceptual and spatial relation skills also are needed to accurately perceive objects viewed from side and rearview mirrors. Depth perception and spatial relation skills are crucial for judging the distance from and speed of other vehicles.

Visuospatial impairments have been reported to be one of the more common deficits that can occur as the result of a stroke, with a prevalence as high as 38% (Pearce, 2005). Gershkoff and Finestone (2009) found that in people who have had a

Table 7.5. Examples of Visual–Perceptual or Processing Deficits in Driving and Community Mobility

Type of Visual Perception or Processing Difficulty	Example of Affected Driving Behaviors	Example of Impact on Alternative Forms of Community Mobility
Depth perception or spatial relations	Difficulty accurately judging or perceiving gap distance when making a lane change	Difficulty walking to a location because the individual may not accurately perceive the depth of curbs or steps
	Difficulty perceiving travel distance between cars or necessary stopping distance	Difficulty accurately perceiving the distance between oneself and traffic when in a crosswalk
	Difficulty perceiving the position of the car in a parking space, resulting in ineffective parking	
Right–left discrimination	Difficulty discriminating right and left in following directions to a location	Difficulty finding a location or describing directions to others because of confusion with right and left turns
Topographical orientation	Difficulty in finding way to and from a location, and he or she may get lost	Confusion or disorientation in both familiar and unfamiliar environments
	Can become disoriented or confused in even a common parking lot or when driving a familiar route	Could easily get lost while walking or become disoriented while using public transportation
Figure–ground discrimination	Difficulty in ability to accurately perceive objects in the environment (pedestrians, vehicles) from the background, especially if similar in color; for example, a person standing at a corner in a gray suit in front of a gray-tone car	Difficulty in ability to safely perceive objects in the environment while walking (e.g., not tripping on a large white rock on a white pavement)

stroke, their performance on a spatial relations task was the most important variable in determining whether they were able to drive safely. Fisk and colleagues (2002) noted that, generally, patients with right-hemisphere strokes perform poorer on performance measures and driving tasks because of the visuospatial impairments that are associated with right-hemisphere damage. Fisk and colleagues (2002) found that stroke survivors reported difficulty when driving alone, parallel parking, driving in heavy traffic, and driving on busy highways. Visual–spatial deficits also have been identified in PD, TBI, and MS (Marinus et al., 2003; McKenna, Cooke, Fleming, Jefferson, & Ogden, 2006; Piras et al., 2003).

Speed of Processing

Speed of processing refers to the speed at which new information can be integrated and retrieved from the memory (Levy, 2005). Working memory is heavily dependent on the speed of processing (Levy, 2005). If an individual has slow reaction time at which information can be processed through working memory, he or she will have difficulty storing that information properly, making it more difficult to retrieve it at a later time.

Speed of processing also influences the rate at which an individual can produce a motor or verbal response to a given stimulus (Bryer, Rapport, & Hanks, 2006). When processing speed is slowed, cumulative delays of street sign recognition, interpretation of the sign's meaning, and initiating the appropriate and desired motor response (e.g., to stop the vehicle) may explain why a known and desired response may in actuality occur too late for safe operation of the vehicle.

When one is driving, visual-processing speed is imperative to be able to process the environmental stimuli and react to unexpected hazards very quickly to remain safe. Numerous studies have examined visual attention and visual processing, finding that they strongly influence the driving performance of older adults (Ball, Owsley, Sloane, Roenker, & Bruni, 1993; Cross et al., 2009; Goode et al., 1998; Owsley et al., 1998). Edwards and colleagues (2009) also found that individuals within their study who had a slowed speed of processing and did not receive speed-of-processing training experienced a more severe decline in driving mobility than those without a delayed processing speed and those with delayed speed of processing who did receive the training. McKnight and McKnight (2000) found a correlation between reaction time (simple and complex) and on-road driving performance.

Typically, a general slowing of the speed of processing occurs with advancing age. Over time, the neurons lose their dendritic branches, which may slow the rate at which information can be communicated (Levy, 2005). This slowed processing speed can be seen in individuals who demonstrate decreased reaction time, dexterity, coordination, and gait speed (Warshawsky-Livne & Shinar, 2002). As previously stated, a delayed speed of processing can affect how someone retrieves information because it may not have been stored appropriately. People who have impaired attention (as in an acquired brain injury) have been known to exhibit delayed processing speed (Bryer et al., 2006).

Alertness, Arousal, and Fatigue

In general, a decreased alertness and arousal level leads to longer reaction times, memory problems, coordination problems, and impaired information processing (Lyznicki, Doege, Davis, & Williams, 1998). An individual's level of alertness and arousal is associated with his or her amount of sleep, internal body clock, time spent on a certain task (especially monotonous tasks), and individual characteristics such as medical conditions (European Road Safety Observatory, 2007). A decreased level of alertness and arousal is generally associated with an increased level of fatigue.

In general, fatigue has been found to affect task performance and result in a loss of task-directed effort (Lyznicki et al., 1998). Although there are various causes for fatigue, the effects are generally the same and include a decreased mental and physical performance capacity (European Road Safety Observatory, 2007).

Sleep apnea is associated with attention and concentration difficulties and increased daytime sleepiness because of hypoxemia and disturbed nocturnal sleep (Dobbs, 2005). In a review of the literature, it was found that there is an increased risk of vehicle crashes in people with sleep apnea. Some drivers minimize their fatigue (either intentionally or by unawareness; Stutts, Wilkins, & Vaughn, 1999) and thereby may fail to recognize when they begin to have difficulties driving because of their sleepiness. Attention, perception, memory, and executive functions that have been determined to be important to driving safety are affected by fatigue and drugs and can result in crashes (Lyznicki et al., 1998).

Medical conditions such as Alzheimer's disease (AD), PD, and MS are known to have symptoms of fatigue or daytime sleepiness associated with them. In a study by Chipchase, Lincoln, and Radford (2003), people with MS reported more fatigue than those without MS. Researchers also found that the drivers with MS admitted to causing significantly more traffic accidents and traffic offenses than the drivers without MS (Knecht, 1977). In Chipchase and colleagues' (2003) study, participants with MS reported that their fatigue affected how they drove, when they drove, and their driving ability.

Excessive daytime sleepiness (with increased wakefulness during the night) is common in AD (Bonanni et al., 2005). Daytime sleepiness or sleep attacks also have been identified in PD (partially because of medication side effects; Hobson et al., 2002; Ondo et al., 2001; Rizzo & Kellison, 2010). This lack of sleep can result in driving safety concerns, as indicated by the finding by Ondo and colleagues (2001) that 22.6% of people with PD sampled who were current drivers reported to have fallen asleep while driving.

Medications can play a big role in arousal while driving. Countless medication bottles have a warning that educates patients that the medication may cause drowsiness (Tyree, 2006). The sedation side effect can greatly influence a person's ability to drive. However, there are a few medications used to treat CNS disorders that act as stimulants and can cause the individual to become overstimulated (Tyree, 2006). It should be noted that many medications allow clients to function (e.g., Sinement for PD, anti-inflammatory medication for arthritis), and they could not perform their ADLs without pharmaceutical intervention. Specific warnings, such as not to drive while on certain medications, need to be monitored carefully.

Insight and Awareness

Insight is the awareness someone has of his or her own physical or mental limitations. Clients with awareness deficits may demonstrate explicit verbal denial of their situation, underestimate the severity of their deficits or disabilities, or fail to make appropriate behavioral accommodations to their situation. Awareness of one's cognitive difficulties is not an all-or-none phenomenon; awareness can be present in varying degrees or levels (Barco, Crosson, Bolesta, Werts, & Stout, 1991; Crosson et al., 1989).

The ability that an individual has to compensate for cognitive deficits is in part dependent on how much awareness that he or she has of the deficits (Barco et al., 1991). Individuals who lack awareness of the consequences of their deficits see little need to compensate for them (as they are unaware of a problem to compensate for) and also are not motivated to use or follow through with strategies introduced to them in a therapy environment. These individuals commonly overestimate their abilities and, when not successful, cannot connect the difficulties with their cognitive changes.

Anstey and colleagues (2005) found that individuals who demonstrate a decreased level of insight may be at higher risk for impaired driving performance and motor vehicle crashes. Researchers also have found that older drivers who have decreased cognitive functioning and do not have an appropriate level of insight may not voluntarily limit or change their driving habits (Carr, Duchek, Meuser, & Morris, 2006). Such individuals (without insight into their limitations) may continue to drive when they are in fact very unsafe to do so.

Many neurological diseases can impair an individual's ability to have insight into the deficits related to the disease process. The more common ones are TBI, stroke (especially with right-hemisphere involvement), and dementia. A lack of awareness has been related to damage to frontal lobe regions and connecting pathways, particularly right-hemisphere involvement (Stuss & Anderson, 2004). In individuals who have survived a stroke, unawareness of cognitive deficits is more prevalent than unawareness of motor deficits resulting from the stroke, with lack of awareness being as high as 42% at discharge (Hartman-Maeir, Soroker, Ring, & Katz, 2002).

Reports have indicated that 30% to 55% of individuals with TBI continue to have awareness deficits for years after their injury (Noe et al., 2005; Prigatano & Altman, 1990). PD also has presented concerns with self-awareness. Individuals with PD have rated themselves as less impaired than corresponding caregiver ratings on ADL functioning (Leritz, Loftis, Crucian, Friedman, & Bowers, 2004). Individuals with dementia may lack insight and not be responsible for driving with limitations they do not recognize (Berger, Rosner, Kark, Bennett, & Medical Society of the State of New York, 2000).

> **Older drivers who have decreased cognitive functioning and do not have an appropriate level of insight may not voluntarily limit or change their driving habits.**

Which Clients With Cognitive Deficits Are Appropriate for Referral for a Comprehensive Driving Evaluation?

Many clinicians and physicians struggle with the issue of when to refer for a comprehensive driving evaluation. Clinicians do not want to "betray" their clients by making a referral or suggesting that driving capability may be in question unless they are certain. Client needs, client safety, public safety, and potential for improvement should be the only considerations for a referral.

Unfortunately, no clear, consistent evidence provides guidance as to *when* a comprehensive driving evaluation and intervention are indicated with individuals affected by cognitive deficits. Each individual's cognitive difficulties, recovery patterns, and prognosis are unique. In addition, it is uncommon for an individual who has a cognitive deficit to have just one area of deficit. Typically, clients with cognitive concerns have issues in several areas of cognitive domain, each to varying degrees.

Thus, the decision of referral is often left to the health care provider or family and is based on clinical reasoning through analysis of the nature of the condition, current health, functional status, insight status, prognosis of the condition, recovery to date, and input from the family and significant others. These are considerations that are commonly taken into account when making the decision of whether or when to refer for a driving assessment.

The advantage of having all occupational therapists address driving and community mobility issues, as a typical part of the assessment of instrumental activities of daily living (IADLs), would greatly benefit society. A referral for an occupational therapy evaluation should include questions about the habits, routines, and goals a client has related to driving and community mobility; when therapists identify cognitive impairments, the client and family should be instructed in how this may interfere with safety in the community. "The conversation" about driving safety, driving cessation, and alternative modes of transportation to support continued participation in community affairs should be a service that occupational therapists offer to all members of society, whenever it is needed. Generalists, then, will face the challenge of deciding when or if a referral for a behind-the-wheel assessment is indicated.

Nature, Duration, and Prognosis Related to Cognitive Impairment

The stability of the client's medical condition is a foundational factor to consider when analyzing his or her potential for safe driving. Before referral for a comprehensive driving evaluation, an individual's medical condition should be stable. The occupational therapist is concerned with the nature of the cognitive deficit, how long this individual has been experiencing cognitive deficits, and the prognosis for improvement. For example, if an individual has unstable seizures, diabetes, or an unstable heart condition, health care providers should not consider a comprehensive driving evaluation until the condition stabilizes. Some states have regulations regarding certain conditions (e.g., waiting time after a seizure before resuming driving), which should be followed.

Individuals with chronic conditions who have experienced cognitive deficits for nearly their entire lives (e.g., developmental disabilities such as cerebral palsy, Asperger's syndrome, or attention deficit disorder) often need to address driving and community mobility at the beginning of the spectrum in terms of learning the skills and safe practices (Monahan, 2009; Monahan & Patten, 2009). Many of these individuals have never independently driven, ridden a bicycle, taken a bus, or crossed a street; consequently, intervention focuses on teaching novice skills. If it is determined that these individuals have the potential to drive, take the bus, ride a bicycle, or use other transportation, they likely will need extensive training time beyond the intensity and time a typical learner would need. Families should be informed of these extended timelines and the associated costs upfront to maintain ethical practices.

Acute Neurological Conditions

Drivers who have an acute onset of a neurological condition (e.g., stroke, TBI) are usually very eager to resume driving. Resuming driving too soon, however, can have disastrous results for the individual and the community. Because there is the potential for recovery from these acute-onset conditions, individuals should complete sufficient therapy to address the deficits and improve deficient skills. Stating a firm time period is not advisable, as each individual's recovery period and pattern are unique and depend on his or her premorbid health status and the location and severity of the neurological trauma.

Comprehensive driving evaluations are costly in time, emotional investment, and fee. Insurance reimbursement for comprehensive driving evaluation and related services is inconsistent. Considering all of the factors, it is generally advisable to wait until the individual has the highest chance of success in passing the comprehensive driving evaluation to avoid having to repeat it or experiencing a result of over-restriction when heeding results of an evaluation conducted too soon. Workers' compensation insurance and vocational rehabilitation are key resources for treatment, as transportation is directly related to the ability to work. Occupational therapists communicate carefully with the team, including case managers, to determine the best time for a comprehensive driving evaluation based on the timing of the individual's recovery and the potential for success.

Progressive Neurological Diseases

Individuals with progressive diseases with cognitive deficits (e.g., AD, PD, MS) have a different situation when considering referral for a comprehensive driving evaluation than those with an acute condition. Many of these individuals may have continued driving with their condition and face decisions about fitness-to-drive and the possibility of driving cessation as their disease progresses. Clinicians, patients, and families should remain vigilant of a deterioration of driving skills, and a comprehensive driving evaluation should be considered once the decline in performance is observed.

If the individual passes the comprehensive driving evaluation, a recommendation to continue driving is considered "temporary" because of the progressive nature of the medical condition, and it is appropriate to have an updated driving assessment (to include the on-road evaluation) in 6 months or if the medical or functional condition shows evidence of decline. Because these conditions are progressive, interventions to improve skills are not effective and driving rehabilitation services largely focus on determining fitness-to-drive and offering suggestions to modify the driving context to remain safe. Aside from a comprehensive driving evaluation to determine driving cessation, signs of obvious concerns include involvement in a crash, near crashes observed by family members or friends, traffic violations, or excessive scrapes and dents on the car (Carr et al., 2006).

Insight and the Effective Use of Compensatory Strategies

As mentioned earlier in this chapter, it is very common in individuals with certain medical conditions (e.g., stroke, TBI, dementia) to have cognitive deficits, which can result in a lack of insight into their cognitive deficits and implications of their cognitive deficits in their daily life. This issue, of course, poses a serious obstacle along the course of recovery. If the medical condition is not progressive, the generalist should attempt interventions to improve insight, ideally before the comprehensive driving assessment. Improved insight leads to improved use and willingness to use compensatory strategies. However, individuals who cannot gain insight into their cognitive deficits are not as likely to benefit from training in compensatory strategies (because they do not see why they need to use them). In such cases, individuals depend on others to compensate for them or environmental modification (Barco et al., 1991).

Subsequently, the occupational therapist needs to ask, "What is the client's insight into his or her cognitive deficits?" and "Has the client been able to effectively use compensatory strategies to compensate for the deficits?" The next question then becomes, "How does this affect a referral for a comprehensive driving evaluation?"

Following, individuals who lack awareness of their cognitive deficits are more apt to be noncompliant with a medical recommendation to not drive because they do not believe they have any cognitive deficits that should interfere with their driving abilities (Carr et al., 2006). Subsequently, because of their lack of awareness of the cognitive deficits, they are not aware of potential safety implications that could result from these deficits. In such cases, the involvement of a family member, significant other, or caregiver and a referral for a comprehensive driving evaluation may be indicated; a referral to the state Department of Motor Vehicles (DMV) also may be indicated to provide evidence of safety concerns that may increase compliance with physician recommendations. Lack of awareness or insight will be discussed later in this chapter in terms of how it impedes intervention success related to driving performance.

Occupational therapists may need to explore the issue of competency of individuals who severely lack insight into their deficits with the primary physician and how it impacts major life decisions and choices. In cases where decision-making capacity is questionable or obviously impaired, it would be imperative to include a family member (e.g., spouse or adult child) when it comes to understanding or enforcing recommendations related to driving.

Client Management of ADLs and IADLs at Home

Knowing what types of activities the client can do independently and what activities the client needs assistance supervision in can be helpful in determining whether a driving or community mobility evaluation is indicated. Driving a motor vehicle, negotiating the intricacies of transit, or traveling through the community by other means are complex IADLs. Safe and successful performance requires the use of several cognitive skills, including judging, sequencing, organizing, prioritizing, identifying, and multitasking (American Occupational Therapy Association, 2008). Other cognitive skills required for safe engagement include complex attention, memory, visual processing, and executive functioning. These same cognitive skills are used in the execution of other ADLs and IADLs and therefore difficulties in complex tasks such as meal preparation, medication management, or paying bills may suggest the presence of difficulties in driving and community mobility as well, warranting an evaluation.

If a client is having significant difficulties carrying out ADLs and IADLs, the clinician should question whether driving is a realistic goal for that individual before adding a health care expense for the family. If a decision about driving and community mobility can be made based on egregious performance in other areas of functioning, this may be preferred, as it saves costs and reduces the risks associated with conducting an on-road evaluation.

Compliance With the Recommendation to Not Drive

One final area of consideration is the current driving status, particularly if the individual has deficits in insight into his or her cognitive difficulties. Is the client currently driving against medical or family recommendations? Drivers who proceed to drive against medical or family recommendations generate substantial conflict with family members who do not allow them to drive. Many families and community resources have identified a variety of suggestions to help address such a concern, including disconnecting the coil wire in the car, disconnecting the car battery, removing a spark plug, hiding the car keys, filing down the car keys, or swapping the keys with keys to another vehicle that is disabled or no longer owned so the driver can still feel like he or she possesses keys (Taylor & Tripodes, 2001).

In circumstances in which the driver has poor insight, a referral for a comprehensive driving evaluation may be indicated, even when it is known that the individual is highly unlikely to pass if other attempts at driving cessation have not been successful. In such cases, the driving evaluator must use good judgment and not put the client (or community) at risk, yet strive to allow the driver to demonstrate erroneous, unsafe driving behaviors as evidence for a driving cessation recommendation. Although not practical in most cases, when a lack of insight is severe, videotaping the on-road evaluation may be instructive to counter the excuses and rationale offered by the driver or family.

The question often is raised as to when or if occupational therapists should consider reporting impaired drivers to the state DMV. To answer this question, one must consider both ethical and legal issues (see Chapter 5). Most ethicists believe it is appropriate to breech confidentiality and report an unsafe driver for the good of the driving public. Every state has its own legal requirements for reporting medically impaired drivers, and states vary according to the reporting mechanism (e.g., voluntary vs. mandatory), confidentiality, and whether civil immunity is granted. It is important to become knowledgeable of the specific laws and statutes in your state.

From an occupational therapist (generalist and specialist) point of view, it would be important as a minimum to communicate any safety concerns to the referring physician. Most states require physician input to make a final decision on driver licensing.

Driving Recommendations and Interventions for Individuals With Cognitive Deficits

Generally, individuals complete a comprehensive driving evaluation with an occupational therapy driver rehabilitation specialist (DRS) and receive a decision of pass, marginal, or fail (Hunt et al., 1997). These outcomes always should include consideration of the individual's unique cognitive deficits, including insight into deficit areas, the disease course, past therapy interventions and effectiveness, the difficulty of the on-road evaluation course in comparison to the client's routine driving, and personality characteristics of the client that may affect driving performance.

Passing a Comprehensive Driving Evaluation in the Presence of Cognitive Deficits

If an individual with cognitive deficits passes a comprehensive driving evaluation (which by definition includes an on-road evaluation), then one may conclude that he or she is safe to drive. However, even if the performance met criteria deemed adequate and safe during the evaluation, the occupational therapist needs to consider the nature of the diagnosis. If the diagnosis is progressive (e.g., dementia, PD, MS), functioning will decline over time and, subsequently, driving performance and safety also will decline. The evaluation may be used as a baseline for comparison against future comprehensive driving evaluations conducted later in the disease process.

Unfortunately, no evidence to support a recommended timeline or interval for follow-up reevaluations currently exists. In light of the lack of evidence, clinicians should collaborate with the driver's primary care physician and consider the individual client's disease progression. Symptom control through medication, other therapeutic interventions, and the anticipated trajectory of the disease course are factors used to decide on reevaluation intervals. These evaluation intervals may be time based (e.g., every 6 months) or can occur following functional or medication changes, or after an exacerbation of a medical illness. This process of establishing a baseline with the anticipation of reevaluations begins to prepare the client and family for driving cessation, should that be the case. Even though most individuals do not wish to discuss driving cessation when they are still capable of driving, it is recommended to help make the transition easier if possible (Adler & Rottunda, 2006).

Failing a Comprehensive Driving Evaluation in the Presence of Cognitive Deficits

If an individual does not pass a comprehensive driving evaluation because of cognitive deficits, the reasons need to be explored and the deficits must be more closely examined in regard to the influence on community mobility safety.

When individuals are no longer capable of driving, they do not cease to require access to the community for shopping, medical care, social participation, and leisure. However, the same deficits that preclude these individuals from driving also will hinder their ability to access alternative forms of transportation. Travelers require intact cognitive skills to decide on a transportation provider, schedule appointments, judge the timing to walk to buses and complete transfers to a destination, manage money to pay for travel, and remain safe in the process.

Clinicians should be aware of area transportation alternatives representing a menu of services from public transit to door-through-door service for a range of performance capabilities; the expected performance for use of those transportation services; service delivery options; and application or eligibility procedures, if applicable. See Chapter 2 for information related to transportation options, travel training, and assistance with eligibility for paratransit.

Knowing the severity of the cognitive or perceptual deficits and how they are affecting function is very important in making recommendations for future driving.

Recommendations Based on Marginal Driving Evaluation Performance in the Presence of Cognitive Deficits

There are occasions when an individual with cognitive deficits makes safety errors on the road test yet does not clearly pass or clearly fail. In such cases, the individual falls into a borderline or marginal recommendation. An example of this may occur if an individual misses a pertinent road sign indicating where to turn on the road evaluation in a novel environment, yet performs well on all other parts of the road test. The individual becomes obviously anxious and needs minimal assistance with problem solving how to get turned around in the unfamiliar environment. This client may demonstrate mild deficits in attention and memory in clinical testing and good executive functioning on various assessments. In such a case, the occupational therapy DRS needs to fully look at the complete evaluation to make a recommendation. Areas of consideration are as follows:

1. What are the cognitive–perceptual deficits that resulted in the questionable performance, and how severe are the deficits?
2. Do these cognitive deficits limit other areas of function?
3. Has the individual had therapy to address the treatment of these deficits? What was the outcome of the therapy?
4. How anxious or nervous was the individual during the assessment, and did this affect the results? Did he or she exhibit awareness of any of the driving difficulties that may have occurred?
5. Was the on-road evaluation similar to the environment the individual typically drives in?
6. Does the individual have the capacity for insight into his or her areas of cognitive difficulties to benefit from further therapy or to follow through with driving restrictions if recommended?
7. Is a repeat comprehensive driving evaluation indicated, either immediately—to contribute additional data before this driving evaluation is considered complete—or as an interval reevaluation conducted at a later date? It is not unreasonable in such "borderline" situations to perform a reevaluation of the road assessment in a more familiar environment or at a date in the not-too-distant future.

Placing Restrictions on a Driver's License

Part of the outcome of the comprehensive driving evaluation is to consider the possibility of driving restrictions and to determine whether restrictions are appropriate for this individual. Restrictions are allowed to be placed on driver's licenses under the jurisdiction of the state licensing authority, and every state has a listing of approved restrictions (accepted restrictions vary by state). Some data suggest that in some medically impaired samples, restricted licenses have been associated with a decreased crash risk (Nasvadi & Wister, 2009).

Common restrictions that are considered for a person with cognitive deficits include, but are not limited to, the following:

• Driving only within a designated-mile radius of his or her home
• Driving only during the daytime
• Driving under certain speed limits or not driving on the interstate.

When restrictions are considered, it also should be considered whether the individual has the capability to adhere to the restriction. Possessing insight into one's deficits is usually important for the driver to be able to successfully follow through with restrictions. If an individual does not have insight into his or her deficits, not only does the person not see a need to use a compensatory strategy, but he or she is equally at risk for not seeing a need to follow through with a restriction. If the driver's memory is severely impaired, he or she may not "remember" to adhere to the restriction. Individuals who lack insight into their condition can become a safety concern not only for family members who try to intervene but also for the community at large, and they likely would not be appropriate candidates for a restricted license.

It is always advisable to confer with the physician and follow state guidelines when considering restricted licenses. More studies are needed on the willingness and ability of occupational therapy DRSs to recommend restricted licenses and the impact on traffic safety.

It is always advisable to confer with the physician and follow state guidelines when considering restricted licenses.

Requiring Interventions Because of Cognitive Deficits

Some individuals can benefit from interventions to improve upon cognitive skills that will lead to safe driving performance. Clinicians should keep in mind two important issues when recommending interventions before a client's return to driving:

1. The client's cognitive skills must be capable of improvement through remediation strategies. This capability includes not only the nature of the diagnosis being amenable to change but also the client possessing the insight and willingness to address the cognitive deficits.
2. The nature of the intervention may not be in the scope or expertise of the DRS. Therefore, referral to a clinician with specialization in cognitive rehabilitation may be the most appropriate means to meet the client's needs.

Interventions to establish or remediate cognitive skills may include strategies to improve attention, memory, or executive functioning. These interventions may be a critical element of an individual's return to driving. Standards of practice described in the literature regarding cognitive rehabilitation should be applied in these cases.

Interventions focused specifically on driving and community mobility, rather than the foundational cognitive skills, are also within the scope of occupational therapy programming for clients with cognitive impairments who have driving and community goals. These interventions typically follow the tradition of typical occupational therapy practice in which the clinician identifies a deficient functional task, provides an opportunity for participation, and grades the activity accordingly to challenge the client while promoting experiences of success. Because of the variability of potential deficits, client driving environments, alternative modes of transportation to be used, and specific client needs, it is difficult to generate an inclusive list of suggested interventions; however, examples of interventions are presented in Table 7.6. Before providing cognitive interventions during on-road training, the following should be considered:

1. How is the client performing in other IADLs? Driving is one of the most complicated IADLs and one with inherent safety risks. It is preferred to work on cognitive deficits in more "safe" situations before driving.

Table 7.6. Examples of Intervention Exercises During On-Road Training

Skill Need	Activity
Divided attention and alternating attention	• Traveling along a moderate-traffic, multilane roadway with several cross streets with instruction to turn at a designated street, thus requiring attention to travel lanes, maintenance of travel speed, and reading of cross-street signage • Holding conversations with client while driving to determine whether he or she has the capability to multitask • Evaluating the client's ability to request the passenger to discontinue conversation while driving when necessary
Short-term memory	• Providing the driver with an address or single nearby destination and allowing him or her to practice and use memory strategies to recall the destination • Using a global positioning system while driving to novel locations
Working memory	• Providing the driver multiple-step directions to a destination and allowing him or her to practice and use memory strategies to successfully complete the route
Problem solving	• Traveling into a known construction or detour area, forcing the driver to resolve an alternate route to the destination
Judgment	• Exiting a parking lot onto a busy road requiring the use of judgment to determine when it is safe to pull out of the parking lot into the flow of traffic
Decision making	• Driving through a large parking lot such as at a mall and requiring the driver to select and commit to a parking space
Flexibility in thinking	• Route planning 3 completely different routes from a starting location to a destination
Planning	• Route planning a trip with 3 stops along the way to the destination
Sequencing	• Making multistep maneuvers such as lane changes, parallel parking, and 3-point turns
Visual scanning	• Traveling through a residential neighborhood with the task of identifying all the mailboxes of a certain color • A more challenging version of this exercise requiring visual scanning further from the path of travel: traveling through a residential neighborhood identifying flags that are typically closer to homes and further from the street

2. Does the individual's diagnosis support the training process? Most progressive diseases involving continued cognitive decline would preclude further on-road training, as described below.
3. Are the client's deficits at a mild level so that it has been determined to be a low safety risk to pursue further training?

Cognition and Community Mobility

Pedestrian Safety

Pedestrian injury is the second leading cause of unintentional injury-related death in children ages 5–14 years in the United States (Nerad, 2005). In 2009, an estimated 13,000 pedestrians were injured, and 244 killed were ages 14 years or younger (NHTSA, 2009b). Children within the 5–9 years of age range are at the most risk because they encounter the most traffic situations and typically are not cognitively able to process and react appropriately to dangerous situations yet (Bart, Katz, Weiss, & Josman, 2008). Typically, children are unable to appropriately judge traffic situations either from a lack of traffic knowledge, limitations in visual–perception skills, increased distractibility, or less-developed motor skills (Bart et al., 2008). Any of these deficits in traffic skills alone or a combination of them can lead to an increased risk for injury or death.

Similarly, Thomson (1991) found two major deficits that children demonstrate compared with adults when crossing the road. The children demonstrated limitations in selecting appropriate sites for safe crossing and deciding when it is safe to cross by judging the flow of traffic. For these reasons, it is suggested that children younger than age 10 should not cross the road without supervision or assistance (Percer, 2009).

On the other end of the age continuum, Langlois and colleagues (1997) found that older adults demonstrated difficulty crossing the road that continued to increase after age 70. The participants of their study identified that they had increased difficulty with crossing the street, having enough time to cross, judging when to cross when a vehicle was turning right, and requiring assistance to cross (Langlois et al., 1997). The participants who identified having difficulty crossing the street generally had a slower walking speed, increased visual deficits, lower mental status scores, and a greater need for assistance with ADLs when compared to the control group of individuals who did not report difficulty crossing the street (Langlois et al., 1997).

Thomson, Tolmie, Foot, and Mclaren (1996) identified four main cognitive abilities required to safely interact with traffic. First, an individual must *detect the presence of traffic*. This involves selective attention, visual acuity and processing, and the coordination of visual and auditory input. An individual also must be able to *make judgments about whether a given site is safe or dangerous*, which incorporates a coordination of past experiences, current given information, and predictions of future consequences. Next, the individual must *make visual timing judgments* that involve determining the speed and direction of a vehicle to provide information about when to cross. Typically, pedestrians interact with two directions or lanes of traffic, so they must coordinate information from different directions. This coordination requires the individual to attend to the various stimuli, retain that information in memory, and integrate the information to make a judgment of when to cross. Finally, *coordination of perception and action* involves relating the time that is available for crossing with the time that the individual requires to cross safely.

Clearly, individuals with any of the cognitive deficits described earlier may have difficulty traveling through the community as pedestrians, particularly when crossing the street. Interventions to address pedestrian concerns may be managed on an individual basis to address a client's cognitive concerns by training in safe pedestrian practices (Bart et al., 2008). Although this approach can benefit an individual client, pedestrian issues are often a community-wide concern and should be addressed from a community- or population-based injury prevention perspective. For example, in a study examining pedestrian-vehicular crashes near schools, it was determined that a programmatic solution such as Safe Routes to School was warranted (Clifton & Kreamer-Fults, 2007).

Although some research suggests that community-based interventions should focus on the built environment of roadways and pedestrian pathways (Clarke, Ailshire, & Lantz, 2009), other studies favor education-focused intervention. Barton, Schwebel, and Morrongiello (2007) found that educating children was an effective practice to prevent pedestrian injuries. The idea of pre-injury education was further strengthened by researchers who discovered that children demonstrated greater distraction and risk when crossing the street while talking on a cell phone (Stavrinos, Byington, & Schwebel, 2009).

Child Passenger Safety

Although there is not a lot of evidence regarding child passenger safety for children with cognitive issues, some guidelines have been published for children with behavioral challenges. The American Academy of Pediatrics (AAP; 1999) published such guidelines, suggesting that if an older child has hyperactivity, autism spectrum disorder, or emotional challenges, he or she may be safest in a seat that cannot be unbuckled by the child. For example, the guidelines include a high-back booster seat that has an internal harness as a potential seating system for these children. Although a 5-point harness is not typically used for a child heavier than 40 pounds, the additional belting can maintain the child in a safe seated position while the vehicle is moving.

Also, the AAP (1999) suggests vests with rear back closure for children whose behavioral challenges may interfere with safe travel. Such vests can be used in cars or school buses (Indiana University School of Medicine, 2010).

The cognitive skills of the child are not the only area of concern for safe transport of children. The cognitive level of the parents is also critical to safe, proper use of child safety seats. The installation and use of child safety seats can be very complex because of the variety of vehicle designs and the types and stages of seats, fastening systems, and harness systems. In fact, a multistate study revealed that 84% of child restraint seats showed critical misuse (Safe Kids USA, 2009).

Parents with cognitive deficits are at a serious disadvantage when using a child safety seat, considering that compliance with its proper use is so difficult for the general public. The reading ability of the installer can be a detriment to using child safety seats properly. Wegner and Girasek (2003) found that the reading level required of parents to read child safety seat installation instructions was too high for effective understanding. The instructions required a 10th-grade reading level on average when approximately 40% of the U.S. adult population is only able to read at the 8th-grade reading level or below (National Center for Education Statistics, 1992).

Additional cognitive deficits in the areas of memory, problem solving, sequencing, and judgment could all limit a parent's ability to properly install and use a child safety seat. For these parents, the risk is too high to manage the seats independently, and it is prudent to take advantage of available resources. It is suggested that a child passenger safety (CPS) technician install the seat and educate the parent in its proper use (see Exhibit 7.1). Ideally, the cognitively impaired parent's occupational therapist is certified as a CPS technician and can grade the learning activity for optimal outcomes (Berres, 2003).

> **If an older child has hyperactivity, autism spectrum disorder, or emotional challenges, he or she may be safest in a seat that cannot be unbuckled by the child.**

Exhibit 7.1. Child Passenger Safety Technician

Health and community practitioners can be certified as child passenger safety (CPS) technicians, earning them the credential of CPS technician. The certification program is coordinated by Safe Kids USA (www.safekids.org) and requires participation in a 4-day course for a total of 32 hours, including classroom instruction, hands-on exercises, and a community safety seat checkup. For more detailed information about National CPS Certification, visit http://cert.safekids.org.

Bicycling

Riding a bicycle requires cognitive and perceptual–motor skills similar to those needed for driving a car. For example, visual-processing skills, decision making, judgment, and spatial awareness are used in the same way that they are used for driving. In addition, there are some skills that are more important when riding a bicycle, such as dynamic balance and kinesthetic awareness.

In a literature review, Wierda and Brookhuis (1991) suggested that there are three levels of subtasks required for riding a bike, based on research by Michon (1985). The first, *strategic level*, is mainly used by older bicyclists such as adolescents and adults. It involves decision making about the purpose, expenses, and benefits of bicycling to a destination versus using other modalities. The second, *maneuvering level*, involves decision making about traffic behavior, such as deciding when to cross, how to avoid obstacles, and the appropriate speed to bicycle safely within a given environment. The final, *control level*, involves the actual bicycling skills, such as balance, speed, pedaling, and shifting gears.

Individuals with cognitive impairment would not likely experience difficulty with the control level of bicycling because the skills are largely based on motor skills. However, those with cognitive impairments may encounter difficulties with the maneuvering and strategic levels because obstacle avoidance, decision making, observance of safety given a specific environment, money management, and route planning are all reliant on executive functioning.

Interventions focused on cycling can span the client spectrum from person to organization to population as with pedestrian interventions. Clinicians may work with individual clients in the early stages of bicycling when they are first learning to ride (Cameron, Shapiro, & Ainsleigh, 2005; Doğru, Önal, & Bek, 2007). However, it is more likely that practitioners addressing bicycling are working with organization- or population-level clients aimed at education about riding and helmet safety (McLaughlin, 2010) or infrastructure design (Neville et al., 2010) for injury prevention.

Summary

It is critical for occupational therapists to relate a client's strengths and weaknesses in cognition to safety issues in community mobility, including driving, pedestrian safety, passenger safety, bicycling, and other forms of transportation. Occupational therapists collect information on a client's habits and routines in regard to community mobility and integrate this information with the client's cognitive status (attention, memory, and executive skills). Occupational therapists are challenged by the content in this chapter to select assessment tools that will provide clients, family members, and other health care professionals with information that provides data that can, at the very least, "start the conversation." In other cases, occupational therapists are challenged to provide the client and family with data that provide evidence of the need for, and ability to participate in, a behind-the-wheel assessment to clarify a client's ability to drive safely.

Determining the safety of a client's ability to drive, in the presence of clinically demonstrated impairments in cognition, involves consideration of many factors. This chapter provides therapists with terminology and examples related to cognitive skills and cognitive impairments that may be used to support the challenging clinical problem-solving process of making a determination about an individual's capacity to drive safely.

References

Adler, G., & Rottunda, S. (2006). Older adults' perspectives on driving cessation. *Journal of Aging Studies, 20*, 227–235.

Akinwuntan, A. E., Feys, H., Baten, G., Arno, P., & Kiekens, C. (2006). Prediction of driving after stroke: A prospective study. *Neurorehabilitation and Neural Repair, 20*, 417–423.

American Academy of Pediatrics. (1999). Transporting children with special health care needs. *Pediatrics, 104*, 988–993.

American Occupational Therapy Association. (2008). Occupational therapy practice framework: Domain and process (2nd ed.). *American Journal of Occupational Therapy, 62*, 625–683. doi:10.5014/ajot.62.6.625

Anstey, K. J., Wood, J., Lord, S., & Walker, J. G. (2005). Cognitive, sensory, and physical factors enabling driving safety in older adults. *Clinical Psychology Review, 25*, 45–65.

Baker, P. T. (2006). Clinical evaluation skills. In J. M. Pellerito (Ed.), *Driver rehabilitation and community mobility: Principles and practice* (pp. 116–140). St. Louis: Mosby.

Ball, K., Owsley, C., Sloane, M. E., Roenker, D. L., & Bruni, J. R. (1993). Visual attention problems as a predictor of vehicle crashes in older drivers. *Investigative Ophthalmology and Visual Science, 34*, 3110–3123.

Barco, P. P., Crosson, B. C., Bolesta, M. M., Werts, D., & Stout, R. (1991). Training awareness and compensation in postacute head injury. In J. S. Kreutzer & P. H. Whehman (Eds.), *Cognitive rehabilitation for persons with traumatic brain injury* (pp. 129–147). Baltimore: Paul H. Brookes.

Bart, O., Katz, N., Weiss, P. L., & Josman, N. (2008). Street crossing by typically developed children in real and virtual environments. *OTJR: Occupation, Participation and Health, 28*, 89–96.

Barton, B. K., Schwebel, D. C., & Morrongiello, B. A. (2007). Brief Report: Increasing children's safe pedestrian behaviors through simple skills training. *Journal of Pediatric Psychology, 32*, 475–480.

Baum, C. M., & Katz, N. (2010). Occupational therapy approach to assessing the relationship between cognition and function. In T. D. Marcotte & I. Grant (Eds.), *Neuropsychology of everyday functioning* (pp. 62–90). New York: Guilford Press.

Bechara, A., Tranel, D., Damasio, H., & Damasio, A. R. (1996). Failure to respond autonomically to anticipated future outcomes following damage to prefrontal cortex. *Cerebral Cortex, 6*, 215–225.

Beers, M., & Berkow, R. (1999). *The Merck manual of diagnosis and therapy* (17th ed.). White-house Station, NJ: Merck Research Laboratories.

Berger, J. T., Rosner, F., Kark, P., Bennett, A. J., & Medical Society of the State of New York. (2000). Reporting by physicians of impaired drivers and potentially impaired drivers. *Journal of General Internal Medicine, 15*(9), 667–672. doi: 10.1046/j.1525-1497.2000.04309.x

Berres, S. (2003, October 20). Keeping kids safe: Passenger restraint systems. *OT Practice, 8*, 13–17.

Boake, C., Francisco, G. E., Ivanhoe, C. B., & Kothart, S. (2000). Brain injury rehabilitation. In R. L. Braddom (Ed.), *Physical medicine and rehabilitation* (pp. 1073–1116). Philadelphia: Saunders.

Boldrini, M., Del Pace, L., Placidi, G. P., Keilp, J., Ellis, S. P., Signori, S., et al. (2005). Selective cognitive deficits in obsessive–compulsive disorder compared to panic disorder with agoraphobia. *Acta Psychiatrica Scandinavica, 111*, 150–158.

Bonanni, E., Maestri, M., Tognoni, G., Fabbrini, M., Nucciarone, B., Manca, M. L., et al. (2005). Daytime sleepiness in mild and moderate Alzheimer's disease and its relationship with cognitive impairment. *Journal of Sleep Research, 14*, 311–317.

Bryer, R. C., Rapport, L. J., & Hanks, R. A. (2006). Determining fitness to drive: Neuropsychological and psychological considerations. In J. M. Pellerito (Ed.), *Driver rehabilitation and community mobility: Principles and practice* (pp. 165–184). St. Louis: Mosby.

Cameron, M. J., Shapiro, R. L., & Ainsleigh, S. A. (2005). Bicycle riding: Pedaling made possible through positive behavioral interventions. *Journal of Positive Behavior Interventions, 7*, 153–158.

Carr, D. B., Duchek, J. M., Meuser, T. M., & Morris, J. C. (2006). Older adult drivers with cognitive impairment. *American Family Physician, 73*, 1029–1036.

Carr, D. B., & Ott, B. R. (2010). The older adult driver with cognitive impairment. *JAMA, 303*, 1632–1641.

Carr, D. B., Schwartzberg, J. G., Manning, L., & Sempek, J. (2010). Medical conditions and medications that may affect driving. In *Physician's guide to assessing and counseling older drivers* (2nd ed., pp. 145–184). Washington, DC: National Highway Traffic Safety Administration.

Chipchase, S. Y., Lincoln, N. B., & Radford, K. A. (2003). A survey of effects of fatigue on driving in people with multiple sclerosis. *Disability and Rehabilitation, 25*, 712–721.

Clarke, P., Ailshire, J. A., & Lantz, P. (2009). Urban built environments and trajectories of mobility disability: Findings from a national sample of community-dwelling American adults (1986–2001). *Social Science Medicine, 69*, 964–970.

Clifton, K. J., & Kreamer-Fults, K. (2007). An examination of the environmental attributes associated with pedestrian–vehicular crashes near public schools. *Accident Analysis and Prevention, 39*, 708–715.

Coeckelbergh, T. R. M., Cornelissen, F. W., Brouwer, W. H., & Kooijman, A. C. (2002). The effect of visual field defects on eye movements and practical fitness to drive. *Vision Research, 42*, 669–677.

Cross, J. M., McGwin, G., Rubin, G. S., Ball, K. K., West, S. K., & Roenker, D. L. (2009). Visual and medical risk factors for motor vehicle collision involvement among older drivers. *British Journal of Ophthalmology, 93*, 400–404.

Crosson, B. C., Barco, P. P., Velozo, C. A., Bolesta, M. M., Cooper, P. V., & Werts, D. (1989). Awareness and compensation in postacute head injury rehabilitation. *Journal of Head Trauma Rehabilitation, 4*(3), 46–54.

Davies, S. J. C., Pandit, S. A., Feeney, A., Stevenson, B. J., Kervin, R. W., Nutt, D. J., et al. (2005). Is there cognitive impairment in clinically "healthy" abstinent alcohol dependence? *Alcohol and Alcoholism, 40*, 498–503.

Dawson, J. D., Anderson, S. W., Uc, E. Y., Dastrup, E., & Rizzo, M. (2009). Predictors of driving safety in early Alzheimer disease. *Neurology, 72*, 521–527.

De Raedt, R., & Ponjaert-Kristofferson, I. (2001). Short cognitive/neuropsychological test battery for first-tier fitness to drive assessment of older adults. *Clinical Neuropsychology, 15*, 329–336.

Deangelis, L. M., & Rosenfeld, S. S. (2010). Tumors: General considerations. In L. P. Rowland & T. A. Pedley (Eds.), *Merritt's neurology* (pp. 371–377). Philadelphia: Lippincott Williams & Wilkins.

Devos, H., Akinwuntan, A. E., Nieuwboer, A., Truijen, S., Tant, M., & De Weerdt, W. (2010). Screening for fitness to drive after stroke: A systematic review and meta-analysis. *Neurology, 76*, 747–756.

Dobbs, A. (1997). Evaluating the driving competence of dementia patients. *Alzheimer Disease and Associated Disorders, 11*(1), 8–12.

Dobbs, B. M. (2005). *Medication conditions and driving: A review of the scientific literature (1960–2000)* (No. DOT-HS-809-690). Springfield, VA: National Technical Information Service.

Doğru, Y. S. S., Önal, Ö., B. Y., & Bek, H. (2007). Teaching how to ride a balance wheeled bicycle to autistic children using the direct instruction method. *Selcuk University Social Sciences Institute Journal, 18*, 245–256.

Duchek, J. M., Carr, D. B., Hunt, L., Roe, C. M., Xiong, C., & Shah, K. (2003). Longitudinal driving performance in early-stage dementia of the Alzheimer type. *Journal of the American Geriatrics Society, 51*, 1342–1347.

Dujardin, K., Donze, A. C., & Hautecoeur, P. (1998). Attention impairment in recently diagnosed multiple sclerosis. *European Journal of Neurology, 5*, 61–66.

Edwards, J., Myers, C., Ross, L. A., Roenker, D. L., Cissell, G. M., & McLaughlin, A. M. (2009). The longitudinal impact of cognitive speed of processing training on driving mobility. *The Gerontologist, 49*, 485–494.

Elliot, R. (2003). Executive functions and their disorders. *British Medical Bulletin, 65*, 49–59.

Engrum, E. S., Lambert, E. W., & Scott, K. (1990). Criterion-related validity of the cognitive behavioral driver's inventory: Brain injured patients versus normal controls. *Cognitive Rehabilitation, 8*, 20–26.

European Road Safety Observatory. (2007). *Fatigue.* Retrieved November 1, 2010, from http://ec.europa.eu/transport/wcm/road_safety/erso/knowledge/Content/55_fatigue/fatigue-2.htm

Fisk, G. D., Owsley, C., & Mennemeier, M. (2002). Vision, attention, and self-reported driving behaviors in community-dwelling stroke survivors. *Archives of Physical Medicine and Rehabilitation, 83,* 469–477.

Fisk, G. D., Owsley, C., & Pulley, L. V. (1997). Driving after stroke: Driving exposure, advice, and evaluations. *Archives of Physical Medicine and Rehabilitation, 78,* 1338–1345.

Galvin, J. E., Roe, C. M., Xiong, C., & Morris, J. C. (2006). Validity and reliability of the AD8 informant interview in dementia. *Neurology, 67,* 1942–1948.

Geldmacher, D. S., & Whitehouse, P. J. (1996). Evaluation of dementia. *New England Journal of Medicine, 335,* 330–336.

Gershkoff, A. M., & Finestone, H. M. (2009). Driving after stroke. In J. Stein, R. L. Harvey, R. F. Macko, C. J. Winstein, & R. D. Zorowitz (Eds.), *Stroke recovery and rehabilitation* (pp. 697–711). New York: Demos Medical Publishing.

Gillen, G. (2009). *Cognitive and perceptual rehabilitation optimizing function.* St. Louis: Mosby.

Goode, K. T., Ball, K. K., Sloane, M., Roenker, D. L., Roth, D. L., & Myers, R. S. (1998). Useful Field of View and other neurocognitive indicators of crash risk in older adults. *Journal of Clinical Psychology in Medical Settings, 5,* 425–440.

Hartman-Maeir, A., Soroker, N., Ring, H., & Katz, N. (2002). Awareness of deficits in stroke rehabilitation. *Journal of Rehabilitation Medicine, 34,* 158–164.

Heilman, K. M., Watson, R. T., & Valenstein, E. (2003). Neglect and related disorders. In K. M. Hilman & E. Valenstein (Eds.), *Clinical neuropsychology* (4th ed., pp. 296–346). New York: Oxford.

Hobson, D. E., Lang, A. E., Martin, W. R. W., Razmy, A., Rivest, J., & Fleming, J. (2002). Excessive daytime sleepiness and sudden-onset sleep in Parkinson disease: A survey by the Canadian Movement Disorders Group. *JAMA, 287,* 455–463.

Hsu, J. (2009). Traumatic brain injury. In E. B. Crepeau, E. S. Cohn, & B. A. B. Schell (Eds.), *Willard and Spackman's occupational therapy* (11th ed., p. 1069–1071). Philadelphia: Lippincott Williams & Wilkins.

Hunt, L. A., Murphy, C. F., Carr, D., Duchek, J. M., Buckles, V., & Morris, J. C. (1997). Reliability of the Washington University Road Test: A performance-based assessment for drivers with dementia of the Alzheimer type. *Archives of Neurology, 54,* 707–712.

Indiana University School of Medicine. (2010). *Children with special health care needs.* Retrieved December 6, 2010, from http://www.preventinjury.org/SNTrestraints.asp

Jones, K., & Harrison, Y. (2001). Frontal lobe function, sleep loss and fragmented sleep. *Sleep Medical Review, 5,* 463–475.

Keller, J., & Stone, K. (2009). Multiple sclerosis. In E. B. Crepeau, E. S. Cohn, & B. A. B. Schell (Eds.), *Willard and Spackman's occupational therapy* (11th ed., pp. 1033–1037). Philadelphia: Lippincott Williams & Wilkins.

Kiosses, D. N., Klimstra, S., Murphy, C., & Alexopoulos, G. S. (2001). Executive dysfunction and disability in elderly patients with major depression. *American Journal of Geriatric Psychiatry, 9,* 269–274.

Knecht, J. (1977). The multiple sclerosis patient as a driver. *Schweizerishe Medizinische Wochenschrift, 107,* 373–378.

Knesek, K. (2009). Cerebrovascular accident. In E. B. Crepeau, E. S. Cohn, & B. A. B. Schell (Eds.), *Willard and Spackman's occupational therapy* (11th ed., pp. 1001–1004). Philadelphia: Lippincott Williams & Wilkins.

Kohlmeyer, K. (2003). Evaluation of performance skills and client factors. In E. B. Crepeau, E. S. Cohn, & B. A. B. Schell (Eds.), *Willard and Spackman's occupational therapy* (11th ed., pp. 365–426). Philadelphia: Lippincott Williams & Wilkins.

Langlois, J. A., Keyl, P. M., Guralnik, J. M., Foley, D. J., Marottoli, R. A., & Wallace, R. B. (1997). Characteristics of older pedestrians who have difficulty crossing the street. *American Journal of Public Health, 87,* 393–397.

Legh-Smith, J., Wade, D. T., & Hewer, R. L. (1986). Driving after stroke. *Journal of the Royal Society of Medicine, 79,* 200–203.

Leritz, E., Loftis, C., Crucian, G., Friedman, W., & Bowers, D. (2004). Self-awareness of deficits in Parkinson disease. *The Clinical Neuropsychologist, 18,* 352–361.

Levy, L. L. (2005). Cognitive aging in perspective: Information processing, cognition, and memory. In N. Katz (Ed.), *Cognition and occupation across the lifespan: Models for intervention in occupational therapy* (2nd ed., pp. 305–325). Bethesda, MD: AOTA Press.

Lidz, C. S. (1987). Cognitive deficiencies revisited. In C. S. Lidz (Ed.), *Dynamic assessments evaluating learning potential* (pp. 444–478). New York: Guilford Press.

Lieb, K., Brucker, S., Bach, M., Els, T., Lücking, C. H., & Greenlee, M. W. (1999). Impairment in preattentive visual processing in patients with Parkinson's disease. *Brain: A Journal of Neurology, 122,* 303–313.

Lincoln, N. B., Radford, K. A., & Nouri, F. M. (2004). *Stroke Drivers Screening Assessment: Revised manual.* Nottingham, England: University of Nottingham.

Lococo, K., & Tyree, R. (2010). *Potentially driver-impairing prescription medications.* Retrieved January 6, 2012, from http://www.medscape.org/viewarticle/725019

Lou, J. Q., & Lane, S. J. (2005). Personal performance capabilities and their impact on occupational performance. In C. H. Christiansen, C. M. Baum, & J. Bass-Haugen (Eds.), *Occupational therapy: Performance, participation, and well-bring* (3rd ed., pp. 268–297). Thorofare, NJ: Slack.

Lundzvist, A., Gerdle, B., & Ronnberg, J. (2000). Neuropsychological aspects of driving after a stroke: In the simulator and on the road. *Applied Cognitive Psychology, 14,* 135–148.

Lyznicki, J. M., Doege, T. C., Davis, R. M., & Williams, M. A. (1998). Sleepiness, driving, and motor vehicle crashes. *JAMA, 279,* 1908–1913.

Marcotte, T. D., Rosenthal, T. J., Roberts, E., Lampinen, S., Scott, J. C., Allen, R. W., et al. (2008). The contribution of cognition and spasticity to driving performance in multiple sclerosis. *Archives of Physical Medicine and Rehabilitation, 89,* 1753–1758.

Marinus, J., Visser, M., Verwey, N. A., Verhey, F. R. J., Middelkoop, H. A. M., Stiggelbout, A. M., et al. (2003). Assessment of cognition in Parkinson's disease. *Neurology, 61,* 1222–1228..

Marottoli, R. A., & Richardson, E. D. (1998). Confidence in, and self-rating of, driving ability among older drivers. *Accident Analysis and Prevention, 30,* 331–336.

Martınez-Aran, A., Vieta, E., Colom, F., Torrent, C., Sanchez-Moreno, J., Reinares, M., et al. (2004). Cognitive impairment in euthymic bipolar patients: Implications for clinical and functional outcome. *Bipolar Disorders, 6,* 224–232.

Mathias, J. L., & Lucas, L. K. (2009). Cognitive predictors of unsafe driving in older drivers: Meta-analysis. *International Psychogeriatrics, 21,* 637–653.

Mayer, S. A., & Badjatia, N. (2010). Trauma: Head injury. In L. P. Rowland & T. A. Pedley (Eds.), *Merritt's neurology* (pp. 479–494). Philadelphia: Lippincott Williams & Wilkins.

McKenna, K., Cooke, D. M., Fleming, J., Jefferson, A., & Ogden, S. (2006). The incidence of visual perceptual impairment in clients with severe traumatic brain injury. *Brain Injury, 20,* 507–518.

McKenna, P., Jefferies, L., Dobson, A., & Frude, N. (2004). The use of a cognitive battery to predict who will fail an on-road driving test. *British Journal of Clinical Psychology, 43,* 325–336.

McKnight, A. J., & McKnight, A. S. (2000, October). *The behavioral contributors to highway crashes of youthful drivers.* Paper presented at the 44th Annual Proceedings of the Association for the Advancement of Automotive Medicine, Chicago.

McLaughlin, K. A. (2010). The effectiveness of a bicycle safety program for improving safety-related knowledge and behavior in young elementary students. *Journal of Pediatric Psychology, 35,* 343–353.

Michon, J. A. (1985). A critical view of driver behavior models: What do we know, what should we do? In L. Evans & R. C. Schwing (Eds.), *Human behavior and traffic safety* (pp. 485–520). New York: Plenum.

Miller, G. (1965). The magical number seven, plus or minus two: Some limits on our capacity for processing information. *Psychological Review, 63,* 81–97.

Milleville-Pennel, I., Pothier, J., Hoc, J., & Mathé, J. (2010). Consequences of cognitive impairments following traumatic brain injury: Pilot study on visual exploration while driving. *Brain Injury, 24,* 678–691.

Monahan, M. (2009). *Driving assessment and training techniques: Addressing the needs of students with cognitive and social limitations behind the wheel.* Bethesda, MD: American Occupational Therapy Association.

Monahan, M., & Patten, K. (2009). *Creating successful transitions to community mobility independence for adolescents: Addressing the needs of students with cognitive, social and behavioral limitations.* Bethesda, MD: American Occupational Therapy Association.

Nasvadi, G. C., & Wister, A. (2009). Do restricted driver's licenses lower crash risk among older drivers? A survival analysis of insurance data from British Columbia. *The Gerontologist, 49,* 474–484.

National Center for Education Statistics. (1992). *National adult literacy survey.* Washington, DC: U.S. Department of Education.

National Highway Traffic Safety Administration. (2009a). *An examination of driver distraction as recorded in NHTSA databases* (No. DOT-HS-811-216). Washington, DC: National Center for Statistics and Analysis.

National Highway Traffic Safety Administration. (2009b). *Traffic safety facts: Children* (No. DOT-HS-811-387). Washington, DC: National Center for Statistics and Analysis.

National Institute of Neurological Disorders and Stroke. (2011). *NINDS dementia information page.* Retrieved December 14, 2011, from http://www.ninds.nih.gov/disorders/dementias/dementia.htm

Neale, V. L. (2005). *An overview of the 100-Car Naturalistic Study and findings.* Retrieved January 5, 2012, from http://www.nhtsa.gov/DOT/NHTSA/NRD/Multimedia/PDFs/Crash%20Avoidance/Driver%20Distraction/100Car_ESV05summary.pdf

Nerad, J. (2005). *Danger in the streets.* Retrieved January 4, 2012, from http://www.drivers.com/article/839

Neville, O., De Bourdeaudhuij, I., Sugiyama, T., Leslie, E., Cerin, E., Van Dyck, D., et al. (2010). Bicycle use for transport in an Australian and a Belgian city: Associations with built-environment attributes. *Journal of Urban Health, 87,* 189–198.

Noe, E., Ferri, J., Caballero, M. C., Villodre, R., Sanchez, A., & Chirivella, J. (2005). Self-awareness after acquired brain injury: Predictors and rehabilitation. *Journal of Neurology, 252,* 168–175.

Nys, G. M., van Zandvoort, M. J., de Kort, P. L., Jansen, B. P., de Haan, E. H., & Kappelle, L. J. (2007). Cognitive disorders in acute stroke: Prevalence and clinical determinants. *Cerebrovascular Disorders, 23,* 408–416.

Olsson, R. H., Jr., Wambold, S., Brock, B., Waugh, D., & Sprague, H. (2005). Visual spatial abilities and fall risk: An assessment tool for individuals with dementia. *Journal of Gerontological Nursing, 31*(9), 45–53.

Ondo, W. G., Vuong, K. D., Khan, H., Atassi, F., Kwak, C., & Jankovic, J. (2001). Daytime sleepiness and other sleep disorders in Parkinson's disease. *Neurology, 57,* 1392–1396.

Ott, B. R., Heindel, W. C., Papandonatos, G. D., Festa, E. K., Davis, J. D., Daiello, L. A., et al. (2008). A longitudinal study of drivers with Alzheimer disease. *Neurology, 70,* 1171–1178.

Owsley, C., Ball, K., McGwin, G., Jr., Sloan, M. E., Roenker, D. L., White, M. F., et al. (1998). Visual processing impairment and risk of motor vehicle crash among older adults. *JAMA, 279,* 1083–1088.

Owsley, C., & McGwin, G., Jr. (2010). Vision and driving. *Vision Research, 50,* 2348–2361.

Pearce, J. M. (2005). Hemianopia. *European Neurology, 53,* 111.

Penades, R., Catalan, R., Salamero, M., Boget, T., Puig, O., & Guarch, J. (2006). Cognitive remediation therapy for outpatients with chronic schizophrenia: A controlled and randomized study. *Schizophrenia Research, 87,* 323–331.

Percer, J. (2009). *Child pedestrian safety education: Applying learning and developmental theories to develop safe street-crossing behaviors* (No. DOT-HS-811-190). Washington, DC: National Highway Traffic Safety Administration.

Piras, M. R., Magnano, I., Canu, E. D., Paulus, K., Satta, W., Soddu, A., et al. (2003). Longitudinal study of cognitive dysfunction in multiple sclerosis: Neuropsychological, neuroradiological, and neurophysiologic findings. *Journal of Neurology, Neurosurgery, and Psychiatry, 74,* 878–885.

Prigatano, G. P., & Altman, I. M. (1990). Impaired awareness of behavioral limitations after traumatic brain injury. *Archives of Physical Medicine and Rehabilitation, 71,* 1058–1064.

Ranney, T. A. (2008). *Driver distraction: A review of the current state-of-knowledge* (No. DOT-HS-810-787). Washington, DC: National Highway Traffic Safety Administration.

Reger, M. A., Welsh, R. K., Stennis-Watson, G., Cholerton, B., Baker, L. D., & Craft, S. (2004). The relationship between neuropsychological functioning and driving ability in dementia: A meta-analysis. *Neuropsychology, 18,* 85–91.

Reitan, R. M. (1958). *Trail Making Test: Manual for administration, scoring, and interpretation.* Indianapolis: Indiana University Medical Center.

Rizzo, M., & Kellison, I. L. (2010). The brain on the road. In T. D. M. I. Grant (Ed.), *Neuropsychology of everyday functioning* (pp. 168–208). New York: Guilford Press.

Robertson, I. H., Ridgeway, V., Greenfield, E., & Parr, A. (1997). Motor recovery after stroke depends on intact sustained attention: A 2-year follow-up study. *Neuropsychology, 11,* 290–295.

Rolls, E. T., Hornak, J., Wade, D., & McGrath, J. (1994). Emotion-related learning in patients with social and emotional changes associated with frontal lobe damage. *Journal of Neurology, Neurosurgery, and Psychiatry, 57,* 1518–1524.

Roth, E. J., & Harvey, R. L. (2000). Rehabilitation of stroke symptoms. In R. L. Braddom (Ed.), *Physical medicine and rehabilitation* (2nd ed., pp. 1117–1160). Philadelphia: Saunders.

Safe Kids USA. (2009). *Car seats, booster, and seat belt safety fact sheet.* Retrieved March 11, 2011, from http://www.safekids.org/our-work/research/fact-sheets/car-seats-booster-and-belt-safety-fact-sheet.html

Schultheis, M. T., Weisser, V., Ang, J., Elovic, E., Nead, R., Sestito, N., et al. (2010). Examining the relationship between cognition and driving performance in multiple sclerosis. *Archives of Physical Medicine and Rehabilitation, 91,* 465–473.

Staplin, L., Gish, K. W., & Wagner, E. K. (2003). MaryPODS revisited: Updated crash analysis and implications for screening program implementation. *Journal of Safety Research, 34,* 389–397.

Stavrinos, D., Byington, K. W., & Schwebel, D. C. (2009). Effect of cell phone distraction on pediatric pedestrian injury risk. *Pediatrics, 123,* 179–185.

Stolwyk, R. J., Charlton, J. L., Triggs, T. J., Iansek, R., & Bradshaw, J. L. (2006). Neuropsychological function and driving ability in people with Parkinson's disease. *Journal of Clinical and Experimental Neuropsychology, 28,* 898–913.

Stuss, D. T., & Anderson, V. (2004). The frontal lobes and theory of mind: Developmental concepts from adult focal lesion research. *Brain Cognition, 55,* 69–83.

Stuss, D. T., Gow, C. A., & Hetherington, C. R. (1992). "No longer Gage": Frontal lobe dysfunction and emotional changes. *Journal of Consulting and Clinical Psychology, 60,* 349–359.

Stutts, J. C., Wilkins, J. W., & Vaughn, B. V. (1999). *Why do people have drowsy driving crashes? Input from drivers who just did.* Retrieved January 5, 2012, from http://www.aaafoundation.org/pd/sleep/pdf

Szlyk, J. P., Myers, L., Zhang, Y. X., Wetzel, L., & Shapiro, R. (2002). Development and assessment of a neuropsychological battery to aid in predicting driving performance. *Journal of Rehabilitation Research and Development, 39,* 483–495.

Taylor, B. D., & Tripodes, S. (2001). The effects of driving cessation on the elderly with dementia and their caregivers. *Accident Analysis and Prevention, 35,* 519–528.

Thomson, J. A. (1991). *The facts about child pedestrian accidents.* London: Continuum International.

Thomson, J. A., Tolmie, A., Foot, H. C., & Mclaren, B. (1996). *Child development and the aims of road safety education: A review and analysis.* London: Department of Transport.

Tyree, R. (2006). Medications, disabilities, and driving. In J. M. Pellerito (Ed.), *Driver rehabilitation and community mobility: Principles and practice* (pp. 185–198). St. Louis: Mosby.

Uc, E. Y., Rizzo, M., Anderson, S. W., Sparks, J. D., Rodnitzky, R. L., & Dawson, J. D. (2007). Impaired navigation in drivers with Parkinson's disease. *Brain: A Journal of Neurology, 130,* 2433–2440.

Uc, E. Y., Rizzo, M., Johnson, A. M., Dastrup, E., Anderson, S. W., & Dawson, J. D. (2009). Road safety in drivers with Parkinson disease. *Neurology, 73,* 2112–2119.

Van Zomeran, A. H., Brouwer, W. H., & Minderhoud, J. M. (1987). Acquired brain damage and driving: A review. *Archives of Physical Medicine and Rehabilitation, 68,* 697–705.

Wang, C., & Carr, D. B. (2004). Older driver safety: A report from the Older Drivers Project. *Journal of the American Geriatrics Society, 52,* 143–149.

Wang, J.-S., Knipling, R. R., & Goodman, M. J. (1996). *The role of driver inattention in crashes: New statistics from the 1995 Crashworthiness Data System.* Retrieved January 5, 2012, from http://www-nrd.nhtsa.dot.gov/departments/Human%20Factors/driver-distraction/PDF/Wang.PDF

Warshawsky-Livne, L., & Shinar, D. (2002). Effects of uncertainty, transmission type, driver age and gender on brake reaction and movement time. *Journal of Safety Research, 33,* 117–128.

Wegner, M. V., & Girasek, D. C. (2003). How readable are child safety seat installation instructions? *Pediatrics, 111,* 588–591.

Whelihan, W. M., DiCarlo, M. A., & Paul, R. H. (2005). The relationship of neuropsychological functioning to driving competence in older persons with early cognitive decline. *Archives of Clinical Neuropsychology, 20,* 217–228.

Wierda, M., & Brookhuis, K. A. (1991). Analysis of cycling skills: A cognitive approach. *Applied Cognitive Psychology, 5,* 113–122.

Withaar, F. K., Brouwer, W. H., & Van Zomeran, A. H. (2000). Fitness to drive in older drivers with cognitive impairment. *Journal of the International Neuropsychological Society, 6,* 480–490.

Wood, J. M., Worringham, C., Kerr, G., Mallon, K., & Silburn, P. (2005). Quantitative assessment of driving performance in Parkinson's disease. *Journal of Neurology, Neurosurgery, and Psychiatry, 76,* 176–180.

Zoltan, B. (2007). *Vision, perception, and cognition* (4th ed.). Thorofare, NJ: Slack.

CHAPTER 8

Vision and Driving

Jennifer Elgin, OTR/L, CDRS; Cynthia Owsley, PhD, MSPH; and Sherrilene Classen, PhD, MPH, OTR/L, FAOTA

Learning Objectives

At the completion of this chapter, readers will be able to

- Recognize the importance of occupational therapists knowing state regulations regarding visual requirements for driving and identify where to locate these regulations;
- Delineate the relevance of vision rehabilitation in relation to driving and the roles and responsibilities of the interdisciplinary vision rehabilitation professional in relation to driving;
- Identify the evidence base of the visual abilities, skills, and function that have been related to safe driving performance and the visual disorders and conditions that have been related to unsafe driving performance;
- Identify the screening procedures as well as the standard clinical assessments, their uses, and the evidence supporting them, as commonly used by occupational therapists in evaluating vision skills, abilities, and function underlying driving performance;
- Recognize the importance of the elements of the comprehensive driving evaluation that are specifically tailored to assessing visually impaired driving from the perspective of a driver rehabilitation specialist specializing in driving and vision issues;
- Identify the outcomes of comprehensive driving evaluation vision rehabilitation interventions and strategies, the evidence supporting the success of these interventions, and the prognosis for successful rehabilitation as these pertain to a variety of visual conditions, from the perspective of a driver rehabilitation specialist specializing in driving and vision issues;
- Delineate the outcome of the rehabilitation process and the available options if driving is no longer possible; and

Key Words

- **age-related macular degeneration**
- **bioptic telescope system**
- **cataract**
- **contrast sensitivity**
- **diabetic retinopathy**
- **disability glare**
- **glaucoma**
- **monocularity**
- **stereoacuity**
- **vision standard**
- **visual acuity**
- **visual field**
- **visual processing speed**

- Identify surgical and medical interventions that may be performed to improve vision and the advances in ophthalmology made in recent years and how these may affect the return to driving.

Introduction

Driving is inarguably a highly visual task. The visual demands of driving are intricate. Controlling a vehicle takes place in a visually cluttered environment and involves the simultaneous use of central and peripheral vision and the execution of primary and secondary tasks (both visual and nonvisual). As the vehicle moves through the environment, the visual world is rapidly changing. The driver often is uncertain as to when and where a critical (and often potentially dangerous) visual event will occur (e.g., vehicle entering roadway, pedestrian walking on roadside, unexpected traffic congestion, traffic light turning from green to yellow).

Visual sensory abilities, such as visual acuity, contrast sensitivity, and light sensitivity throughout the visual field, are important in the detection, discrimination, recognition, and identification of objects and events during driving. Yet by themselves, visual sensory abilities are not exclusively sufficient for understanding the role of vision in driving. Other types of visual skills, such as divided attention, visual processing speed, motion perception, and visual search and scanning abilities, are also critical to driving performance.

Regulatory and Ethical Issues

When applying for a driver's license in most jurisdictions around the world, a visual acuity screening test is used to identify candidates who meet some minimum level of visual acuity, which is often called the jurisdiction's *vision standard*. The purpose of this screening test is to ensure that licensed drivers have a prespecified level of vision (or better) and to screen out applicants who have poor vision (i.e., vision that is not good enough to meet the standard). There is a wide range of visual acuity standards across U.S. states and in other countries, but most fall into the range of 20/30 to 20/60 visual acuity as measured by a letter identification chart (American Association of Motor Vehicle Administrators, 2006; American Medical Association, 2003; Peli & Peli, 2002).

Some jurisdictions measure visual acuity in both eyes when used together, and others measure it for each eye separately. If drivers do not meet the standard, in some jurisdictions they are denied licensure outright. However, in other jurisdictions, there is an opportunity to go through additional screening or road tests to demonstrate good visual or driving skills. In still other jurisdictions, there is an opportunity to obtain a letter from an ophthalmologist or optometrist stating that the vision impairment is not a threat to driver safety, and on the basis of this letter, the jurisdiction may allow licensure. Thus, it is important to understand that there are wide variations in vision screening policies throughout the United States and the world.

For this reason, occupational therapists working in the area of driving evaluation and rehabilitation need to understand the laws and policies of the jurisdictions in which they practice and in which their clients live and may want to drive. They can obtain this information from the governmental agency that manages driver licensing in that jurisdiction. These state-based agencies have a variety of names in the United States (e.g., Department of Motor Vehicles, Motor Vehicle Administration, Department of Public Safety), but regardless of name, this information is publicly available through the state government. Most U.S. states now have Web sites that provide this information for easy access by the public and health care providers.

Screening and Rescreening

In essentially all jurisdictions in the United States and many other countries, visual acuity screening takes place when one initially applies for a license, usually when one is a young adult or teenager. In many but not all jurisdictions, visual acuity is periodically rescreened when applying for license renewal (Grabowski & Morrisey, 2001). The states that have rescreening programs vary widely in the organization and implementation of these programs (e.g., age at which rescreening is implemented, how many years between rescreening).

It is also important to point out that some U.S. states do not have any rescreening policies. That is, once visual acuity is screened as part of the initial license application (usually when one is young), it is not screened again by the license office unless a physician or other health care provider brings an impairment or medical condition to the licensing office's attention.

Once again, occupational therapists need to understand whether their jurisdictions have rescreening policies and, if so, what they are. If practicing in a state that has no rescreening policy, or a policy that does not screen drivers until they reach a very advanced age, the occupational therapist who is managing the care of a person with significant vision impairment needs to recognize that the licensing office will have no way of knowing that the person's visual acuity has dropped below the vision standard unless a health care provider (or other person such as a family member or neighbor) reports the person to the licensing authority.

Screening brings us to the issue of reporting persons with medical conditions or functional impairments to the jurisdiction's licensing authority. In states that have a medical advisory board, the board typically works closely with the licensing office to address these cases. Some states have mandatory reporting laws that specify that a health care provider must report patients or clients who have medical conditions or functional impairments that could threaten safe driving; some states have mandatory reporting laws for specific medical conditions only, not just any medical condition. Other states encourage or allow for voluntary reporting from health care providers but do not mandate it. It is important for occupational therapists to know the laws and policies of the states in which they practice.

Whether health care providers should report patients or clients who have vision impairment that could threaten safe driving to the licensing authority is viewed as somewhat controversial among some health care communities. Some professionals have cited reporting as a violation of a patient's privacy rights and a potential breach of health care provider–patient confidentiality (see Chapter 5). Others have argued that one must balance the mobility needs and privacy rights of the client against the need to maintain public safety, that is, protecting the public from drivers with visual impairment who could cause injury or death on the road because of impaired driving skills. Some states have enacted laws to protect health care providers, who may report drivers with medical conditions such as vision impairment that pose a threat to driver safety, from litigation that is based on a purported violation of health care privacy laws. The American Occupational Therapy Association (AOTA) does not have an official policy on reporting but encourages therapists to be knowledgeable of their state laws and practice and to act accordingly.

Most jurisdictions also have what is termed a *visual field standard*, which is usually expressed as some minimum extent of vision across the horizontal or vertical visual field or both.

Most jurisdictions also have what is termed a *visual field standard,* which is usually expressed as some minimum extent of vision across the horizontal or vertical visual field or both. Extent is usually expressed in degrees of visual angle from fixation or through fixation from one side of the field to the other. Some jurisdictions have specific policies about the field extent when both eyes are open (the binocular field), whereas others are silent or not specific about this issue. Another challenge in interpreting the visual field standard provided by licensing policies is that there are many methodologies for measuring visual field extent, and what method is used will influence screening test results.

Regardless of potential confusions in interpreting the visual field standard, occupational therapists should familiarize themselves with the visual field standard in the jurisdiction in which they practice. Whenever there are perceived ambiguities in the definition of the visual field standard or in the appropriate screening methods, therapists should address any questions to the head administrator in the jurisdiction's licensing office or medical advisory board.

Color vision is tested when one applies for a personal license in more than 40 U.S. states. In addition, the ability to respond properly to color traffic signals is a requirement for a commercial vehicle license in the United States (Decina, Breton, & Staplin, 1991). The reason for testing color vision in both personal and commercial licensing is not because it is widely held that color vision deficiency elevates the risk for crash involvement but rather, to ensure that drivers can obey color traffic control devices and other color signals on the road (e.g., taillights; Heath & Schmidt, 1959).

Multidisciplinary Approach

In providing driving evaluation and rehabilitation services to clients with visual impairment, occupational therapists work closely with ophthalmologists, optometrists, and other vision rehabilitation professionals who refer clients to them. Ophthalmologists and optometrists provide key information about ocular diagnosis, treatment history, and prognosis, including whether the eye condition and vision impairment are likely to be progressive as opposed to stable. In addition, their examination notes will offer important information about the client's visual sensory status (e.g., visual acuity, visual field sensitivity).

Ophthalmologists, optometrists, and vision rehabilitation specialists will provide some people with visual impairment with assistive devices such as magnifiers or telescopes to facilitate the use of their residual vision. In particular, vision rehabilitation specialists may have already worked with the client in developing strategies and accommodations to perform the visual activities of daily living (ADLs), other than driving. These professionals can provide valuable insights to the occupational therapist who may focus on driving assessment and rehabilitation.

For persons with visual impairment, often the very first conversation they have about driving fitness is with their ophthalmologist or optometrist, and thus many patients with visual impairment will want their eye care specialist to continue to participate in the driving conversation. Neurologists and neurosurgeons treat patients with visual impairments that arise from brain injury (e.g., stroke, trauma, tumor) and also may refer a client to occupational therapy for a comprehensive driving evaluation (CDE).

Although internists and family physicians do not focus on vision care per se, they manage the overall health of the patient, which includes eye health, and it is not uncommon for these providers to suggest a CDE or rehabilitation for patients with vision impairment. Internists and family physicians are often very familiar with the client as well as the family, given longstanding doctor–patient relationships, and can assist in facilitating a patient's acceptance of the occupational therapist's recommendation regarding driving.

For occupational therapists providing driving evaluation and rehabilitation services, the care plan will benefit greatly from a multidisciplinary approach, drawing on the broad expertise of the physicians (e.g., ophthalmologists, neurologists, internists, family physicians), optometrists, other rehabilitation specialists, and other health care providers who participate in the care of the client's vision issues and functional task performance.

Vision Impairment and Driver Safety and Performance

Many types of vision impairment exist, but this chapter focuses on those that are most commonly encountered by occupational therapists providing driving evaluation and rehabilitation services and that also present the most often mentioned functional ramifications of visual pathway diseases and conditions. Many medical conditions and diseases can cause vision impairment. In older adult drivers, the most common include cataract, age-related macular degeneration (AMD), glaucoma, diabetic retinopathy (DR), and brain injury resulting from cerebral vascular accident (CVA) or stroke.

Most conditions cause several types of vision impairment. For example, cataract causes decreased acuity and contrast sensitivity, increased glare problems, and depressed light sensitivity throughout the visual field. Glaucoma causes peripheral visual field loss but in its later stages also can cause visual acuity and contrast sensitivity impairment in central vision.

Although these conditions can occur at any age, they are relatively uncommon in young adults. Common causes of vision impairments in young adults include retinal degenerations (e.g., Stargardt's disease, retinitis pigmentosa, photoreceptor dystrophies), ocular albinism, albinism, optic atrophy, optic nerve hypoplasia, and injury. *Nystagmus* (rapid, involuntary, repetitive eye movements) is often a feature of visual disorders that are congenital or emerge early in development.

For persons with any of these medical conditions, the functional manifestation of vision impairment varies widely, with some individuals with the condition having minor visual deficits and others having moderate or severe deficits. Thus, it is important not to conclude that just because a driver has one of these eye conditions, his or her vision impairment necessarily hampers driving. First, the visual impairment may be minor to moderate and not reach the threshold at which it interferes with task performance during driving. Second, the driver may have developed compensatory strategies that offset how the impairment affects performance.

Visual Acuity

Visual acuity, the ability to resolve detail, is the ubiquitous visual screening test used by licensing agencies for the determination of driving fitness. The use of visual acuity screening for initial and periodic relicensure for driving has face validity. It is the choice of ophthalmologists and optometrists when assessing the integrity and health of the visual system and is the primary visual function evaluated during a CDE. In addition, road signs in the United States are designed on the basis of sight distances assuming that drivers have at least 20/30 binocular visual acuity (Federal Highway Administration, 2003). Drivers with acuity worse than that level are likely to have difficulty reading highway signage (e.g., speed limit signs, stop signs, exit signs on the interstate) at distances deemed safe for making vehicle control decisions (e.g., lane changes, turns, exiting; Schieber, 2004). Thus, requiring that licensed drivers have visual acuity at the 20/30 level or better enhances the likelihood that drivers can read highway signs well in advance of the time they need to make decisions and execute motor responses.

However, many drivers with visual impairment are likely to restrict their driving to highly familiar routes where the roadway characteristics and the signage along the way are well known. On one hand, there may be no serious safety threat from a driver in this scenario—with 20/80 visual acuity, for example—in depending on the signage and the detailed features of the road, because the route is very familiar. On the other hand, this driver may be less likely to identify a new sign well in advance to act upon it or may have problems seeing small obstacles in the road (Higgins, Wood, & Tait, 1998).

Visual Acuity and Collision Risk

Most research has indicated that impairments in visual acuity are not related to motor vehicle collision involvement, and of those studies that have found associations between acuity and collision involvement, these associations are very weak (Charman, 1997; Owsley & McGwin, 1999, 2010). Therefore, visual acuity testing is a very poor screening test for identifying drivers who are likely to crash in subsequent years. Although these visual acuity screening tests will ensure that drivers can identify signage at safe stopping distances, they will not ensure that an individual is a safe driver from a visual standpoint.

It is useful to consider why visual acuity screening tests are not related to crash risk. Visual acuity–related driving skills (e.g., sign recognition) may not be crucial to the safe operation of a vehicle in most on-road circumstances. Reading signage may be important for route planning, but it may not be critical for collision avoidance.

Another consideration is that visual acuity testing does not measure the visual skills most critical for the safe operation of a motor vehicle. Visual acuity tests were originally designed for the clinical diagnosis and monitoring of eye disease and do not by themselves reflect the visual complexity of the driving task. Guiding a vehicle along a roadway and through intersections involves the simultaneous use of central and peripheral vision and primary and secondary task demands, all in the midst of a visually cluttered environment in which critical events occur with little or no advance warning. Visual acuity screening tests generally do not include these stimulus features and in fact seek to minimize distractions and secondary task demands. Acuity is typically evaluated under high-contrast and luminance conditions, whereas driving encompasses wide-ranging contrast and luminance levels.

Finally, stationary visual acuity test targets do not represent the motion-based driving environment. It is possible that drivers with severe visual acuity impairment have simply been removed from the road, which would be particularly true in states that require vision rescreening at the time of license renewal. A related issue is the fact that drivers with vision impairment may voluntarily restrict or stop driving (Ball et al., 1998; Freeman, Munoz, Turano, & West, 2006).

It is important to know a client's visual acuity. First, visual acuity testing indicates whether the client is likely to meet the jurisdiction's vision standard. Second, it indicates whether he or she will likely be able to read signage at a safe stopping distances. Third, it reveals whether the client will be successful at small road hazard avoidance. However, simply knowing a client's visual acuity will not help one to understand his or her motor vehicle collision risk unless the visual acuity impairment is so severe (e.g., 20/500) that safe driving is out of the question on common-sense grounds. Assessment, intervention, and implications of the impact of acuity impairments are discussed further in later sections of this chapter.

Visual Field (Peripheral Vision)

Research has suggested that serious visual field impairment elevates motor vehicle collision risk, yet little is known about how severe the field loss has to be and what areas of the visual field need to be impaired for field loss to threaten driver safety. One often-quoted study on California drivers reported that drivers with severe binocular field loss (i.e., field loss in both eyes) had significantly raised motor vehicle collision and violation rates compared with those without any loss (Johnson & Keltner, 1983). A similar finding was reported in a study on Maryland drivers (Rubin et al., 1999).

Two studies on drivers with glaucoma (which causes peripheral vision impairment) who had at least moderate to severe vision impairment indicated that those drivers were more likely to be involved in collisions than those who had normal visual fields or minor impairment (Haymes, LeBlanc, Nicolela, Chiasson, & Chauhan, 2007; McGwin et al., 2005). However, not all studies have shown an association between visual field impairment and motor vehicle collision involvement (Owsley & McGwin, 2010). Thus, much remains unknown and is deserving of further research. Studies on driving performance in which visual field restriction was simulated with occluding goggles have suggested that visual field impairment compromises some aspects of driving performance (e.g., identification of road signs, avoidance of obstacles, reaction time) but not other aspects of driving performance (e.g., speed estimation, stopping distance; Wood, Dique, & Troutbeck, 1993; Wood & Troutbeck, 1992).

Despite these observations that drivers with visual field defects exhibit impaired driving performance in some maneuvers, a cautionary remark must be made that large individual differences exist in which some drivers with such impairments may have no more of an on-road performance problem than drivers with normal sight (Bowers, Peli, Elgin, McGwin, & Owsley, 2005; Elgin et al., 2010; Racette & Casson, 2005; Wood et al., 2009). For example, homonymous hemianopia is a severe visual-field defect occurring when field loss is evident in the same relative position in visual space in each eye. This condition results from postchiasmal damage to the visual pathways, with the most common etiology being stroke and other causes including traumatic brain injury (TBI) and tumor. When the homonymous defect occurs in one-half of the visual field, it is called *homonymous hemianopia;* when it occurs in one quadrant of the visual field, the defect is called *homonymous quadrantanopia.*

Individuals with hemianopic or quadrantanopic field defects, regardless of the cause or prognosis, are considered unsafe to drive in many jurisdictions around the world and are prohibited from licensure. However, there is little to no evidence to support this policy. Research recently showed that some drivers with hemianopia and quadrantanopia have on-road driving skills that are indistinguishable from drivers of the same age who have normal visual fields (Elgin et al., 2010; Wood et al., 2009). The study also found that what distinguishes good drivers with hemianopia and quadrantanopia from those with impaired driving skills is that the good drivers appear to compensate by making more head and eye movements toward the blind side of their visual field (Wood et al., 2011). They also have more stable lane-keeping skills and fewer sudden braking episodes.

Because there is such wide variability in driving skills in individuals with significant visual field impairment such as hemianopia and quadrantanopia, individual assessments of driving skills are recommended rather than the denial of driving licensure. It is also worth pointing out that some clients with hemianopia and quadrantanopia and impaired driving performance may not have insight into their problems on the road (Parker et al., 2011). In essence, Parker et al. (2011) showed that there can be drivers with hemianopia with serious driving performance problems who do not report such problems when asked whether they have any difficulty with various driving situations.

Therefore, it remains the responsibility of the occupational therapist to take the client factors (e.g., presence or absence of self-awareness as it relates to hemianopia) and how they affect driving into consideration. This information can be solicited via an interview with the client, talking with stakeholders (e.g., a family member), or a discussion group on the effects of hemianopia on driving. If the occupational therapist notes that self-awareness may be lacking, client or family education must be pursued.

Contrast Sensitivity

At press time, spatial contrast sensitivity is not currently used as a licensing requirement in any U.S. state. *Contrast* is a physical dimension referring to the light–dark transition (or difference) at a border or an edge of an image that delineates the existence of a pattern or object (Owsley, 2003). The amount of contrast a person needs to see an object is called *contrast threshold*. In clinical care and clinical research settings, contrast threshold is usually expressed as contrast sensitivity, in which sensitivity is simply the reciprocal of threshold. Thus, persons with low thresholds are said to have high sensitivity and those with high thresholds to have low sensitivity.

In an assessment of contrast sensitivity as a screening test at licensure renewals in California, those who failed the screening test were more likely to incur future crashes than those who passed (Hennessy, 1995; Hennessy & Janke, 2009). Contrast sensitivity deficits are common in older adults with cataract. Research has indicated that for older drivers with clinically significant cataract, contrast sensitivity impairment was strongly associated with a recent crash history (Owsley, Stalvey, Wells, Sloane, & McGwin, 2001). The association was twice as strong when both eyes were impaired than when only one eye was impaired. Furthermore, the researchers found that cataract surgery and intraocular lens (IOL) insertion in this same cohort (which improved their vision) reduced their risk of future crash involvement by 50% compared with those in the cohort who did not elect cataract surgery (Owsley et al., 2002).

In terms of driving performance, research has further shown that for older drivers with cataract, cataract surgery improves driving performance, an effect that is mediated by improvement in contrast sensitivity after surgery (Wood & Carberry, 2004, 2006). These driving performance results parallel the driver safety benefits (e.g., reduced crash rate) of cataract surgery described in the previous paragraph. Further evidence supporting the key role of contrast sensitivity in driving performance comes from both on-road and simulator studies of drivers with Parkinson's disease (PD), which also can cause contrast sensitivity impairment (Amick, Grace, & Ott, 2007; Classen et al., 2009, 2011; Uc, Rizzo, Anderson, et al., 2009; Uc, Rizzo, Johnson, et al., 2009; Worringham, Wood, Kerr, & Silburn, 2006).

Visual Processing Speed and Divided Attention

Slowing in the processing of visual information, in which especially in a situation where one must divide attention between two or more tasks, is one of the strongest risk factors for unsafe driving (i.e., increased risk of crash involvement) in older drivers (Owsley et al., 1998). The Useful Field of View (UFOV®) task is a method for measuring visual processing speed under divided-attention conditions (Ball, Edwards, & Ross, 2007; Edwards et al., 2005, 2006). The UFOV task estimates the minimum target duration needed by an observer to detect or discriminate targets presented in central vision, while localizing a simultaneously presented peripheral target (Figure 8.1).

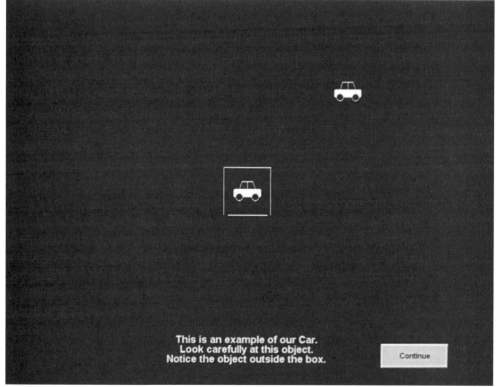

Figure 8.1. Task 2 of the Useful Field of View.

Note. Provided by Visual Awareness Research Group, Inc., Hoover, AL. Used with permission.

The association between slowed visual processing speed and crash involvement has been shown to be independent of other factors that elevate crash risk (e.g., visual sensory impairment, medical comorbidities, cognitive status) and is the strongest visual risk factor for crash involvement in older drivers in population-based studies (Cross et al., 2009; Owsley et al., 1998; Rubin et al., 1999). These research findings have prompted several jurisdictions to examine the feasibility of using a processing speed, divided-attention task as a way to screen older drivers when they apply for routine relicensure (Ball et al., 2006; Hennessy & Janke, 2009). These studies on the UFOV have implied that visual attention and visual processing speed are critical considerations in the evaluation of safe driving skills and may be better screening tests than visual sensory tests (e.g., visual acuity) for identifying crash-prone older drivers.

Visual processing speed and divided attention have also been associated with driving performance problems on the road. When evaluated on a closed-road course, those older drivers with divided-attention deficits were less likely to detect and recognize signs and pedestrians and needed more time to complete the course (Wood et al., 1993). In a study on drivers with hemianopia or quadrantanopia, those who exhibited slowed visual processing speed in a divided-attention task were rated as having vehicle control problems by trained back-seat evaluators masked to the driver health and functional characteristics (Wood et al., 2009).

Several studies have shown that drivers seen at rehabilitation clinics because of dementia (e.g., Alzheimer's disease [AD]) or brain injury (stroke) were at higher risk of failing an on-road driving test administered by a driver rehabilitation specialist (DRS) if they performed poorly on the UFOV test (Classen et al., 2009, 2011; Cushman, 1996; Duchek, Hunt, Ball, Buckles, & Morris, 1998; Edwards et al., 2006; Mazer, Korner-Bitensky, & Sofer, 1998; Myers, Ball, Kalina, Roth, & Goode, 2000). (*Please note:* The studies listed here have used the UFOV in different ways. Some have used the UFOV Subtest 2 only, whereas others have reported on each individual UFOV subtest score. Readers are referred to the studies referenced earlier to make further determinations of which score of the UFOV was used to make predictions.)

Monocularity

A question that arises when discussing vision and driving is whether one needs two eyes to drive. Two eyes provide for a wider visual field than a single eye, are necessary for stereoscopic depth perception, and also make possible binocular summation (the increased visual sensitivity of the visual system when using two eyes as opposed to one). The definition of *monocularity* varies widely in research on monocular drivers, ranging from denoting a total absence of function in one eye to one eye having impaired vision below some cut-point with respect to some aspect of visual function (usually visual acuity).

Research on the safety and performance of drivers with monocularity is largely devoted to studies on commercial drivers (e.g., truck, delivery vehicle, taxi, bus). With respect to drivers of personal vehicles, most jurisdictions visually screen drivers on both eyes or consider only the better-seeing eye when persons apply for licensure. Thus, the question of licensure of monocular individuals for personal driving may not practically arise very often because many jurisdictions screen acuity with both eyes together (thus they would never know if the person was monocular).

There appears to be widespread acceptance that one eye is sufficient for safe driving of a personal vehicle because research has never proven otherwise. However, in the United States, interstate truck drivers must have visual acuity of 20/40 or better in each eye, which has stimulated research examining whether requiring good acuity in both eyes for interstate truck drivers is really supported by data.

For example, a study in California (Roger, Ratz, & Janke, 1987) examined the 2-year crash and conviction rates of thousands of heavy-vehicle operators, including a subgroup of drivers who had visual impairments. Drivers with visual impairments (those with 20/40 visual acuity or worse in the worse eye) had significantly more total crashes and convictions than did drivers without impairments. Driving exposure did not differ in the two groups.

However, another study examined the visual and driving performances of monocular and binocular commercial drivers and found no differences with respect to visual search, lane placement, clearance judgment, gap judgment, hazard detection, and information recognition (McKnight, Shinar, & Hilburn, 1991). Drivers with monocularity were less adept than drivers with binocularity in sign-reading distance in both daytime and nighttime driving, which is consistent with what is known about *binocular summation* (input from two eyes is better than from either eye alone when the two eyes have similar vision) and *binocular inhibition* (when the vision in one eye is much worse than the other, the vision with both eyes is worse than the better-seeing eye). The authors concluded that although drivers with monocularity have some reductions in certain driving functions compared with drivers with binocularity, differences in the performance of most day-to-day driving functions were not apparent. A limitation of this study is that the definitions of monocular versus binocular drivers were not clearly stated.

The importance of good vision in both eyes for commercial drivers of heavy trucks also may be called into question by a study (Maag, Vanasse, Dionne, & Laberge-Nadeau, 1997) of commercial vehicle drivers who received waivers of the federal vision requirements (Federal Highway Administration, 1996), that is, the waiver allowed for drivers who had worse than 20/40 visual acuity in one or both eyes. The severity of the vision impairment, and the extent to which it involved both eyes and a single eye, was not described in the report. The crash rates of drivers in the waiver program as of 1995, adjusted for self-reported miles traveled, were compared with the crash rates of heavy trucks provided by the 1994 General Estimates System of the National Highway Traffic Safety Administration. The waiver group's crash rate was not higher than that of the national reference group, nor were the waiver group's crashes more severe (Maag et al., 1997).

Caution is needed in generalizing the results of studies on commercial drivers to drivers of personal vehicles. Commercial drivers have very high levels of driving exposure compared with noncommercial drivers of personal vehicles because they are on the road almost continuously during their workday, logging more miles per day than many drivers of personal vehicles cover in a week. Routes routinely involve traffic congestion, multiple stops, parking, and back-up maneuvers. The visual challenges of commercial driving are arguably more intense than those of personal-use driving, and the visual requirements for commercial driving may not be wholly transferrable to personal driving.

Other Aspects of Vision

With respect to *stereoacuity* (depth cues made available through binocular vision), several studies on commercial drivers have reported that commercial motor vehicle drivers with impaired stereoacuity were at elevated risk for motor vehicle collisions (Maag et al., 1997), or once in a crash, their crashes tended to be more severe (as measured by the total number of crash-related victims) than those of drivers who had normal stereoacuity (Dionne, Desjardins, Laberge-Nadeau, & Maag, 1995; Laberge-Nadeau et al., 1996). As mentioned earlier, studies on commercial drivers may not be generalizable to drivers of personal vehicles because the former have very high driving exposure under often dense traffic conditions. Large studies on older drivers that examined deficits in stereoacuity as a risk factor for future motor vehicle collision involvement found no association (Owsley et al., 1998; Rubin et al., 1999). Stereoacuity may be more relevant for the driver's interactions with the dashboard (e.g., seeing controls or gauges) than for understanding crash risk. In general, the impact of binocular-vision disorders on driving has not been comprehensively addressed in research to date.

Research has confirmed that drivers with color deficiencies have longer reaction times to traffic control devices with color signals and are also likely to make more color confusions than persons with normal color vision (Atchison, Pendersen, Dain, & Wood, 2003; Vingrys & Cole, 1988). However, in naturalistic driving, the critical cues on the road typically can be obtained through multiple sources of information (e.g., luminance, position, pattern). Thus, it is not surprising that the literature has largely supported no link between color deficiencies and vehicle crash involvement (Atchison et al., 2003; Vingrys & Cole, 1988).

It is also important to emphasize that most drivers with color deficiency are not color blind; rather, they have a reduced ability to discriminate color. Because of the overwhelming wealth of evidence, it is reasonable to conclude that color vision deficiency by itself does not increase crash risk in personal or commercial drivers, although in some circumstances it may affect the performance of interpreting traffic control devices and other color-coded signals if other cues (e.g., luminance, position, pattern) are not sufficiently informative.

Motion perception has a great deal of face validity to the driving task because the vehicle, and thus the driver, is moving through the roadway environment. There has been little research on how impairments in motion processing may affect driving performance and safety. Researchers found that older drivers with elevated motion thresholds had difficulties in detecting signs and hazards and took longer to complete the course (Wood, 2002), and they had worse performance evaluations as assessed by raters specialized in on-road evaluation (Wood, Anstey, Kerr, Lacherez, & Lord, 2008). For older adults with AD, impairment in motion thresholds was a strong predictor of collisions in the driving simulator (Rizzo, Reinach, McGehee, & Dawson, 1997). Research has not linked motion perception to increased crash risk on the road.

Disability glare, an increased sensitivity to glare, has been discussed as a serious threat to the safety of older drivers, but studies have not confirmed this notion (Ball, Owsley, Sloane, Roenker, & Bruni, 1993; Owsley et al., 1998, 2001). This failure to find an association between glare and road safety may be attributed to methodological difficulties in defining *glare* and in measuring a complex phenomenon (e.g., discomfort glare, disability glare) as well as to a poor understanding of what people mean when they say they have glare problems.

Occupational Therapy Clinical Evaluation and Treatment of Visual Function

Occupational therapists involved in traditional clinical practice have an important role to play in identifying declines or limitations in the visual functioning of a client. If an occupational therapist identifies a visual deficit and the client is driving, the next step may be to refer the client to a DRS for further evaluation. If the client is not actively driving, a similar referral may be solicited to ensure that the client has a comprehensive community mobility plan developed.

Because driving is a highly visual task, vision screening conducted as an essential component of any generalist's clinical evaluation may flag the at-risk driver in need of further evaluation. Vision screening conducted during a CDE often includes tests for distance acuity, contrast sensitivity, visual fields, depth perception, and visual processing speed regardless of diagnosis or the reason for referral. Occupational therapists involved in driver evaluation should have a good understanding of visual function and its relationship to driving (see the overview provided earlier and in Owsley & McGwin, 2010).

Clients may be referred to the occupational therapist generalist and the DRS from sources other than eye care providers. Such professionals may include primary care physicians, internists, neurologists, neurosurgeons, and vocational rehabilitation counselors, and thus the client may not have had a recent comprehensive eye examination. For example, a visual field assessment performed by the occupational therapist during a driving assessment may reveal previously unidentified vision impairment, such as homonymous hemianopia or quadrantanopia. Whenever the occupational therapist identifies visual dysfunction that is not discussed or mentioned in referral chart notes, the client should be referred to an ophthalmologist or optometrist for diagnostic follow-up.

The purpose of an in-clinic evaluation is to conduct a battery of visual, cognitive, and motor assessments to screen for functional abilities important to safe driving. This evaluation is a critical part of a CDE because it provides information needed to make decisions about the client's readiness to perform the on-road evaluation. For example, when a client is referred for a CDE after a TBI, stroke, or other type of brain injury, and the scores on the in-clinic evaluation indicate the client is at significant risk for a crash, the on-road assessment should not be completed until the client undergoes additional rehabilitation and improvement in functional abilities important for safe driving. This point may be debated by some who believe that every client referred for a driving evaluation should receive an on-road evaluation, but the safety of the occupational therapist, client, and other road users must take priority, postponing the on-road evaluation if necessary.

Because of the progressive nature of their conditions, rehabilitation of essential skills for driving may not be an option for patients who have been diagnosed with a progressive, neurodegenerative disease affecting visual and cognitive functions (e.g., AD, PD, or Huntington's disease), especially if their scores on in-clinic screening assessments indicate that they are at high risk for motor vehicle collision

Because of the progressive nature of their conditions, rehabilitation of essential skills for driving may not be an option for patients who have been diagnosed.

involvement. For some clients, driving cessation and community mobility alternatives should be discussed without requiring an on-road evaluation.

Evidence-based clinical assessments are a necessary part of the CDE because they provide the occupational therapist with crucial information about client factors. The occupational therapist combines these data with information on the client's medical conditions, comorbidities, medication use, driving habits, crash history, and functional abilities and then makes a decision about whether an on-road evaluation is appropriate.

Assessment of Visual Acuity

As explained earlier in this chapter, there is no strong evidence linking visual acuity and motor vehicle collisions; nevertheless, visual acuity must be included in evaluations because nearly all jurisdictions have licensing requirements that specify that visual acuity can be no worse than a certain level to be eligible for licensure.

Distance acuity, a component of visual acuity, can be measured with many different apparatuses. The familiar acuity chart, often called the *Snellen chart* (Precision Vision, LaSalle, IL), is probably the most recognized eye chart, with the big "E" on the top line, but there are many types of acuity chart designs used in clinics throughout the United States and elsewhere. The Early Treatment of Diabetic Retinopathy Study letter chart (Ferris, Kassoff, Bresnick, & Bailey, 1982) is frequently used to measure distance acuity in clinical research settings, including studies on driving (Precision Vision, LaSalle, IL). When measuring visual acuity for the purposes of a CDE, one should obtain measurements for each eye separately (OD or right eye; OS or left eye) and both eyes together (OU). Acuity charts are available in electronic and wall-mounted formats.

Clients who do not meet the legal visual acuity requirements to drive in their state should not be taken on an on-road evaluation (unless the jurisdiction has given special legal approval for the evaluation). If the client has a diagnosed vision condition that is being monitored by an ophthalmologist or optometrist, a referral for low vision evaluation and potential rehabilitation is appropriate before on-road testing is pursued any further. (Low-vision evaluations typically are conducted by ophthalmologists or optometrists who specialize in low vision assessment and rehabilitation.) The vision rehabilitation specialist may prescribe assistive optical devices to improve the functional performance of the client with visual impairment. If the occupational therapist has a client with vision impairment and without a diagnosis in the medical history or referral notes, a referral for a comprehensive eye exam is necessary to determine the etiology and potential treatment options of the vision impairment.

Assessment of Contrast Sensitivity

It is important to obtain information on the client's contrast sensitivity because research has shown that impaired contrast sensitivity increases crash risk and impairs driving performance (Owsley et al., 2001, 2002; Wood & Carberry, 2006). The Pelli–Robson Contrast Sensitivity test (Pelli, Robson, & Wilkins, 1988) is a commonly used method for measuring contrast sensitivity and consists of a wall-mounted chart. Other contrast sensitivity charts include the Optec 2500 or 5500 visual analyzer machine (Stereo Optical, Chicago, IL) and the Mars chart (Precision Vision, La Salle, IL), which is a handheld chart. The LEA Low Contrast eye charts

(Richmond Products, Albuquerque, NM) measure visual acuity under low-contrast conditions, which is not a measure of contrast sensitivity but will provide information on how low environmental illumination impairs visual acuity. The Driving Health Inventory (Transanalytics Health and Safety Services, Quakertown, PA) includes a brief computerized screening of contrast sensitivity.

At present there are no state driving standards regarding contrast sensitivity. Research has shown a strong relationship between contrast sensitivity impairment and crash risk (Owsley et al., 2001, 2002; Wood & Carberry, 2006), and therefore the occupational therapist conducting the CDE should consider the client's contrast sensitivity when making decisions about conducting an on-road evaluation. The clients with impairment should be educated about the possible causes of contrast sensitivity impairment and the risk of crash.

In older drivers, cataract is a common cause of contrast sensitivity impairment. If cataract surgery and IOL insertion are deemed appropriate by an ophthalmologist and elected by the client, patients can experience an often dramatic improvement in contrast sensitivity (as well as in visual acuity).

If the cause of contrast sensitivity impairment is unknown because the client has not had a recent comprehensive eye exam, a referral should be made to an ophthalmologist or optometrist, regardless of severity. If the cause is known and there is no option for improvement, the recommendation should be no driving for those clients with severe impairment (1.20 logMAR units or less on the Pelli–Robson; Owsley et al., 2002). Those with moderate impairment can be taken on an on-road evaluation, and if they pass, the occupational therapist should discuss restricted driving and the use of alternate routes, such as avoiding interstates, night driving, high-traffic roads, and unprotected intersections.

Assessment of Visual Field (Peripheral Vision)

Visual field loss can occur as a result of many medical conditions. Stroke, TBI, brain tumor, multiple sclerosis, DR, glaucoma, and retinitis pigmentosa are among some of the more common causes. During a comprehensive eye exam, eye care professionals typically test the central 24°–30° radius of the visual field on a Humphrey® Field Analyzer (HFA; Carl Ziess Meditec, Dublin, CA) or similar visual field testing apparatus. These visual field instruments typically measure light sensitivity (i.e., how bright a small target has to be before a person indicates he or she sees it). However, visual field areas more peripheral than the central 30° radius field are also appropriate when assessing the visual field for driving, and they could be more relevant given that in driving it is important to detect obstacles moving into the roadway scene as early as possible.

Examples of visual field assessments that include mid- to far peripheral vision are the 120-point HFA screening test and the Goldmann perimetry test (Haag Streit USA, Mason, OH). Most visual field tests used clinically are monocular, with each eye tested separately, but the occupational therapist, whose focus is on functional ability, may find that a binocular visual field test such as the binocular Esterman test (also available on the HFA) is more useful for understanding what the client is seeing while driving because both eyes are used together when driving (Esterman, 1982). The merging of monocular field tests (sometimes called the *integrated visual field*) is another option for screening. These tests mentioned are considered the gold-standard tests used by eye care professionals and can be administered by occupational therapists when trained appropriately. There are many other options that are less expensive and easier to administer, including the Keystone vision screener (Mast Concepts, Reno, NV) and vision testers by Stereo Optical such as the Optec 2500 or 5500 (which includes contrast sensitivity slides) and Visual Analyzer (Stereo Optical Co. Inc., Chicago).

Clearly, it is beyond the scope of the occupational therapy generalist to identify or administer the above-mentioned tests. What is important is that the generalist is able to identify a visual field problem, perhaps by observing the client in a functional setting, and then make referrals for appropriate evaluation and follow-up.

Clients must meet the visual field requirements for driving in their state before an on-road evaluation can be completed. Those who have a visual field impairment can be taken for an on-road evaluation if they meet the visual field requirements in their jurisdiction and are not experiencing any functional impairment. A DRS usually makes such determinations. However, the generalist will play a role in identifying clients who are experiencing functional difficulties (e.g., identifying objects in the environment, especially on the side of their visual field defect, sometimes called a *cut*). Such clients should be referred for a comprehensive low vision evaluation with specific integrated vision testing before being given an on-road evaluation.

Several rehabilitation options exist for patients with homonymous field loss who wish to return to driving. That being said, in some jurisdictions, a person with field cuts is prohibited from driving and may not be allowed to use compensatory techniques for driving. The DRS can introduce the client to options such as panoramic rear-view mirrors, blind-spot mirrors, prisms (in conjunction with the eye care specialist), and scanning training to increase head and eye movement. Scanning can expand the visual field with just head or eye movement, but often the patient may need training to become an efficient scanner.

Generalists can help with executing aspects of the treatment plan, such as designing a graded therapeutic activity program that may include paper-and-pencil tasks, computer-based activities, scan courses, and Dynavision training (described next). It is critical that the therapeutic programs include activities that go beyond a midline, tabletop (or computer screen) format and incorporate activities that challenge a client's scanning skills for all instrumental activities of daily living (IADLs) that require a client to respond to visual stimuli in all areas of the visual field.

Prisms are sometimes prescribed by low vision specialists for patients with visual field loss. These prisms shift images from the missing field into the intact field. Research on visual field loss and driving with prisms is very limited, with research on prisms thus far focused on their ability to expand the visual field (Bowers, Keeney, & Peli, 2008), not the driving outcome. At present, no research has suggested that prisms are an effective rehabilitation technique for improving driving performance in persons with homonymous hemianopia or that prisms are superior to scanning training in improving driving performance.

Assessment of Visual Processing, Scanning, and Attention

Dynavision

Another device often used during a CDE is the Dynavision (Dynavision International, West Chester, OH). The Dynavision can be used for both screening and training of visual scanning skills, visual attention, and peripheral vision awareness.

The Dynavision D2 records reaction times in each quadrant of the visual field that provides objective assessment of a client's scanning skills. For clients with homonymous field loss, increased reaction time in quadrants in the missing fields indicates reduced compensation for the field loss (Warren, 2011).

Previous research on the Dynavision has been limited; the research that does exist has primarily focused on its use as a training device rather than as a screening tool. This test combined with clinical observation can provide valuable information about how well clients with visual field loss are using increased head and eye movement to compensate for it.

The visual demands of driving require more skills than intact visual sensory functions, such as good acuity and intact peripheral visual fields, because controlling a vehicle requires paying attention to multiple stimuli in a cluttered, dynamic, and constantly changing environment. Drivers must have the skills to quickly and visually process what is happening to react appropriately to unexpected events in a timely fashion. Screening for impaired visual information–processing speed and ability to divide attention is an essential part of an evidence-based CDE.

As mentioned earlier in this chapter, an extensive body of research has supported the correlation between processing speed impairment and crash risk, but not all assessments for measuring processing speed have been tested in research settings. When choosing which screening assessments to include in a CDE, one must consider the evidence supporting the use of the assessment as it relates to driving ability and its appropriateness for each client on the basis of diagnosis and functional ability.

Useful Field of Vision Test

The UFOV test measures visual processing speed (Subtest 1) under divided attention (Subtest 2) and selective attention (Subtest 3) conditions. It has considerable evidence behind it, indicating that poor UFOV divided-attention scores are associated with increased crash risk and impaired driving performance.

The UFOV should not be used with clients who have significant visual field loss or visual acuity of less than 20/70 (Owsley, Ball, & Keeton, 1994), because one cannot identify the location of a peripheral target presented at any duration if one has severe loss in that peripheral field region. Furthermore, one must have sufficient visual acuity to be able to detect and discriminate the test's targets presented in central vision.

The UFOV test is not affected by motor reaction time, and therefore the score is not affected by any motor impairment. The resulting score is an index of the fastest presentation of the test target where the client is able to correctly identify it most of the time. Those who have poor UFOV scores will require a longer time to identify the targets, and those who have good UFOV scores require very brief presentation times to identify the targets.

Trail Making Test

The Trail Making Test, Parts A and B (Reitan, 1958), is a neuropsychological instrument used to assess speed of visual search, attention, mental flexibility, and motor functioning (Spreen & Strauss, 1991). Trails B measures the ability to deal with multiple stimuli and visual search, a skill that is important in driving (Goode et al., 1998). This test may not be valid with clients who have difficulty with writing tasks because of motor impairment.

Goode et al. (1998) examined the crash reports of 239 drivers for the 5 years preceding the study. Of those drivers, 115 had not been involved in an at-fault crash, and 124 had been involved in one or more at-fault crashes. Even though the cutoff for this test is 180 seconds, this study found that the noncrash participants had a mean score of 124.81 seconds on Trails B and the crash participants had a mean score of 147.35 seconds.

This is a relatively inexpensive paper-and-pencil test that provides an opportunity to observe the client's visual search patterns. If the client's search pattern is disorganized or exhibits a pattern indicative of hemi-inattention or neglect, further testing should be conducted. The Bells Test (Gauthier, DeHaut, & Joanette, 1989), Clock Test (Shulman, Shedletsky, & Silver, 1986), or Line-Bisection (Schenkenberg, Bradford, & Ajax, 1980) are paper-and-pencil tests often used to further assess scanning if inattention is suspected.

Brain Injury Visual Assessment Battery for Adults

The Brain Injury Visual Assessment Battery for Adults (Warren, 1998) assessment manual includes many cancellation tests as well as instructions for making a scan course for evaluation and training. This assessment, in addition to clinical observation, provides valuable information about how well clients with visual field loss are compensating for such losses.

All the measurements from the earlier-mentioned sections generally are made with the client wearing his or her habitual optical (spectacle or contact lens) correction for distant activities. If the client reports that he or she does not wear glasses or contact lenses to drive, the testing should be completed without glasses or contact lenses. However, if the client has difficulty with the vision tests, he or she should be asked to put on glasses or contacts to continue the tests. Often clients will not realize how much better their vision is with glasses or contacts, which can be a great opportunity to educate them about what they can see with and without their glasses or contacts and possibly improve their driving ability.

Rehabilitation Options

The DRSs at the University of Alabama at Birmingham established a protocol in which clients who demonstrated severe impairment in visual-processing speed on at least two evidence-based screening tests (e.g., the Trails B, UFOV) at the time of initial evaluation would not be taken for an on-road evaluation. (Table 8.1 provides examples of clients with diagnoses and functional profiles who should not be taken out for an on-road evaluation.) However, if the client does not have a progressive disease, rehabilitation options can be discussed. These options might include UFOV training, which improves processing speed and divided-attention skills in some clients (Ball, Edwards, & Ross, 2007). It has been shown to transfer to safer on-road behaviors (Roenker, Cissell, Ball, Wadley, & Edwards, 2003) and to reduce crash risk (Ball, Edwards, Ross, & McGwin, 2010). Other practice-based rehabilitation strategies may include training on Dynavision, playing Wii™ (Nintendo of America, Redmond, WA) games such as tennis or baseball, and playing speed-based computer games.

Table 8.1. Examples of Clients Who Should Not Undergo an On-Road Evaluation

Diagnosis	Visual Acuity	Contrast Sensitivity	UFOV Task 2 (seconds)	Trails B (seconds)	Dynavision	Client's Self-Report of Functional Impairment	Clinical Observation	On-Road Assessment
Alzheimer's disease	20/30 OD 20/25 OS	1.65 OU	420 s	318.20 s	NA	No memory loss and no difficulty with any driving situations	Short-term memory loss, difficulty understanding and following directions, family reports client got lost driving to the grocery store	No BTW and alternative transportation should be discussed
Cataract	20/80 OD 20/60 OS	1.10 OD 1.20 OS	250 s	128.38 s	NA	Avoids driving at night due to difficulty but no recent crashes	Normal memory function; cognitive skills normal for age	No BTW and referral to ophthalmologist for comprehensive eye examination; reevaluate if cataract surgery is performed
CVA with left homonymous hemianopia	20/20 OD 20/20 OS	1.65 OD 1.65 OS	NA	260.14 s	Slowed score in the left hemi-field	Has not driven since CVA and has been bumping into walls, cabinet doors, and so on, on the leftside	Does not scan to left at all and does not understand impairment	No BTW and referral to a low vision specialist; may qualify for BTW following rehabilitation

Note. BTW = behind-the-wheel evaluation, CVA = cardiovascular accident, NA = not applicable, OD = right eye, OS = left eye, OU = both eyes, Trails B = Trail Making Test Part B, UFOV = Useful Field of View.

Another therapeutic strategy to increase a client's awareness of problems with information processing speed and divided attention is to engage a client in timed computerized activities (such as those available on Lumosity.com, Positscience.com, or Cognitivelabs.com), establish a baseline on timed performance, and then have the client perform the same task while talking and answering questions (even simple biographical or current events questions).

The effectiveness of these practice-based rehabilitation strategies to improve driving skills has not yet been empirically demonstrated. Studies should be conducted to test the efficacy and effectiveness of such strategies over time. In the meantime, clinicians may use strategies such as exposure to this form of training to increase awareness of divided-attention problems. As the client improves or heals, the therapist considers benchmarks indicating readiness, prompting retesting or referral for the CDE.

Implications of Visual Impairments for On-Road Evaluations

Clients with in-clinic evaluation results that satisfy the minimum requirements for driving (which varies by state) are given the opportunity to complete the second portion of the CDE, called the *on-road evaluation,* before any determination about driving skills is made. Although significant impairment of contrast sensitivity, visual fields, visual information–processing speed, and divided attention may indicate that the client is at risk for a crash, the absence or degree of such impairments does not necessarily guarantee that the client may exhibit safe driving skills when behind the wheel. The on-road evaluation should be client centered, occupation based, and conducted in the client's context. The settings and equipment vary broadly, from an in-clinic interactive simulator to an evaluation vehicle equipped with an instructor brake.

The *narrated drive* is an assessment strategy that provides the occupational therapist with critical information about what the client is viewing as the car moves down the road. It should capture the client's context (i.e., the client is encouraged to verbally describe or narrate what he or she sees relevant to the driving scene). Responses may yield information pertaining to the colors of the traffic lights, four-way stops, two-way stops, yielding, one-way roads, construction zones, school zones, pedestrian crossings, speed limits, brake lights or left- and right-turn signals of lead vehicles, pedestrians, and other objects in the road. This strategy provides an opportunity for the occupational therapist to capture content-rich and driving-specific information from the client's own observation through his or her narrated descriptions. Such information may further inform the occupational therapist of the client's functional capacity to drive safely.

Many evaluators choose to begin the on-road evaluation in a parking lot and progress to more complicated traffic areas, such as roads characterized by high-density traffic traveling at higher speeds. Ideally, if the client reports that he or she drives to the grocery store, bank, church, and restaurant, then these should be the prime destinations traveled to during the on-road evaluation. To optimize the evaluation procedure and to observe natural driving behaviors, only absolutely essential information should be given verbally to the client. Directions such as "at the next traffic light, take a right" give the client information that a traffic light, stop sign, intersection, and so on are ahead, and prepare the client to take the necessary action. This is information that the evaluator will want the client to recognize without any cues. Directions such as "now drive me to your favorite grocery store" allow the client to make all the decisions, and the evaluator will be able to observe when and if the client responds appropriately to the traffic lights, stop signs, and intersections.

Depending on the client factors (e.g., glare sensitivity, slowed processing speed), the occupational therapist can structure the on-road evaluation to allow for optimal safety and performance of the client. If adaptations were necessary to accommodate the driver during the on-road evaluation, then these must be recommended as safety strategies and discussed with the client or family after the drive. Clients with decreased visual function may report that they only drive in familiar areas. If this is the case, the on-road evaluation should be conducted in areas familiar to the client. If the client reports that he or she frequently drives in unfamiliar areas but always uses a global positioning system (GPS), the evaluator should integrate the use of a GPS for driving in an unfamiliar area.

Implications of Decreased Visual Acuity

During an on-road evaluation for a client with decreased visual acuity who does not use adaptive equipment, the evaluator should incorporate routes that will require the client to identify traffic lights, road signs, stop-and-go traffic, and lane changes. These clients may not see the color of traffic lights in advance, necessitating them to react suddenly when they become aware of the situation. Evaluators also may observe that these clients have difficulty seeing lane markings, driving in and out of shade, and maintaining lane control on roads without a center line. These drivers will likely report having difficulty driving at night and driving on high-traffic roads (McGwin, Chapman, & Owsley, 2000). If the client has difficulty noticing details, a bioptic telescope system may be helpful even if the client's acuity impairment is not below the legal limits for driving. Driving with a bioptic telescope is described in more detail later in this chapter.

Implications of Impairments in Contrast Sensitivity

Contrast sensitivity impairment can decrease the visibility of objects in the roadway environment, and in general the visual scene looks washed out, with objects either invisible or, if visible, perceived to be without distinct borders. Clients with contrast sensitivity impairment may report more difficulty making unprotected left turns (McGwin et al., 2000), so the on-road evaluation should include many opportunities for such drivers to execute this maneuver. Education about avoiding traffic situations, especially left turns against oncoming traffic, should be discussed. The occupational therapist also may recommend to the client and help him or her to find alternative and safer routes on which to travel.

Implications of Visual Field Impairment

If clients with visual field impairment or loss exhibit adequate scanning skills in the clinic, the on-road evaluation should be extensive to ensure these skills carry over in the driving environment. The evaluator should pay close attention to lane position while driving with clients with visual field impairment. This is a skill that is often difficult for these drivers, especially when driving on the interstate. One possible explanation is that the driver does not have objects available within his or her intact or remaining visual field to anchor oneself in space (e.g., houses, trees, curbs), which makes it difficult for the driver to scan and keep the car in its lane (Bowers, Mandel, Goldstein, & Peli, 2010; Wood et al., 2011). The evaluator must stay vigilant in continuously checking the client's head and eye movements. Wood et al. (2011) found that drivers with visual field loss (hemianopia) who made more head and eye movements to the blind side were more likely to be rated as safe drivers.

Implications of Slowing in Visual Information–Processing Speed

Clients with impairment in visual-processing speed and divided attention will have difficulty reacting quickly when encountering unexpected events. They also may have difficulty judging the speed and distance of other cars. These drivers may be prone to crashes or near misses when turning left, especially at busy intersections that require drivers to pay attention to simultaneously occurring events. During the on-road evaluation, the occupational therapist must pay close attention to the client's reactions to brake lights and directional signals, traffic lights, and changes in traffic flow. Asking a client with decreased processing speed and impaired divided attention to follow a map of the route, instead of giving verbal directions, may be challenging for the client and elicit rich information for evaluation purposes. The evaluator may engage in casual conversation during the drive to examine how the client can divide his or her attention.

However, evaluators should maintain the ethical principles of beneficence and nonmaleficence and never knowingly put a client at risk or set him or her up for failure. For example, clients with decreased processing speed should not drive on the interstate during the behind-the-wheel evaluation; likewise, they should agree to avoid high-speed roads if continued driving is recommended. High speeds and night driving both require quick reactions, and these situations should be avoided if decreased processing speed is detected.

Bioptic Telescope System

As of August 2009, 39 states allow persons with low vision to drive with a *bioptic telescope system (BTS)*. Each state, though, has different rules for driving with a BTS. A BTS is a miniature telescope mounted into regular lenses above the client's line of sight (Figure 8.2). The regular lens is sometimes referred to as the *carrier lens*.

Many types of bioptic systems exist, which may be either Keplerian or Galilean magnification styles of telescopes. *Keplerian telescopes* use a combination of lenses and prisms to produce the widest field of view and sharpest edge-to-edge image possible. *Galilean telescopes* are smaller, lighter weight, and less complicated, but they produce a smaller field of view. A 3× Keplerian telescope may provide up to a 15° field of view (Figure 8.3), and a 3× Galilean telescope provides a 5° to 11° field of view (Figure 8.4). A BTS can also be fixed focus for driving only or focusable for use during other ADLs. The low vision eye care specialist (ophthalmologist or optometrist with specialized training in low vision assessment and rehabilitation) may provide the client with a choice of which BTS to use and accommodate user preferences. Other specialists make specific recommendations on the basis of their medical opinions of what is needed as a result of their evaluations.

One primary role of the occupational therapist is to train the client.

One primary role of the occupational therapist is to train the client to use the BTS to optimize his or her participation in IADLs, including the possibility of driving. The occupational therapist who provides these services should seek and obtain specialized training in low vision. Before initiating driving training, the occupational therapist should make every effort to fully understand what the client sees through his or her particular type of BTS. The fitting of the telescopes can be altered between the time the system is dispensed and when the client comes in for training.

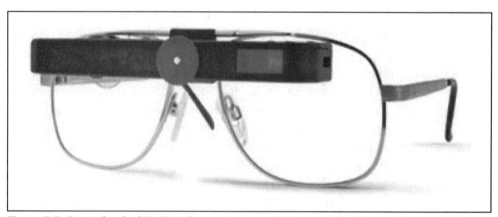

Figure 8.2. Example of a bioptic telescope mounted into a regular lens and spectacle frame.
Note. Provided by Ocutech, Chapel Hill, NC. Used with permission.

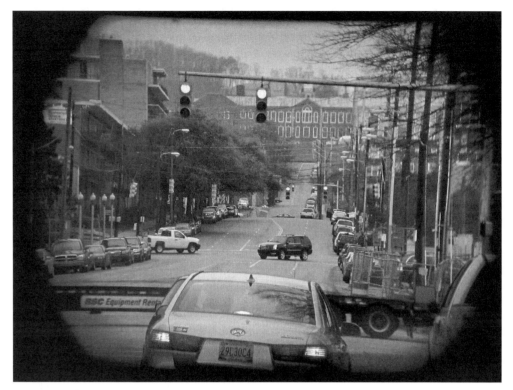

Figure 8.3. Street view through a 4X Keplerian telescope.
Note. Provided by Ocutech, Chapel Hill, NC. Used with permission.

For example, the client may drop the system on a hard surface and bend the frame, sit on the system, or attempt bending the nosepiece for comfort. Any of these actions will affect how the BTS fits.

The driver dependent on this device must be knowledgeable and aware of how to ensure optimal adjustment. A collaborative relationship with the low vision eye care specialist who prescribed the BTS is essential because the specialist's expertise and skills are often needed in concert with the training provided by the therapist.

To be successful in bioptic driving, the client must first be proficient in the use of the BTS. Many factors, not just the client's vision, influence the successful use of the BTS. For example, the bioptic should be appropriate for the client and its intended use and must fit correctly. Many clients are so motivated to drive that they fail to report difficulties experienced with the BTS to the prescribing physician. When the client comes for training, the occupational therapist must have an open dialogue with the client and ask questions that will reveal problems with the BTS affecting functional performance.

Most clients will be fit with a *monocular telescope* (a telescope above one eye, usually the eye with better acuity). One survey found that 88% of drivers using a BTS reported using a monocular telescope (Bowers, Apfelbaum, & Peli, 2005). Very few clients are fitted in *binocular telescopes* (a telescope in front of each eye). If a client is fitted with binocular telescopes, the occupational therapist should ensure that the client is not experiencing double vision. Some clients will not realize that they should be seeing only one image. The occupational therapist also should observe the client's head position when looking through the carrier lens (Figure 8.5). The client's head

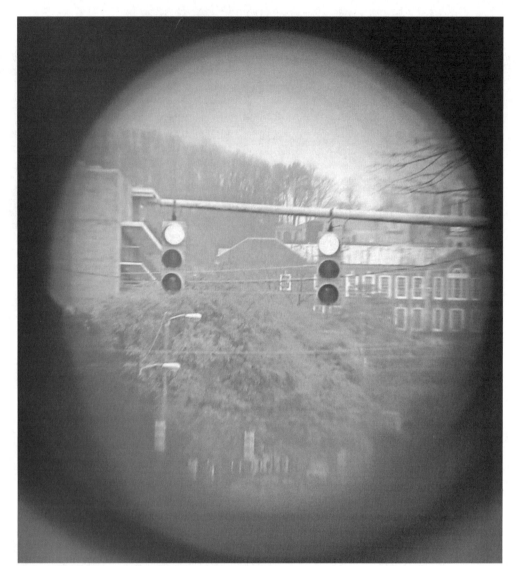

Figure 8.4. Street view through a Galilean telescope.
Note. Provided by Ocutech, Chapel Hill, NC. Used with permission.

should not be tilted back to view through the carrier lens. The telescope should not block the pupil when looking straight ahead, and the client should have to tilt the head down slightly to look into the telescope (Figure 8.6). The occupational therapist may provide practice opportunities to the client to alternate viewing through the telescope and the carrier lens several times to establish this skill. If the client reports any difficulty seeing through the BTS, the therapist should refer the client back to the low vision eye care specialist for further adjustments before training begins.

The client should practice using the BTS in the clinic with guidance from the occupational therapist at first to ensure that he or she is using the proper technique to view through the telescope. If the client practices without instruction, he or she may use it improperly and acquire bad habits. The client must feel comfortable driving without the BTS because the carrier lens will be used for 95% of the driving task. The client must be able to locate traffic lights, road signs, pedestrians, obstacles, and potential threats with the carrier lens and use the telescope only to see details.

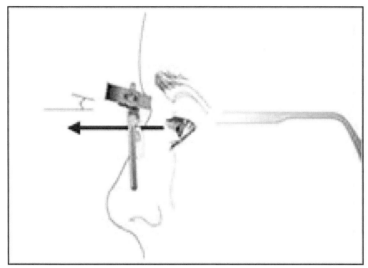

Figure 8.5. Head position while looking through a carrier lens.
Note. Provided by Ocutech, Chapel Hill, NC. Used with permission.

A client who is unable to see sufficiently through the carrier lens and who uses the bioptic only to spot details is generally not a good candidate for driving. Clients who have been diagnosed with albinism, ocular albinism, nystagmus, Stargardt's disease, and optic atrophy are typically good candidates for bioptic driving.

Clients typically want to begin driving as soon as they receive the BTS, but many hours of nondriver training should be completed first to ensure proficiency in the general use of the BTS. Some states have regulations regarding the hours of training needed with a DRS before attempting licensure with bioptic lenses. Training can be achieved in many ways in the clinic. At first the training should be focused on spotting stationary objects. Clients should practice using the carrier lens to search for objects and then switch to the telescope to identify the object. This technique is called *dipping* or *spotting* because the client tilts the head downward slightly and looks into the telescope. The dip should not exceed 2 s. If the desired

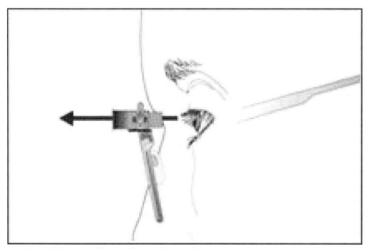

Figure 8.6. Head position while looking through a telescope.
Note. Provided by Ocutech, Chapel Hill, NC. Used with permission.

object is not found within this time, the client should find the object again in the carrier lens and then try to spot with the telescope. Part of the training is conducted outdoors where glare is encountered and where a variety of stationary and moving objects are to be spotted. The therapist may instruct the client to identify traffic lights, oncoming cars, pedestrians, and road signs (e.g., yield, stop, one way, right-lane turn only) from a standing position. Clients also may be challenged, as a passenger in the car, to improve spotting while the vehicle is traveling at various speeds before the client would be offered an opportunity for on-road training.

Although the BTS is not used for tracking during driving, this is a useful technique for practice. The therapist should instruct the client to locate a particular vehicle and track it as it comes toward and passes him or her. Such practice helps the client learn how objects look at different distances.

Once the client is successfully using the bioptic in everyday activities, training should shift to more client-centered and occupation-based activities. There are many community occupation-based activities that can be used in training, such as shopping in a grocery or electronics store. If a store has motorized carts, the client can practice using the device while shopping with the cart. The therapist also should educate family members on the use of the BTS to enhance their understanding of how the system works. Although BTS driving is not allowed in the state of Florida, **Adaptive Mobility Services** in Orlando offers a 3-day hands-on course for occupational therapists to learn how to provide bioptic training. Occupational therapists are encouraged to search for training courses in their specific areas.

Options If Driving Is No Longer Possible

The strategies as discussed in the previous section are designed to promote driving as safely as possible for clients with visual impairment, and for as long as possible. However, at times the occupational therapist will have to make the decision to recommend driving cessation. Chapter 2 deals extensively with the strategies as well as interventions necessary to facilitate clients' continued and independent community mobility if they no longer drive, as well as addressing the community mobility needs of those who have never driven. Chapter 4 addresses the psychosocial issues related to driving cessation.

An in-depth discussion of the resources for promoting independence in community mobility for those with low vision or for those who are blind is beyond the scope of this chapter. However, readers are encouraged to build up a referral network of adjunct professionals who may appropriately manage the client's needs that cannot be met by the occupational therapist in the general setting or by the DRS. Readers also are directed to the **American Foundation for the Blind, Lighthouse International,** or similar state and local organizations for a list of resources that may benefit clients in independence in community mobility.

The occupational therapy intervention for persons who can no longer drive follows the same process as described in *Occupational Therapy Practice Framework: Domain and Process* (2nd ed.; AOTA, 2008). As such, the occupational therapist will do the following:

- Determine the client's readiness to discuss alternative mobility and transportation options

- Determine the client's capacities and limitations pertaining to the use of such options
- Select, test, and adopt, with the client and his or her family or support system, the most appropriate options
- Train the client to increase his or her competence and confidence to use the options in a graded environment
- Use simple tasks initially (e.g., learning how to use a bus schedule)
- Advance to the most comprehensive tasks (e.g., taking a bus trip to a location in the community)
- Grade supervision from full supervision initially to no supervision eventually.

These strategies are, at best, clinical practice strategies. Much research is still needed to find and implement evidence-based intervention strategies to address transitioning from driving to nondriving and to the efficacy or effectiveness of the use of alternative transportation options in the community to meet the clients' mobility needs.

Other Issues in Managing Clients With Ocular Diseases and Conditions

When a person with visual impairment presents to the occupational therapist in any clinical setting, it is important for the therapist to realize that the future course of the client's vision impairment could take several paths. For example, clients with optic atrophy, optic nerve hypoplasia, or Stargardt's disease often reach a plateau in the level of their impairment in that the impairment ceases to become progressively worse or does so only modestly as they go through adulthood. In other words, their vision will have some stability over time. These conditions are more commonly seen in clients who present to the driving clinic as young adults, because these are congenital or early life–onset conditions.

Clients with retinitis pigmentosa (RP) may also present as young adults or teenagers because this is an inherited, early life–onset condition. Unfortunately, for most patients with RP, the vision impairment grows progressively worse, first affecting the periphery and then finally robbing the client of central vision as well. At present, there are no proven effective treatments for RP, for significantly arresting its progression, for restoring vision, or for preventing this inherited disease, although efforts to develop treatments are a research area of high priority.

For the occupational therapist addressing driving with a client with a progressive, degenerative condition such as RP, it is imperative to plan for and encourage the client to participate in ongoing, periodic evaluations of his or her driving abilities (if the client is indeed still driving) as the course of the disease progresses. As with any progressive disease, an essential responsibility of the occupational therapist is to include preparation for the day when the client's visual abilities will no longer support safe driving, and thus driving cessation will be necessary. This dialogue should include a discussion and possible referral to specialists trained in alternative transportation options for persons with low vision to ensure the primary goal of maintained independence in community mobility.

There are many eye conditions, particularly later adulthood–onset conditions, in which vision impairment can grow worse as time passes. Fortunately, in many of these conditions, there are treatment options for slowing the disease's progression, or in some cases reversing the impairment and restoring vision to a normal or near-normal level. The rest of this section will discuss these conditions and current interventions used by ophthalmologists to slow or prevent vision loss or to restore vision. Following are three organizations for more information on these eye conditions or to further explore any of the interventions mentioned.

- **American Academy of Ophthalmology (one.aao.org/ce/default.aspx)**
- **National Eye Institute (www.nei.nih.gov/health)**
- Lighthouse International (www.lighthouse.org).

Cataract

Age-related *cataract*, the increased opacity of the crystalline lens occurring in late adulthood, is a highly treatable condition for most people. Cataract surgery, in which the crystalline lens is surgically removed and replaced by an IOL, is the most common surgical procedure covered by Medicare performed on older adults in the United States (Grossman & Edson, 2002). It is a highly effective procedure for improving visual acuity and contrast sensitivity, and for many older adults, these improvements lead to normal or near-normal vision.

Cataract surgery is one of the safest surgical procedures, has a very low complication rate, and is performed as an outpatient procedure, minimizing personal burden. The power of the IOL selected and inserted by the ophthalmologist brings the patient's vision to its best distance correction or approximates it. Most patients will still require spectacles for near-vision activities, such as reading, because the eye cannot accommodate (focus) to different distances. However, multifocal IOLs have been developed that allow for multiple planes of focus, which can support both near and distance visual activities. The downside of multifocal IOLs is that the contrast of the image formed by the lens is reduced (thus reducing a patient's contrast sensitivity); some patients are not bothered by this, whereas others are. Single-focus lenses are still very popular as a result. In recent years, considerable effort has been devoted to developing and evaluating accommodating IOLs (i.e., IOLs that allow the eye an adjustable focus for different distances, so that spectacle correction is not needed).

The occupational therapist conducting a CDE on an older client with contrast sensitivity or acuity impairment who reports that he or she has not had cataract surgery should refer the client to an ophthalmologist for a comprehensive eye examination (if the client has not had one in the past year). Contrast sensitivity or acuity impairment can be caused by conditions other than cataract, but cataract is the most common cause in older persons who have not yet had cataract surgery. If the client reports problems seeing the roadway environment, reading highway signs, and driving at night, cataract could very well be the culprit causing these visibility problems.

Because cataract surgery is safe, effective, and covered by most insurance plans (including Medicare), it is a realistic option for restoring vision in a rather straightforward way. Research has demonstrated that cataract surgery reduces crash risk by 50% (Owsley et al., 2002) and improves driving performance (Wood

& Carberry, 2006), so this is an evidence-based strategy for improving driver safety and performance in persons with vision impairment because of cataract.

Age-Related Macular Degeneration

AMD is the most common cause of irreversible vision impairment in the United States (Friedman, O'Colmain, et al., 2004). AMD is a degenerative disease of the *macula* (the area of the retina used for central vision) in which photoreceptors malfunction and can eventually die. *Photoreceptors* are the neural cells in the retina where vision starts. That is, they are responsible for transducing light energy from the world into neural impulses that begin the process of sending information about images to the brain. Therefore, if photoreceptors do not function well or die, the process of vision cannot begin or begins in a degraded way. Recent research has shown that AMD is most likely caused by a complex interplay between genetics (there are genes that predispose one to the disease) and the environment (e.g., smoking increases the risk for the disease; Schmidt et al., 2006).

There are currently several proven treatments for AMD. For persons with intermediate stages of AMD, taking high levels of an oral formulation of antioxidants (e.g., vitamin C, vitamin E, beta carotene) and zinc can reduce the risk of developing advanced AMD. However, there is no evidence that this formulation prevents AMD in those currently free from AMD or prevents further progression of the disease once someone has its earliest stages. An ongoing, nationwide study is examining whether other supplements, namely lutein, zeathanthin, long-chain omega-3 fatty acids, and eicosapentaenoic acid, also reduce the risk for advanced AMD; study results are not yet available (National Eye Institute, 2011).

A treatment for the advanced form of AMD called *exudative AMD*, or *wet AMD*, is photodynamic therapy (PDT). In exudative AMD, there is a proliferation of leaky blood vessels in the macula that causes photoreceptor dysfunction and death and, thus, vision loss. In PDT, a dye is injected into the eye, where it flows into these abnormal blood vessels. A special type of cold laser light is directed at the vessels, which activates the dye and destroys the aberrant vessels.

Since the emergence of the anti-vascular endothelial growth factor or anti-VEGF treatments, PDT is not as commonly used to treat exudative AMD as it used to be. However, researchers are focusing on potentially further improving treatment for exudative AMD by combining the PDT and anti-VEGF approaches.

The anti-VEGF treatments developed during the past decade are now the commonly used and accepted treatments for exudative AMD. Anti-VEGF treatments, which are injected into the eye, target VEGF, a protein involved in blood vessel formation, and inhibit new blood vessel growth. Two commonly used treatments are ranibizumab and bevacizumab. Another anti-VEGF treatment is pegaptinib sodium, which is used much less frequently since the development of ranibizumab and bevacizumab. Clinical trials have shown that ranibizumab and bevacizumab prevent further vision loss in patients who have exudative disease, and in some patients, visual acuity exhibited sustained improvement to the level that some patients reported that they could return to driving. Although not yet confirmed on a population basis, some have predicted that the very severe vision loss that often accompanies exudative AMD may not be the case for many AMD

AMD is the most common cause of irreversible vision impairment in the United States.

patients in future years, given the positive treatment effects of ranibizumab and bevacizumab.

Although these treatments are not cures for the disease and do not restore vision to normal nondisease levels, there is evidence that they slow the progression of the vision impairment. This may mean that AMD patients will have more years of driving potential because their visual acuity will not fall below the vision standard for licensure as rapidly as it might if these anti-VEGF treatments were not available.

Currently, there are no proven treatments for the other advanced form of AMD, geographic atrophy. In addition, there are no proven strategies for preventing AMD altogether or for arresting its earliest progression. Of course, smoking cessation is an appropriate measure, to reduce the risk not only for AMD but also many other chronic health conditions. Developing and evaluating AMD treatments is a very active area of research around the world. Research is focusing on many approaches, including new anti-VEGF strategies, anti-inflammatory treatments, radiation therapy, vascular stabilization through inhibiting platelet-derived growth factor, inhibiting the complement system, and gene therapy.

In evaluating driving fitness in persons with AMD, the occupational therapist should be aware of several issues. First, AMD disease severity—whether one has early, intermediate, or advanced disease—is not necessarily closely related to the severity of vision impairment. An older adult can retain relatively good visual acuity (i.e., within the vision standard for licensure) even when he or she is well into the intermediate phase of AMD. Thus, in a CDE, the emphasis is on what visual abilities the client has, not on his or her level of disease severity.

Second, it is very useful to communicate with the clients with AMD's ophthalmologist or optometrist, which includes requesting the chart notes, referral or follow-up letters, or phone conversation records. This communication will give the therapist information about recent treatment interventions or planned treatments for the patient in the near future (e.g., further anti-VEGF treatment), which could slow disease progression or even restore vision. Perhaps visual acuity does not meet the visual standard for the jurisdiction at the CDE visit, but given a course of AMD treatment planned for the very near future, there might be a good chance of improved acuity for the client.

Third, as mentioned earlier, moderate to severe visual acuity impairment does not often occur until late-stage disease. However, there are other aspects of vision that can be impaired early on in the disease, such as visibility problems under poor lighting or at night and impaired contrast sensitivity. Reports of night driving difficulty by a patient with AMD are associated with impaired light sensitivity under darkened conditions as measured in the clinic (Scilley et al., 2002). Thus, measuring visual acuity or contrast sensitivity under low luminance conditions may be a good way for the occupational therapist to uncover a potential visibility problem the patient faces on the road.

Fourth, because those with AMD will be older adults, it is also important to screen cognitive skills; information processing speed is known to decrease in late adulthood and may indicate a need to consider self-imposed driving restrictions. The ability of a client with AMD to adopt compensatory strategies on the road that help cope with reduced visibility could be affected by his or her cognitive status.

Fifth, because some clients with AMD seen for driving assessment will have significant vision impairment, it is important that in-clinic testing materials for cognitive screening have large enough characters that the client can actually see them well enough to respond.

Finally, although the BTS could theoretically be useful for drivers with AMD who do not meet the vision standard, existing studies and reports on BTS driving have rarely reported on BTS use by drivers with AMD; these reports mostly focus on BTS use by young or middle-aged adults with early-onset eye diseases (Bowers et al., 2005; Park, Unatin, & Park, 1995). Future research will need to probe why more drivers with AMD do not use the BTS intervention option.

Glaucoma

Glaucoma is the second leading cause of vision loss among adults in the United States and is the leading cause in African Americans (Friedman, Wolfs, et al., 2004). *Glaucoma* is a progressive disease of the optic nerve, characterized by changes in the structure of the *optic disk* (where ganglion cell axons from the retina exit the eye and form the optic nerve), thinning of the retinal nerve fiber layer, and loss of visual function beginning in the peripheral visual field. In end-stage glaucoma, central vision also is affected, including loss in visual acuity. The most common type of glaucoma is primary open-angle glaucoma.

The most common treatment for glaucoma is pharmacologically lowering intra-ocular pressure (IOP) by instilling eye drops (American Health Assistance Foundation, 2011). Several eye drop medications can be used, including prostaglandin-like compounds, beta blockers, alpha-agonists, carbonic anhydrase inhibitors, miotic or cholinergic agents, and epinephrine compounds. There are also oral medications (carbonic anhydrase inhibitors), but these are less commonly used. Although research has demonstrated that the use of IOP-lowering drops can slow the progression of the disease for many patients and prevent vision loss, there is no known cure for the disease. Once the optic nerve is damaged in glaucoma, the damage cannot be reversed.

Much research is ongoing to develop better treatments and preventive strategies for glaucoma. One line of work is looking at whether neuroprotective agents can be developed to effectively protect the optic nerve from degenerative damage because of glaucoma.

For some persons with glaucoma, eye drop and oral medications are ineffective in lowering pressure or too difficult for the patient to tolerate because they can cause unpleasant ocular or systemic side effects. In these situations, ophthalmologists can recommend surgical options to reduce IOP. Laser surgery is one option, namely a procedure called *trabeculoplasty*, in which the laser is used to open up clogged drainage canals and help the *aqueous humor* (fluid in the eye) drain more easily. In most cases, trabeculoplasty lowers IOP. It is a brief in-clinic procedure lasting 10–20 minutes and is performed after an eye drop anesthetic. If neither eye drops nor trabeculoplasty is successful in reducing IOP, another procedure called a *trabeculectomy* may be performed as outpatient surgery. In this procedure, a filter or pathway is created in the *sclera* (white part of the eye) so that the aqueous humor can freely leave. Other surgical procedures to lower IOP in glaucoma continue to be developed and evaluated, including drainage implants.

Although visual field impairment is one criterion for primary open-angle glaucoma diagnosis, the degree of this field impairment can vary drastically from very minor to severe with extensive light sensitivity loss. Because the visual fields of the two eyes overlap extensively, visual field loss in one eye or both eyes does not necessarily mean that the binocular field is impaired, which is why binocular field assessment is critical when the occupational therapist is doing a driving assessment with a client with glaucoma. Even in cases of binocular field loss, the driver with glaucoma may have developed scanning strategies to compensate for areas in which the binocular field is impaired. If scanning strategies appear to be deficient in drivers with glaucoma who have binocular field loss, participation with the Dynavision or other scanning training protocols could be an appropriate intervention to try with these clients.

Therapists need to be aware of the visual field standards in the jurisdictions in which they work, so that they can ensure that their recommendations to patients for driving are consistent with what is legally allowable by the state. Because visual field loss can be progressive in some patients with glaucoma, the therapist also should communicate with the ophthalmologist treating the patient in the event the visual field loss grows more severe, in which case another CDE could be in order.

Diabetic Retinopathy

DR is a common sight-threatening complication of both Type 1 and Type 2 diabetes. DR is the leading cause of acquired blindness in the adult population in the United States (Kempen et al., 2004). Early disease is called *nonproliferative DR* and is the most common form of the condition. In this condition, blood vessels in the retina become weak and bulging *(microaneurysms),* can cause blood to leak into the retina, and may lead to swelling in retinal nerve fibers (a condition called *diabetic macular edema).* Advanced DR is characterized by the formation of new, aberrant blood vessels in the retina, which is called *proliferative DR.* These vessels are also weak and prone to causing a hemorrhage into the vitreous (middle part of the eye). Scar tissue can form that increases the risk for retinal detachment. DR also can be associated with the development of glaucoma, in which the IOP in the eye increases as the normal outflow of fluid in the eye is impeded.

Diabetes also is associated with an increased risk of cataract. DR impairs visual acuity and contrast sensitivity in central vision but can also create areas of light sensitivity loss throughout the retina (called *scotomas).* In its most severe form, it can cause total blindness in an eye. Blood sugar levels that are out of control and elevated are the primary cause of DR. Research has demonstrated that when persons with diabetes maintain good glucose control, their risk for DR is significantly reduced. Thus, a primary strategy for preventing DR or slowing progression is good glucose control.

The longer one has diabetes, the higher the risk for acquiring the condition. A patient with diabetes may not be aware that DR is developing because its symptoms are silent, that is, at first the person may not experience symptoms of eye or visual problems. However, an ophthalmologist or optometrist can detect DR through a comprehensive eye exam, which is why physicians recommend that their patients with diabetes seek comprehensive eye examinations every 1–3 years, depending on the patient's individual clinical profile. To prevent DR, in addition to maintaining good blood sugar control, patients are recommended to seek treatment for hypertension and high cholesterol and stop smoking.

There are no treatments that can cure DR, but there are treatments that can slow disease progression. Photocoagulation through laser treatment can be effective. A surgical procedure called *vitrectomy* is useful if there has been vitreous hemorrhage, which impedes the formation of a retinal image. In vitrectomy, the vitreous gel inside the eye is removed. There is a great deal of ongoing research on new treatments for DR, including the use of anti-VEGF drugs (discussed earlier in the "Age-Related Macular Degeneration" section) that inhibit new vessel formation and have the potential for improving visual acuity or slowing its impairment over time.

As mentioned earlier, impairments in visual acuity, contrast sensitivity, and light sensitivity throughout the visual field are common visual functional consequences of diabetes. Thus, the occupational therapist managing a CDE for a patient with diabetes will want to screen these visual functions, regardless of whether there is a confirmed diagnosis of retinopathy complications when the patient first arrives for the driving assessment. It is also important for the therapist to recognize that not only does diabetes have ocular manifestations, but it is a systemic disease with ramifications for physical function and cognitive functioning, and these skill sets should be screened as well. In addition, if glucose control is poor (as suggested by chart notes from the referring physician or by client self-report), the occupational therapist has the added challenge of discussing with the patient how this situation could negatively affect awareness and the execution of safe driving behaviors behind the wheel.

Summary

On the basis of knowledge of the eye diseases, medical interventions, and potential outcomes, an important message for the occupational therapist is to realize that the future course of the client's vision impairment could take several paths. Such trajectories may include

1. Clients experiencing vision impairments growing progressively worse with no proven effective treatment (e.g., retinitis pigmentosa);
2. Clients with eye conditions (e.g., optic atrophy, optic nerve hypoplasia, Stargardt's disease) that in many cases may reach a plateau at which the level of impairment ceases to become progressively worse or does so only modestly as they go through adulthood; or
3. Clients with eye conditions (e.g., cataract, AMD, glaucoma, DR) with later-adulthood onset, in which vision impairment can grow worse as time passes.

It is also important to realize that there are treatment options for slowing the disease's progression or, in some cases (e.g., cataract), reversing the impairment and restoring vision to a normal or near-normal level.

Apart from understanding the eye diseases, their treatments, and their outcomes, the occupational therapist is encouraged to always be knowledgeable about the visual requirements for driving as they pertain to the representative jurisdiction and to have a close, collegial, and collaborative relationship with the ophthalmologist or other eye care professional treating the clients. The therapist should make referrals to the eye care professionals on an as-needed basis, and certainly if the client has one of the major eye conditions discussed and has not had an eye examination in the past year. The therapist should evaluate clients for baseline visual and driving function and discuss with the patient how his or her underlying condition could negatively affect awareness and execution of safe driving behaviors behind the wheel.

Therapists should encourage clients to participate in ongoing, periodic evaluations of their driving abilities (if they are indeed still driving) as the course of their disease progresses. Part of working with the client with progressive irreversible eye impairment must include preparation for the day when the client's visual abilities will likely not support safe driving, and thus driving cessation will be necessary. This conversation must include a discussion of transitioning from driving to the use of alternative transportation options for the client to maintain independence in community accessibility and mobility and to enjoy societal participation. **Appendix 8.A.** lists vision-related resources for driving and community mobility.

Finally, although advances in the treatment of eye conditions are enabling clients to experience outcomes that may slow disease progression, prevent diseases, or stop reoccurrence of the diseases (see Appendix 8.B), much is still unknown about the impact of medical and surgical interventions on independent and safe driving performance. This paucity of knowledge opens reasonable clinical practice or research opportunities for occupational therapists to work, collaboratively, with vision specialists to examine the essential client and contextual factors underlying the ability to drive safely or to use alternative transportation options independently. (Appendix 8.B. describes a personal account of advances in ophthalmology.) When such efficacy and effectiveness studies are conducted, occupational therapists will be perfectly positioned to implement evidence-based intervention strategies to enhance the community accessibility and mobility of clients with visual disorders.

References

American Association of Motor Vehicle Administrators. (2006). *State vision requirements for license to drive.* Retrieved April 13, 2006, from www.aamva.org/NR/rdonlyres/4C38EEE9-5DC7-449C-A496-15757A99C3F6/0/SummaryOfMedicalAdvisoryBoardPractices1.pdf

American Health Assistance Foundation. (2011). *Glaucoma treatment.* Retrieved January 29, 2012, from www.ahaf.org/glaucoma/treatment/common

American Medical Association. (2003). *Physician's guide to assessing and counseling older drivers.* Chicago: Author.

American Occupational Therapy Association. (2008). Occupational therapy practice framework: Domain and process (2nd ed.). *American Journal of Occupational Therapy, 62,* 625–683. doi: 10.5014.ajot.62.6.625

Amick, M. M., Grace, J., & Ott, B. R. (2007). Visual and cognitive predictors of driving safety in Parkinson's disease patients. *Archives of Clinical Neuropsychology, 22,* 957–967.

Atchison, D. A., Pendersen, C., Dain, S., & Wood, J. M. (2003). Traffic signal color recognition is a problem for both protan and deutan color-vision deficients. *Human Factors, 45,* 495–503.

Ball, K., Edwards, J., & Ross, L. (2007). The impact of speed of processing training on cognitive and everyday functions. *Journals of Gerontology, Series B: Psychological Sciences and Social Sciences 62,* 19–31.

Ball, K., Edwards, J. D., Ross, L. A., & McGwin, G., Jr. (2010). Cognitive training decreases motor vehicle collision involvement of older drivers. *Journal of the American Geriatrics Society, 58,* 2107–2113.

Ball, K., Owsley, C., Sloane, M. E., Roenker, D. L., & Bruni, J. R. (1993). Visual attention problems as a predictor of vehicle crashes in older drivers. *Investigative Ophthalmology and Visual Science, 34,* 3110–3123.

Ball, K., Owsley, C., Stalvey, B., Roenker, D. L., Sloane, M., & Graves, M. (1998). Driving avoidance and functional impairment in older drivers. *Accident Analysis and Prevention, 30,* 313–322.

Ball, K., Roenker, D., Wadley, V., Edwards, J., Roth, D., McGwin, G., Jr., et al. (2006). Can high-risk older drivers be identified through performance-based measures in a Department of Motor Vehicles setting? *Journal of the American Geriatrics Society, 54,* 77–84.

Bowers, A. R., Apfelbaum, D. H., & Peli, E. (2005). Bioptic telescopes meet the needs of drivers with moderate visual acuity loss. *Investigative Ophthalmology and Visual Science, 46,* 66–74.

Bowers, A. R., Keeney, K., & Peli, E. (2008). Community-based trial of peripheral prism visual field expansion for hemianopia. *Archives of Ophthalmology, 126,* 657–664.

Bowers, A. R., Mandel, A. J., Goldstein, R. B., & Peli, E. (2010). Driving with hemianopia, II: Lane position and steering in a driving simulator. *Investigative Ophthalmology and Visual Science, 51,* 6605–6613.

Bowers, A., Peli, E., Elgin, J., McGwin, G., & Owsley, C. (2005). On-road driving with moderate visual field loss. *Optometry and Vision Science, 82,* 657–667.

Charman, W. N. (1997). Vision and driving—A literature review and commentary. *Ophthalmic and Physiological Optics, 17,* 371–391.

Classen, S., McCarthy, D. P., Shechtman, O., Awadzi, K. D., Lanford, D. N., Okun, M. S., et al. (2009). Useful Field of View as a reliable screening measure of driving performance in people with Parkinson's disease: Results of a pilot study. *Traffic Injury Prevention, 10,* 593–598.

Classen, S., Witter, D., Lanford, D. N., Okun, M. S., Rodriguez, R. L., Romrell, J., et al. (2011) Usefulness of screening tools for predicting driving performance in people with Parkinson's disease. *American Journal of Occupational Therapy, 65,* 519–588. doi.10.5014/ajot.2011.001073

Cross, J. M., McGwin, G., Jr., Rubin, G. S., Ball, K. K., West, S. K., Roenker, D. L., et al. (2009). Visual and medical risk factors for motor vehicle collision involvement among older drivers. *British Journal of Ophthalmology, 93,* 400–404.

Cushman, L. A. (1996). Cognitive capacity and concurrent driving performance in older drivers. *IATSS Research, 20,* 38–45.

Decina, L. E., Breton, M. E., & Staplin, L. (1991). *Visual disorders and commercial drivers* (Report No. DTFH61-90-C-0093). Washington, DC: Federal Highway Administration, Office of Motor Carriers.

Dionne, G., Desjardins, D., Laberge-Nadeau, C., & Maag, U. (1995). Medical conditions, risk exposure, and truck drivers' accidents: An analysis with count data regression models. *Accident Analysis and Prevention, 27,* 295–305.

Duchek, J. M., Hunt, L., Ball, K., Buckles, V., & Morris, J. C. (1998). Attention and driving performance in Alzheimer's disease. *Journals of Gerontology, Series B: Psychological Sciences, and Social Sciences, 53,* 130–141.

Edwards, J., Ross, L., Wadley, V., Clay, O., Crowe, M., Roenker, D., et al. (2006). The Useful Field of View test: Normative data for older adults. *Archives of Clinical Neuropsychology, 21,* 275–286.

Edwards, J. D., Vance, D. E., Wadley, V. G., Cissell, G. M., Roenker, D., & Ball, K. (2005). The reliability and validity of Useful Field of View test scores for older adults. *Journal of Clinical and Experimental Neuropsychology, 27,* 529–543.

Elgin, J., McGwin, G., Wood, J., Vaphiades, M., Braswell, R., DeCarlo, D., et al. (2010). Evaluation of on-road driving in people with hemianopia and quadrantanopia. *American Journal of Occupational Therapy, 64,* 268–278. doi: 10.5014/ajot.64.2.268.

Esterman, B. (1982). Functional scoring of the binocular field. *Ophthalmology, 89,* 1226–1234.

Federal Highway Administration, Office of Motor Carrier Standards. (1996). *The seventh monitoring report on the drivers of commercial motor vehicles who receive vision waivers.* Washington, DC: U.S. Department of Transportation.

Federal Highway Administration. (2003). *Manual on uniform traffic control devices, 2003 edition, revision 1.* Washington, DC: U.S. Department of Transportation.

Ferris, F. L., Kassoff, A., Bresnick, G. H., & Bailey, I. (1982). New visual acuity charts for clinical research. *American Journal of Ophthalmology, 94,* 91–96.

Freeman, E. E., Munoz, B., Turano, K. A., & West, S. K. (2006). Measures of visual function and their association with driving modification in older adults. *Investigative Ophthalmology and Visual Science, 47,* 514–520.

Friedman, D. S., O'Colmain, B. J., Munoz, B., Tomany, S. C., McCarty, C., de Jong, P. T., et al. (2004). Prevalence of age-related macular degeneration in the United States. *Archives of Ophthalmology, 122,* 564–572.

Friedman, D. S., Wolfs, R. C., O'Colmain, B. J., Klein, B. E., Taylor, H. R., West, S., et al. (2004). Prevalence of open-angle glaucoma among adults in the United States. *Archives of Ophthalmology, 122,* 532–538.

Gauthier, L., DeHaut, F., & Joanette, Y. (1989). The Bells Test: A quantitative and qualitative test for visual neglect. *International Journal of Clinical Neuropsychology, 11,* 49–54.

Goode, K. T., Ball, K. K., Sloane, M., Roenker, D. L., Roth, D. L., Myers, R. S., et al. (1998). Useful field of view and other neurocognitive indicators of crash risk in older adults. *Journal of Clinical Psychology in Medical Settings, 5,* 425–440.

Grabowski, D. C., & Morrisey, M. A. (2001). The effect of state regulations on motor vehicle fatalities for younger and older drivers: A review and analysis. *Milbank Quarterly, 79,* 517–545.

Grossman, M., & Edson, M. (2002). *Natural eye care.* Retrieved January 29, 2012, from www.visionworksusa.com/cataract_chapter.htm

Haymes, S. A., LeBlanc, R. P., Nicolela, M. T., Chiasson, L. A., & Chauhan, B. C. (2007). Risk of falls and motor vehicle collisions in glaucoma. *Investigative Ophthalmology and Visual Science, 48,* 1149–1155.

Heath, G. G., & Schmidt, I. (1959). Signal color recognition in color defective observers. *American Journal of Optometry and Archives of the American Academy of Optometry, 36,* 421–437.

Hennessy, D. F., & Janke, M. K. (2009). *Clearing a road to driving fitness by better assessing driving wellness: Development of California's prospective three-tier driving center assessment system* (Report No. CAL-DMV-RSS-05-215). Sacramento: California Department of Motor Vehicles, Research and Development Section.

Higgins, K. E., Wood, J., & Tait, A. (1998). Vision and driving: Selective effect of optical blur on different driving tasks. *Human Factors, 41,* 224–232.

Johnson, C. A., & Keltner, J. L. (1983). Incidence of visual field loss in 20,000 eyes and its relationship to driving performance. *Archives of Ophthalmology, 101,* 371–375.

Kempen, J. H., O'Colmain, B. J., Leske, M. C., Haffner, S. M., Klein, R., Moss, S. E., et al. (2004). The prevalence of diabetic retinopathy among adults in the United States. *Archives of Ophthalmology, 122,* 552–563.

Laberge-Nadeau, C., Dionne, G., Maag, U., Desjardins, D., Vanasse, C., & Ekoe, J.-M. (1996). Medical conditions and the severity of commercial motor vehicle drivers' road accidents. *Accident Analysis and Prevention, 28,* 43–51.

Maag, U., Vanasse, C., Dionne, G., & Laberge-Nadeau, C. (1997). Taxi-drivers' accidents: How binocular vision problems are related to their rate and severity in terms of the number of victims. *Accident Analysis and Prevention, 29,* 217–224.

Mazer, B. L., Korner-Bitensky, N. A., & Sofer, S. (1998). Predicting ability to drive after stroke. *Archives of Physical Medicine and Rehabilitation, 79,* 743–750.

McGwin, G., Jr., Chapman, V., & Owsley, C. (2000). Visual risk factors for driving difficulty among older drivers. *Accident Analysis and Prevention, 32,* 735–744.

McGwin, G., Jr., Xie, A., Mays, A., Joiner, W., DeCarlo, D., Hall, T., et al. (2005). Visual field defects and the risk of motor vehicle collisions among patients with glaucoma. *Investigative Ophthalmology and Visual Science, 46,* 4437–4441.

McKnight, A. J., Shinar, D., & Hilburn, B. (1991). The visual and driving performance of monocular and binocular heavy-duty truck drivers. *Accident Analysis and Prevention, 23,* 225–237.

Myers, R. S., Ball, K. K., Kalina, T. D., Roth, D. L., & Goode, K. T. (2000). Relation of Useful Field of View and other screening tests to on-road driving performance. *Perceptual and Motor Skills, 91,* 279–290.

National Eye Institute. (2011). *Age-related eye disease study 2 (AREDS2).* Retrieved June 28, 2012, from http://www.nei.nih.gov/areds2

Owsley, C. (2003). Contrast sensitivity. *Ophthalmology Clinics of North America, 16,* 171–177.

Owsley, C., Ball, K., & Keeton, D. (1994). Relationship between visual sensitivity and target localization in older adults. *Vision Research, 35,* 579–587.

Owsley, C., Ball, K., McGwin, G., Jr., Sloane, M. E., Roenker, D. L., White, M. F., et al. (1998). Visual processing impairment and risk of motor vehicle crash among older adults. *JAMA, 279,* 1083–1088.

Owsley, C., & McGwin, G., Jr. (1999). Vision impairment and driving. *Survey of Ophthalmology, 43,* 535–550.

Owsley, C., & McGwin, G., Jr. (2010). Vision and driving. *Vision Research, 50,* 2348–2361.

Owsley, C., McGwin, G., Jr., Sloane, M. E., Wells, J., Stalvey, B. T., & Gauthreaux, S. (2002). Impact of cataract surgery on motor vehicle crash involvement by older adults. *JAMA, 288,* 841–849.

Owsley, C., Stalvey, B. T., Wells, J., Sloane, M. E., & McGwin, G., Jr. (2001). Visual risk factors for crash involvement in older drivers with cataract. *Archives of Ophthalmology, 119,* 881–887.

Park, W. L., Unatin, J., & Park, C. K. (1995). A profile of the demographics, training and driving history of the telescopic drivers in the state of Michigan. *Journal of the American Optometric Association, 66,* 274–280.

Parker, W., McGwin, G., Jr., Wood, J., Elgin, J., Vaphiades, M., Kline, L., et al. (2011). Self-reported driving difficulty by persons with hemianopia and quadrantanopia. *Current Eye Research, 36,* 270–277.

Peli, E., & Peli, D. (2002). *Driving with confidence: A practical guide to driving with low vision.* River Edge, NJ: World Scientific Press.

Pelli, D. G., Robson, J. G., & Wilkins, A. J. (1988). The design of a new letter chart for measuring contrast sensitivity. *Clinical Vision Sciences, 2,* 187–199.

Racette, L., & Casson, E. J. (2005). The impact of visual field loss on driving performance: Evidence from on-road driving assessments. *Optometry and Vision Science, 82,* 668–674.

Reitan, R. (1958). The relation of the Trail Making Test to organic brain damage. *Journal of Consulting Psychology, 19,* 393–394.

Rizzo, M., Reinach, S., McGehee, D., & Dawson, J. (1997). Simulated car crashes and crash predictors in drivers with Alzheimer disease. *Archives of Neurology, 54,* 545–551.

Roenker, D. L., Cissell, G. M., Ball, K. K., Wadley, V. G., & Edwards, J. D. (2003). Speed-of-processing and driving simulator training result in improved driving performance. *Human Factors, 45,* 218–233.

Roger, P. N., Ratz, M., & Janke, M. K. (1987). *Accident and conviction rates of visually impaired heavy-vehicle operators.* Sacramento: California Department of Motor Vehicles, Research and Development Section.

Rubin, G. S., Keyl, P. M., Munoz, B., Bandeen-Roche, K., Huang, G. H., West, S. K., et al. (1999). The association of vision, cognition, and attention with crashes in an older American population: SEE Study. *Investigative Ophthalmology and Visual Science, 40*(Suppl.), S387.

Schenkenberg, T., Bradford, D. C., & Ajax, E. T. (1980). Line bisection and unilateral visual neglect in patients with neurologic impairment. *Neurology, 30,* 509–517.

Schieber, F. (2004). Highway research to enhance safety and mobility of older road users. In *Transportation in an aging society: A decade of experience* (Conference Proceedings 27, pp. 125–154). Washington, DC: National Academies Press.

Schmidt, S., Hauser, M. A., Scott, W. K., Postel, E. A., Agarwal, A., Gallins, P., et al. (2006). Cigarette smoking strongly modifies the association of LOC387715 and age-related macular degeneration. *American Journal of Human Genetics, 78,* 852–864.

Scilley, K., Jackson, G. R., Cideciyan, A. V., Maguire, M. G., Jacobson, S. G., & Owsley, C. (2002). Early age-related maculopathy and self-reported visual difficulty in daily life. *Ophthalmology, 109,* 1235–1242.

Shulman, K. I., Shedletsky, R., & Silver, I. L. (1986). The challenge of time: Clock-drawing and cognitive function in the elderly. *International Journal of Geriatric Psychiatry, 1,* 135–140.

Spreen, O., & Strauss, E. (1991). *A compendium of neuropsychological tests.* New York: Oxford University Press.

Uc, E. Y., Rizzo, M., Anderson, S. W., Dastrup, E., Sparks, J. D., & Dawson, J. D. (2009). Driving under low-contrast visibility conditions in Parkinson disease. *Neurology, 73,* 1103–1110.

Uc, E. Y., Rizzo, M., Johnson, A. M., Dastrup, E., Anderson, S. W., & Dawson, J. D. (2009). Road safety in drivers with Parkinson disease. *Neurology, 73,* 2112–2119.

Vingrys, A. J., & Cole, B. L. (1988). Are colour vision standards justified for the transport industry? *Ophthalmic and Physiological Optics, 8,* 257–274.

Warren, M. (1998). *Brain Injury Visual Assessment Battery for Adults test manual.* Birmingham, AL: VisAbilities Rehab Services.

Warren, M. (2011). Intervention for adults with vision impairment from acquired brain injury. In M. Warren & E. A. Barstow (Eds.), *Occupational therapy interventions for adults with low vision* (pp. 403–448). Bethesda, MD: AOTA Press.

Wood, J. M. (2002). Age and visual impairment decrease driving performance as measured on a closed-road circuit. *Human Factors, 44,* 482–494.

Wood, J. M., Anstey, K. J., Kerr, G. K., Lacherez, P. F., & Lord, S. (2008). A multidomain approach for predicting older driver safety under in-traffic road conditions. *Journal of the American Geriatrics Society, 56,* 986–993.

Wood, J. M., & Carberry, T. P. (2004). Older drivers and cataracts: Measures of driving performance before and after cataract surgery. *Transportation Research Record: Journal of the Transportation Research Board, 1865,* 7–13.

Wood, J. M., & Carberry, T. P. (2006). Bilateral cataract surgery and driving performance. *British Journal of Ophthalmology, 90,* 1277–1280.

Wood, J. M., Dique, T., & Troutbeck, R. (1993). The effect of artificial visual impairment on functional visual fields and driving performance. *Clinical Vision Science, 8,* 563–575.

Wood, J. M., McGwin, G., Jr., Elgin, J., Vaphiades, M. S., Braswell, R. A., DeCarlo, D. K., et al. (2009). On-road driving performance by persons with hemianopia and quadrantanopia. *Investigative Ophthalmology and Visual Science, 50,* 577–585.

Wood, J., McGwin, G., Jr., Elgin, J., Vaphiades, M., Braswell, R., DeCarlo, D., et al. (2011). Hemianopic and quadrantopic field loss, eye and head movements, and driving. *Investigative Ophthalmology and Visual Science, 52,* 1220–1225.

Wood, J. M., & Troutbeck, R. (1992). Effect of restriction of the binocular visual field on driving performance. *Ophthalmic and Physiological Optics, 12,* 291–298.

Worringham, C., Wood, J. M., Kerr, G., & Silburn, P. (2006). Predictors of driving assessment outcome in Parkinson's disease. *Movement Disorders, 21,* 230–235.

Appendix 8.A. Vision-Related Resources

- *Occupational Therapy Interventions for Adults With Low Vision,* edited by Mary Warren, MS, OTR/L, SCLV, FAOTA, and Elizabeth A. Barstow, MS, OTR/L, SCLV (available from AOTA at http://myaota.aota.org/shop_aota/ prodview.aspx?TYPE=D&PID=724&SKU=1252). As the U.S. population continues to age, occupational therapy practitioners must be prepared to address the increasing low vision needs of clients, helping them to maintain a good quality of life. This comprehensive text provides an occupational therapy approach to all aspects of low vision, from evaluation to intervention and rehabilitation.

- *University of Alabama at Birmingham Graduate Certificate in Low Vision Rehabilitation* (more information at www.uab.edu/ot/low-vision-rehabilitation-graduate-certificate). The Graduate Certificate in Low Vision Rehabilitation is a practice-oriented certificate degree program to prepare occupational therapists to provide comprehensive, competent intervention to adults with visual impairment from age-related eye diseases and brain injury. The program is designed for occupational therapists already working in low vision rehabilitation, those interested in starting low vision rehabilitation programs, and those just interested in expanding their practice skills.

- *Early Treatment of Diabetic Retinopathy Study Distance Visual Acuity Chart* (available at www.precision-vision.com).

- *Mars Letter Contrast Sensitivity Test* (available at www.marsperceptrix.com).

- *LEA Numbers Low Contrast Flipchart* (available at www.good-lite.com).

- *Pelli–Robson Letter Contrast Sensitivity Chart* (available at www.psych. nyu.edu/pelli/pellirobson).

- *Adaptive Mobility Sources,* Florida (www.adaptivemobility.com).

- *Age-Related Eye Disease Study 2* (www.nei.nih.gov/areds2). AREDS–2 is a multicenter, randomized trial study to determine whether a modified combination of vitamins and minerals can further slow the progression of vision loss from age-related macular degeneration.

- *American Foundation for the Blind* (www.afb.org). The American Foundation for the Blind promotes independent and healthy living for individuals with vision loss, broadens access to technology, improves the information and tools available to the professionals who work with individuals with blindness or visual impairment, and advocates on behalf of the rights and interests of Americans with vision loss.

- *Lighthouse International* (www.lighthouse.org). Lighthouse International works to prevent vision loss and treat and empower those with visual impairment gain independence.

- *American Academy of Ophthalmology* (www.aao.org). This association represents eye physicians and its Web site contains resources to educate the public on eye diseases and conditions.

- *National Eye Institute* (http://www.nih.gov/about/almanac/organization/NEI.htm). Part of the National Institutes for Health, the National Eye Institute conducts and supports research, training, health information dissemination, and other programs related to blinding eye diseases, visual disorders, mechanisms of visual function, preservation of sight, and the special health problems of individuals with visual impairment or blindness.

- *Snellen Chart* (available at www.precision-vision.com/index.cfm/category/114/snellen-eye-charts.cfm).
- *Optec 2500 or 5500 Visual Analyzer* (available at www.stereooptical.com/products/vision-testers/optec-5500).
- *Driving Health Inventory* (available at www.transanalytics.com/researchApplication.htm)
- *Humphrey Field Analyzer* (available at www.meditec.zeiss.com/88256D E3007B916B/0/8E8B485E8FF2B16EC125789D0047AF9E/$file/perimetry-brochure.pdf).
- *Goldmann Perimetry Test* (available at www.haag-streit.com/products/perimetry.html).
- *Keystone Vision Screener* (available at www.keystoneview.com/index.php?option=com_virtuemart&Itemid=106&lang=en).
- *Dynavision* (available at http://www.dynavisiond2.com/index.php).
- *Bioptic Telescope* (available at www.ocutech.com).
- *Keplerian Telescope* (available at http://www.ocutech.com/Products/VES-MINI/).

Appendix 8.B. A Personal Perspective and Introduction to Advances in Ophthalmology

Sherrilene Classen, PhD, MPH, OTR/L

Introduction

Vision is essential for driving—without the ability to see, one simply cannot drive. When vision is impaired because of uncorrected or undetected age-related or medical conditions, drivers are a risk to themselves, their passengers, pedestrians, and other road users.

The science to improve vision is rapidly evolving through the discoveries of new technologies (e.g., eye trackers to pinpoint gaze and saccade activity); interventions such as wavefront-guided refractive surgery for the correction of far- or near-sightedness; and therapeutic applications such as new drug treatments (e.g., bivacizumab, ranibizumab) for the management of age-related macular degeneration (AMD). Concurrently, research is emerging on the efficacy or effectiveness of these leading-edge approaches.

Competency in conducting visual assessments requires staying current with advances in vision evaluation and treatment. The rapid progress in ophthalmology advancements has exceeded the base knowledge that most practitioners have acquired in the occupational therapy curriculum—that is, basic knowledge on the anatomy of the visual system, major impairments or diseases of the eye, and exposure to visual acuity and visual field deficits. Some occupational therapists may have been exposed to specialty courses addressing *low vision rehabilitation*, such as the one offered through the Graduate Certificate in Low Vision Rehabilitation at the University of Alabama, Birmingham (UAB), whereas others may have acquired skills in *vision rehabilitation*, in which the aim is mainly to provide rehabilitation for those with a loss of visual acuity or impairment in the visual fields. Finally, others may have been exposed to *vision therapy*, an approach designed to remediate underlying vision disorders, including neurosensory or neuromuscular functions (Rosenfeld, 2011). However, many occupational therapists may not have acquired additional knowledge on the advancements in vision since graduating from their occupational therapy training.

The main purpose of this appendix is to introduce occupational therapists to advances in ophthalmology, as I observed during a year-long knowledge enhancement project to better understand the visual system and its relationship to driving. During 2011, I completed a course "Understanding and Managing Visual Deficits: A Guide for Occupational Therapists," presented by Mitchell Scheiman, OD, FCOVD, and engaged in week-long visitations with experts in the field, including Cynthia Owsley, PhD, at UAB and Peter Rosen, MD, board-certified ophthalmologist, University of California–San Diego. I attended conferences, including those of the Association for Research in Vision Ophthalmology (Fort Lauderdale, FL) and of the Vision Sciences Society (Naples, FL). I visited with scientists such as Dr. Wiebo Brouwer from the University Medical Center, Groningen, the Netherlands, and Dr. Hannes Devos from De Katolieke University, Leuven, Belgium. Both of these scientists are studying neurological conditions, including those conditions that impair the visual system and its related effect on driving performance. I also participated in expert research panels (Dementia and Driving, International Psychogeriatric Conference, the Hague, the Netherlands); engaged in scholarly discussions with Ergun Uc, MD, board-certified neurologist, University of Iowa, and expert on visual impairment in people with Parkinson's disease; and attended and delivered a presentation at the Eye and the Auto International Conference (Detroit, MI). These experiences

- Enabled me to have a better understanding of the complexities of the visual system and how it affects driving,
- Left me with many visual system questions still to be answered, and
- Imprinted on me the importance of sharing information that is difficult to obtain in one lecture or one continuing education session with occupational therapy colleagues.

I share the advances in ophthalmology I observed, with the disclaimer that I am not an ophthalmologist or vision expert but rather a rehabilitation scientist and occupational therapist intrigued by the richness and complexity of the visual system.

Overview

In a systematic literature review, Bourne (2011) estimated that the global burden of those with significant visual impairment because of conditions such as cataract, glaucoma, uncorrected refractive error, macular degeneration, and other eye diseases (e.g., trachoma, vitamin A deficiency, external injury, diabetic retinopathy (DR) and other retinopathies, and external ocular injuries) accounted for about 45.7 million people. In the United States, about 30% of people experience some form of visual impairment, and this number is expected to increase because of the aging of the population as well as the growing global pandemic of Type 2 diabetes and its associated secondary effects on vision (Wong, 2011). It is realistic to expect that such visual impairments will affect the independent and safe driving performance of adults and the community mobility of all groups in the population.

Major biological, genetic, genomic, medical, and surgical advances are currently being investigated, tested, or implemented that may revolutionize this decade for people with low vision or those who are blind. Although these approaches have a strong biomedical orientation and mainly pertain to body function and structure, occupational therapists may appreciate knowledge of these techniques to better understand treatment options for their clients. Moreover, some of these techniques may make the difference between impaired and functional vision, and thus between dependence and independence in driving and community mobility. I must note that many of these approaches have not been tested empirically to make clear their relationship with driving performance or community mobility.

Medical and Surgical Advances

Refractive error includes *myopia* (nearsightedness), *hyperopia* (farsightedness), and *astigmatism* (blurred vision). The global prevalence of refractive errors has been estimated to be 800 million to 2.3 billion people (World Health Organization, 2009). Significant advances have been made in the screening, early detection, diagnosis, and treatment of refractive error. Treatment of refractive error, which may potentially influence many aspects of independent and safe mobility, is prescribing *wavefront-guided corrective lenses* (not invasive) or performing *wavefront-guided refractive surgery* (invasive) (Kensick, Brown, & Ginsburg, 2007). Essentially, wavefront technologies improve optometric and surgical results by optimizing retinal image quality and reducing optical blur through eliminating or reducing high-order aberrations. This improvement is especially essential for clients with high-order aberrations in which vision is not adequately compensated for with conventional lower-order spectacles.

Advances in Diagnosing Eye Diseases

The diagnosis and early detection of posterior eye diseases (e.g., glaucoma, retinopathy, AMD) are now possible through the use of advanced technologies such as *confocal scanning laser ophthalmoscopy (SLO;* Webb, Hughes, & Delori, 1987) and *high-resolution time and frequency domain optical coherence tomography (HD–OCT).* Confocal SLO is a retinal imaging technique that uses laser light to illuminate the retina and to generate high-contrast images through optical slicing techniques. Confocal SLO provides images of the multilayered retina to detect abnormalities (Webb et al., 1987).

HD–OCT uses principles of light interferometry, that is, shining a laser light into the eye to generate cross-sectional images of the eye to observe preclinical and clinical disease progression. HD–OCT does not require contact with the tissue and as such is noninvasive (Arevalo, Krivoy, & Fernandez, 2009). HD–OCT is therefore a client-friendly technique that has the advantage of imaging and quantitatively analyzing retinal thickness, nerve fiber layer, and optic nerve structures with good reproducibility. These technologies have revolutionized the analysis of internal eye structures. They have also made it possible for ophthalmologists to correlate the structural and accompanying functional changes in the eye for early detection and to follow the progression of disease patterns.

Advances in Treating Eye Diseases

Cataract

Cataract, the most common cause of blindness, can be detected with routine eye-care visits and corrected with surgery. Surgery techniques include *intraocular lens* (IOL) *implants*, using monofocal or multifocal lenses. An intraocular lens is a prosthetic lens implant that is placed in the eye after a cataract is removed. These lenses are made of plastic or silicone and stay permanently in the eye after removal of the eye's natural crystalline lens, a structure inside the human eye that helps focus light onto the retina, much like the lens of a camera would do. IOLs may be either monofocal or multifocal (Improve Your Vision, 2009).

Monofocal lenses have a single zone of clear focus, usually set for excellent distance vision but requiring the use of reading glasses for near tasks, such as reading or sewing. *Multifocal lenses* have several zones of clear vision and allow for both distance and near correction (Improve Your Vision, 2009). These surgical techniques restore lost vision and allow people to maintain their independence in driving and community mobility.

Diabetic Retinopathy

Diabetes affected 246 million people worldwide in 2007, and a 55% increase is projected by 2025, with potentially 380 million people being affected worldwide (Wong, 2011). It is estimated that 30%–50% of this global population will have (Wong, 2011). *DR*, damage to the retina owing to complications of diabetes mellitus, is a common sight-threatening complication of diabetes, both Type 1 and Type 2, and is the leading cause of acquired blindness in the adult population in the United States.

New advances in slowing the progression of the disease include applying selective *wavelength laser treatment*. Such laser treatments resolve the retinal thickening and absorb the *hard exudates* (fluid that has exuded out of a tissue or its capillaries because of injury or inflammation). In DR, the microcirculatory problems in the retina of people with diabetes can cause retinal ischemia, which results in physiological processes that may cause the creation of new blood vessels in the retina and elsewhere in the eye, heralding changes that may threaten the sight. *Anti-vascular endothelial growth factor* (anti-VEGF) agents, treatments given to inhibit angiogenesis (growth of new blood vessels from preexisting vessels), may be efficacious in treating DR. Although treatment advances are evident, progress has been slowed by scientists not fully understanding the pathogenetic mechanisms (Lansingh, 2011).

Age-Related Macular Degeneration

Treatments for *AMD*, a medical condition that usually affects older adults and results in a loss of vision in the macula or center of the visual field because of damage to the retina, include those aimed at surgical correction and medications. The surgical procedure includes *macular translocation*, which involves detaching a portion of the retina and relocating it to a healthier place in the eye. Progress in medical treatments to preserve vision includes applying anti-VEGF treatments (previously discussed) through *vitreous injections*. This method inhibits new blood vessel growth *(angiogenesis).*

In a Phase 3 clinical study, Rosenfeld et al. (2006) reported that monthly intra-vitreal injection of ranibizumab led to a significant increase in the level of mean visual acuity compared with sham injections. They concluded that ranibizumab is very effective in the treatment of minimally classic or wet AMD with low rates of ocular adverse effects. In follow-up studies, the effectiveness of two drugs, biva-cizumab and ranibizumab, was determined to be equally promising in decreasing the risk of hemorrhages in the eye and in maintaining the integrity of eye health (Williams, 2011).

Other Advances

Neuroprotection

Neuroprotection entails the mechanisms and strategies used to protect against neu-ronal injury or degeneration of cells in the central nervous system as a result of chronic neurodegenerative processes or disease (Whitcup, 2008). Some strategies or mechanisms may include free radical trappers or scavengers, anti-excitotoxic agents (preserving nerve cells damaged by substances such as glutamate), apoptosis (programmed cell death) inhibitors, anti-inflammatory agents, neurotrophic factors (nerve growth factors that regulate the growth, differentiation, and survival of cer-tain neurons in the peripheral and central nervous systems), or gene therapy.

The goal of neuroprotection is to limit neuronal dysfunction or death after injury and to attempt to maintain the highest possible integrity of cellular interactions in the brain, resulting in an undisturbed neural function. There is a wide range of neu-roprotection products available or under investigation in eye health. For example, much attention has been focused on neuroprotection as a strategy in therapies for glaucomatous optic neuropathy as a means of preserving retinal ganglion cells and their axonal projections (Marcic, Belyea, & Katz, 2003). However, from a review of the current status of neuroprotection in ophthalmic disease, Danesh-Meyer and Levin (2009) concluded that "almost all clinical studies of neuroprotection in neurologic and ophthalmologic disease so far have failed to show efficacy, despite encourag-ing preclinical studies" (p. 186). More optimistically, Whitcup (2008) concluded that "properly designed clinical trials with validated endpoints will yield the most useful information on the neuroprotective effects of therapy, and may provide new treat-ment options to prevent the loss of neurologic function, including vision" (p. 323).

Genomics

Genomics uses large-scale sequencing and genotyping, molecular diagnostics, and gene identification to understand and manipulate gene regulation for enhanced vision function. Genetics, however, provides insight into the human genome and the molecular structure and function of genes (Gabriel, 2011). For example, gene therapy may be useful for suppressing tumor genes to help treat cancers of the eye. Research on tumor suppressor genes continues to shed light on the molecular pathophysiology of ophthalmic tumors and will increasingly yield diagnostic and therapeutic applications. Genetic testing and gene-based therapies can be applied in a targeted way to address disease identification and management (Gabriel, 2011). Gene therapy, as such, is producing a paradigm shift for the management of visual diseases.

Epigenetics

Epigenetics is the study of changes in the *phenotype* (appearance) or gene expression caused by mechanisms other than changes in the underlying DNA sequence (Kowluru, 2011). Epigenetic changes modify chromatin without affecting the DNA sequence, and these stable and heritable covalent modifications can lead to phenotypic variability and susceptibility to disease (Kowluru, 2011). Using epigenetic approaches may help reveal useful markers and environmental factors associated with eye diseases that could facilitate the development of new diagnostic and treatment strategies for many sight-threatening diseases.

Optogenetics

Optogenetic methods are based on using genetic and molecular approaches to selectively target the light-sensitive proteins in cell populations in vivo (Boyden, 2011). Activation of light in these light-sensitive proteins is selective and limited only to those cells expressing the proteins. This selectivity, along with the light-sensitive proteins' fast temporal kinetics of light activation, has opened new ways to probe the cellular and circuitry organization of the nervous system and its relation to behavior (Boyden, 2011). Optogenetic technologies, such as optogenetic retina implants, are emerging at a rapid pace with animal and human studies in progress for the restoration of vision (Roska, 2011). Optogenetics is an exciting technology with a huge potential for restoring vision in those who were previously classified as blind through diagnoses such as retinitis pigmentosa.

Summary

I have reviewed the advances in ophthalmology as I observed them during a year-long knowledge enhancement project to better understand the visual system, current progress and future advances, and its potential implications for continued driving. As such, I introduced occupational therapy colleagues to novel strategies, procedures, treatments, and surgeries in the field of ophthalmology. It is my hope that I have shared knowledge that is otherwise difficult to come by through traditional continuing education courses.

Advances in the discussed medical and surgical methods allow ophthalmologists to better diagnose, treat, and manage disease severity and progression. Yet it is still unclear how these cutting-edge techniques correlate with increases in functional ability. Clinicians and researchers in ophthalmology are expanding efforts to amplify their understanding of how to assess visual performance in relation to task performance. This integration of science with function opens plausible opportunities for occupational therapists and researchers to work collaboratively with medical professionals such as ophthalmologists, bioengineers, and neuroscientists in areas of translational research.

Occupational therapists can contribute particularly by assessing the essential client factors and environmental factors within the context of an ophthalmological intervention and, as such, helping the vision specialist to get a better sense of how the client may be functioning within his or her context. Likewise, the occupational therapist may be instrumental in assessing, intervening, and reporting on the underlying (visual and other) abilities to enable safe driving or independence in community mobility. With the advancements in ophthalmology, and being a member of the multidisciplinary vision team, the occupational therapist is perfectly positioned to participate in effectiveness studies conducted to examine how advances in ophthalmology may enhance function in clients. Finally, in concert with the vision team, occupational therapists may develop, test, and implement additional intervention strategies to enhance the visual abilities underlying driving or independence in community mobility.

Indeed, these advances in ophthalmology hold the potential for occupational therapists to embrace vision as a core function and to participate in developments to make occupational therapy a needed service, especially pertaining to driving and community mobility.

Acknowledgments

I appreciate the insights, knowledge, and editorial help of Peter Rosen as I was writing this piece; all the scientists, ophthalmologists, optometrists, neurologists, and other vision and driving researchers who have contributed richly to my knowledge; and the University of Florida for awarding me with the Faculty Enhancement Opportunity to be able to more deeply study vision and driving-related issues.

References

Arevalo, J. F., Krivoy, D., & Fernandez, C. F. (2009). How does optical coherence tomography work? Basic principles. In J. F. Arevalo (Ed.), *Retinal angiography and optical coherence tomography* (pp. 217–222). New York: Springer.

Bourne, R. R. (2011, May). *Global burden of visual impairment and blindness: The systematic review process and findings.* Paper presented at the annual meeting of the Association for Research in Vision and Ophthalmology, Fort Lauderdale, FL.

Boyden, E. (2011, May). *Optogenetics: Tools for controlling neurocircuits with light.* Paper presented at the annual meeting of the Association for Research in Vision and Ophthalmology, Fort Lauderdale, FL.

Danesh-Meyer, H. V., & Levin, L. A. (2009). Neuroprotection: Extrapolating from neurologic diseases to the eye. *American Journal of Ophthalmology, 148,* 186–191.

Gabriel, S. (2011, May). *Current technologies and the future of genomics research.* Paper presented at the annual meeting of the Association for Research in Vision and Ophthalmology, Fort Lauderdale, FL.

Improve Your Vision. (2009). *Eye glossary.* Retrieved September 29, 2011, from www.improveyourvision.com/understanding-vision/eye-glossary.html

Kensick, J., Brown, M. C., & Ginsburg, A. (2007, May). *Improvement of night driving visibility detection with wavefront-guided spectacle lenses.* Poster presented at the annual meeting of the Association for Research in Vision and Ophthalmology, Fort Lauderdale, FL.

Kowluru, R. A. (2011, May). *Epigenetics modifications and ocular diseases.* Special interest group presented at the annual meeting of the Association for Research in Vision and Ophthalmology, Fort Lauderdale, FL.

Lansingh, V. C. (2011, May). *Training of cataract surgery to meet the expected needs.* Paper presented at the annual meeting of the Association for Research in Vision and Ophthalmology, Fort Lauderdale, FL.

Marcic, T. S., Belyea, D. A., & Katz, B. (2003). Neuroprotection in glaucoma: A model for neuroprotection in optic neuropathies. *Current Opinion in Ophthalmology, 14,* 353–356.

Rosenfeld, P. J., Brown, D. M., Heier, J. S., Boyer, D. S., Kaiser, P. K., Chung, C. Y., et al. (2006). Ranibizumab for neovascular age-related macular degeneration. *New England Journal of Medicine, 355,* 1419–1431.

Rosenfeld, S. (2011). Vision and occupational therapy: Terminology, tips, and trends. *OT Practice, 16*(15), 7–11.

Roska, B. (2011, May). *Targeting optogenetic tools to strategically important retinal cell types in retinal degeneration to restore visual function.* Paper presented at the annual meeting of the Association for Research in Vision and Ophthalmology, Fort Lauderdale, FL.

Vision and Driving   219

Webb, R. H., Hughes, G. W., & Delori, F. C. (1987). Confocal scanning laser ophthalmoscope.
    Applied Optics, 26, 1492–1499.
Whitcup, S. M. (2008). Clinical trials in neuroprotection. *Progress in Brain Research, 173*,
    323–335.
Williams, D. F. (2011, May). *How do the results of the CATT trial affect the use of anti-VEGF
    agents in DME?* Paper presented at the annual meeting of the Association for Research in
    Vision and Ophthalmology, Fort Lauderdale, FL.
Wong, T. (2011, May). *Diabetic retinopathy: Major research advances and gaps to translating such
    research.* Paper presented at the annual meeting of the Association for Research in Vision
    and Ophthalmology, Fort Lauderdale, FL.
World Health Organization. (2009). *Disease and injury country estimates.* Retrieved
    September 29, 2011, from www.who.int/healthinfo/global_burden_disease/estimates_
    country/en/index.html

CHAPTER 9

Occupational Therapy Driving Evaluation: Using Evidence-Based Screening and Assessment Tools

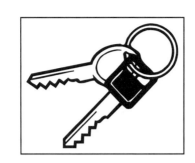

Sherrilene Classen, PhD, MPH, OTR/L, FAOTA;
Anne Dickerson, PhD, OTR/L, FAOTA; and
Michael D. Justiss, PhD, OTR

Learning Objectives

At the completion of this chapter, readers will be able to

- Delineate measurement theory, its application, and its importance according to the main principles of measurement as it relates to driving;
- Recognize the importance of collecting general demographic, driving habits, and driving history information;
- Identify the standard clinical assessments, their uses, and the evidence supporting them as commonly used by occupational therapists in evaluating driving knowledge, skills, and abilities;
- Recognize the importance of the behind-the-wheel component and the information it contributes to the overall driving evaluation; and
- Identify types, uses, and evidence of self-report tools that may inform clinical decision making for continuation of driving and use of community mobility.

Introduction

This chapter provides occupational therapists with basic background information on measurement theory as it relates to driving and an introduction to the *comprehensive driving evaluation (CDE)*. Specifically, the CDE consists of various components (e.g., self-report, interview, family or caregiver report, clinical assessment, behind-the-wheel evaluation) that affect the occupational therapist's eventual decision regarding continuation of driving and the use of community mobility options. As such, this chapter clarifies the distinctions among the different assessments and types of assessments, the domains of functional performance assessed, and the evidence supporting the use of individual assessments.

Key Words

- bias
- closed-course evaluation
- comprehensive driving evaluation
- descriptive instrument
- error
- evaluative instrument
- item response theory
- naturalistic driving
- nonstandardized instrument
- open-road evaluation
- predictive instrument
- receiver operating characteristic curve
- reliability
- simulator sickness
- standardized instrument
- validity

Measurement

Measurement, in its simplest form, is defined as the rules for quantifying a classification of certain attributes or characteristics (Law, 1987). The assignment of a quantifiable value makes possible a mathematical evaluation of the construct being measured in a standardized way so that comparisons across individuals or groups of individuals can be made.

In the case of a driving performance test, measurement allows a therapist to assign values to a driving performance outcome and to make comparisons between people undergoing the same test. Generally three types of instruments exist in measurement: (1) descriptive, (2) evaluative, and (3) predictive.

Generally three types of instruments exist in measurement: (1) descriptive, (2) evaluative, and (3) predictive.

- *Descriptive instruments* use items to describe individuals within groups and to characterize the differences between individuals on the attribute being measured. This information can be used by the therapist to assess the specific characteristics of an individual to determine whether and what type of intervention is needed. An example of a descriptive instrument is the Dementia Rating Scale (Morris, 1993) discussed in this chapter (see **Table 9.1** for Web site).
- *Evaluative instruments* use criteria or items to measure an individual over time. The most appropriate characteristics included in an evaluative instrument are associated with those that can be sensitive to change within an individual. The Simulator Sickness Questionnaire (Kennedy, Lane, Berbaum, & Lilienthal, 1993) discussed later in this chapter is an example of an evaluative measure.
- *Predictive instruments* use criteria to classify individuals to predict a certain trait in comparison to set criteria. For example, a predictive tool can measure driving performance in an older adult to predict whether that individual will be able to successfully return to driving. The Useful Field of View (UFOV®; Edwards et al., 2006), discussed later in this chapter, is an example of a predictor instrument. Predictive tools are often used as screening instruments.

It is not just the type of instrument that is important but also the operational issues related to the instrument. Such considerations may be related to the format (e.g., paper-and-pencil, computer-administered), cost, and orientation of the test (e.g., invasive or not, degree of cooperation required). Likewise, the clinical utility or usefulness must be considered. This includes time to complete the test, scoring procedures, and training required to administer the test. Occupational therapists need to make decisions regarding which test to use on the basis of the specific needs for their clients (descriptive, evaluative, or predictive) and the aforementioned practical and logistical considerations. Our next topic—whether the tools are standardized, are validated with research, or are nonstandardized tools—is an important consideration when making decisions on skills and performances underlying driving safety.

Standardized vs. Nonstandardized Instruments

A *standardized instrument* is one that has undergone extensive development and typically provides a user manual detailing the process of development, protocol for administration, procedure for scoring, and rules for interpretation. Descriptive and predictive instruments should provide normative data as a reference from which

Table 9.1. Driving Assessments

Assessment	Source	Description	Related Evidence
Vision or Visual–Perceptual Assessments			
Clock test	Clock drawing available at www.medicine. mcgill.ca/strokengine-assess/PDF/ CDTSampleCircle.pdf Instructions provided in Manos & Wu (1994) (No commercial materials needed)	The client is asked to reproduce the face of a clock set to a specific time. This may detect difficulties with visual–spatial skills, visual perception, selective attention, memory, abstract thinking, and executive functioning.	Manos (1999) Juby et al. (2002)
Color perception (Ishihara color test)	Widely available from vendors such as Precision Vision: precision-vision.com/index.cfm/ category/67/color-vision-tests.cfm?CFID= 18398261&CFTOKEN=fff8c663a468b309- 45315EC9-E97B-1D3B-BA3520783553A1A3 Also available in the Optec Functional Vision Analyzer: www.stereooptical.com/products/ slide-packages	A test for red or green color deficiencies was first published in 1917 by Dr. Shinobu Ishihara.	Owsley et al. (1991) Owsley & McGwin (1999)
Contrast sensitivity	Varied tests of contrast sensitivity including the Pelli–Robson (Janke & Eberhard, 1998) are available from vendors such as Precision Vision: precision-vision.com/index.cfm/ category/10/contrast-eye-charts.cfm Contrast sensitivity slides also available for the Optec Functional Vision Analyzer: www. stereooptical.com/products/slide-packages www.nhtsa.gov/people/injury/olddrive/ safe/02a.htm	A contrast sensitivity test measures how well people can discern objects with fuzzy, poorly defined edges or low-contrast objects that may be only slightly brighter or darker than their surroundings, which is important to night driving.	Bowers et al. (2005) Janke (2001) Janke & Eberhard (1998) McCarthy & Mann (2006) Owsley et al. (1999) Owsley et al. (2002) Stav et al. (2008)
Depth perception	Available in the Optec Functional Vision Analyzer: www.stereooptical.com/products/ slide-packages	This is the ability to perceive the environment in three dimensions and to understand the distance of objects in relation to each other. It is created by stereopsis, the two eyes working together to view objects in the environment. For more information, see Wong et al. (2002).	Margolis et al. (2002) Owsley et al. (1991) Owsley & McGwin (1999) Racette & Casson (2005)
Glare recovery	Available in certain models of the Optec Functional Vision Analyzer: www. stereooptical.com/products/vision-testers/ optec-5000	This assesses vision impairment and how quickly a person recovers vision after exposure to a bright light source.	Ball et al. (1993) Owsley et al. (1991)
Letter and number cancellation (Cancel H tests)	Details on letter and number cancellation tests can be found in Lezak et al. (2004) Cancel H test forms can be obtained from Bob Uttl, Psychology Department, Oregon State University; 204C Moreland Hall, Corvallis, OR 97331-5303, or e-mail bob. uttl@orst.edu	This assesses visual scanning and selective attention as a client scans a grouping of letters and has to select and draw a hash mark through the targeted letter (H).	Eby et al. (2009) Richardson & Marottoli (2003)
Motor-Free Visual Perception Test	Colarusso & Hammill (2003) Available from AOTA at http://myaota.aota.org/ shop_aota/prodview.aspx?TYPE=D&PID=27 9&SKU=1387 or from Western Psychological Services at http://portal.wpspublish. com/portal/page?_pageid=53,69183&_ dad=portal&_schema=PORTAL	This assesses an individual's visual perception ability in the domains of spatial relationships, visual closure, visual discrimination, visual memory, and figure ground. No motor involvement is needed to make a response.	Ball et al. (2006) Mazer et al. (1998)

(Continued)

Table 9.1. Driving Assessments *(cont.)*

Assessment	Source	Description	Related Evidence
Ocular movement	Slides for testing phorias available in the Optec Functional Vision Analyzer: www.stereooptical.com/products/slide-packages	Ocular movement is assessed, including ocular range of motion, convergence, divergence, saccades, and the vertical and lateral phorias.	Gutman & Schonfeld (2009)
Optec Functional Vision Analyzer	Stereo Optical: www.stereooptical.com/products/vision-testers/functional-vision-analyzer	This assesses a variety of visual skills by providing a series of illuminated slides addressing areas such as depth perception, acuity, contrast sensitivity, phorias, glare recovery, color perception, and recognition.	Classen et al. (2011) Stav et al. (2008)
Symbol Digit Modalities Test	Western Psychological Services: http://portal.wpspublish.com/portal/page?_pageid=53,69289&_dad=portal&_schema=PORTAL	This assesses neurocognitive function underlying many substitution tasks including attention, visual scanning, and motor speed. It is a timed test in which clients are asked to match numbers to a series of symbols according to a reference key (paper and pencil).	Schanke & Sundet (2000) Schultheis et al. (2010)
Useful Field of View (UFOV)	Visual Awareness: www.visualawareness.com/Pages/whatis.html UFOV Subtest 2 included in both the DrivingHealth Inventory and the Roadwise Review, TransAnalytics Health & Safety Services; Staplin, Lococo et al. (2003); www.drivinghealth.com/screening.htm	A three-part computer-based cognitive assessment is used to determine crash risk. It assesses (1) central vision loss and cognitive processing speed, (2) divided attention, and (3) selective attention. After completing the three tests, clients are categorized according to a 5-point rating scale ranging from very low to very high crash risk.	National Institute on Aging/National Institutes of Health: Useful Field of View Test for Older Drivers: http://aging.senate.gov/award/nih22.pdf Visual Awareness (publications on UFOV): www.visualawareness.com/Pages/publications.html
Visual acuity (Snellen chart)	Precision Vision: http://precision-vision.com/index.cfm/category/9/acuity-charts-high-contrast.cfm Visual acuity slides also included in Optec Functional Vision Analyzer: www.stereooptical.com/products/slide-packages	A wall chart is available for testing static acuity at varied distances.	Edwards et al. (2008) Janke (2001) Janke & Eberhard (1998) Margolis et al. (2002) McCarthy & Mann (2006) Stav et al. (2008)
Visual field	Tests include the Goldmann and Esterman perimetry tests Visual field testing included in Optec Functional Vision Analyzer: www.stereooptical.com/products/vision-testers	Visual field is considered the range of view that a person can see as he or she looks ahead, without eye or head movements, and is tested to determine whether the field is restricted. For more information on testing, see Gutman and Schonfeld (2009).	Bowers et al. (2005) Coeckelbergh et al. (2002) Owsley & McGwin (1999) Racette & Casson (2005)

Cognition, Memory, and Executive Function Skill

Assessment of motor and process skills	Fisher (2006) Users must be trained through a course (testing materials included) and complete a calibration testing; for details, see www.ampsintl.com/AMPS/index.php	This is an observational measure of the quality of performance for completing an ADL; it uses standardized ADL tasks.	Dickerson et al. (2011)

Table 9.1. Driving Assessments *(cont.)*

Assessment	Source	Description	Related Evidence
Clinical Dementia Rating	Available at http://alzheimer.wustl.edu/cdr/aboutcdr.htm	This is a 5-point scale that categorizes levels of dementia, based on domains of cogntion and functional performance: memory, orientation, judgment and problem solving, community affairs, home and hobbies, and personal care. The scale ranges from normal cognition to severe dementia.	Carr & Ott (2010) Duchek et al. (2003) Morris (1993)
Cognitive Behavioral Driving Inventory	More information available at www.neuroscience.cnter.com/pss/cbdi.html	This is a computer-based neurocognitive battery validated for the population with traumatic brain injuries and designed to assess cognitive and behavioral skills required for driving.	Engum, Lambert et al. (1990) Bouillon et al. (2006)
Cognitive Linguistic Quick Test	Helm-Estabrooks (2001) Available at Pearson Assessments: www.pearson assessments.com/HAIWEB/Cultures/en-us/Productdetail.htm?Pid=015-8328-000	This is an assessment battery of five cognitive domains (attention, memory, executive functions, language, and visual–spatial skills) developed for adults with neurological impairment. It includes a clock drawing test.	Parashos et al. (2009)
DriveABLE	DriveABLE Assessment Centres (1998) More information available at www.driveable.com/index.php/about-driveable	This is a two-part standardized evaluation to determine driver competence: the computer-based DriveABLE cognitive assessment tool and the DriveABLE on-road evaluation.	Dobbs (1997, 2005)
Maze Navigation Test	Whelihan et al. (2001)	This paper-and-pencil tracing activity was found to be correlated with on-road driving performance. It is not timed.	Devos et al. (2007) Ott et al. (2003) Whelihan et al. (2005)
Mini-Mental State Exam	Folstein et al. (1975, 2010) Available at PAR: www4.parinc.com/Products/Product.aspx?ProductID=MMSE-2	This is a brief assessment of cognitive function that includes domains of comprehension, reading, writing, drawing tasks, arithmetic, memory, and orientation.	Iverson et al. (2010) Marottoli & Richardson (1998)
Montreal Cognitive Assessment	Available at www.mocatest.org Development described in Nasreddine et al. (2005)	This is a brief assessment of cognitive function that includes the domains of memory recall, visual–spatial abilities, and executive function. It includes a clock drawing test.	Crizzle (2011)
Neurobehavioral Cognitive Status Examination (Cognistat)	Both paper and computerized versions available at www.cognistat.com	Available in paper and computer-based formats, Cognistat is a brief neurocognitive assessment that includes the domains of consciousness, orientation, attention span, language, constructional ability, memory, calculation, and reasoning or judgment.	Matsuda & Saito (2004) Mysiw et al. (1989) Petzold et al. (2010) Unsworth et al. (2005)
Rules of the road and sign recognition	Free online version of multiple-choice tests (5 tests, 30 questions each) available at USA Traffic Signs: www.usa-traffic-signs.com/Test_s/50.htm State departments of motor vehicles are the best sources for state-specific and current road rules and sign guides.	These assess areas of symbolic recognition, reasoning, and judgment pertaining to driving rules and statutes.	Carr et al. (1998) MacGregor et al. (2001) Stav et al. (2008) Uc et al. (2005)

(Continued)

Table 9.1. Driving Assessments *(cont.)*

Assessment	Source	Description	Related Evidence
Short Blessed Test	Katzman et al. (1983) Example at Washington University: http://mybraintest.org/dl/ShortBlessedTest_WashingtonUniversityVersion.pdf	This is a brief 6-item assessment used to differentiate cognitive function related to dementia. It assesses domains of memory, orientation, and concentration.	Stutts (1998) Trobe et al. (1996)
Trail Making Test: Part A and Part B	Reitan (1958) Details on Trails A and Trails B can be found in Lezak et al. (2004) Test online at www.granddriver.net/data/media/docs/Ulowa_trailMaking.pdf and www.tbi-impact.org/cde/mod_templates/12_F_08_TMT.pdf	This is a paper-and-pencil assessment that measures cognitive flexibility, motor control, perceptual complexity, visual scanning, and executive function.	Ball et al. (2006) Classen et al. (2009) Stav et al. (2008)
Wechsler Digit Symbol	Wechsler (1939) Available at http://www.pearsonassessments.com/HAIWEB/Cultures/en-us/Productdetail.htm?Pid=015-8980-808 Details on the Wechsler Digit Symbol test can be found in Lezak et al. (2004)	This is a subtest from the Wechsler Adult Intelligence Scale measured as part of the processing speed index: visual perception, motor and mental speed, and visual–motor coordination.	Molnar et al. (2006)
Motor Skills Assessment			
Brake reaction timer	Various models including the RT-2S Brake Reaction Time Tester as used by Dickerson et al. (2008) Available at www.deltaintegration.com/brakingresponsetimemonitor.html and www.vericomcomputers.com	This is a measure of the time required to move the foot from accelerator to brake in response to a single stimulus (red light). Options are available to expand to complex or choice reaction times responding to multiple stimuli requiring choice of response (see Vericom).	Dickerson et al. (2008)
Finger to nose, toe tap	Demonstrations of these screenings can be found at http://library.med.utah.edu/neurologicexam/html/coordination_normal.html	These timed motor coordination tests for upper and lower extremities are neurological screenings that detect dysmetria and reflect cerebellar deficits leading to diminished coordination.	Stav et al. (2008)
Get Up and Go (GUG) **Timed Up and Go (TUG)**	GUG: Mathias et al. (1986) TUG: Shumway-Cook et al. (2000) Available at www.unmc.edu/media/intmed/geriatrics/nebgec/pdf/frailelderlyjuly09/toolkits/timedupandgo_w_norms.pdf	The TUG is a timed performance of getting up from a chair, walking 3 m, turning around, and walking back to sit down again—as an indicator of fall risk. The TUG was derived from the GUG, which is an observational rating of fall risk using a scale ranging from 1 to 5.	Dawson et al. (2010)
Rapid Pace Walk	Marottoli et al. (1994)	This is a timed clinical test in which clients are instructed to walk (10 ft each up and back as fast as the participant feels safe and comfortable); it is used as a measure for postural instability and gait disturbance.	Classen, Witter et al. (2011) Marottoli et al. (1994) Stav et al. (2008)

Table 9.1. Driving Assessments *(cont.)*

Assessment	Source	Description	Related Evidence
Range of motion, strength	Marottoli et al. (1994) Stav et al. (2008) Hunter-Zaworski (1990)	Gross range of motion and strength are assessed for the neck, trunk, and upper and lower extremities. For example, strength and range of motion are determined using manual muscle testing of shoulder abduction, grasp, hip flexion, knee flexion, and knee extension: categorized as good (full resistance and full range of motion) versus fair or poor (less than full resistance or range of motion).	Stav et al. (2008)
Composite Batteries			
Assessment of Driving Related Skills	Carr et al. (2010) Available at www.nhtsa.gov/staticfiles/traffic_tech/tt389.pdf	This assessment battery addresses the domains required for safe driving: vision, cognition, and motor function.	McCarthy & Mann (2006) Posse et al. (2006)
DrivingHealth Inventory	Available at www.drivinghealth.com/screening.htm (TransAnalytics Health & Safety Services)	This computer-based assessment battery assesses the domains of vision, cognition, and motor function as they pertain to increased crash risk. More information is available at www.drivinghealth.com.	Edwards et al. (2008) Staplin, Lococo et al. (2003)
Occupational Therapy Driver Off-Road Assessment	Unsworth (2011) Available from AOTA: http://myaota.aota.org/shop_aota/prodview.aspx?TYPE=D&PID=87188032&SKU=1261	This battery of assessments allows practitioners to find clients' strengths and weaknesses and pinpoint areas on which to focus during rehabilitation without going on the road.	Unsworth (2011)
On-Road Evaluations			
Closed route	Not a commercially available assessment but rather a method to increase the objectivity of the assessment process; see related evidence	Performance is measured in a contained off-road environment typically with tasks or demands relating to car controls and car handling or maneuvers.	Odenheimer et al. (1994)
Open road with fixed route	Not a commercially available assessment but rather a method to increase the objectivity of the assessment process; see related evidence	Using a fixed-route course design, drivers are tested under the same environmental or infrastructure conditions (e.g., single or double lanes, fixed or signalized intersections), allowing some control over performance variance attributed to roadway components.	Bédard et al. (2008) Di Stefano & Macdonald (2003) Hunt et al. (1997) Justiss et al. (2006) Richardson & Marottoli (2003) Shechtman et al. (2010)
Naturalistic	Not a commercially available assessment but rather a method to increase the objectivity of the assessment process; see related evidence	With unimpeded or unrestricted driving under real-world conditions without the presence of an evaluator, data collection may be through car devices or videotaping.	100-car naturalistic driving study by Dingus et al. (2006)
Instrumented vehicle	Not a commercially available assessment but rather a method to increase the objectivity of the assessment process; see related evidence	Instrumentation may include multiple video feeds of the driver and the surrounding environment, as well as vehicle kinematics (e.g., speed, steering wheel movement), collected via installed electronics and sensors. For further details, see Rizzo et al. (2002).	Classen et al. (2007) Dawson et al. (2010)

(Continued)

Table 9.1. Driving Assessments *(cont.)*

Assessment	Source	Description	Related Evidence
Simulators			
Driving simulators	Available from the following vendors: DriveSafety: www.drivesafety.com EcaFaros: www.ecafaros.com STISim: www.stisimdrive.com Virage: www.viragesimulation.com/English.htm	Interactive, computer-based programs simulate the activity of driving. These may range in cost and size from a table-mounted computer screen with video-game controller (steering and pedals) to a fully integrated vehicle cab with "wrap-around" screen for fuller embeddedness in the driving experience.	Shectman et al. (2007, 2008, 2009) Stern & Schold-Davis (2006)
Simulator Sickness Questionnaire	Kennedy et al. (1993)	This questionnaire measures symptoms of simulator sickness. Awareness of symptoms can help with implementation of mitigation strategies as described in Classen, Bewernitz, & Shechtman (2011).	Classen & Owens (in press)
Self-Reports and Self-Assessments			
AAA Roadwise Review	Available from AAA's Foundation for Driver Safety: www.roadwisereview.com Also available as a CD from regional AAA offices	This is a self-administered, computer-based screening tool designed to help seniors measure mental and physical abilities required of safe driving.	Bédard et al. (2011) Staplin & Dinh-Zarr (2006)
Driving Habits Questionnaire	Available from the University of Alabama–Birmingham: www.eyes.uab.edu/tools/DHQ.pdf	The development was described in Owsley et al. (1999). This instrument captures information about the types of avoidance behaviors that are often identified as compensatory strategies by older drivers.	Ball et al. (1998)
SAFER Driving: The Enhanced Driving Decisions Workbook	This workbook was refined into a Web-based tool: www.um-saferdriving.org/firstPage.php	The development was described in Eby et al. (2003). This workbook looks at driving knowledge and skill as well as health conditions and medication.	Eby et al. (2008)
Safe Driving Behavior Measure (SDBM)	The items of the SDBM are available in Classen, Wen, Velozo, Bédard, Brumback, et al. (2012) and Classen, Wen, Velozo, Bédard, Winter, et al. (2012)	The development was described in Classen et al. (2010). The 68-item SDBM has driver and caregiver versions addressing demographics, driving habits, and driving behaviors.	Classen, Wen, Velozo, Bédard, Brumback et al. (2012) Classen Wen, Velozo, Bédard, Winter et al. (2012) et al.

Note. ADL= activity of daily living; AOTA= American Occupational Therapy Association. Studies cited under "Related Evidence" include but are not limited to driving studies and do not constitute an expansive list of all studies. Likewise, vendors listed are representative of some, but not inclusive of all, possible vendors. Table created by Sandra Winters. Used with permission.

the study participants' comparisons can be made. When reported in peer-reviewed journals, research shows that the quality of the instruments has been critically appraised. Occupational therapists need to search for signs of bias, such as referral sources, the characteristics of the sample on the basis of the demographic data, whether the evaluator was blinded to the participants, the appropriateness of the statistical techniques used, and the claims made in terms of the generalizations to the population (Law, 1987).

Validity

Further, psychometric evaluation must be made by considering *external validity* (i.e., can generalizations be made to the general population?) and *internal validity* (i.e., does the instrument measure what it is supposed to measure?) as well as reliability. *Validity* pertains to the accuracy of measurement and can be subdivided into two functions: (1) how the instrument looks, which includes reports on *face validity* (i.e., does it overall look as though the instrument is measuring what it is supposed to measure?) and *content validity* (i.e., has the instrument been rated by expert reviewers?) and (2) how the instrument acts, which includes *construct validity*, or how the instrument compares with other instruments measuring the same construct (convergent) or different constructs (divergent) as well as *criterion validity* (concurrent or predictive) of the instrument when compared with a criterion or gold standard measure.

Further, it is important to discern whether the measurement tool can capture change over time (also called *responsiveness*). For example, will an instrument that detects functional deficits in the early stages of dementia also be adequate to use (i.e., responsive) during the later stages of dementia?

Reliability

Reliability pertains to the reproducibility of the results and the amount of variation measured that is real and not the result of error. Reliability therefore includes concepts related to consistency of the same rater (*intrarater reliability*), consistency among different raters (*inter-rater reliability*), or internal consistency in the test (*test–retest reliability;* Streiner & Norman, 2003).

Error

Error is associated with a reduction in reliability and can appear as *random error* (inconsistencies that cannot be predicted causing error) or *systematic error* (the same type of error that occurs during testing because of a design flaw) among observations, in participants, among instruments, or over time. Test–retest and rater reliability (intra- and inter-) are very important considerations for evaluative or predictive instruments, whereas internal consistency is most important for descriptive instruments (Law, 1987).

Receiver Operating Characteristic Curve

The *receiver operating characteristic (ROC) curve* is a plot of the rate of true positives (true hits or sensitivity) against the rate of false positives (true misses or 1-specificity) resulting from application of many arbitrarily chosen cutoff points of the predictor test (Portney & Watkins, 2000). Therefore, the ROC curve demonstrates the effectiveness of using different cutoff values and reveals the optimal cutoff value for the predictor test. ROC curves allow one to determine the predictive or criterion validity of a test as actually measured against a gold-standard outcome.

In the case of driving, the on-road test is considered the gold standard (Di Stefano & Macdonald, 2005), and any of the aforementioned measures may be the predictor test. If the area under the curve (AUC), an index of discriminability, is statistically significant, then further attention can be paid to the other measures, such as sensitivity, specificity, positive predictive value, and negative predictive value.

Sensitivity is the predictor test's ability to obtain a positive test when the condition really exists (a true positive). An example is whether the predictor test suggests the participant will be failing the on-road test, and this prediction is then verified by the actual outcome of the on-road test. *Specificity* is the predictor test's ability to obtain a negative result when the condition is really absent (a true negative).

For example, the predictor test might suggest that the participant should pass, and the result is then verified by the participant passing the on-road test (Portney & Watkins, 2000). *Positive predictive value* is the probability of the participant, given a certain cut-point on the predictor test, to fail the on-road evaluation, whereas *negative predictive value* is the probability of the participant, given a cut-point on the predictor test, to pass the on-road test. It is important to note that the number of false positives (those who receive a passing score but fail the road test) and false negatives (those who receive a failing score but pass the road test) and thus the sensitivity and specificity values change with the cutoff value. The formula for calculating these values is well described in the Portney and Watkins (2000) text.

Occupational therapists are encouraged to observe ROC curves for tests used to predict on-road outcomes. For example, Classen et al. (2009) showed that in a pilot study with patients with Parkinson's disease (PD), the UFOV risk index's score of 3 (range = 1–5) emerged, compared with a battery of other screening tests, as the optimal test for passing the on-road test. The 3-point cutoff value yielded sensitivity of 87%, specificity of 82%, and AUC = 92% (SE = 0.61, p = .002). Similarly, the UFOV Subtest 2 (divided attention) optimum cutoff value for passing the on-road test is 223 ms (range = 16–500 ms), sensitivity of 87.5%, specificity of 81.8%, and AUC = 91% (SE = 0.73, p = .003), whereas the UFOV Subtest 3 (selected attention) optimal cutoff value is 273 ms (range = 16–500 ms), sensitivity of 75%, specificity of 72.7%, and AUC = 87% (SE = 0.81, p = .007). The authors concluded that the UFOV may be a superior screening measure (compared with other measures of disease, cognition, and vision) for predicting on-road driving performance, but its rigor must be verified in a larger sample of people with PD (Classen et al., 2009).

Item Response Theory

Although validity testing can improve a tool's utility, acceptability, and item relevance, traditional methods have limitations when the goal is the development of accurate items to precisely and objectively estimate a person's function. For example, a precise and objective measurement of driving function requires assessing the difficulty a person has with driving situations of differing complexity, such as parking and merging. Therefore, in addition to traditional measurement methods addressing validity, use of an Item Response Theory (IRT) approach offers advantages (Bond & Fox, 2007).

IRT is a measurement model that relates item difficulty for a measure to person ability, thereby enabling more precise measurement (Bond & Fox, 2007). IRT has been used in driving studies to develop driving scales and to analyze behaviors observed in on-road testing (Kay, Bundy, Clemson, & Jolly, 2008; Myers, Paradis, & Blanchard, 2008). In constructing a measure using IRT, behaviors representing the construct under consideration (e.g., safe driving) are outlined on a continuum of item difficulty for people with a greater or lesser capacity. Items are designed with a range and specificity to maximally separate people on the basis of ability. For example, we propose that people who are not safe drivers would report having difficulty with relatively easy items such as staying in their designated lane when driving. Conversely, people who are safer drivers will consistently accomplish easy items and may only report difficulty with hard items such as controlling their cars on a snowy road. Therefore, given such benefits of IRT as obtaining increased precision, the IRT method becomes particularly useful when measuring a functional behavior such as driving.

Moreover, using IRT one may determine rater effects: a function of *severity* or *leniency*, defined as the tendency that a rater assigns ratings consistently lower or higher than other raters (Myford & Wolfe, 2004). In addition to item difficulties and person abilities, the Many Facets Rasch Model (MFRM) includes and calibrates an additional parameter (the rater) and provides, in relation to the other parameters (item or person), its fit statistics (Bond & Fox, 2007). Therefore, the MFRM can detect the potential erratic responses of raters and rater severity.

Demographic Information

An important aspect of the CDE is the creation of the driver's occupational profile. Age, gender, medical history, medical conditions, medication use, and driving habits may affect driver safety.

Age, gender, medical history, medical conditions, medication use, and driving habits may affect driver safety.

Age

Age should not be a sole factor for determining driver safety. However, age has been identified as a risk factor for crashes. For instance, the two age cohorts with the highest traffic fatality rates are teenage and older drivers (> age 65; National Highway Traffic Safety Administration [NHTSA], 2009c). Older drivers are more likely to be involved in vehicle-to-vehicle and intersection crashes than younger drivers but have fewer alcohol-related crashes (Eby, Trombley, Molnar, & Shope, 1998). Research has demonstrated a low mileage bias with these crash rates, meaning drivers traveling shorter distances are at greater risk for crashes than those traveling longer distances, regardless of age (Hakamies-Blomqvist, Raitanen, & O'Neill, 2002; Langford, Methorst, & Hakamies-Blomqvist, 2006). Older drivers tend to naturally curtail their driving and are believed to be overrepresented in these crash rates (Langford et al., 2006).

However, a more recent report by NHTSA (2009b) revealed national crash data identifying behaviors and situations associated with increased crash risk for older adults. The report indicated that drivers ages 60–69 had crash rates similar to middle-aged adults; however, drivers ages 70–79 had crash involvement ratios higher than average and drivers ages 80 or older were at very high crash risk, especially at intersections with flashing signals or yield signs.

Age-related declines in driving-related skills (vision, cognition, and sensorimotor function) are well documented (Di Stefano & Macdonald, 2003; Eby et al., 1998; Perryman & Fitten, 1996). With increasing age comes an increase in the prevalence of comorbid conditions (e.g., dementia, stroke, cataracts) that may affect driving skills.

Gender

Recent studies have shown that older women, compared with older men, are more susceptible to injuries from motor vehicle crashes. In 1999, the rates for motor vehicle–related injury were twice as high for older men than for older women (Stevens & Dellinger, 2002), but the proportions of fatalities are higher among women (Baker, Falb, Voas, & Lacey, 2003). Older women tend to stop driving prematurely, stop for different reasons than men, show less confidence in driving behaviors, self-regulate more, have different attitudes, and give up driving earlier and for less specific reasons (Classen, Shechtman, Joo, Awadzi, & Lanford, 2011; Rosenbloom & Herbel, 2009). Therefore, older women emerge as a high-risk group, needing interventions to improve their safe driving. Older women may also be at risk for social isolation and being homebound with decreased community participation, requiring interventions to overcome these issues.

Medical History and Conditions

A detailed medical history will provide information about health conditions (status and progression) as well as identify medications that may potentially impair driving performance. A detailed review of the literature (1960–2000) that captures the impact of medical conditions on driving performance can be found through the NHTSA Web site. The report is divided into 15 sections ranging from specific disease states (e.g., cardiovascular, nervous system) to the aging driver and effects of medication or anesthesia (Dobbs, 2005).

Medical conditions can therefore serve as red flags that a client's driving performance may be impaired (Dobbs, 2005). For instance, a client with cataracts will likely have impaired visual acuity and contrast sensitivity, resulting in a higher crash risk (Owsley & McGwin, 1999; Owsley, Sekuler, & Siemsen, 1983; Owsley, Stalvey, Wells, & Sloane, 1999). A client who is hypertensive may present with impaired cognitive functioning such as decreased attention, memory, and executive function (Waldstein, 1995). A hypertensive state can result in a cerebrovascular accident (CVA) or stroke. The trauma to the brain from either an ischemic or a hemorrhagic event can greatly affect all driving-related skills.

Other conditions such as sleep disorders (e.g., narcolepsy, sleep apnea) can affect a driver's state of arousal and responsiveness. Drivers with sleep apnea are 2–3 times more likely to be in a motor vehicle crash than healthy controls (Aldrich, 1989; Findley et al., 1995).

 These are but a few examples of medical conditions that may affect driver safety, and readers are referred to the ***Physician's Guide to Assessing and Counseling Older Drivers*** (Carr, Schwartzberg, Manning, & Sempek, 2010) for more comprehensive reading. In addition, NHTSA's (2009a) ***Driver Fitness Medical Guidelines*** provides licensing agencies with guidelines for making decisions about a person's fitness to drive on the basis of his or her specific medical condition.

Medications

Antidepressants, antihistamines, and benzodiazepines are examples of drug classifications that can impair driving safety. The use of tricyclic antidepressants impairs psychomotor ability, as demonstrated by a decrease in lane-keeping stability and an increase in overall crash risk (Leveille et al., 1994; Ray, Gurwitz, Decker, & Kennedy, 1992). Similarly, the use of benzodiazepines for anxiety and insomnia can cause sedation and drowsiness. Use of these medications is associated with an increased risk of vehicle crashes (Golombok, Moodley, & Lader, 1988; Hemmelgarn, Suissa, Huang, Boivin, & Pinard, 1997).

Older adults with comorbid conditions often will have extensive medication regimens to address a variety of symptoms. Taking multiple prescription medications can result in polypharmacy, which may increase the probability of adverse drug–drug interactions that can further complicate driver function.

Driving Habits

Driving habits can provide insight into behavioral aspects of performance and safety. As previously mentioned, older drivers often self-regulate their driving to reduce the task demands of this dynamic activity. They will drive slower, travel shorter distances, and avoid complex or challenging environments such as driving in poor weather conditions or in high traffic density (Stav, Justiss, Belchior, & Lanford, 2006).

The **Driving Habits Questionnaire** (DHQ; Owsley et al. 1999) is an instrument that captures information about these types of avoidance behaviors that are often identified as compensatory strategies to adjust for declining skill. The DHQ has been used in research and with drivers with vision and attention impairments. These drivers reported more avoidance behaviors than unimpaired drivers (Owsley et al., 1999). The DHQ also was used in a study that found that older drivers who had an at-fault crash within the past 5 years were more likely to avoid complex driving situations (Ball et al., 1998).

Clinical Assessment Tools

The complex IADL of driving demands the integration of visual, perceptual, cognitive, motor, and integrative (executive) skills. It seems obvious that individuals with significant impairments in any one of these areas would need to cease driving until appropriate rehabilitation is complete, but the problem with this rationale is that many of the actual components of driving are so well learned over years of experience that they are easy to execute in a familiar environment. Thus, both the individual being assessed and the assessor may identify the individual as having adequate skills in a familiar, benign context.

The challenge is that even with familiar contexts, driving occurs in a dynamic environment that can create demands on the individual to make a critical executive decision within a fraction of a second. This is one of the reasons that standardized assessments need to be used. In the clinical assessment context, there is also a unique potential to use driving simulation methods as efficient and cost-effective driving evaluation tools.

The decision of what clinical assessment tools to use is not easy. First, a comprehensive set of measures is needed to cover all the areas of vision, perception, cognition, and motor function that enable safe driving. For each assessment tool, there should be solid evidence linking the tool to outcomes of driving performance and, ideally, to safety. Although evidence-based studies are increasing, there is still much work to be done in this area. There is no specific tool available that can provide clinicians with a definitive determination about a client's ability to drive safely in all situations.

In the next section, we discuss only some of the tools that are commonly used by driver rehabilitation specialists (DRSs) as well as the empirical evidence, or lack of it, underlying them. Table 9.1 describes selected driving-related assessments, cites evidence supporting their use, and gives information on obtaining them.

Vision

The fundamental role of vision in driving is to distinguish safety-relevant objects and markings from their background. With poor vision, drivers are slower to acquire or may miss altogether the critical information needed for path guidance, navigation, hazard recognition, and crash avoidance. Fortunately, the most important aspects of the visual sensory aspect for driving—contrast sensitivity, acuity, and visual fields—can be evaluated quickly and reliably in the therapist's office.

Visual Acuity

Most licensing authorities use visual acuity as the first level of screening in a driving evaluation. This is usually true for the occupational therapist doing a driving evaluation as well. Using the Snellen chart ("E" chart with letters) or the Optec Functional Vision Analyzer (Stereo Optical Co., Chicago), visual acuity is evaluated to determine whether the individual meets the state guidelines. For binocular visual acuity, 20/40 is the most common standard, although some states have low vision programs that allow people to drive up to 20/70 acuity. A person with 20/70 acuity would need to be at 20 ft to read what a person with normal acuity (20/20) could read at 70 ft. Naturally, if an individual's vision can be improved with corrective lenses to meet the guidelines, one can drive with a restriction of wearing glasses on the license.

The research evidence is clear that visual acuity is not linked to driving outcomes when corrected to more than 20/70 (Edwards et al., 2008; Janke, 2001; Janke & Eberhard, 1998; Margolis et al., 2002; McCarthy & Mann, 2006; Stav, Justiss, McCarthy, Mann, & Lanford, 2008). An individual whose vision with lenses can be corrected only to 20/200 vision is considered legally blind and should generally not be considered further for driving privileges, unless the person shows very good potential for low vision rehabilitation, including the use of bioptic telescope lenses for driving. (See Chapter 8 for more information on vision.)

Contrast Sensitivity

The closely related measure of contrast sensitivity differs from acuity in that the test stimuli are not objects with well-defined edges, nor do they appear in sharp contrast to their background (e.g., black letters on a white background). Instead, a *contrast sensitivity test* measures how well an individual can discern objects with fuzzy, poorly defined edges, or low-contrast objects that may be only slightly brighter or darker than their surroundings. This aspect of vision is critical to see the edge of the road when there is no painted line, to make out a curb or object in the road or a pedestrian in dark clothing at night, and to drive safely in rain or fog.

Contrast sensitivity is tested using special eye charts with contrasts ranging from high to low. There is abundant evidence to demonstrate that poor contrast sensitivity is associated with poorer outcomes on driving measures (Bowers, Peli, Elgin, McGwin, & Owsley, 2005; Janke, 2001; Janke & Eberhard, 1998; McCarthy & Mann, 2006; Owsley et al., 1999, 2002; Stav et al., 2008). Thus, contrast sensitivity should be a definitive component of driving assessment, especially for the older driver, because contrast sensitivity is known to become progressively more impaired with advancing age, beginning as early as the mid-40s. The Optec Functional Vision Analyzer often is used for contrast sensitivity as well as the Pelli–Robson Contrast Sensitivity Chart (Haag-Streit/Reliance Medical Products, Mason, OH).

Visual Field

Visual field is considered the range of view that an individual can see as he or she looks ahead, without eye or head movements, and is usually tested to evaluate whether there is a reduction in the area the individual can see. Central vision is where the receptors for discrimination of details are the greatest, with peripheral vision mainly capturing movement. The normal range is about 60° nasally, 100° temporally, 60° above, and 75° below the horizontal axis.

Central vision is where Racette and Casson (2005) found that the extent of the field loss may be related to driver fitness, that is, drivers with larger visual field loss were more likely to be unsafe drivers than individuals with smaller field loss, but there were large individual differences. Although overall the location of the loss did not influence driving performance, individuals with left hemifield and diffuse visual loss in the right hemifield seem to be associated with impairments.

In the case of visual field cuts, an on-road assessment seems to be essential to determine fitness to drive because peripheral and other visual field cuts can negatively affect safe driving, especially with maneuvers that require a wide field of view (Bowers et al., 2005). However, as with depth perception, it may be possible for drivers with visual field impairment to adapt their viewing behaviors by increasing scanning (Coeckelbergh, Brouwer, Cornelissen, van Wolffelaar, & Kooijamn, 2002), and it is likely that individuals with naturally occurring restriction from eye disease develop compensatory mechanisms over time (Owsley & McGwin, 1999). Thus, for sudden-onset field cuts, the additional evaluation of visual attention, cognition, and others will be critical, and training might be considered.

There are commercially available devices to precisely measure field cut, but most occupational therapists screen for visual field deficits using a pencil or stick. The clinician can stand in front or behind, asking the client to stare ahead, and present the stimulus (stick), asking the client to identify when and where he or she first perceives the stimulus. Clients who have a diagnosis that indicates there may be the potential for scotomas or other significant visual field impairments should be referred to an ophthalmologist or optometrist with a specific request for peripheral field assessments.

Ocular Movement

Occupational therapists typically complete an assessment of ocular movement, including ocular range of motion, convergence, divergence, saccades, gaze stability, and the vertical and lateral phorias. Readers may obtain detailed directions on evaluating acuity, peripheral field, and oculomotor skills in other texts, including *Screening Adult Neurologic Populations: A Step-by-Step Instruction Manual* by Gutman and Schonfeld (2009).

Depth Perception

Depth perception is the ability to perceive the environment in three dimensions and to understand the distance of objects in relation to each other. Depth perception is readily yielded by *stereopsis,* the use of the two eyes viewing the environment on the basis of retinal disparity (Wong, Woods, & Peli, 2002). Obviously, this is a critical skill for driving, because one needs to be able to calculate distance, location of other vehicles, and gap between vehicles. However, a variety of clues assist individuals with perception of distance, including *motion parallax* (the effect in which nearby things pass quickly and far-off objects appear stationary), motion from changing object sizes, perspective, relative size, and familiar size.

A novice driver who lacks depth perception will need significant practice to learn the perspectives of vehicles as well as the experiences of relative sizes on roadways. Experienced drivers who go from binocular vision to monocular vision will learn quickly, because objects in the driving environment are familiar, and they are able to use the other clues for judging depth (Racette & Casson, 2005). Thus, the assessment of depth perception using visual tests (e.g., Optec) or online will be important for drivers and, in particular, new drivers. However, no studies have shown that poor depth perception alone leads to increased crash risk (Margolis et al., 2002; Owsley, Ball, Sloane, Roenker, & Bruni, 1991; Owsley & McGwin, 1999; Racette & Casson, 2005).

Color Perception

About 7% of the U.S. population is unable to distinguish the different wavelengths of colors, particularly among the greens and reds (Lezak, Howieson, & Loring, 2004). Even for an individual with color deficiency, there are other clues to perceive the state of a traffic signal, for example, the position of the illuminated signal face. Because there is no evidence that color deficiency is linked to unsafe driving (Owsley & McGwin, 1999; Owsley et al., 1991), DRSs might consider eliminating this from the vision testing and not test it simply because it is included in some of the standard visual testing packages.

Glare Recovery

The high beam of an oncoming motor vehicle has a blinding effect and can decrease visibility. This glare forms a veil of luminance, which scatters light in the eye and reduces the contrast (and thus the visibility) of a target against the background. The total amount of glare exposure determines the length of recovery.

There is clear evidence that glare recovery—the amount of time it takes to recover vision—increases with age, with older adults often taking up to 6 times longer to recover than young adults (Collins, 1989; Collins & Brown, 1989), which is often the reason older adults decrease driving at night. Individuals with cataracts or glaucoma or who have undergone radial keratectomy or photorefractive keratectomy also often have more difficulty with night vision (Owsley & McGwin, 1999).

However, older drivers with glaucoma actually have a crash rate that is 40%–50% lower than those without glaucoma when adjusted for demographic, medical, and visual functional characteristics. This seemingly conflicting phenomenon is likely because the drivers with glaucoma self-regulate to avoid potentially challenging driving situations (McGwin et al., 2004). Because glare recovery has not been related to crash outcomes in studies (Ball, Owsley, Sloane, Roenker, & Bruni, 1993; Owsley et al., 1991), it may be evaluated selectively.

Visual–Perceptual Assessments

Useful Field of View

The UFOV test (Visual Awareness Group, Punta Gorda, FL) was specifically designed and developed by Ball and colleagues to evaluate how aging affects processing speed and attention, especially in relationship to driving. Ball and colleagues have conducted extensive research relating the scores of the UFOV to various measures related to unsafe driving and crashes or citations (Ball et al., 1993, 2006; Myers et al., 2000; Owsley et al., 1991).

UFOV is a computer-based assessment that may be administered with a touch screen or a mouse. It has three subtests that measure (1) processing speed, (2) divided attention, and (3) selective attention. Subtest 1, *processing speed,* consists of discriminating whether a car or truck figure was briefly presented on the screen, in central vision. The exposure duration is decreased on successive trials. Subtest 2, *divided attention,* includes this same discrimination but also requires the test taker to identify in which of eight locations around the edge of the screen a second figure was simultaneously presented. Subtest 3, *selective attention,* adds clutter to the screen while requiring the same responses as Subtest 2, namely, "Which figure was shown in the center of the screen?" and, "Where was the other figure shown at the edge of the screen?" In each subtest, there are multiple trials, and as the test progresses, the speed of presentation increases and decreases in steps until the program finds the shortest exposure duration at which the patient can meet a criterion for response accuracy.

In a review of vision impairment and driving, Owsley and McGwin (1999) claimed that in drivers with Alzheimer's disease (AD), the UFOV is one of the best predictors of crash involvement in a simulator and poor on-the-road performance. The second subtest, divided attention, has been most often used in research studies because of its high correlation to the UFOV total score; it is the best predictor of (at-fault) crash involvement (Owsley et al., 1998). UFOV Subtest 2 is included as part of the Roadwise Review and the DrivingHealth Inventory.

In a prospective cohort study of approximately 2,000 older drivers at the Maryland Motor Vehicle Administration field sites, it was found that working memory (cued recall), Trails B, the Motor-Free Visual Perception Test (MVPT), and UFOV Subtest 2 were all significant predictors of future at-fault crashes (Ball et al., 2006). More recently, independent researchers have supported this finding. Specifically, Classen and colleagues (Classen et al., 2009; Classen, Witter, et al., 2011) found that the UFOV (except for Subtest 1) is the best test to predict on-road outcomes in individuals with PD compared with the MMSE (Folstein, Folstein, & McHugh, 1975), Rapid Pace Walk, and Unified Parkinson Disease Rating Scale (Fahn, Marsden, Calne, & Goldstein, 1987).

Motor-Free Visual Perceptual Test

The MVPT (Colarusso & Hammill, 2003) assesses visual–perceptual ability without motor involvement and was designed as a screening tool. This test has been used to measure spatial relationships, visual closure, visual discrimination, visual memory, and figure ground. The MVPT has been used in multiple studies to determine whether it is associated with poor driving outcomes. In its principal application to driving, only the visual closure component has been used in which the individual selects from four alternative line drawings with missing information to say which could be completed to match an example figure. Most studies have shown a relationship to poor performance in driving (Ball et al., 2006; Mazer, Korner-Bitensky, & Sofer, 1998).

The MVPT is now in its third edition (Colarusso & Hammill, 2003); the revised version includes more test stimuli, but the earlier version with fewer test plates has the most evidence linking it to driving outcomes (i.e., visual closure). In a review, Oswanski et al. (2007) suggested that the combination of the MVPT and Clock Test provided an accurate screening tool for senior drivers, but different approaches may be needed for other specific diagnostic groups. This was supported by a recent study among drivers with multiple sclerosis in which the Symbol Digit Modalities Test (Wechsler, 1997) and not the MVPT was the strongest predictor for collision and traffic violation (Schultheis et al., 2010).

Wechsler Digit Symbol

The Digit Symbol test is a neuropsychological test contained in the Wechsler Adult Intelligence Scale (Wechsler, 1997). The task involves the substitution of a symbol for a matched number for nine pairs. The individual is given a paper with squares below a list of numbers and asked to fill in the appropriate number for the matched symbols. The task is timed for 90 s, and clients are asked to perform as quickly and accurately as possible.

Because the test is based largely on processing speed, it is sensitive to brain damage, depression, and particularly dementia, although it is not sensitive to location of the brain damage (Lezak, Howieson, & Loring, 2004). However, it is also important to recognize that age effects are prominent with processing speed. Slowing of processing speed can be exhibited as early as age 30, and after age 60, the raw scores of this assessment drop sharply (Wechsler, 1997). Thus, the Digit Symbol test will not necessarily predict specific skills with driving. Accordingly, researchers (Molnar, Patel, Marshall, Man-Son-Hing, & Wilson, 2006) found no correlation of Digit Symbol findings to on-road testing in their systematic review.

Symbol Digit Modalities Test

The Symbol Digit Modalities Test (SDMT; Western Psychological Services, Torrance, CA) is related to the Digit Symbol test but reverses the presentation of the material so that the symbol is presented and the client writes in the corresponding number. The advantage of the SDMT over the digit span is that the client can also report the numbers orally. In fact, Lezak et al. (2004) recommended giving both written and oral administrations to compare the two response modalities.

As with many other screening tools, the SDMT is effective in differentiating early dementia and other brain injuries, but there is inconsistent evidence of the direct link to driving performance. In a study with multiple sclerosis (Schultheis et al., 2010), it was found to be the strongest predictor of on-road performance demonstrating processing speed. However, this study also indicated that the Trails B and MVPT–Revised were not significant predictors of driving performance among people with multiple sclerosis, contrary to other studies. In contrast, in a study with community-living older adults (Richardson & Marottoli, 2003), the SDMT was not correlated with on-road performance. In another study comparing neuropsychological assessments with on-road performance of patients with brain injury, both the Trail Making Test and SDMT discriminated between the outcomes of drivers (Schanke & Sundet, 2000).

Clock Test

The Clock Test (e.g., Manos & Wu, 1994) is a widely used cognitive screen in geriatric practice. It is sensitive to focal lesions and evaluates visual–perceptual and visual–spatial abilities as well as language, working memory, and executive functions (Lezak et al., 2004). There are more than a dozen administration and scoring systems with suggested cutoffs and interrater reliability scores that show great sensitivity to AD both with and without the MMSE (see Lezak et al., 2004). Perhaps the most widely used one by rehabilitation specialists is the predrawn circle with directions to set the hands to 10 min past 11:00 (Manos & Wu, 1994).

Researchers (Eby, Molnar, & Kartje, 2009) who reviewed the literature on clock drawing found mixed results among the studies. As mentioned earlier, Oswanski et al. (2007) found both the MVPT (Colarusso & Hammill, 2003) and clock drawing to be significant predictors of on-road driving. The diversity of the task and variable in scoring protocols may make it difficult to correlate with outcomes, but a qualitative observation of performance on this test may assist in screening for cognitive deficits and visual field cuts.

Letter or Number Cancellation

Letter or number cancellation tests were established in 1974 with 9 variations to evaluate for visual inattention and specific lesions of the brain (Lezak et al., 2004). The basic test consists of 6 lines of 52 characters with 18 of the target characters randomly interspersed in the lines. Results are evaluated by the time and number of omissions.

Uttl and Pilkenton-Taylor (2001) demonstrated that there is an age-related decline in speed of performance but no age-related differences in the spatial distribution of cancellation errors. Although Eby et al. (2009) reported mixed results in relation to driving, Richardson and Marottoli (2003) found that visual attention, tested by a number cancellation task, accounted for the greatest amount of variance and was associated with more than half of the specific driving maneuvers required of the older drivers in the study. However, they also found that executive function (Trails B) and visual memory were closely related.

The Bells Test (Gauthier, Dehaut, & Joanette, 1989) is a variation of this type of visual scanning and selected attention tool in which the client is asked to find 35 bells that are embedded among 264 distractors.

Cognition, Memory, and Executive Function Skills

Clinical Dementia Rating

The Clinical Dementia Rating (CDR; Morris, 1993) is an instrument that characterizes the level of cognitive and functional performance in individuals who are at risk, suspected of, or have been diagnosed with AD or other dementing disorders. The user rates six domains (memory, orientation, judgment and problem solving, community affairs, home and hobbies, personal care) on a 5-point scale with the scoring algorithm representing the severity level of dementia. According to the scale, CDR of 0 represents *no dementia*; 0.5, *possible dementia*; 1, *mild*; 2, *moderate*; and 3, *severe*. The information necessary to make the decision is based on a semistructured interview of the client and a reliable informant.

The CDR was created and widely researched at the Alzheimer's Disease Research Center, Washington University, and training through protocols has established good reliability (Morris, 1997). Several studies have found significant correlations between CDR and simulated driving, self-reported crashes, and driver records of citations (Carr & Ott, 2010; Duchek et al., 2003). Thus, although driving specialists may not assign the CDR rating without proper training, it certainly can and should be used to assist in determining the probability of a person's risk for unsafe driving.

Accordingly, in a recent systematic review of the literature (Iverson et al., 2010), a group of experts invited by the American Academy of Neurology evaluated the literature and found strong evidence that the CDR is useful for identifying individuals at risk for unsafe driving. A sample algorithm (in the publication) for evaluating driving competence and risk management using the CDR may be a useful tool for driving specialists when considering drivers with dementia.

The CDR has been used primarily by physicians and advanced practice nurses. However, other health professionals have demonstrated good reliability in administering the CDR after training (Morris et al., 1997). Individual health professionals and researchers can access free training to use the protocol. To access the system and related documentation, go to http://alzheimer.wustl.edu, click on the Clinical Dementia Rating link in the Education Menu, and then follow the instructions to access the training modules. Full training requires 6–9 hr, but this training can be broken up over multiple sittings. This system is made possible through funding from the National Institute on Aging.

Trail Making Test Part A and Part B

The Trail Making Test Part A (Trails A) and Trail Making Test Part B (Trails B; Reitan, 1958) are used to test visual scanning with a motor component (Lezak et al., 2004; Shum, McFarland, & Bain, 1990). Trails A requires the individual to trace and connect the numbers from 1 to 25 that are scattered on a standard-sized sheet of paper. Trails B adds to the task difficulty (divided attention) by requiring the individual to switch from numbers to letters so that he or she goes from 1 to A, A to 2, 2 to B, and so forth. The individual is required to join the letters and numbers with a pencil as quickly as possible.

Both Trails A and B are timed. Trails A and B typically are completed with paper and pencil, but now computer programs are available with touch screens. With intact function, the two parts of the Trail Making Test should take less than 5 min, with Trails A taking an average of 29 s and Trails B taking an average of 75 s. Deficits become quite evident when Trails A takes more than 78 s and Trails B takes more than 273 s (Lezak et al., 2004).

Although a few studies link Trails A with driving outcomes, it is most often used as a warm up for the more complex Trails B. Specifically, Trails A allows the participant to become familiar with the sequential search aspects of this test protocol before introducing the divided–attention component in Trails B. Using times for Trails B without first doing Trails A will likely skew the driving specialist's assessment results because the standard procedure is using both parts.

Trails B has been used extensively in comparing driving outcomes and has been shown to be significantly related to other driving measures such as on-road driving, simulated driving, and crashes (Ball et al., 2006; Kantor, Mauger, Richardson, & Unroe, 2004; Richardson & Marottoli, 2003). However, studies have shown that Trails B is not as strongly linked to other driving measures (McCarthy & Mann, 2006; Stav et al., 2008). Although the number of seconds is used as the evidence in most studies, when an individual is having difficulty with the task, careful observation also will provide information about the quality of his or her mistakes to provide information about his or her deficits, specifically on visual scanning and tracking and mentally following a sequence (Lezak et al., 2004).

Mini-Mental State Examination

The MMSE (Folstein et al., 1975) has been the most widely used brief screening tool for cognitive impairment, either alone or as a component of other protocols (Lezak et al., 2004). The original MMSE was composed of 11 questions that covered orientation, registration, attention, calculation, recall, language, and visual–spatial perception that took 5–10 min to administer. The maximum score is 30 with scores less than 24 indicative of cognitive impairment.

A new standard version, the MMSE–2™ with a user's guide (Folstein, Folstein, White, & Messer, 2010), has been developed to expand its usefulness in populations with milder forms of cognitive impairment as well as using alternative forms (Blue and Red) to decrease the possibility of practice effects. Permission is required to use the MMSE–2.

There is now also a MMSE–2: BV (Brief Version) that takes 5 min; MMSE–2: SV (Standard Version) that takes 10–15 min, which is equivalent in questions to the former version; and the MMSE–2: EV (Expanded Version) that takes 20 min to avoid ceiling effects. Permission is also required to use these three versions.

The MMSE has been used as a measure of cognitive function in many studies (Marottoli et al., 1998; Trobe, Waller, Cook-Flannagan, Teshima, & Bieliauskas, 1996). Typically, lower scores are associated with unsafe driving abilities as well as for failing on-the-road examinations, but it has not been useful for predicting driving outcomes. Even in early studies, the specificity and sensitivity of the MMSE was not found to be sufficient for effective prediction (Fox, Bowden, Bashford, & Smith, 1997; Odenheimer et al., 1994). Accordingly, the Iverson et al. (2010) systematic review concluded that a MMSE score of less than 24 may be useful in identifying people at risk for unsafe driving, but data are conflicting in terms of correlations between MMSE scores and driving performance.

Short Blessed Test

The Short Blessed Test (SBT; Katzman et al., 1983) is also a screening tool for cognitive impairment, similar to the MMSE (Folstein et al., 1975). For many driving evaluators, it has become the tool of choice, because there is less risk of practice skills than with older versions of the MMSE. The SBT is a 6-item test, validated for cognitive impairment, that discriminates among mild, moderate, and severe cognitive deficits (Katzman et al., 1983). Items include orientation of year, month, and time. A memory task of a name and address is included as well as counting backward from 20 and repeating the months in reverse order. It has weighted scores for a total score of 28.

As with the MMSE, lower scores on the SBT are related to decreased cognitive outcomes and do not necessarily have a direct relationship with driving outcomes (Stutts, 1998; Trobe et al., 1996). However, when there is clear cognitive impairment evident on these assessments, particularly when the screening tools indicate moderate to severe dementia, it is very likely the individual should not be driving, and a CDE is unwarranted.

Montreal Cognitive Assessment

The Montreal Cognitive Assessment (MoCA; Nasreddine et al., 2005) was developed as a brief screening tool for mild cognitive impairment, and it evaluates multiple domains of cognitive function. It is a one-page, 30-point test that takes about 10–15 min to administer. Specifically, it includes tasks of short-term memory; visual–spatial (clock drawing and cube copying); executive function (modified trail making, phonemic fluency, verbal abstraction); attention, concentration, and working memory (serial subtraction, digits forward and back, target detection); language (naming animals, sentence repetition); and orientation to time (Ismail, Rajji, & Shulman, 2009). It has been translated into multiple languages and has three versions to avoid learning effects.

Nasreddine et al. (2005) compared individuals with mild cognitive impairment and normal controls using the MMSE (Folstein et al., 1975) and MoCA. This study established a cutoff score of 26 of 30 for normal cognition and reported sensitivity scores of 90% and specificity of 87% (Nasreddine et al., 2005). However, in a relatively recent systematic review, Lonie, Tierney, and Ebmeier (2009) noted that the MoCA, as well as other cognitive screening tools, lacks test–retest reliability for 6- to 12-month intervals, which is clinically relevant.

The MoCA, like the MMSE and the SBT (Katzman et al., 1983), is a tool used by a practitioner to screen for cognitive deficits. This is a critical concept for the occupational therapist. A cognitive screen identifies specific cognitive deficits. However, these screening tools do not identify the specific condition underlying the cognitive deficits or make reliable inferences about the course and eventual outcome of cognitive impairment (Lonie et al., 2009). More important, only one of these tools is necessary to make a driving decision when the score shows severe cognitive impairment, although additional support from other assessments may be useful.

Maze Navigation Test

The Maze Navigation Test (MNT; Whelihan, DiCarlo, Camparetto, & Donovan, 2001) is an assessment measure relatively recently applied to driving. Based on the Porteus Mazes (Porteus, 1959), its mazes were designed as a measure of executive functioning with the intention of applying the results to activities such as driving. The MNT consists of a sample and 8 progressively more complex paper-and-pencil mazes that are completed, with both the time for completion and the number of errors recorded. Normative data are available for older age groups for completion time and number of errors. Age is correlated with time but not with errors (Whelihan et al., 2001).

In a study of individuals with early-stage cognitive dementia, the MNT was found to be significantly related to driving ability, as measured by an on-road assessment (Whelihan, DiCarlo, & Paul, 2005). Ott and colleagues (2003) have used a computerized maze assessment, also based on the Porteus Mazes, to evaluate driving outcomes of individuals with early dementia. The results of their study indicated that although Porteus Maze (Porteus, 1959) time and Trails B (Reitan, 1958) time were both correlated with the driving scores, only the maze's drawing time was predictive of the driving outcome in a multivariate regression analysis. Thus, the MNT, an executive assessment, may be a valuable tool for driving evaluators to consider.

Neurobehavioral Cognitive Status Examination

The Neurobehavioral Cognitive Status Examination (Cognistat; Kiernan, Mueller, Langston, & Van Dyke, 1987) is a cognitive assessment that has been widely used in rehabilitations settings. It uses a screening and metric system that covers the general areas of level of consciousness, orientation, and attention span as well as ability areas of language, constructional ability, memory, calculation skills, and reasoning or judgment. Rather than being a global assessment, it provides a profile of cognitive status in the domains of functioning.

As early as 1989 (Mysiw, Beegan, & Gatens, 1989), it demonstrated sensitivity to impairment, similar to that of the MMSE, in orientation and memory, and the calculations and judgment outcomes were related to functional measures. In a more recent study, functional competency of people with mild AD was largely predicted from the Cognistat scores for orientation, abstract thinking, and psychomotor speed (Matsuda & Saito, 2004), which suggests that it would be a good screening tool for a functional task such as driving.

However, with the exception of one review study, no studies have linked the outcome of the Cognistat to driving. Regardless, with the numerous studies on the Cognistat's Web site that illustrate its usefulness as a screening tool, clinicians might consider using this tool.

Assessment of Motor and Process Skills

The Assessment of Motor and Process Skills (AMPS; Fisher, 2006) is an observational assessment tool based on the MFRM (Item Response Theory), as discussed earlier in this chapter. The AMPS is designed to evaluate the *quality* of an individual's performance while completing a familiar instrumental activity of daily living (IADL), such as making a salad. The evaluator observes and scores an individual on at least two tasks, observing how the individual moves objects and himself or herself in the environment as well as how he or she plans, organizes, and executes the tasks. Two scales, 16 motor items and 20 process items, are scored using a 4-point scale ranging from deficit to effective performance. The MFRM model allows the evaluator to select familiar tasks, from easy to difficult, which allows the tool to be used with a variety of client abilities.

To use the computer analysis for obtaining ratio-level data output, the evaluator must be "standardized" within the MFRM, that is, trained and calibrated in use of the AMPS. Although these practicalities might be considered a barrier to ease of administration, the AMPS is a tool developed by an occupational therapist and designed specifically for occupational therapy. Additionally, it has significant validity and reliability studies that support its use in all practice areas.

In relation to driving, Dickerson, Reistetter, and Trujillo (2010) have shown a significant relationship between the process scale from the performance assessment and whether the driver passed, failed, or needed restrictions from a CDE. The evidence has suggested that the AMPS, as an occupational therapy performance measure, is an evidence-based assessment tool for determining at-risk drivers. It also supports other studies indicating that cognitive issues are more important than motor issues in identifying unsafe drivers.

Recently, Dickerson, Reistetter, Schold Davis, and Monohan (2011) used this evidence to create an **algorithm for appropriate referral** to DRSs by general practice occupational therapists. Considering that the AMPS is a tool to observe IADLs, the authors emphasize that general occupational therapists can use their observational skills and activity analysis while observing complex IADLs to identify at-risk drivers with or without a standardized assessment. Specifically, the algorithm encourages therapists to use their current evaluations to make a determination of who needs to cease driving, who is likely safe to resume driving, and who needs further assessment. However, the value of the AMPS is clearly the data output at the measurement level of ratio. Thus, the AMPS could potentially be a specific occupational therapy–designed assessment tool that is used with specific cutoff scores for safe and unsafe driving; further research needs to be done.

Cognitive Linguistic Quick Test

The Cognitive Linguistic Quick Test (CLQT; Helm-Estabrooks, 2001) was developed by a speech–language pathologist as a quick tool to identify deficits in attention, memory, executive function, language, and visual–spatial skills of adults with neurological impairment. It consists of 10 tasks, similar to components of several other cognitive assessments (e.g., symbol cancellation, mazes, clock drawing). It can be administered in 15–30 min with scoring an additional 10–15 min, with the advantage of four nonlinguistic tasks that speech–language therapists can use with clients with aphasia.

In the development of the CLQT, four studies were used to form two sets of normal cutoff scores (ages 18–69 and 70–89) for the tasks, cognitive domains, and overall cognitive performance (Helm-Estabrooks, 2001). In a follow-up study, Helm-Estabrooks (2002) supported evidence that the CLQT may be helpful in use with clients with aphasia, because the study supported the contention that it is impossible to predict cognition based on language test scores if the individual has aphasia.

In a more recent study (Parashos, Johnson, Erickson-Davis, & Wielinski, 2009), the CLQT was compared with the MMSE in a study of 93 individuals with PD. Not surprisingly, the CLQT was found to be superior to the MMSE in providing cognitive domain–specific information, but no studies have used the CLQT associated with driving outcomes. It would seem that the CLQT could be used as a screening tool, much like other cognitive screens for driving, but there is no evidence that it is superior to others, except in the case of clients with aphasia.

Cognitive Behavioral Driving Inventory

The Cognitive Behavioral Driving Inventory (CBDI; Engum, Cron, Hulse, Pendergrass, & Lambert, 1988) was developed as a computerized neuropsychological test battery to assess cognitive and behavioral skills necessary for safe driving. It was specifically designed for individuals with brain injury. The actual administration consists of both computerized and standardized psychometric tasks scores entered into the computer program so that a report is produced with the client's strengths, weaknesses, and a visual field reaction time map. There is a recommendation of pass or fail on driving ability. The standardized psychometric tests include raw scores from the Picture Completion and Digit Symbol (Weschler, 2008) and Trail Making Test (Reitan, 1958). Measurement of visual fields is necessary, but brake reaction times are optional for the testing.

The computer-based testing consists of four components of Bracy's Computer Assisted Cognitive Rehabilitation (Bracy, 1985) and requires the client to use a joystick to respond to visual output on the screen as quickly as possible with visual discrimination, scanning, and attention skills. The software calculates a General

Driver's Index, the average of the 27 individual scores and scatter variances. Clients are classified as passing, borderline, or failing (Bouillon, Mazer, & Gelinas, 2006).

The CBDI has been standardized (Engum, Cron, et al., 1988; Engum, Lambert, Womac, & Pendergrass, 1988) and has internal reliability scores and test scores related to on-road performance (Engum, Cron, et al., 1988; Engum, Lambert, & Scott, 1990). Another validity study also compared a psychologist's score of the CBDI and a driving instructor's pass-or-fail decision and found significant correlation between outcomes (Engum, Lambert, & Bracy, 1990). A more recent study by occupational therapy researchers comparing the CBDI with other assessments and driving results found that the CBDI scores were significantly worse for those who failed the on-road test (Bouillon et al., 2006). However, the sensitivity was 62% and the specificity 81%, with positive predictive values of 73% and negative values of 71%, leading these researchers to the conclusion that scores on the CBDI are not sufficient to replace a driving evaluation. Further, Bouillon et al. (2006) emphasized that it was only predictive of those with right CVAs or traumatic brain injuries (TBIs), hypothesizing that the CBDI does not specifically evaluate all the important deficits in clients.

DriveABLE

DriveABLE (Dobbs, 1997) was developed as a product and service to identify and assess a driver with medical impairments in his or her ability to drive safely. There are two basic components of the system. The DriveABLE Cognitive Assessment Tool (DriveABLE Assessment Centres, 1998) is a touch-screen computer program with 6 programmed subtests. Each subtest measures different component skills, including measure reaction time, attentional fields, attention shifting, decision making, executive functions, and hazard identification. Upon completion, the program generates a report with client information, task scores, and the predicted fail probability of the on-road assessment on the basis of a complex algorithm from previous research by the developers (Dobbs, 1997; Dobbs, Heller, & Schopflocher, 1998).

The second product is the standardized On-Road Driving Assessment, reported to be designed and standardized for the medically compromised driver (www.driverable.com). The standardized road course has specific performance evaluation criteria that provides frequency and severity of driving errors in a report that summarizes the results and allows for a recommendation of driving continuance.

In a recent study, Korner-Bitensky and Sofer (2009) suggested that the DriveABLE screen was predictive of clients who would fail an on-road driving test. However, this study was retrospective of clients who were already referred for a driving evaluation, which would affect the positive predictive values of the screening tool for the general population of older adults. At this point, there is not enough evidence, independent of the for-profit developers, to determine whether DriveABLE has the sensitivity and specificity to be used as an exclusive tool with older adults, as advertised.

Rules of the Road and Sign Recognition

There are so many variations of tests to evaluate knowing rules of the road or traffic sign recognition that it is difficult to evaluate the efficiency of this kind of assessment. In one study (Stav et al., 2008), knowing rules of the road and sign recognition were not strongly related to performance. However, in two studies of individuals with dementia, differences in performance on traffic sign recognition were evident when compared with performance of individuals without dementia (Carr, LaBarge, Dunnigan, & Storandt, 1998; Uc, Rizzo, Anderson, Shi, & Dawson, 2005). Further, MacGregor, Freeman, and Zhang (2001) found that the traffic sign recognition test distinguished between accident and nonaccident groups ages 65 years or older. However, the sensitivity and specificity were not strong enough to devise a cut-point that was acceptable.

It would seem that, just as with other cognitive measures, when the individual is very impaired, failure on the sign recognition test is evident, but it will not be a general predictor of on-road performance.

Summary

In summary, it is clear that cognition is a large component of driving. In relation to dementia, Table 9.2 illustrates the range of dementia: mild, moderate, and severe based on the CDR (Carr & Ott, 2010). The table was developed on the basis of CDR results of members of the 1000 Honolulu Heart Study (Curb & Curb, 2002), their driving histories, and collaborating data from other studies. In the Honolulu study, no one was driving at the moderate-to-severe level (CDR = 2.0), 60%–70% of the individuals at the mild level (CDR = 1.0) were nondrivers, and 30% were not driving (CDR = 0.5). If one examines the scores of the other cognitive assessments in Table 9.2, it demonstrates that it may not be as important what cognitive assessment is used, but that one is used and linked to the appropriate evidence.

It is critical for practitioners to use an evidence-based cognitive assessment to determine how to address driving with the client.

In other words, it is critical for practitioners to use an evidence-based cognitive assessment to determine how to address driving with the client. If the client has moderate to severe dementia, driving is not an option for mobility, and it needs to be addressed if either the client or the family indicates plans to return. If the cognitive assessment indicates a mild or questionable level of dementia, the practitioner needs to pursue performance-based evaluations to examine the client's abilities more discriminately. In terms of which cognitive assessments to use, the critical key is to ensure that there is appropriate evidence for determining cognitive function, whether the assessment is the MMSE (Folstein et al., 1975), the SBT (Katzman et al., 1983), the MoCA (Nasreddine et al., 2005), or others. Further, it is critical to understand that most of the cognitive tools by themselves and listed here are cognitive screening tools and should not be used individually to determine fitness to drive, except in the cases of severe cognitive impairment, such as in the severe stages of AD.

Motor Skills Assessment

Occupational therapists are clearly versed and competent in the physical assessment of their clients. Typically the DRS will complete a functional assessment of both upper and lower extremities. In cases of disorders that are approached from more of a biomechanical perspective, such as spinal cord injury, individual measurements of range of motion and manual muscle testing are indicated to determine the level of adaptations that may be needed for the motor vehicle. In the case of neurological disorders, such as multiple sclerosis, it is not the individual measurements or manual muscle testing that is critical but an overall functional mobility assessment needed as for any IADL.

With aging older adults, the complexity of psychomotor, visual–perceptual, and cognition interactions make teasing out the individual components difficult. There

Table 9.2. Clinical Description of Dementia Severity Levels

Clinical Measure of Dementia Severity	No Dementia (CDR = 0)	Questionable or Very Mild Dementia (CDR = 0.5)	Mild Dementia (CDR = 1.0)	Moderate to Severe Dementia (CDR = 2.0)
For the dementia specialist: CDR	No memory loss or inconsistency; memory loss fully oriented; judgment intact; function intact; personal care intact	Consistent slight forgetfulness; slight difficulty with orientation or judgment; slight impairment in community activities or home activities; personal care intact	Memory loss interferes with everyday activities; geographic disorientation; moderate impairment in judgment; mild but definite impairment of community or home activities; needs prompting for personal care	Severe memory loss; severe difficulty with time relationships and judgment; no longer independent in activities; only simple chores preserved; needs assistance in personal effects
For the clinician:				
Short Blessed Test	1.2 (1.9)[a]	4.8 (5.9)[b]	15.4 (5.2)[c]	18.5 (5.5)[c]
Mini-Mental State Exam	28.9 (1.3)[c]	23.1 (2.5)[d]	20 (3.9)[c]	16.1 (4.7)[c]
For the neuro-psychologist:				
Logical memory	8.8 (2.9)[a]	4.3 (2.7)[e]	1.9 (1.7)[e]	1.5 (2.3)[f]
Block design	30.1 (8.6)[a]	22.2 (9.8)	12.0 (9.6)	3.2 (6.6)[g]
Digit symbol	45.6 (11.5)[a]	31.7 (13.6)	17.0 (13.3)[e]	8.3 (8.7)[g]
Trailmaking A	40.9 (20.0)[a]	70.2 (39.2)[e]	108.3 (50.5)[e]	Score too low
Benton copy	9.6 (.88)[a]	9.1 (1.6)[e]	7.3 (2.7)[e]	Score too low

Note. Numbers represent average scores for the levels of dementia, depending on the assessment tool. Based on samples that average ~75 years of age and ~14 years of education. CDR = Clinical Dementia Rating.

From *Data to Decision: What Physicians Want in a Driving Rehabilitation Report*, by A. Dickerson, E. Schold Davis, and D. Carr, 2010. Used with permission of the authors.
[a]Johnson et al. (2009).
[b]Hunt et al. (1997).
[c]Morris et al. (1989).
[d]Nourhashemi et al. (2007).
[e]Balota et al. (1998).
[f]Hill et al. (1992).
[g]Kemper et al. (1993).

may be functional motor assessments that could be done, but there is still limited evidence about how the decrease of motor ability alone affects driving performance. However, in one study, there was a clear relationship between limited neck rotation and driving performance (McPherson, Ostrow, & Shaffron, 1989), whereas other studies have not found this to be true (Janke & Eberhard, 1998).

Brake Reaction Timer

Grabowski and Morrisey (2001) identified three major areas of concern with regard to older drivers' physical abilities: (1) declining vision, (2) decreasing cognitive abilities, and (3) diminishing psychomotor skills. Although psychomotor skills may be primary, all three areas affect the brake reaction timing. The slowing of movement with age includes

- Failure to use advance preparatory information
- Slowness in processing information
- Slowness in responding to information

- Difficulty with task complexity
- Inability to regulate speed (Stelmach & Nahom, 1992).

Additionally, as task difficulty or complexity increases, age-related slowing also increases (Marottoli & Drickamer, 1993), although practice can mediate declines (Salthouse, 1993). Thus, the measuring of brake reaction time performance in older adults is complex.

There is no question that slowing of brake reaction rates is found with increasing age (Green, 2000; Summala, 2000). Older drivers have on average been found to respond from 0.1 to 0.3 s slower than other adult drivers (Green, 2000); however, simple reaction time may not relate to real-world driving environment (Marottoli & Drickamer, 1993).

Although most researchers have agreed that simple brake reaction time is not closely related to driving performance, there is some evidence in support of its utility. In a study by Myers et al. (2000), reaction time was related to the outcome on a driving test, but it did not have as strong a relationship as the UFOV. Additionally, other researchers linked reaction time with the MMSE (Folstein et al., 1975) for a model to predict on-the-road performance (Kantor et al., 2004). It may be that a simple brake reaction timer (no longer manufactured but often still used) is an effective screening tool for psychomotor performance. It will clearly differentiate those who are too impaired to drive safely, but it does not have the ability to differentiate those at higher psychomotor skills.

One advantage of the simple brake reaction timer is that it does have good face validity with clients, particularly older adults. Additionally, when observing the client performing the task, the qualitative observation of understanding and following directions is useful for the therapist. In effect, it is a subjective cognitive screen. Most DRSs (Dickerson, 2011) use the simple brake reaction timer developed years ago by AAA, affectionately known as the "blue box," even though it has not been manufactured or maintained for almost a decade. In recent studies, it has been fairly clear that the blue box does not accurately reflect simple reaction time tests (Dickerson et al., 2008; Nguyen, Hau, & Bartlett, 2000), and other reaction timers are available, such as the Model RT–2S from Advanced Therapy Products (Glen Allen, VA).

Rapid Pace Walk

The Rapid Pace Walk (Marottoli et al., 1994) measures the amount of time it takes an individual to walk back and forth 10 ft, assessing lower limb mobility, trunk stability, postural control, and balance. In a prospective study of older adults, those individuals who took more than 7 s to complete the Rapid Pace Walk were twice as likely to experience an adverse traffic event.

In two other studies (McCarthy & Mann, 2006; Stav et al., 2008), the Rapid Pace Walk showed a strong correlation for the domain of motor performance and differentiating between those who passed and failed an on-road evaluation, and it held up as an independent predictor of passing or failing an on-road course in people with PD (Classen, Witter, et al., 2011). The Classen, Witter, et al. (2011) study with people with PD illustrates a good example of a specific assessment tool being appropriately linked to a specific diagnostic category because of expected symptoms or behaviors.

Get Up and Go and Timed Up and Go

The Get Up and Go (GUG; Mathias, Nayak, & Isaacs, 1986) test was developed to assess an individual's risk for falls. Similar to the Rapid Pace Walk, the seated individual is asked to get up, walk 10 ft, and come back to the chair. In one study related to driving (Dawson, Uc, Anderson, Johnson, & Rizzo, 2010), significant age differences existed, but the GUG was not an individual predictor of driving safety among older drivers.

Similarly, the Timed Up and Go (TUG; Shumway-Cook, Brauer, & Woollacott, 2000) is a timed instrument with three conditions in which the client is asked to (1) get up, walk 3 m, and sit down; (2) complete the walking task counting backward from a random number between 20 and 100; and (3) complete the walking task holding full cup of water.

Research (Shumway-Cook et al., 2000) has indicated that the TUG is a sensitive and specific measure for identifying older adults who are at risk for falls and decreased mobility, but most driving research studies have used the Rapid Pace Walk rather than GUG or TUG, so there are no direct correlations. However, as with any screening tool, all three tools can offer a qualitative evaluation of the client's physical capacities that might be needed for driving.

Composite Batteries

Considering the complexity of driving, it is clear that there is likely not one assessment that can be used to evaluate all the knowledge and skills to determine whether an individual is able to continue driving, to learn to drive, or to learn the accommodations needed for driving. DRSs recognize this and thus use an array of assessments to measure cognition, vision–perception, and motor skills as well as driving knowledge and competencies. There is no consensus on what composes the best array for the CDE, but several batteries are recognized as good screening batteries.

Assessment of Driving Related Skills

The Assessment of Driving Related Skills (ADReS; Carr et al., 2010) was developed by a consensus panel of driving safety experts who worked in conjunction with the American Medical Association (AMA). The tests selected, which cover the three key functions of vision, cognition, and motor or somatosensory function, were chosen from the available functional tests on the basis of ease of use, availability, amount of time to complete, and quality of information provided.

Through the *Physician's Guide to Assessing and Counseling Older Drivers* (Carr et al., 2010), AMA has recommended that physicians adopt the ADReS battery to screen their older adults as to their driving abilities. Within the guide, the ADReS is thoroughly described, evidence is offered in terms of the selected tests, and materials to complete the battery are made readily available. Specifically, the battery includes testing visual fields by confrontation, visual acuity by the Snellen eye chart, an adopted version of the clock drawing task, Trails B (Reitan, 1958), muscle strength, and neck and extremity range of motion.

However, the test battery as a whole has not been validated using driving outcomes either in primary care practice settings or in samples of drivers with dementia. In a 2006 study, McCarthy and Mann did find that the ADReS was successful in identifying individuals who failed an on-road evaluation. However, it lacked sensitivity, in that it recommended further evaluation for most participants in the study.

Driving Health Inventory

The DrivingHealth® Inventory (DHI) is a computer-based (PC only) screening protocol (TransAnalytics Health and Safety Services, Quakertown, PA) that includes 2 measures of visual ability, 2 measures of physical ability, and 4 measures of perceptual–cognitive ability. The vision measures, which are high- and low-contrast acuity, were identified in research by the California Department of Motor Vehicles as critical to driving (Janke, 1994). The physical measures include lower limb strength and mobility as well as head and neck flexibility. The perceptual–cognitive measures include working memory (using the three-word cued recall test from the MMSE, "bed–apple–shoe"), visual–spatial ability (the MVPT or visual closure subtest; Colarusso & Hammill, 2003), visual search with divided attention (the Trail Making Test; Reitan, 1958), and visual information–processing speed with divided attention (UFOV Subtest 2; Edwards et al., 2006).

The physical and perceptual–cognitive measures reflect the specific tests that were significant predictors of at-fault crash risk in the Maryland Older Driver Study (Staplin, Gish, & Wagner, 2003). Initially, the Gross Impairments Screening battery, or GRIMPS, was developed from the Maryland Older Drivers Study (Staplin & Lococo, 2003; Staplin, Lococo, Gish, & Decina, 2003), but the DHI has since replaced the GRIMPS.

The DHI's computer-based protocol provides a standardized test administration lasting about 30 min. Results categorize performance in terms of no deficit, mild deficit, or serious deficit on each individual measure of functional ability noted earlier. Although the DHI screens a comprehensive set of functional abilities needed to drive safely, scores are not combined across measures, because a serious deficit in any one measure is reason for a more in-depth assessment by a DRS. The cut-points for categorizing the degree of deficit were derived from the odds-ratio analyses described in Staplin, Lococo, et al. (2003). DHI test results are presented in a text report and graphic summary that includes feedback about the implications of a patient's scores for safe driving (see Figure 9.1). More information about the DrivingHealth Inventory and the research behind it is available at its Web site (www.drivinghealth.com).

4Cs

The 4Cs is an interview-based screening intended to be used by health care practitioners modeled after screenings for alcoholism (O'Connor, Kapust, Lin, Hollis, & Jones, 2010). The interview or direct observation is focused on four domains: (1) crash history, (2) family concerns, (3) clinical conditions, and (4) cognitive function. Each domain is scored from 1 to 5 for a total score ranging from 4 to 16, with specific criteria for each point. The scores on the four domains are added to obtain the total score, with a higher number indicating a higher risk of unsafe driving.

In this initial study, in three of the four domains, three groups of drivers characterized by unsafe, marginal, and safe were significantly different as measured by a clinical driving assessment and on-road assessment. The ROC curve for fail or marginal versus pass was good (AUC = 0.812), but there was no separation between

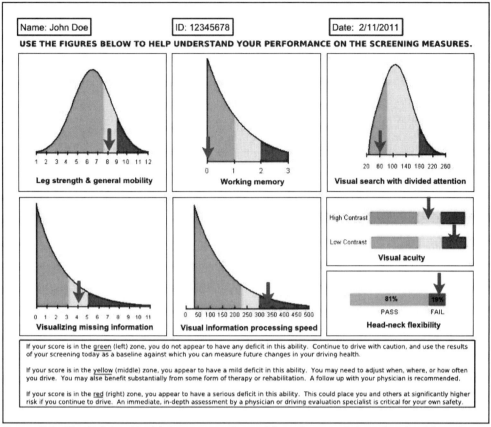

Figure 9.1. The Driving Health Inventory places drivers in one of three levels of function for each measure.

Note. Data from Janke (1994); Staplin, Gish, and Wagner (2003); and Staplin, Lococo, Gish, and Decina (2003). Figure provided by L. Staplin. Used with permission.

fail and marginal (O'Connor et al., 2010). However, it certainly has potential as a screening tool for a busy primary care office, and the scoring criteria and calculation are easy.

Occupational Therapy Driver Off-Road Assessment

The Occupational Therapy Driver Off-Road Assessment (OT–DORA; Unsworth, 2011) was developed by a group of Australian occupational therapists as a standardized assessment battery (Krishnasamy & Unsworth, 2011; Unsworth, Pallant, Russell, Germano, & Odell, 2010). The group did an extensive literature review and work to determining what assessments could be done efficiently as a pre-assessment battery before the on-road component.

The OT–DORA has two categories: (1) the core assessments and (2) optional assessments, if they are clinically indicated. The core assessments include a visual acuity test (the Snellen chart or an equivalent), a visual confrontation test, a test of proprioception of the lower limb, the Berg Balance Scale (Berg, Wood-Dauphinee, Williams, & Gayton, 1989), the Motoricity Index (Collin & Wade, 1990, a motor sequences screen, and 4 assessments developed by the OT–DORA group. These are the Road Law and Road Craft Test (RLRCT; Unsworth et al., 2010), the OT Drive

Home Maze Test (Krishnasamy & Unsworth, 2011), the Simulated Accelerator–Brake Test (Haughton & Unsworth, 2008), and the Right Heel Pivot Test (Unsworth, 2008), of which the latter two do not have published evidence in the literature.

The Drive Home Maze Test (Krishnasamy & Unsworth, 2011) is proposed to test executive function, attention, and visual–constructive skills by having the individual complete a pencil-and-paper maze. The individual's time and number of crossing lines are counted. In their preliminary study, there was a strong positive relationship between the time it took to complete the maze and the percentage of risk of failing the on-road test. The RLRCT is a 15-item test of road laws and knowledge of what to do in driving situations. Unsworth et al. (2010) used Rasch analysis to examine the RLRCT and found, with the limitation of one item, that it achieved good fit for older adults, but it was not clearly associated with whether an individual failed or passed a road test.

The OT–DORA has been revised to be used by practitioners in the United States and Canada. However, it will continue to need research done by Unsworth and her colleagues as well as independent researchers to determine the utility and validity of this and other screening batteries.

Considerations in Use of Common Tools

In 2005, Unsworth, Lovell, Terrington, and Thomas reviewed the common tools used in the clinical component of the comprehensive driving assessment in Australia. The criteria selected for the review included that the assessment (1) had to be in at least one cited peer-reviewed journal, (2) could be completed within 50 min by an occupational therapist, and (3) measured not just reaction time. The selected tools were evaluated on the criteria of prevalence of use (in Australia and internationally), length or ease to complete, method of administration (self or interviewer required), ease of scoring, whether it was created specifically for driving, evidence of reliability and validity, and cost. Each criterion was weighted by scores of 1 to 2, or 1 to 3 for total scores.

Using an arbitrary breakpoint, Unsworth et al. (2005) considered the MMSE (Folstein et al., 1975), Trails A and B (Reitan, 1958), and Rey–Osterrieth Complex Figure Text (a neuropsychological assessment for visual–spatial abilities, memory, attention, and executive functions; Bennett-Levy, 1984) as assessments to be worthy of inclusion in the clinical assessment component of the CDE. As recognized in the study, the three assessments scored well because of their longevity and frequency of use, not because they were linked to outcomes, and none of these were developed specifically for driving. Accordingly, such a review needs to be taken in context, because it adds little evidence of appropriate use of tools for safe driving.

On-Road Evaluation

The on-road driving evaluation and subsequent evaluator judgment of safety (e.g., pass, fail) has been described as the criterion standard for evaluating driver competence (Hunt et al., 1997; Justiss, Mann, Stav, & Velozo, 2006; Odenheimer et al., 1994). *On-road* can be divided into contextually variable levels: *closed road* and *on road* (or *open road*). The closed-road context usually consists of a no-traffic or limited-traffic area such as a parking lot or closed-road circuit that provides a safe venue for drivers to orient themselves to the vehicle's controls and perform basic maneuvers in preparation for driving (on road) on conventional roadways (Stav, 2004).

Each context provides challenges for achieving a reliable and valid approach for determining driver safety. Inability to control for environmental conditions such as traffic density, weather, other drivers' behaviors, and roadway conditions (e.g., construction) may increase evaluator error (Hunt et al., 1997), supporting the criticism that the final judgment (pass or fail) may be unfair or too subjective. In this section, we will review the reliability and validity of methods that improve the objectivity of traditional closed-road and on-road procedures as well as discuss non-traditional methods such as the use of instrumented vehicles to measure naturalistic driving and driving simulators.

Closed-Road Assessment

A closed-road course provides a safe and controllable environment for an evaluator to observe a client's ability to safely operate a motor vehicle. In practice, a DRS may use a closed-road course to screen whether a client can adequately demonstrate basic understanding of vehicle controls (e.g., adjust mirrors, don or doff the seat belt, turn the ignition, shift gear) as well as perform basic maneuvers (e.g., backing up, turning left or right, parking; Stav et al., 2006). Often, based on evaluator judgment (clinical reasoning), observation of deficits in this area may guide the practitioner to discontinue the evaluation if the client is unable to safely perform these tasks under highly controlled conditions. Evaluator judgment of driver competence, even when supported by professional experience and direct observation of performance, may be criticized as being too subjective. Methods have been developed to reliably measure driver performance in both closed- and on-road environments to provide validation of driving outcomes (e.g., pass or fail).

Researchers have recognized that driving is a dynamic and complex activity, largely because of environmental influences (e.g., other drivers, road conditions). Therefore, performance measured in a closed- or off-road environment will be different from performance on the open road. Each environmental condition has unique characteristics and observable behaviors.

Odenheimer and colleagues (1994) designed a performance-based driving evaluation that provides a quantified measure of driving skill in both closed- and on-road environments (review of on-road outcomes is discussed later in this chapter). The closed-road course consists of items related to general familiarity with 21 vehicle features and controls (e.g., seat belts, signals, ignition, pedals) and is scored for seven maneuvering tasks (e.g., driving straight, turning, parking). These performance items are scaled as pass or fail (1 vs. 0 point) and summed for a total closed-course score. Passing of an item (1) is determined when the driver is able to perform that particular task (error free) on the basis of predetermined operational definitions of *task success*. An example for seat belts is "identifying and properly donning seat belt without prompting."

These methods demonstrated good interrater reliability ($r = .84$) and internal consistency ($r = .78$). The main outcome for this process is still to determine whether a client is safe to continue to drive. This study used the criterion standard of evaluator judgment after an on-road assessment that was scaled as pass, marginal, or fail (global rating). A moderate correlation between the closed-road course performance score and the global rating was observed ($r = .44$, $p < .05$). See Table 9.3 for summary of related assessment methodologies.

Table 9.3. Reliability and Validity Summary for On-Road Assessments

Study	Description	Reliability	Validity
Washington University Road Test (Hunt et al., 1997)	Standardized on-road test ($n = 123$); participants with dementia (mild, very mild, control)	**Interrater reliability** Global rating between investigators (occupational therapist), Cronbach's $\alpha = .96$; global rating between investigator and instructor, Cronbach's $\alpha = .85$ **Test–retest reliability** Quantitative score, $k = .76$; global rating, $k = .53$	High correlation between quantitative score and global rating ($r = .60$, $p < .001$) **Concurrent validity** Inclusion of DMV road test items
New Haven Study (Richardson & Marotolli, 2003)	Standardized on-road test ($n = 35$); quantified road performance scores	**Internal consistency** Cronbach's $\alpha = .88$ **Interrater reliability** Intraclass correlation coefficient (ICC = .99)	**Construct validity** Moderate correlation with visual attention ($r = .43$), visual memory ($r = .40$), and executive functioning ($r = -.38$) **Concurrent validity** Use of existing DMV road test
Performance-Based Driving Evaluation (Odenheimer et al., 1994)	Standardized performance-based road test ($n = 30$); closed- and in-traffic road scores	**Interrater reliability** Closed course = .84; in traffic = .74 **Internal consistency** Cronbach's α, closed course = .78; in traffic = .89	Correlation between driving score and global rating, in traffic ($r = .74$, $p < .01$); closed course ($r = .44$, $p < .05$) **Construct validity** Correlation with MMSE ($r = .72$), traffic signs ($r = .69$), visual memory ($r = .50$), verbal memory ($r = .37$), Trails A ($r = .33$), complex reaction time ($r = .58$); all age adjusted
DriveABLE (Dobbs et al., 1998)	Computer screen followed by an on-road exam		**Predictive validity** (road test) 68% pass–fail outcome for older adults with cognitive impairment **Predictive validity** (screen) *Sensitivity* 94% accuracy for predicting failure of road test *Specificity* 98% accuracy for predicting failure of road test
Behind-the-Wheel Evaluation (Galski et al., 1992)	Study comparing on-road performance to cognitive function, simulated driving ($n = 35$)		**Correlation of street index** *Cognition* Trails A ($r = .42$, $p < .05$), figure test change score ($r = .44$, $p < .01$), maze test ($r = .43$, $p < .05$), visual form discrimination ($r = -.56$, $p < .001$), double letter cancellation ($r = -.57$, $p < .001$), block design ($r = .60$, $p < .001$) *Simulator* Signal errors ($r = -.64$, $p < .001$), threat recognition ($r = .69$, $p < .001$) *Lot behaviors* Following directions ($r = -.59$), slow response ($r = -.68$), inattention ($r = -.71$), distractibility ($r = -.72$); all $ps < .001$
Driver Performance Measure (Justiss et al., 2006)	Development of standardized methods for BTW assessment; fixed route, 45–60 min, structured scoring protocol; quantified value 0–1.00 range (percentage score)	**Interrater reliability** ICC = .94 **Test–retest** ICC = .95 **Internal consistency** Cronbach's $\alpha = .94$	**Criterion validity** (performance score vs. 4-point GRS) $r = .84$, $p < .001$ Regression model accounting for 44% of the variance in GRS: retained UFOV rating, contrast sensitivity slide B, Rapid Pace Walk, and MMSE (Stav et al., 2006)

Table 9.3. Reliability and Validity Summary for On-Road Assessments *(cont.)*

Study	Description	Reliability	Validity
Open-Road Assessment (Mallon & Wood, 2004)	Standardized road test to assess the validity of directed and self-directed navigational instructional components		**Criterion validity** $r = .76$, $p < .001$
Sum of Maneuvers (Shechtman et al., 2010)	Standardized BTW assessment with quantified value of performance (SMS 0–273); categorical pass–fail outcome	Significant differences in SMS ($F = 29.9$, $df = 1$, $p <= .001$) between drivers who passed the driving test and those who failed	SMS cutoff = 230/273; sensitivity (0.91) and specificity (0.87)

Note. BTW = behind-the-wheel; DMV = Department of Motor Vehicles (Bureau of Motor Vehicles in some states); ICC = intraclass correlation coefficient; GRS = global rating score; MMSE = Mini-Mental State Examination; SMS = Sum of Maneuvers; UFOV = Useful Field of View.

Another driving study used comparable methods to measure closed-road and on-road driving performance (Galski, Bruno, & Ehle, 1992). Similar to Odenheimer et al. (1994), Galski et al. (1992) created a "Lot Index" or score to quantify closed- or off-road driving behaviors (familiarity with vehicle controls). Certain lot behaviors (e.g., following directions, slow response) contributed significantly toward 93% of the explained variance in the on-road driving performance outcome.

These results support the use of a closed- or off-road segment of the CDE to be used for determining driver competence or safety. Closed-road driving performance can provide valuable information for guiding DRSs regarding whether they should proceed to the open road. The different techniques used to quantify observed performance provide the structured methodology or standardized procedures that minimize evaluator error and improve reliability, and one hopes, the predictive validity of the closed-road assessment for determining on-road performance. Similar performance observation techniques are also used for the on-road assessment.

> **Closed-road driving performance can provide valuable information for guiding DRSs regarding whether they should proceed to the open road.**

On-Road Assessment

As opposed to the relative safety of the closed-road driving assessment, the addition of environmental or contextual factors for the on-road evaluation can complicate methods of in-vehicle assessment and subsequent determination of safety. Testing on a closed course provides a safe environment by limiting exposure to the unpredictable and confounding behavior of other drivers but limits the ability to assess how a driver might respond in a real-world or potentially hazardous situation.

How a driving course is designed can influence this exposure. On-road assessment methodologies can use a fixed-route or variable-route course design. Although the latter may be a more occupationally centered (ecologically valid) approach, it lacks the experimental control needed for determining the reliability of the assessment procedures or the validity of the outcome measure (driving performance and safety).

Course Design

The fixed-route course design has been identified as a foundation for reliable and valid assessment of driving performance (Di Stefano & Macdonald, 2003; Hunt et al., 1997; Justiss et al., 2006; Richardson & Marottoli, 2003). By guiding drivers through the same environmental or infrastructure conditions (e.g., single or double lanes, fixed or signalized intersections), the evaluator can provide some control over performance variance attributed to roadway components. Similarly, a carefully developed course can be designed to control for the probability of unexpected or challenging events, which are necessary for determining driver responsiveness to potentially hazardous situations (Justiss et al., 2006). If a course is too easy (e.g., little to no traffic or challenges), it becomes difficult to differentiate between good and poor drivers, because all can perform adequately under the course conditions. The same is true for an overly challenging course. Therefore, inappropriate route design can result in poor sensitivity for determining driving competence (Di Stefano & Macdonald, 2005).

Recommendations for course design parameters were developed from an international consensus conference on driver safety (Korner-Bitensky, Gelinas, Man-Son-Hing, & Marshall, 2005; Stephens et al., 2005). It has been suggested that a progressively complex, fixed-route course of approximately 45–60 min would provide adequate environmental exposure to the driver for an evaluator to determine performance competence (e.g., pass or fail). This evaluator judgment or global rating of competence after an on-road assessment has been described as the criterion standard for measuring driver performance. This outcome may be a dichotomous pass–fail or may vary between ordinal levels of performance such as pass–marginal–fail. Although the global rating is a subjective interpretation of overall driving performance, researchers have developed standardized methods to quantify evaluator observations to validate this decision (Mazer et al., 2003; Roenker, Cissell, Ball, Wadley, & Edwards, 2003).

Measuring On-Road Performance

Different quantitative methods to assess on-road driving performance have been explored. Some studies use methods to count driving errors (Mazer et al., 2003; Roenker et al., 2003), and others use more elaborate scoring mechanisms that scale individual driving components (Galski, Bruno, & Ehle, 1993; Hunt et al., 1997; Justiss et al., 2006; Mallon & Wood, 2004; Odenheimer et al., 1994).

A behavioral model describes driving as a complex task that is hierarchically controlled across three levels: strategic, tactical, and operational (Michon, 1985; Ranney, 1994). The *strategic* or *planning* level reflects general goal formation including trip planning and selecting a route and its alternatives. The *tactical* level reflects the navigational influences of the selected route, such as turns, curves, and traffic. The *operational* level involves the ability to control the vehicle given the environmental or situational influences (Ranney, 1994).

Researchers using this hierarchical approach have developed task analysis strategies that evaluate the tactical and operational levels of driving to more objectively measure performance (Di Stefano & Macdonald, 2003; Hunt et al., 1997; Justiss et al., 2006; Richardson & Marottoli, 2003). Types of driving maneuvers (e.g., turning left or right, changing lanes) can be identified and quantified on a fixed-route course.

Each driving maneuver has associated behaviors that reflect the ability to control the vehicle safely through the environment (e.g., steering, braking, visual scanning). Rating the performance quality of this human–machine–environment interaction across a progressively complex road course provides a quantifiable and standardized method for objectively determining driving safety. For example, during a left turn (tactical maneuver), an evaluator may note a driver's inability to maintain consistent steering (operational control) during the turn. Different scoring techniques may be applied to either level of observation. This behavioral hierarchy of the driving task (strategic, tactical, and operational) provides a theoretical foundation for understanding and quantifying the components of this dynamic IADL.

As mentioned earlier, a quantified score could be a total frequency of driving errors or a summed total of maneuver scores based on predetermined, operational definitions of *task success*. These scoring algorithms are used to establish the reliability and validity for on-road assessment procedures. For example, Odenheimer et al. (1994) rated each maneuver (left turn, right turn, etc.) as a 1 *(pass)* or 0 *(fail)* on the basis of observed performance. These maneuver scores were summed for a total performance score.

This numerical value is often used to establish interrater and test–retest (stability) reliability. Criterion validity is established when these numerical values of overall driving performance are correlated with the evaluator's global rating of safety (e.g., pass or fail). Recent research has established valid cut-points for these quantified values of driver performance with adequate sensitivity and specificity for determining who should pass and who should fail the behind-the-wheel assessment (Bédard, Weaver, Dārzin, & Porter, 2008; Shechtman, Awadzi, Classen, Lanford, & Joo, 2010).

The design of the road course combined with an established scoring algorithm provides the structure to satisfy the research and practice needs when determining driver competence. Table 9.3 provides some examples of research studies that provide reliability and validity characteristics of standardized on-road evaluation procedures. For greater detail, please see full references in the "References" section at the end of this chapter.

Instrumented Vehicles and Naturalistic Driving Studies

Although there have been advances in on-road evaluation procedures for improving objectivity and reliability, there are still some limitations to the ecological validity of these methods. Fixed-route courses provide the foundation for greater experimental control, but verbally guiding a driver through a designated route can influence a driver's performance and limit choice or decision-making behaviors (Mallon & Wood, 2004).

The term *naturalistic driving* refers to unimpeded or unrestricted driving under real-world conditions, with no influence from an evaluator. There is a distinct shift in the performance outcome evaluated under these conditions: vehicle crashes. Data from an instrumented vehicle may provide more crash detail than routine crash outcomes commonly used as part of larger epidemiological studies of crash risk. They are often a result of police report after the incident has occurred and based on preliminary estimates of crash reconstruction characteristics. Contributing factors such as fatigue or distracted behavior may be difficult to ascertain.

100-Car Naturalistic Driving Study

The 100-Car Naturalistic Driving Study (Dingus, Neale, Klauer, Petersen, & Carroll, 2006) was designed to capture driving behavior, performance, fatigue, impairment, error in judgment, risk taking, aggressiveness and traffic violations, and so on through data recorded from an instrumented vehicle. Over approximately 12–13 months, these researchers captured 2 million vehicle miles and about 43,000 driving hours of data on 241 primary and secondary drivers.

Instrumentation from the vehicle included multiple video feeds of the driver and the surrounding environment, as well as vehicle kinematics (e.g., speed, steering wheel movement). The driver was also instructed to push a button (on the installed instrumentation) whenever there was a close call or an incident; researchers then were able to analyze what was happening in the car and in the environment before the close call. This detailed information enabled the researchers to study the relationships among these variables and crashes, near crashes, and other incidents.

A data acquisition system was mounted in the trunk of the subject vehicle and integrated with the variety of sensor streams that created a recording "bubble" or field around the vehicle using both video and radar. The in-cab and exterior sensor apparatus was designed to be unobtrusive to both the driver and outside vehicles so as not to have any undue influence on behavior or impede the driver's visual field.

Results indicated that 78% of crashes and 65% of near crashes were the result of driver inattention. The most prevalent form of driver inattention was secondary task engagement with electronic devices (cell phones), followed by passenger-related distraction (talking). Crashes tended to occur at lower speeds and were attributed to the environment (e.g., weather) and precrash behavior by the driver. Not surprisingly, drivers who were not facing forward had longer brake response times, and 81% of rear-end collisions occurred when the lead vehicle was stopped. Results also indicated that in many cases, braking alone was not enough to avoid a collision.

This information may provide a foundation for driver training strategies to improve crash avoidance behaviors (steering responsiveness) and the use of more complex or choice reaction times for predicting crash risk. These data also provide valuable information for the development of vehicle countermeasures such as advance warning systems and active safety systems to minimize or mitigate vehicle crashes. As these systems become more prevalent in modern vehicles, the driving evaluator should be aware of how these countermeasures may influence driver behavior.

Instrumented Driving and Dementia

Also using instrumented driving, Eby and colleagues (2009) designed a study to investigate the feasibility of using vehicle instrumentation to monitor the driving performance of older adults with early-stage dementia. Driving behaviors from the group with dementia were compared with the behaviors of older drivers without dementia (control) over a 1-month period. Although the drivers with dementia drove shorter distances to fewer locations and avoided nighttime and highway driving, they became lost more often than the control group.

There was no significant difference between the control group and the individuals with early-stage dementia when examining safety issues. There are several explanations for not finding safety differences, with the most likely being the fact that all of the drivers with early-stage dementia had to pass an on-road test before enrollment in the study. Thus, a driving specialist found the drivers "safe" a month before implementation and instrumentation was needed for longer than 1 mo to measure decreasing abilities.

Avoidance behaviors and becoming lost are often ascertained by the occupational therapist during the occupational profile through self-report mechanisms. With a client population that has cognitive impairment, the reliability of self-reported driving behavior may be suspect and require informant (caregiver) confirmation if available. The use of vehicle instrumentation can provide an objective approach to monitor driver behaviors that may place the individual at risk.

Simulators

Types and Configurations. Driving simulators use computer-based technology to create the impression of driving a vehicle (Stern & Schold Davis, 2006). Examples of current developers of simulators include STISim (Systems Technology, Hawthorn, CA), DriveSafety (DriveSafety, Inc., Murray, UT), and GlobalSim (GlobalSim, Inc., Draper, UT) simulation. However, other manufacturers and models are available on the market.

Simulators may vary from desktop configurations using one to three computer monitors to cab configurations with life-sized graphics (Figure 9.2). They may be fixed based, as displayed in Figures 9.2 and 9.3, in which the simulator does not move during the scenarios, or motion based, in which the simulator moves in

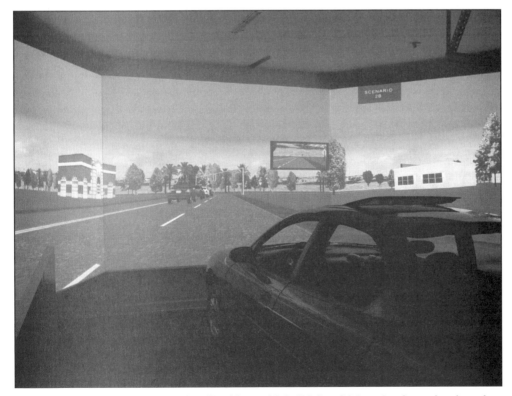

Figure 9.2. The STISim M500W is a fixed-base, high-fidelity driving simulator developed and marketed by Systems Technology, Inc., of Hawthorn, CA.

Note. Provided by S. Classen. Used with permission.

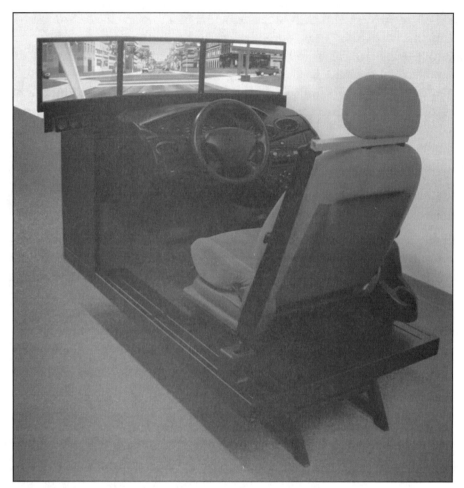

Figure 9.3. The DriveSafety DS–250a is a compact, nonimmersive driving simulation system optimized for use in clinical settings.

Note. Provided by S. Classen. Used with permission.

conjunction with scenario actions. The cost varies on the basis of graphics resolution and motion-based features. For example, high-fidelity simulators with high resolution and fast refresh rates may vary from $25,000 to more than $100,000 (Stern & Schold Davis, 2006).

Some simulators may be bought with premade scenarios, and others provide the opportunity to create one's own scenarios. Before purchasing a simulator, the buyer needs to be sure that the fidelity of the simulator scenarios and simulator are guaranteed by the manufacturers.

Advantages. Occupational therapists use driving simulators to provide a safe alternative to on-road evaluations because driving errors and crashes made in a simulator pose little risk to the physical or emotional well-being of the participants. For example, Stern and Schold-Davis (2006) used a simulator in occupational therapy clinical practice to remediate participants' performance skills (e.g., visually scanning the environment) and patterns (e.g., checking the right lane before merging).

Additional benefits of using a simulator, rather than on-road evaluation, to assess driving performance in the research or clinical setting include opportunity to create an impression of driving a vehicle in a virtual world with minimal physical space requirements. Studies are highly reproducible and cost-effective, and factors (e.g., weather, day vs. night, or fog vs. sunshine) can be modified through programming, for example, a participant driving in sunshine, rain, or snow. If standardized procedures are used (e.g., use of scenarios with fidelity), objective data can be collected through the kinematics data collection system (vehicle output data; e.g., headway or following distance or number of red light offenses) of the simulator. In the current absence of turn-key scenarios (ready-made scenarios to be used), occupational therapists will require the use of a technical support person to help with obtaining, reading, and interpreting the kinematics data.

Additionally, the simulator provides a low-risk and high-benefit situation in which high-risk groups can be studied or trained behind the wheel. Participants can drive different scenarios (e.g., residential area, city, or rural driving scenes) in a matter of minutes. One also can tailor driving situations that are sensitive to people with specific driving impairments, for example, for those with decreased peripheral vision. All tests can be conducted under objective and repeatable conditions.

Driving simulators have been used to assess the driving performance skills of participants who are potentially unsafe in a car (e.g., those with a moderate to severe TBIs), to examine the use of in-vehicle technologies such as lane departure warning systems, and to determine the participant's interaction with the environment such as negotiating intersections incorporating highway design guidelines (Shechtman, Classen, Awadzi, & Mann, 2009; Shechtman et al., 2007, 2008).

Limitations

Limitations to the use of simulators include that they are a representation of reality, but not reality itself. Although absolute validity was found in one study, ecological validity (i.e., relevance to real-world driving) is still being questioned (Shechtman et al., 2009). Graphics may be experienced as cartoonlike and thus not be representative of the real driving experience. Creating customized scenarios for the simulator is time consuming, is labor intensive, and requires the skill set of a computer scientist or programmer.

However, the biggest limitation, potentially, pertains to the experience of *simulator adaptation syndrome,* also called *simulator sickness (SS),* which is physical discomfort experienced when "driving" a simulated vehicle because of incompatible signals from visual, auditory, and motion systems. SS affects the driver in the absence of true motion and shares many of the same symptoms as motion sickness (Hettinger, Berbaum, Kennedy, Dunlap, & Nolan, 1990). Such symptoms range from cold sweats, restlessness, pallor, and nausea to excessive salivating and vomiting. Sensory Conflict Theory explains that the brain interprets sensory messages of movement as inharmonious or "noxious" among the ocular, motor, and kinesthetic systems (Reason & Brand, 1975). This noxious response elicits action from the autonomic nervous system.

In an evidence-based literature review on the determinants of SS, the authors used the *Occupational Therapy Practice Framework* (American Occupational Therapy Association, 2008) to organize the review (Classen, Bewernitz, & Shechtman, 2011). Using the American Academy of Neurology's classification criteria (Edlund, Gronseth, So, & Franklin, 2004), they extracted data from 10 (of 19) studies and assigned each a class of I to IV, with Class I indicating the highest level of evidence.

Although no Class I studies were found, the authors deduced that client factors—that is, older clients (> age 70) and being female, as well as context or environment factors such as scenario design and duration; simulator configuration; number of exposures; number of curves and turns; and calibration of the brake, steering, and other vehicle components—are probably increasing the rates of SS. The authors also found that activity demands such as *vection* (perception of movement without moving), speed of driving, and postural instability (as determined by postural sway) possibly contribute to SS.

Because no Class I studies exist that specify which factors are predictive (or not) of SS, occupational therapists need to take these mentioned factors into consideration as those that can probably or possibly predict SS. Simulator mitigation strategies (discussed next) can be implemented to curtail the effects of the exposures.

Simulator Sickness Mitigation Strategies

Mitigation strategies are important to prevent the onset or to minimize the experience of SS. One of the first strategies to prevent SS is to screen for the client's propensity. A good tool for this is the Simulator Sickness Questionnaire (SSQ; Kennedy, Fowlkes, Berbaum, & Lilienthal, 1992; see Exhibit 9.1). The SSQ can be administered as a baseline or as a screen before deciding whether the client can use

Exhibit 9.1. Simulator Sickness Questionnaire

SSQ Symptom	Nausea Score	Nausea Weight	Oculomotor Score	Oculomotor Weight	Disorientation Score	Disorientation Weight
General discomfort		1		1		0
Fatigue		0		1		0
Headache		0		1		0
Eyestrain		0		1		0
Difficulty focusing		0		1		1
Increased salivation		1		0		0
Sweating		1		0		0
Nausea		1		0		1
Difficulty concentrating		1		1		0
Fullness of head		0		0		1
Blurred vision		0		1		1
Dizzy (eyes open)		0		0		1
Dizzy (eyes closed)		0		0		1
Vertigo		0		0		1
Stomach awareness		1		0		0
Burping		1		0		0
Total						

Note. Participants report the degree to which they experience each of the above symptoms; 0 = *none*, 1 = *slight*, 2 = *moderate*, 3 = *severe*. Scoring: Weighted scale scores: Multiply Nausea × 9.54, Oculomotor × 7.58, Disorientation × 13.92. Total SSQ score = add the three scale scores × 3.74.
From "Simulator Sickness Questionnare: An Enhanced Method for Quantifying Simulator Sickness," by R. S. Kennedy, N. E. Lane, K. S. Berbaums, and M. G. Lilienthal, 1993, *International Journal of Aviation Psychology, 3*. Copyright © 1993 by Laurence Erlbaum. Used with permission.

the simulator. It can be used frequently with the client while on the simulator drive so that comparisons can be made.

The SSQ rates 16 symptoms across three domains: (1) oculomotor, (2) disorientation, and (3) nausea. Participants report the degree to which they experience each symptom on a scale ranging from 0 to 3, with 0 = *none*, 1 = *slight*, 2 = *moderate*, and 3 = *severe*. The scoring uses a weighted-scale score and requires one to multiply the score on the nausea domain by 9.54, that on the oculomotor domain by 7.58, and that on the disorientation domain by 13.92. The total SSQ score is derived by adding the three scale scores and then multiplying the sum by 3.74.

Clients also need to be informed about diet before scheduling a simulator session. Eating a low-fat diet, abstaining from alcohol or caffeine, and having carbohydrate-rich snacks the night before simulator testing tends to be effective in relieving motion sickness and, based on our research experience, also SS (Centers for Disease Control and Prevention, 2011). A Reliefband, a Food and Drug Administration–approved unit to curtail the onset of SS available at most drugstores, may be offered before the drive if the participant is susceptible to SS (e.g., has a history of motion sickness).

All participants must be offered an opportunity to drive an acclimation scenario, which usually contains elements of a straight drive, without detailed environments and reduced visual stimuli. The objective is to get the participant comfortable in the drive and to get used to the dynamics of the simulator. Acclimation drives vary from 5–15 min.

Participants must be observed during the drive by a trained evaluator who knows the signs and symptoms of SS and who will not hesitate to terminate the drive if the participant is experiencing discomfort. Participants who are experiencing mild discomfort may be allowed to rest, be offered snacks and ginger ale, or quit. From our simulator study experiences, we have also learned that keeping all right turns to the end of the drive, allowing for constant airflow by having a fan blowing on the dashboard of the car cab, and keeping the temperature in the testing room at about 70° F help to minimize the SS symptoms. Additionally, occupational therapists are encouraged to work with the manufacturer to ensure optimal calibration among the steering wheel, brake, and transmission and to use systems that render a minimum refresh rate (smoothness of the visually displayed scenarios) of about 100 Hz. Finally, based on the literature, a triscreen desktop configuration providing about 110° field of view, compared with a single desktop or a 180° field of view configuration yielded the least amount of SS among participants (Park et al., 2004).

Validity and Reliability of the Driving Simulator

The validity of the simulator test is very important to help provide a rationale for clinical decisions to determine fitness to drive or interventions to improve driving performance. Likewise, reliability of the simulator (test–retest) and reliability between evaluators (interrater) using the system are equally important.

In an evidence-based validity study, Shechtman et al. (2009) replicated real-world intersections in the driving simulator (STISIM M500W, Systems Technology Inc., Hawthorne, CA) and assessed the number and type of driving errors committed by the same 39 participants while negotiating a right and a left turn both on the road and in the simulator. They found no significant interactions between the type of vehicle (road vs. simulator) and the type of turn (right vs. left) for any of the driving errors, indicating that the same trends exist between driving errors made on the road and in the simulator and thus suggesting relative validity (same direction or magnitude of effects) in the simulator. They also found no significant differences between the road and the simulator for lane maintenance, adjustment to stimuli, and visual scanning errors, indicating absolute validity (same numerical values) for these types of errors.

The findings suggest early support for external validity for the driving simulator used in this study, indicating that the results of assessing driving errors when negotiating turns in the simulator can be generalized or transferred to the road under the same testing conditions. A follow-up study with a larger sample size is needed to establish whether driving performance in the simulator is predictive of driving performance on the road.

Bédard, Parkkari, Weaver, Riendeau, and Dahlquist (2010) examined the validity and reproducibility of simulator-based driving evaluations. First, they examined correlations among Trails A and B (Lezak et al., 2004; Shum, McFarland, & Bain, 1990), demerit (lost) points for simulated drives, and simulator-recorded errors. With one exception, correlations ranged from .44 ($p = .103$) to .83 ($p = .001$) between the Trail Making Test and the simulated drive. Then correlations were examined among Trails A, UFOV (Edwards et al., 2006), and demerit points for simulated drives; correlations ranged from .50 to .82 (all $ps < .001$). The correlation between demerit points for on-road and simulated drives was .74 ($p = .035$). They examined reproducibility of simulator assessments using the playback function of the simulated drive and determined that the intraclass correlation coefficients ranged from .73 to .87 (all $ps < .001$). These results suggest that simulators could be used with reasonable validity and reliability to facilitate the evaluation of fitness to drive.

Simulator technology is providing opportunities for future applications in clinical practice and research because of advantages and usefulness. However, more studies are needed that provide empirical data on driving performance outcomes using specific simulators and specific populations. Currently, the evidence is promising, but the data may not be sufficient to suggest that simulators may be used to assess fitness to drive in complex, borderline clinical cases.

Self-Report

Valid self-report measures may hold multiple benefits for users, including being freely available, having little or no cost, being used in the privacy of one's own home, providing immediate feedback to the user, and providing opportunity for increasing one's knowledge and for potentially changing one's behaviors.

Bias

An underlying concern with using self-reports to assess driving performance is the bias underlying self-report. For example, people confident about their driving may be more likely to complete a driving self-report, which is referred to as *selection bias* (Zhou & Lyles, 1997). Alternatively people may infuse *social desirability bias,* meaning that respondents are answering the questions according to how they would like to be perceived, typically by understating undesirable behavior (Lajunen & Summala, 2003). Other forms of bias that may influence valid and reliable ratings are *recall bias,* the ability to accurately remember facts pertaining to the question (Fowler, 1995), and *rater bias,* pertaining to the consistency of the person completing the self-report. For example, researchers reported that older adults tended to overrate their driving ability compared with the results of a driving evaluator (Marottoli & Richardson, 1998).

From a research perspective, these issues need to be addressed by using modern statistical adjustments that account for anticipated response bias, by obtaining a proxy report in addition to self-report, and by using measures that are validated against a gold standard criterion measure (Sundstrom, 2005, 2008).

Tools

Among available self-report tools, we discuss three designed for older drivers. Those measures are the **Driving Decisions Workbook** (Eby, Molnar, Shope, Vivoda, & Fordyce, 2003), the computer-based **Roadwise Review** (AAA, 2004), and the Safe Driving Behaviors Measure (Classen et al., 2010; Winter et al., 2011).

Strengths of the measures include assessment of driving that includes medical conditions and medication use (*Driving Decisions Workbook*), measurement of physical and cognitive abilities predictive of at-fault crashes among drivers ages 65 and older (*Roadwise Review*), and education for drivers about risk factors and strategies for driving safely (*Driving Decisions Workbook* and *Roadwise Review*). Only the *Driving Decisions Workbook* development entailed comparison with a criterion measure to determine the influence of self-report bias (e.g., social desirability).

The *Driving Decisions Workbook* and *Roadwise Review* both incorporated focus group feedback from stakeholders during measure development (Eby et al., 2003; Staplin & Dinh-Zarr, 2006). The *Driving Decisions Workbook* designed with an educational focus (i.e., emphasizing safety knowledge such as driving strategies) is 37 pages long, and each page has between 1 and 6 questions. The workbook is designed for people to work through at their own pace, following their own interests. It also contains a question-and-answer section to obtain more information, and participants averaged 30 min to complete it (Eby et al., 2003). Current research is ongoing to develop a computerized version.

The computer-based *Roadwise Review* takes approximately 40 min to complete, may be challenging for older adults with low computer fluency to use, and requires the assistance of another person to complete the noncognitive measures (Staplin & Dinh-Zarr, 2006).

Classen and colleagues (2010) developed a self-report Safe Driving Behavior Measure (SDBM; now called the **Fitness-To-Drive Screening Measure**) for older drivers and their family members or caregivers. On completion, use of these measures will position occupational therapists to accurately determine a driver's level of safe driving through a description of observable driving behaviors, and an entry point to assess the client's level of safe driving from which a rehabilitation intervention can be planned. The assessment has three sections: A, demographic profile; B, driving history profile; and C, driving behaviors. For Section C, based on the past 3 mo of driving, the individual rates his or her difficulty in executing a variety of driving tasks, on a scale ranging from *very difficult* to *not difficult*. The final score represents the reported level of difficulty for an individual across all the items behaviors (Classen et al., 2010).

In the SDBM, the researchers used Rasch analysis to turn the ordinal data into equal-interval data and express that with a unit of measure called a *logit* (log-odds unit). Acceptable face validity and content validity have been established. Psychometric testing results have been promising, and the construct validity results are encouraging (Classen, Wen, et al., 2012). Preliminary inter-rater reliability results (*n* = 80 drivers, 2 evaluators, 80 family members or caregivers) showed a significantly moderate agreement between the evaluators and family members or caregivers, but not between the drivers. Rater effects were found between the evaluator and the caregiver, with the evaluator being the more severe rater.

Although research is ongoing, these findings have implications for family members or caregivers to rate their loved one's (the older driver's) driving behaviors, closer to the evaluators' ratings (Classen, Wen, et al., 2012). In this way, family members or caregivers may present the occupational therapist, generalist, or specialist with information for clinical interpretation and intervention.

Self-report tools are useful for raising awareness about declining skills underlying the task of driving. They are also appropriate for starting the conversation about continued driving, referring the client for a Dementia Rating Scale, or considering driving cessation. These assessments traditionally have not been developed to be predictive of on-road performance or crashes.

Conclusion

Occupational therapists must be more discriminating in their search for tools with evidence to support their use. Therapists should look for sensitivity and specificity studies that support the use of the tool with populations to determine who might be at risk for safe driving.

Standardized assessment tools provide occupational therapists with opportunities to objectively evaluate their client's strengths and weaknesses in the skills needed for safe driving and community mobility. Using these tools not only provides therapists with information for clinical reasoning, it also provides concrete data for clients and family members to use in understanding a client's strengths and limitations. In addition, the use of standardized tools provides a medium for effective communication among therapists and professionals in other fields and in the community.

A key aspect for occupational therapists is to ensure that they use a tool as it was intended. For example, the UFOV (Edwards et al., 2006) demonstrates good predictive validity for driving, but it is adapted and separated for use in the DHI and the *Roadwise Review*, so therapists should not assume that these adapted versions are predictive.

In addition to the standardized assessments tools described in this chapter, there are clearly tools that are used that are not standardized or do not have the evidence to back their usefulness. More research needs to be done, particularly in terms of driver simulation and on-road assessment. In the meantime, though, occupational therapists must use their observational skills, knowledge of activity analysis, and clinical reasoning to address this critical IADL of driving. There is much therapists can contribute from their interactions with clients doing other complex tasks that use the same underlying skills.

Occupational therapists are encouraged to use standardized assessment tools in the evaluation process, carefully considering which tools to select. Wisely selected tools that span the abilities of vision, cognition, and motor skills should be comprehensive but not duplicative. Only one cognitive screening is necessary, for example, and the TUG (Shumway-Cook et al., 2000) may be enough rather than a full assessment of strength and range of motion. Therapists also must collaborate together in considering the impact of impairments in visual, cognitive, and motor skills on driving and community mobility, so that clients receive the most effective and efficient assessment and intervention, avoiding excessive cost. See **Appendix 9.A** for more assessment-related resources.

References

Aldrich, M. S. (1989). Automobile accidents in patients with sleep disorders. *Sleep, 12,* 487–494.

American Automobile Association. (2004). *Roadwise review*. Heathrow, FL: AAA Public Affairs.

American Occupational Therapy Association. (2008). Occupational therapy practice framework: Domain and process (2nd ed.). *American Journal of Occupational Therapy, 62,* 625–683. doi: 10.5014.ajot.62.6.675

Baker, T. K., Falb, T., Voas, R., & Lacey, J. (2003). Older women drivers: Fatal crashes in good conditions. *Journal of Safety Research, 34,* 399–405.

Ball, K. K., Owsley, C., Sloane, M. E., Roenker, D. L., & Bruni, J. R. (1993). Visual attention problems as a predictor of vehicle crashes in older drivers. *Investigative Ophthalmology and Visual Science, 34,* 3110–3123.

Ball, K. K., Owsley, C., Stalvey, B. T., Roenker, D. L., Sloane, M. E., & Graves, M. (1998). Driving avoidance and functional impairment in older drivers. *Accident Analysis and Prevention, 30,* 313–322.

Ball, K. K., Roenker, D. L., Wadley, V. G., Edwards, J. D., Roth, D. L., McGwin, G., et al. (2006). Can high-risk older drivers be identified through performance-based measures in a department of motor vehicles setting? *Journal of the American Geriatrics Society, 54,* 77–84.

Balota, D. A., Storandt, M., McKeel, D. W., & Morris, J. C. (1998). Relating anatomy to function in Alzheimer's disease. *Neurology, 50,* 979–985.

Bédard, M., Parkkari, M., Weaver, B., Riendeau, J., & Dahlquist, M. (2010). Assessment of driving performance using a simulator protocol: Validity and reproducibility. *American Journal of Occupational Therapy, 64,* 336–340. doi: 10.5014/ajot.64.2.336

Bédard, M., Riendeau, J., Weaver, B., & Clarkson, A. (2011). Roadwise review has limited congruence with actual driving performance of aging drivers. *Accident Analysis and Prevention, 43,* 2209–2214.

Bédard, M., Weaver, B., Dārzin, P., & Porter, M. M. (2008). Predicting driving performance in older adults: We are not there yet! *Traffic Injury Prevention, 9,* 336–341.

Bennett-Levy, J. (1984). Determinants of performance on the Rey–Osterrieth Complex Figure Test: An analysis, and a new technique for single-case assessment. *British Journal of Clinical Psychology, 23,* 109–119.

Berg, K., Wood-Dauphinee, S., Williams, J. I., & Gayton, D. (1989). Measuring balance in the elderly: Preliminary development of an instrument. *Physiotherapy Canada, 41,* 304–311.

Bond, T. G., & Fox, C. M. (2007). *Applying the Rasch model: Fundamental measurement in the human sciences* (2nd ed.). Mahwah, NJ: Erlbaum.

Bouillon, L., Mazer, B., & Gelinas, I. (2006). Validity of the Cognitive Behavioral Driver's Inventory in predicting driving outcome. *American Journal of Occupational Therapy, 60,* 420–427. http://dx.doi.org/10.5014/ajot.60.4.420

Bowers, A., Peli, E., Elgin, J., McGwin, G., Jr., & Owsley, C. (2005). On-road driving with moderate visual field loss. *Optometry and Vision Science, 82,* 657–667.

Bracy, O. L. (1985). Cognitive rehabilitation: A process approach. *Cognitive Rehabilitation, 4,* 10–17.

Carr, D. B., LaBarge, E., Dunnigan, K., & Storandt, M. (1998). Differentiating drivers with dementia of the Alzheimer type from healthy older persons with a traffic sign naming test. *Journals of Gerontology, Series A: Biological Sciences and Medical Sciences, 53,* 135–139.

Carr, D. B., & Ott, B. R. (2010). The older adult driver with cognitive impairment. *JAMA, 303,* 1632–1641.

Carr, D. B., Schwartzberg, J. G., Manning, L., & Sempek, J. (2010). *Physician's guide to assessing and counseling older drivers.* Washington, DC: National Highway Traffic Safety Administration.

Centers for Disease Control and Prevention. (2011). *Travelers' health.* Retrieved January 16, 2011, from wwwnc.cdc.gov/travel/yellowbook/2012/chapter-2-the-pre-travel-consulta-tion/motion-sickness.htm

Classen, S., Bewernitz, M., & Shechtman, O. (2011). Driving simulator sickness: An evidence-based review of the literature. *American Journal of Occupational Therapy, 65,* 179–188. doi: 10.5014/ajot.2011.000802

Classen, S., McCarthy, D. P., Shechtman, O., Awadzi, K. D., Lanford, D. N., Okun, M. S., et al. (2009). Useful Field of View as a reliable screening measure of driving performance in people with Parkinson's disease: Results of a pilot study. *Traffic Injury Prevention, 10,* 593–598.

Classen, S., & Owens, A. B. (in press). Simulator sickness among returning combat veterans with mild traumatic brain injury and/or post-traumatic stress disorder *Advances in Trans-portation Studies: An International Journal.*

Classen, S., Shechtman, O., Joo, Y., Awadzi, K. D., & Lanford, D. N. (2011). Traffic violations vs. driving errors: Implications for older female drivers. *In Women's issues in transporta-tion: Vol. 2.* (pp. 55–63). Washington, DC: Transportation Research Board.

Classen, S., Shechtman, O., Stephens, B., Davis, E., Justiss, M., Bendixen, R., et al. (2007). The impact of roadway intersection design on driving performance of young and senior adults. *Traffic Injury Prevention, 8,* 69–77.

Classen, S., Wen, P., Velozo, C., Bédard, M., Brumback, B., Winter, S. M., et al. (2012). Rater reliability and rater effects of the Safe Driving Behavior Measure. *American Journal of Occupational Therapy, 66,* 69–77. doi: 10.5014/ajot.2012.002261

Classen, S., Wen, P., Velozo, C. A., Bédard, M., Winter, S. M., Brumback, B., et al. (2012). Psy-chometrics of the Self-Report Safe Driving Behavior Measure for Older Adults. *American Journal of Occupational Therapy, 66,* 233–241. doi: 10.5014/ajot.2012.001834

Classen, S., Winter, S. M., Velozo, C. A., Bédard, M., Lanford, D., Brumback, B., et al. (2010). Item development and validity testing for a Safe Driving Behavior Measure. *American Journal of Occupational Therapy, 64,* 296–305. doi: 10.5014/ajot.64.2.296

Classen, S., Witter, D. P., Lanford, D. N., Okun, M. S., Rodriguez, R. L., Romrell, J., et al. (2011). Usefulness of screening tools for predicting driving performance in people with Parkinson's disease. *American Journal of Occupational Therapy, 65,* 579–588. doi: 10.5014/ajot.2011.001073

Coeckelbergh, T. R. M., Brouwer, W. H., Cornelissen, F. W., van Wolffelaar, P., & Kooijamn, A. C. (2002). The effect of visual field defects on driving performance: A driving simula-tor study. *Archives of Ophthalmology, 120,* 1509–1516.

Colarusso, R. P., & Hammill, D. D. (2003). *Motor-Free Visual Perception Test–3.* Los Angeles: Western Psychological Services.

Collin, C., & Wade, D. (1990). Assessing motor impairment after stroke: A pilot reliability study. *Journal of Neurology, Neurosurgery, and Psychiatry, 53,* 576–579.

Collins, M. J. (1989). The onset of prolonged glare recovery with age. *Ophthalmic and Physiological Optics, 9,* 368–371.

Collins, M. J., & Brown, B. (1989). Glare recovery and age related maculopathy. *Clinical Vision Sciences, 4,* 145–153.

Crizzle, A. M. (2011). *Self-regulatory driving behaviour, perceived abilities and comfort level of older drivers with Parkinson's disease compared to age-matched healthy controls.* Unpublished dissertation, University of Waterloo, Ontario.

Curb, J., & Curb, J. (2002). *Honolulu heart study.* Bethesda, MD: National Heart, Lung, and Blood Institute. Retrieved February 2, 2012, from www.clinicaltrials.gov/ct2/show/study/NCT00005123

Dawson, J. D., Uc, E. Y., Anderson, S. W., Johnson, A. M., & Rizzo, M. (2010). Neuropsychological predictors of driving errors in older adults. *Journal of the American Geriatrics Society, 58,* 1090–1096.

Devos, H., Vandenberghe, W., Nieuwboer, A., Tant, M., Baten, G., & De Weerdt, W. (2007). Predictors of fitness to drive in people with Parkinson disease. *Neurology, 69,* 1434–1441.

Dickerson, A. E. (2011, November). *Fitness to driver appraisals: How does the driving rehabilitation specialist evaluate older adults with dementia?* Paper presented at the Gerontological Society of America Conference, Boston.

Dickerson, A. E., Reistetter, T., Parnell, M., Robinson, S., Stone, K., & Whitley, K. (2008). Standardizing the RT–2S Brake Reaction Time Tester. *Physical and Occupational Therapy in Geriatrics, 27,* 96–106.

Dickerson, A. E., Reistetter, T., Schold Davis, E., & Monohan, M. (2011). Evaluating driving as a valued instrumental activity of daily living. *American Journal of Occupational Therapy, 65,* 64–75. doi: 10.5014/ajot.2011.09052

Dickerson, A. E., Reistetter, T., & Trujillo, L. (2010). Using an IADL assessment to identify older adults who need a behind-the-wheel driving evaluation. *Journal of Applied Gerontology, 29,* 494–506.

Dickerson, A. D., Schold Davis, E., & Carr, D. (2010, September). *From data to decision: What physicians want in a driving rehabilitation report.* Paper presented at the Association of Driving Rehabilitation Specialists Annual Conference, Kansas City, MO.

Dingus, T. A., Neale, V. L., Klauer, S. G., Petersen, A. D., & Carroll, R. J. (2006). The development of a naturalistic data collection system to perform critical incident analysis: An investigation of safety and fatigue issues in long-haul trucking. *Accident Analysis and Prevention, 38,* 1127–1136.

Di Stefano, M., & Macdonald, W. (2003). Assessment of older drivers: Relationships among on-road errors, medical conditions and test outcome. *Journal of Safety Research, 34,* 415–429.

Di Stefano, M., & Macdonald, W. (2005). On-the-road evaluation of driving performance. In J. M. Pellerito (Ed.), *Driver rehabilitation and community principles and practice* (pp. 255–274). St. Louis: Elsevier/Mosby.

Dobbs, A. R. (1997). Evaluating the driving competence of dementia patients. *Alzheimer Disease and Associated Disorders, 11,* 8–12.

Dobbs, A. R. (2005, June). The development of a scientifically based driving assessment and standardization procedures for evaluating medically at-risk drivers. In *Proceedings of the 15th Canadian Multidisciplinary Road Safety Conference* (pp. 1–16). Ottawa, ON: Canadian Association of Road Safety Professionals.

Dobbs, A. R., Heller, R. B., & Schopflocher, D. (1998). A comparative approach to identify unsafe older drivers. *Accident Analysis and Prevention, 30,* 363–370.

Dobbs, B. M. (2005). *Medical conditions and driving: A review of the literature (1960–2000).* Washington, DC: U.S. Department of Transportation.

DriveABLE Assessment Centres. (1998). *DriveABLE competence screen and road test.* Edmonton, Alberta: Author.

Duchek, J., Carr, D., Hunt, L., Roe, C., Xiong, C., Shah, K., et al. (2003). Longitudinal driving performance in early-stage dementia of the Alzheimer type. *Journal of the American Geriatrics Society, 51,* 1342–1347.

Eby, D. W., Molnar, L. J., & Kartje, P. S. (2008). SAFER driving: Self-screening based on health concerns. *The Gerontologist, 47,* 86.

Eby, D. W., Molnar, L. J., & Kartje, P. S. (2009). *Maintaining safe mobility in an aging society.* New York: CRC Press.

Eby, D. W., Molnar, L. J., Shope, J. T., Vivoda, J. M., & Fordyce, T. A. (2003). Improving older driver knowledge and self-awareness through self-assessment: The driving decisions workbook. *Journal of Safety Research, 34,* 371–381.

Eby, D. W., Trombley, D. A., Molnar, L. J., & Shope, J. T. (1998). *The assessment of older drivers' capabilities: A review of the literature* (No. UMTRI-98-24). Ann Arbor: University of Michigan, Transportation Research Institute.

Edlund, W., Gronseth, G., So, Y., & Franklin, G. (2004). *American Academy of Neurology clinical practice guideline process manual.* St. Paul, MN: American Academy of Neurology.

Edwards, J. D., Leonard, K. M., Lunsman, M., Dodson, J., Bradley, S., Myers, C. A., et al. (2008). Acceptability and validity of older driver screening with the DrivingHealth® Inventory. *Accident Analysis and Prevention, 40,* 1157–1163.

Edwards, J. D., Ross, L. A., Wadley, V. G., Clay, O. J., Crowe, M., Roenker, D. L., et al. (2006). The Useful Field of View test: Normative data for older adults. *Archives of Clinical Neuropsychology, 21,* 275–286.

Engum, E. S., Cron, L., Hulse, C. K., Pendergrass, T. M., & Lambert, W. (1988). Cognitive Behavioral Driver's Inventory. *Cognitive Rehabilitation, 6,* 34–50.

Engum, E. S., Lambert, W., & Bracy, O. L. (1990). *Manual for the Cognitive Behavioral Driver's Inventory.* Indianapolis, IN: Psychological Software Service.

Engum, E. S., Lambert, W., & Scott, K. (1990). Criterion-related validity of the Cognitive Behavioral Driver's Inventory: Brain-injured patients versus normal controls. *Cognitive Rehabilitation, 8,* 20–26.

Engum, E. S., Lambert, W., Womac, J., & Pendergrass, T. M. (1988). Norms and decision making rules for the Cognitive Behavioral Driver's Inventory. *Cognitive Rehabilitation, 6,* 12–18.

Fahn, S., Marsden, C. D., Calne, D. B., & Goldstein, M. (Eds.). (1987). *Recent developments in Parkinson's disease, Vol. 2* (pp. 153–163, 293–304). Florham Park, NJ: Macmillan Health Care Information.

Findley, L., Unverzagt, M., Guchu, R., Fabrizio, M., Buckner, J., & Suratt, P. (1995). Vigilance and automobile accidents in patients with sleep apnea or narcolepsy. *Chest, 108,* 619–624.

Fisher, A. G. (2006). *Assessment of Motor and Process Skills: User's manual, Vol. 2.* Fort Collins, CO: Three Star Press.

Folstein, M. F., Folstein, S. E., & McHugh, P. R. (1975). "Mini-Mental State": A practical method for grading the cognitive state of patients for the clinician. *Journal of Psychiatric Research, 12,* 189–198.

Folstein, M. F., Folstein, S. E., White, T., & Messer, M. A. (2010). *Mini-Mental State Exam–2, User's guide* (2nd ed.). Lutz, FL: PAR.

Fowler, F., Jr. (1995). *Improving survey questions: Design and evaluation.* Thousand Oaks, CA: Sage.

Fox, G. K., Bowden, S. C., Bashford, G. M., & Smith, D. S. (1997). Alzheimer's disease and driving: Prediction and assessment of driving performance. *Journal of the American Geriatrics Society, 45,* 949–953.

Galski, T., Bruno, R. L., & Ehle, H. T. (1992). Driving after cerebral damage: A model with implications for evaluation. *American Journal of Occupational Therapy, 46,* 324–332. doi: 10.5014.ajot.46.4.324

Galski, T., Bruno, R. L., & Ehle, H. T. (1993). Prediction of behind-the-wheel driving performance in patients with cerebral brain damage: A discriminant function analysis. *American Journal of Occupational Therapy, 47,* 391–396. doi: 10.5014.ajot.47.5.391

Gauthier, L., Dehaut, F., & Joanette, Y. (1989). The Bells Test: A quantitative and qualitative test for visual neglect. *International Journal of Clinical Neuropsychology, 11,* 49–54.

Golombok, S., Moodley, P., & Lader, M. (1988). Cognitive impairment in long-term benzodiazepine users. *Psychological Medicine, 18,* 365–374.

Grabowski, D. C., & Morrisey, M. A. (2001). The effect of state regulations on motor vehicle fatalities for younger and older drivers: A review and analysis. *Milbank Quarterly, 79,* 517–545.

Green, M. (2000). "How long does it take to stop?" Methodological analysis of driver perception–brake times. *Transportation Human Factors, 2,* 195–216.

Gutman, S. A., & Schonfeld, A. B. (2009). *Screening adult neurologic populations: A step-by-step instruction manual* (2nd ed.). Bethesda, MD: AOTA Press.

Hakamies-Blomqvist, L., Raitanen, T., & O'Neill, D. (2002). Driver ageing does not cause higher accident rates per km. *Transportation Research Part F: Traffic Psychology and Behaviour, 5,* 271–274.

Haughton, R., & Unsworth, C. A. (2008). *Development of the simulated brake test.* Unpublished manual, La Trobe University, Melbourne, Victoria, Australia.

Helm-Estabrooks, N. (2001). *Cognitive Linguistic Quick Test.* San Antonio, TX: Psychological Corporation.

Helm-Estabrooks, N. (2002). Cognition and aphasia: A discussion and a study. *Journal of Communication Disorders, 35,* 171–186.

Hemmelgarn, B., Suissa, S., Huang, A., Boivin, J. F., & Pinard, G. (1997). Benzodiazepine use and the risk of motor vehicle crash in the elderly. *JAMA, 278,* 27–31.

Hettinger, L. J., Berbaum, K. S., Kennedy, R. S., Dunlap, W. P., & Nolan, M. D. (1990). Vection and simulator sickness. *Military Psychology, 2,* 171–181.

Hill, R. D., Storandt, M., & Labarge, E. (1992). Psychometric discrimination of moderate senile dementia of the Alzheimer type. *Archives of Neurology, 49,* 377–380.

Hunt, L. A., Murphy, C. F., Carr, D., Duchek, J. M., Buckles, V., & Morris, J. C. (1997). Reliability of the Washington University Road Test: A performance-based assessment for drivers with dementia of the Alzheimer type. *Archives of Neurology, 54,* 707–712.

Hunter-Zaworski, K. M. (1990) T-intersection simulator performance of drivers with physical limitations. *Transportation Research Record, 1281,* 11–15.

Ishihara, S. (1917). *Tests for Color Blindness.* Tokyo: University of Tokyo.

Ismail, Z., Rajji, T. K., & Shulman, K. J. (2009). Brief cognitive screening instruments: An update. *International Journal of Geriatric Psychiatry, 25,*111–120.

Iverson, D. J., Gronseth, G. S., Reger, M. A., Classen, S., Dubinsky, R. M., & Rizzo, M. (2010). Practice parameter update: Evaluation and management of driving risk in dementia: Report of the Quality Standards Subcommittee of the American Academy of Neurology. *Neurology, 74,* 1316–1324.

Janke, M. (1994). *Age-related disabilities that may impair driving and their assessment* (Pub. No. RSS-94-156). Sacramento: California Department of Motor Vehicles.

Janke, M. K. (2001). Assessing older drivers—Two studies. *Journal of Safety Research, 32,* 43–74.

Janke, M. K., & Eberhard, J. W. (1998). Assessing medically impaired older drivers in a licensing agency setting. *Accident Analysis and Prevention, 30,* 347–361.

Johnson, D. K., Storandt, M., Morris, J. C., & Galving, J. E. (2009). Longitudinal study of the transition from healthy aging to Alzheimer disease. *Archives of Neurology, 66,* 1254–1259.

Juby, A., Tench, S., & Baker, V. (2002). The value of clock drawing in identifying executive cognitive dysfunction in people with a normal Mini-Mental State Examination score. *Canadian Medical Association Journal, 167,* 859–864.

Justiss, M. D., Mann, W. C., Stav, W. B., & Velozo, C. (2006). Development of a behind-the-wheel driving performance assessment for older adults. *Topics in Geriatric Rehabilitation, 22,* 121–128.

Kantor, B., Mauger, L., Richardson, V. E., & Unroe, K. T. (2004). Analysis of an older driver evaluation program. *Journal of the American Geriatrics Society, 52,* 1326–1330.

Katzman, R., Brown, T., Fuld, P., Peck, A., Schechter, R., & Schimmel, H. (1983). Validation of a short orientation-memory-concentration test of cognitive impairment. *American Journal of Psychiatry, 140,* 734–739.

Kay, L., Bundy, A., Clemson, L., & Jolly, N. (2008). Validity and reliability of the on-road driving assessment with senior drivers. *Accident Analysis and Prevention, 40,* 751–759.

Kemper, S., LaBarge, E., Ferraro, R., Cheung, H., & Storandt, M. (1993). On the preservation of syntax in Alzheimer's disease. *Archives of Neurology, 50,* 81–86.

Kennedy, R. S., Fowlkes, J. E., Berbaum, K. S., & Lilienthal, M. G. (1992). Use of a motion sickness history questionnaire for prediction of simulator sickness. *Aviation, Space, and Environmental Medicine, 63,* 588–593.

Kennedy, R. S., Lane, N. E., Berbaum, K. S., & Lilienthal, M. G. (1993). Simulator Sickness Questionnaire: An enhanced method for quantifying simulator sickness. *International Journal of Aviation Psychology, 3,* 203–220.

Kiernan, R. J., Mueller, J., Langston, J. W., & Van Dyke, C. (1987). The Neurobehavioral Cognitive Status Examination: A brief but differentiated approach to cognitive assessment. *Annals of Internal Medicine, 107,* 481–485.

Korner-Bitensky, N., Gelinas, I., Man-Son-Hing, M., & Marshall, S. (2005). Recommendations of the Canadian Consensus Conference on driving evaluation in older drivers. In W. Mann (Ed.), *Community mobility: Driving and transportation alternatives for older persons* (pp. 123–144). Binghamton, NY: Haworth Press.

Korner-Bitensky, N., & Sofer, S. (2009). The DriveABLE competence screen as a predictor of on-road driving in a clinical sample. *Australian Occupational Therapy Journal, 56,* 200–205.

Krishnasamy, C., & Unsworth, C. A. (2011). Normative data, preliminary inter-rater reliability and predictive validity of the Drive Home Maze Test. *Clinical Rehabilitation, 25,* 88–95.

Lajunen, T., & Summala, H. (2003). Can we trust self-reports of driving? Effects of impression management on driver behaviour questionnaire responses. *Transportation Research Part F: Traffic Psychology and Behaviour, 6,* 97–107.

Langford, J., Methorst, R., & Hakamies-Blomqvist, L. (2006). Older drivers do not have a high crash risk—A replication of low mileage bias. *Accident Analysis and Prevention, 38,* 574–578.

Law, M. (1987). Measurement in occupational therapy: Scientific criteria for evaluation. *Canadian Journal of Occupational Therapy, 54,* 133–138.

Leveille, S. G., Buchner, D., Koepsell, T., McCloskey, L., Wolf, M. E., & Wagner, E. H. (1994). Psychoactive medications and injurious motor vehicle collisions involving older drivers. *Epidemiology, 5,* 591–598.

Lezak, M. D., Howieson, D. B., & Loring, D. W. (2004). *Neuropsychological assessment* (4th ed.). New York: Oxford University Press.

Lonie, J. A., Tierney, K. M., & Ebmeier, K. P. (2009). Screening for mild cognitive impairment: A systematic review. *International Journal of Geriatric Psychiatry, 24,* 902–915.

MacGregor, J. M., Freeman, D. H., & Zhang, D. (2001). A traffic sign recognition test can discriminate between older drivers who have and have not had a motor vehicle crash. *Journal of the American Geriatrics Society, 49,* 466–469.

Mallon, K., & Wood, J. M. (2004). Occupational therapy assessment of open-road driving performance: Validity of directed and self-directed navigational instructional components. *American Journal of Occupational Therapy, 58,* 279–286.

Manos, P. J. (1999). Ten-point clock test sensitivity for Alzheimer's disease in patients with MMSE scores greater than 23. *International Journal of Geriatric Psychiatry, 14,* 454–458.

Manos, P. J., & Wu, R. (1994). The ten-point Clock Test: A quick screen and grading method for cognitive impairment in medical and surgical patients. *International Journal of Psychiatry in Medicine, 24,* 229–244.

Margolis, K. L., Kerani, R. P., McGovern, P., Songer, T., Cauley, J. A., & Ensrud, K. E. (2002). Risk factors for motor vehicle crashes in older women. *Journals of Gerontology, Series A: Biological Sciences and Medical Sciences, 57,* 186–191.

Marottoli, R. A., Cooney, L. M., Jr., Wagner, R., Doucette, J., & Tinetti, M. E. (1994). Predictors of automobile crashes and moving violations among elderly drivers. *Annals of Internal Medicine, 121,* 842–846.

Marottoli, R. A., & Drickamer, M. A. (1993). Psychomotor mobility and the elderly driver. *Clinics in Geriatric Medicine, 9,* 403–411.

Marottoli, R. A., & Richardson, E. D. (1998). Confidence in, and self-rating of, driving ability among older drivers. *Accident Analysis and Prevention, 30,* 331–336.

Marottoli, R. A., Richardson, E. D., Stowe, M. H., Miller, E. G., Brass, L. M., Cooney, L. M., Jr., et al. (1998). Development of a test battery to identify older drivers at risk for self-reported adverse driving events. *Journal of the American Geriatrics Society, 46,* 562–568.

Mathias, S., Nayak, U. S., & Isaacs, B. (1986). Balance in elderly patients: The "get-up and go" test. *Archives of Physical Medicine and Rehabilitation, 67,* 387–389.

Matsuda, O., & Saito, M. (2004). Functional competency and cognitive ability in mild Alzheimer's disease: Relationship between ADL assessed by a relative/carer-rated scale and neuropsychological performance. *International Psychogeriatrics, 17,* 275–288.

Mazer, B., Korner-Bitensky, N., & Sofer, S. (1998). Predicting ability to drive after stroke. *Archives of Physical Medicine and Rehabilitation, 79,* 743–750.

Mazer, B. L., Sofer, S., Korner-Bitensky, N., Gelinas, I., Hanley, J., & Wood-Dauphinee, S. (2003). Effectiveness of a visual attention retraining program on the driving performance of clients with stroke. *Archives of Physical Medicine and Rehabilitation, 84,* 541–550.

McCarthy, D. P., & Mann, W. C. (2006). Sensitivity and specificity of the Assessment of Driving-Related Skills older driver screening tool. *Topics in Geriatric Rehabilitation, 22,* 139–152.

McGwin, G., Mays, A., Joiner, W., Decarlo, D. K., McNeal, S., & Owsley, C. (2004). Is glaucoma associated with motor vehicle collision involvement and driving avoidance? *Investigative Ophthalmology and Visual Science, 45,* 3934–3939.

McPherson, K., Ostrow, A., & Shaffron, P. (1989). *Physical fitness and the aging driver.* Washington, DC: AAA Foundation for Traffic Safety.

Michon, J. A. (1985). A critical view of driver behavior models: What do we know, what should we do? In E. L. Evans & R. Schwing (Eds.), *Human behavior and traffic safety* (pp. 485–520). New York: Plenum.

Molnar, F. J., Patel, A., Marshall, S. C., Man-Son-Hing, M., & Wilson, K. G. (2006). Clinical utility of office-based cognitive predictors of fitness to drive in persons with dementia: A systematic review. *Journal of the American Geriatrics Society, 54,* 1809–1824.

Morris, J. C. (1993). The Clinical Dementia Rating (CDR): Current version and scoring rules. *Neurology, 43*, 2412–2414.

Morris, J. C. (1997). Clinical Dementia Rating: A reliable and valid diagnostic and staging measure for dementia of the Alzheimer type. *International Psychogeriatrics, 9*(Suppl. S1), 173–176.

Morris, J. C., Ernesto, C., Schafter, K., Coasts, M., Leon, S., Sano, M., et al. (1997). Clinical Dementia Rating training and reliability in the multicenter studies. *Neurology, 48*, 1508–1510.

Morris, J. C., Heyman, A., Mohs, R. C, Hughes, J. P., Van Belle, G., Fillenbaum, G., et al. (1989). The Consortium to Establish a Registry for Alzheimer Disease (CERAD). *Neurology, 39*, 1159–1165.

Myers, A. M., Paradis, J. A., & Blanchard, R. A. (2008). Conceptualizing and measuring confidence in older drivers: Development of the day and night driving comfort scales. *Archives of Physical Medicine and Rehabilitation, 89*, 630–640.

Myers, R. S., Ball, K. K., Kalina, T. D., Roth, D. L., & Goode, K. T. (2000). Relation of Useful Field of View and other screening tests to on-road driving performance. *Perceptual and Motor Skills, 91*, 279–290.

Myford, C. M., & Wolfe, E. W. (2004). Detecting and measuring rater effects using many-facet Rasch measurement: Part II. *Journal of Applied Measurement, 5*, 189–227.

Mysiw, W., Beegan, J. G., & Gatens, P. F. (1989). Prospective cognitive assessment of stroke patients before inpatient rehabilitation. *American Journal of Physical Medical and Rehabilitation, 68*, 168–171.

Nasreddine, Z. S., Phillips, N. A., Bédirian, V., Charbonneau, S., Whitehead, V., Collin, I., et al. (2005). The Montreal Cognitive Assessment (MoCA): A brief screening tool for mild cognitive impairment. *Journal of the American Geriatrics Society, 53*, 695–699.

National Highway Traffic Safety Administration. (2009a). *Driver fitness medical guidelines* (No. DOT-HS-811-210). Washington, DC: Author.

National Highway Traffic Safety Administration. (2009b). *Identifying behaviors and situations associated with increased crash risk for older drivers* (No. DOT-HS-811-093). Washington, DC: Author.

National Highway Traffic Safety Administration. (2009c). *Traffic safety facts 2009 data* (No. DOT-HS-811-391). Washington, DC: Author.

Nguyen, T., Hau, R., & Bartlett, J. (2000). Driving reaction time before and after anterior cruciate ligament reconstruction. *Knee Surgery, Sports Traumatology, Arthroscopy, 8*, 226–230.

Nourhashemi, F., Ousset, P. J., Gillette-Guyonnet, S., Cantet, C., Andrieu, S., & Vellas, B. (2007). A 2-year follow-up of 233 very mild (CDR 0.5) Alzeimer's disease patients (REAL. FR cohort). *International Journal of Geriatric Psychiatry, 23*, 460–465.

O'Connor, M. G., Kapust, L. R., Lin, B., Hollis, A. M., & Jones, R. N. (2010). The 4Cs (crash history, family concerns, clinical condition, and cognitive functions): A screening tool for the evaluation of the at-risk driver. *Journal of the American Geriatrics Society, 58*, 1104–1108.

Odenheimer, G. L., Beaudet, M., Jette, A. M., Albert, M. S., Grande, L., & Minaker, K. L. (1994). Performance-based driving evaluation of the elderly driver: Safety, reliability, and validity. *Journals of Gerontology, Series A: Biological Sciences and Medical Sciences, 49*, 153–159.

Oswanski, M. F., Sharma, O. P., Raj, S. S., Vassar, L. A., Woods, K. L., Sargent, W. M., et al. (2007). Evaluation of two assessment tools in predicting driving ability of senior drivers. *American Journal of Physical Medicine and Rehabilitation, 86*, 190–199.

Ott, B. R., Heindel, W. C., Whelihan, W. M., Caron, M. D., Piatt, A. L., & DiCarlo, M. A. (2003). Maze test performance and reported driving ability in early dementia. *Journal of Geriatric Psychiatry and Neurology, 16*, 151–155.

Owsley, C., Ball, K., McGwin, G., Sloane, M. E., Roenker, D. L., White, M. F., et al. (1998). Visual processing impairment and risk of motor vehicle crash among older adults. *JAMA, 279*, 1083–1088.

Owsley, C., Ball, K., Sloane, M. E., Roenker, D. L., & Bruni, J. R. (1991). Visual/cognitive correlates of vehicle accidents in older drivers. *Psychology and Aging, 6*, 403–415.

Owsley, C., & McGwin, G. (1999). Vision impairment and driving. *Survey Ophthalmology, 43*, 535–550.

Owsley, C., McGwin, G., Sloane, M. E., Wells, J., Stalvey, B. T., & Gauthreaux, S. (2002). Impact of cataract surgery on motor vehicle crash involvement by older adults. *JAMA, 288*, 841–849.

Owsley, C., Sekuler, R., & Siemsen, D. (1983). Contrast sensitivity throughout adulthood. *Vision Research, 23,* 689–699.

Owsley, C., Stalvey, B. T., Wells, J., & Sloane, M. E. (1999). Older drivers and cataract: Driving habits and crash risk. *Journals of Gerontology, Series A: Biological Sciences and Medical Sciences, 54,* 203–211.

Parashos, S. A., Johnson, M. L., Erickson-Davis, C., & Wielinski, C. L. (2009). Assessing cognition in Parkinson disease: Use of the Cognitive Linguistic Quick Test. *Journal of Geriatric Psychiatry and Neurology, 22,* 228–234.

Park, G., Rosenthal, T. J., Allen, R. W., Cook, M. L., Fiorentino, D., & Viire, E. S. (2004). Simulator sickness results obtained during a novice driver training study. *Proceedings of the 48th Annual Human Factors Ergonomics Society, 2,* 2652–2656

Perryman, K. M., & Fitten, L. J. (1996). Effects of normal aging on the performance of motor-vehicle operational skills. *Journal of Geriatric Psychiatry and Neurology, 9,* 136–141.

Petzold, A., Korner-Bitensky, N., Rochette, A., Teasell, R., Marshall, S., & Perrier, M. J. (2010). Driving poststroke: Problem identification, assessment use, and interventions offered by Canadian occupational therapists. *Topics in Stroke Rehabilitation, 17,* 371–379.

Porteus, S. D. (1959). *The Maze Test and clinical psychology.* Oxford, UK: Pacific Books.

Portney, L., & Watkins, M. P. (2000). *Foundations of clinical research: Applications to practice* (2nd ed.). Upper Saddle River, NJ: Prentice Hall Health.

Posse, C., McCarthy, D. P., & Mann, W. C. (2006). A pilot study of interrater reliability of the Assessment of Driving-Related Skills: Older driver screening tool. *Topics in Geriatric Rehabilitation, 22,* 113–120.

Racette, L., & Casson, E. J. (2005). The impact of visual field loss on driving performance: Evidence from on-road driving assessments. *Optometry and Vision Science, 82,* 668–674.

Ranney, T. A. (1994). Models of driving behavior: A review of their evolution. *Accident Analysis and Prevention, 26,* 733–750.

Ray, W. A., Gurwitz, J., Decker, M. D., & Kennedy, D. L. (1992). Medications and the safety of the older driver: Is there a basis for concern? *Human Factors, 34,* 33–47.

Reason, J. T., & Brand, J. J. (1975). *Motion sickness.* New York: Academic Press.

Reitan, R. M. (1958). Validity of the Trail Making Test as an indicator of organic brain damage. *Perceptual and Motor Skills, 8,* 271–276.

Richardson, E. D., & Marottoli, R. A. (2003). Visual attention and driving behaviors among community-living older persons. *Journals of Gerontology, Series A: Biological Sciences and Medical Sciences, 58,* 832–836.

Rizzo, M., Jermeland, J., & Severson, J. (2002). Instrumented vehicles and driving simulators. *Gerontechnology, 1,* 291–296.

Roenker, D. L., Cissell, G. M., Ball, K. K., Wadley, V. G., & Edwards, J. D. (2003). Speed-of-processing and driving simulator training result in improved driving performance. *Human Factors, 45,* 218–233.

Rosenbloom, S., & Herbel, S. (2009). The safety and mobility patterns of older women. *Public Works Management and Policy, 13,* 338–353.

Salthouse, T. A. (1993). Speed mediation of adult age differences in cognition. *Psychology and Aging, 29,* 722–738.

Schanke, A. K., & Sundet, K. (2000). Comprehensive driving assessment: Neuropsychological testing and on-road evaluation of brain-injured patients. *Scandinavian Journal of Psychology, 41,* 113–121.

Schultheis, M. T., Weisser, V., Ang, J., Elovic, E., Nead, R., Sestito, N., et al. (2010). Examining the relationship between cognition and driving performance in multiple sclerosis. *Archives of Physical Medicine and Rehabilitation, 91,* 465–473.

Shechtman, O., Awadzi, K. D., Classen, S., Lanford, D. N., & Joo, Y. (2010). Validity and critical driving errors of on-road assessment for older drivers. *American Journal of Occupational Therapy, 64,* 242–251. http://dx.doi.org/10.5014/ajot.64.2.242

Shechtman, O., Classen, S., Awadzi, K. D., & Mann, W. (2009). Comparison of driving errors between on-the-road and simulated driving assessment: A validation study. *Traffic Injury Prevention, 10,* 379–385.

Shechtman, O., Classen, S., Stephens, B., Bendixen, R., Belchior, P., Sandhu, B., et al. (2007). The impact of intersection design on simulated driving performance of young and senior adults. *Traffic Injury Prevention, 8,* 78–86.

Shechtman, O., Classen, S., Stephens, B., Davis, E., Awadzi, K. D., & Mann, W. (2008). The impact of roadway intersection design on simulated driving performance of younger and older adults during recovery from a turn. *Advances in Transportation Studies: An International Journal,* 7–20.

Shum, D. H. K., McFarland, K. A., & Bain, J. D. (1990). Construct validity of eight tests of attention: Comparison of normal and closed head injured samples. *Clinical Neuropsychologist, 4,* 151–162.

Shumway-Cook, A., Brauer, S., & Woollacott, M. (2000). Predicting the probability for falls in community-dwelling older adults using the Timed Up & Go test. *Physical Therapy, 80,* 896–903.

Staplin, L., & Dinh-Zarr, T. B. (2006). Promoting rehabilitation of safe driving abilities through computer-based clinical and personal screening techniques. *Topics in Geriatric Rehabilitation, 22,* 129–138.

Staplin, L., Gish, K., & Wagner, E. (2003). MaryPODS revisited: Updated crash analysis and implications for screening program implementation. *Journal of Safety Research, 34,* 389–397.

Staplin, L., & Lococo, K. (2003). *Model driver screening and evaluation program: Guidelines for motor vehicle administrators* (Report No. DOT-HS-809-581). Washington, DC: National Highway Traffic Safety Administration.

Staplin, L., Lococo, K., Gish, K., & Decina, L. (2003). *Model Driver Screening and Evaluation Program final technical report, Vol. 2: Maryland Pilot Older Driver Study* (Report No. DOT-HS-809-583). Washington, DC: National Highway Traffic Safety Administration.

Stav, W. B. (2004). *Driving rehabilitation: A guide for assessment and intervention.* San Antonio, TX: Psychological Corporation.

Stav, W., Justiss, M., Belchior, P., & Lanford, D. (2006). Clinical practice in driving. *Topics in Geriatric Rehabilitation, 22,* 153–161.

Stav, W. B., Justiss, M. D., McCarthy, D. P., Mann, W. C., & Lanford, D. N. (2008). Predictability of clinical assessments for driving performance. *Journal of Safety Research, 39,* 1–7.

Stelmach, G. E., & Nahom, A. (1992). Cognitive-motor abilities of the elderly driver. *Human Factors, 34,* 53–65.

Stephens, B. W., McCarthy, D. P., Marsiske, M., Shechtman, O., Classen, S., Justiss, M., et al. (2005). International Older Driver Consensus Conference on Assessment, Remediation and Counseling for Transportation Alternatives: Summary and recommendations. *Physical and Occupational Therapy in Geriatrics, 23,* 103–121.

Stern, E., & Schold Davis, E. (2006). Driving simulators. In J. M. Pellirito (Ed.), *Driver rehabilitation and community mobility: Principles and practice* (pp. 223–235). St. Louis, MO Elsevier/Mosby.

Stevens, J. A., & Dellinger, A. M. (2002). Motor vehicle and fall related deaths among older Americans 1990–98: Sex, race, and ethnic disparities. *Injury Prevention, 8,* 272–275.

Streiner, D. L., & Norman, G. R. (2003). Devising the items. In *Health measurement scales: A practical guide to their development and use* (pp. 15–27). Oxford, UK: Oxford University Press.

Stutts, J. C. (1998). Do older drivers with visual and cognitive impairments drive less? *Journal of the American Geriatrics Society, 46,* 854–861.

Summala, H. (2000). Brake reaction times and driver behavior analysis. *Transportation Human Factors, 2,* 217–226.

Sundstrom, A. (2005). *Self-assessment of knowledge and abilities* (No. EM No 54). Umeå, Sweden: Umeå University.

Sundstrom, A. (2008). Self-assessment of driving skill—A review from a measurement perspective. *Transportation Research Part F: Traffic Psychology Behavior, 11,* 1–9.

Trobe, J. D., Waller, P. F., Cook-Flannagan, C. A., Teshima, S. M., & Bieliauskas, L. A. (1996). Crashes and violations among drivers with Alzheimer disease. *Archives of Neurology, 53,* 411–416.

Uc, E. Y., Rizzo, M., Anderson, S. W., Shi, Q., & Dawson, J. D. (2005). Driver landmark and traffic sign identification in early Alzheimer's disease. *Journal of Neurology, Neurosurgery, and Psychiatry, 76,* 764–768.

Unsworth, C. A. (2008). *Development of the Right Heel Pivot Test.* Unpublished manual, La Trobe University, Melbourne, Victoria, Australia.

Unsworth, C. A. (2011). *OT–DORA: Occupational Therapy Driver Off-Road Assessment Battery.* Bethesda, MD: AOTA Press.

Unsworth, C. A., Lovell, R. K., Terrington, N. S., & Thomas, S. A. (2005). Review of tests contributing to the occupational therapy off-road driver assessment. *Australian Occupational Therapy Journal, 52,* 57–74.

Unsworth, C. A., Pallant, J. F., Russell, K. J., Germano, C., & Odell, M. (2010). Validation of a test of road law and road craft knowledge with older or functionally impaired drivers. *American Journal of Occupational Therapy, 64*, 306–315. doi: 10.5014. ajot.64.2.306

Uttl, B., & Pilkenton-Taylor, C. (2001). Letter cancellation performance across the adult life span. *Clinical Neuropsychologist, 15*, 521–530.

Waldstein, S. R. (1995). Hypertension and neuropsychological function: A lifespan perspective. *Experimental Aging Research, 21*, 321–352.

Wechsler, D. (1939). *The measurement of adult intelligence.* Baltimore: Williams & Wilkins.

Wechsler, D. (1997). *WAIS–III administration and scoring manual.* San Antonio, TX: Psychological Corporation.

Wechsler, D. (2008). *Weschler Adult Intelligence Scale–Revised.* London: Pearson.

Whelihan, W. M., DiCarlo, M. A., Comparetto, T., & Donovan, M. (2001). *The maze Navigation Test: Normative data and preliminary psychometric properties.* Poster presented at the Annual Meeting of the National Academy of Neuropsychology, Chicago.

Whelihan, W. M., DiCarlo, M. A., & Paul, R. H. (2005). The relationship of neuropsychological functioning to driving competence in older persons with early cognitive decline. *Archives of Clinical Neuropsychology, 20*, 217–228.

Winter, S. M., Classen, S., Bédard, M., Lutz, B., Velozo, C. A., Lanford, D. N., et al. (2011). Focus group findings for the self-report Safe Driving Behavior Measure. *Canadian Journal of Occupational Therapy, 78*, 72–79.

Wong, B. P. H., Woods, R. L., & Peli, E. (2002). Stereoacuity at distance and near. *Optometry and Vision Science, 79*, 771–778.

Zhou, M., & Lyles, R. W. (1997). Self-selection bias in driver performance studies. *Transportation Research Record: Journal of the Transportation Research Board, 1573*, 86–90.

Appendix 9.A. Assessment-Related Resources

- **Driving Decisions Workbook:** go to http://deepblue.lib.umich.edu/ bitstream/2027.42/1321/2/94.135.0001.001.pdf for a PDF of the full workbook.
- **Dementia Rating Scale:** see www.alz.washington.edu/NONMEMBER/cdr2. html for a description
- **National Highway Traffic and Safety Administration:** a detailed literature review on medical conditions and driving performance is found at www.nhtsa.gov/people/injury/research/MedicalusCondition_Driving/ Medical%20Cond%20809%20690-8-04_Medical%20Cond%20809%20 690-8-04.pdf
- **Roadwise Review:** http://www.roadwisereview.com
- **Driving Habits Questionnaire:** www.eyes.uab.edu/tools/DHQ.pdf
- **Optec Functional Vision Analyzer:** www.stereooptical.com
- **Glare recovery:** sdhawan.com/ophthalmology/glare.html
- **Clock drawing:** http://www.psychiatrictimes.com/cognitive-impairment/ content/article/10168/54386
- **Trail Making Tests A and B:** www.tbi-impact.org/cde/mod_templates/ 12_F_08_TMT.pdf
- **Cognistat exam:** www.cognistat.com
- **Driving Health Inventory:** www.drivinghealth.com
- **Drivers 65+ Self-Rating Form:** http://www.aaafoundation.org/quizzes/ index.cfm?button-driver55

CHAPTER 10

Use of Adaptive Equipment to Compensate for Impairments in Motor Performance Skills and Client Factors

Anne Hegberg, MS, OTR/L, CDRS

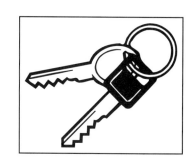

Learning Objectives

At the completion of this chapter, readers will be able to

- Appreciate the range of adaptive equipment and vehicle modification options available, from simple (mechanical) to complex (high tech);
- Differentiate equipment that is appropriate for general occupational therapists to explore with clients from the more complex equipment and modifications (directly involving the control of a moving vehicle) that require the skill and expertise of a driver rehabilitation specialist;
- Identify key elements to consider as criteria to justify referral to a driver rehabilitation specialist; and
- Identify the roles and importance of the multidisciplinary team when exploring and prescribing adaptive equipment or vehicle modifications.

Introduction

Occupational therapists in a generalist setting (e.g., schools, rehabilitation centers, continuous care communities) may be the first professionals to identify clients who could benefit from driver rehabilitation services. Considering the limited number of driving programs in each state and the locations of programs in primarily urban areas, many individuals may never realize their potential as drivers or benefit from vehicle modifications or adaptive equipment (e.g., easing the burden associated with transportation, including loading a scooter, transferring from wheelchair to passenger seat, applying safety restraints). If general-practice occupational therapists are unaware of what driver rehabilitation programs offer, they can appropriately refer their clients to occupational therapy specialists.

Key Words

- **adaptive equipment**
- **driver rehabilitation**
- **driver–vehicle fit**
- **driving controls**
- **mobility device storage**
- **predrive**
- **primary driving controls**
- **secondary driving controls**
- **securement**
- **teritiary driving controls**
- **transfer seat**
- **vehicle entry**
- **wheelchair accessibility**

Practitioner's Reflection 10.1. Joe

Joe is a 34-year-old with a spinal cord injury resulting in paraplegia. He has completed his rehabilitation elsewhere and is referred for a driver evaluation. Joe arrives at the evaluation in his ultra-lightweight, rigid-frame wheelchair. Because of his size and decreased trunk balance, he requires assistance to transfer and is planning to drive from his wheelchair. The design of the wheelchair (rigid frame) and the low back are not compatible with driving for two reasons: First, there is no power lock-down for the wheelchair, and second, the low back does not provide adequate support for the dynamics of driving. Joe's insurance paid for the wheelchair, as prescribed during his inpatient rehabilitation, and he is not eligible for another wheelchair for 5 years. His hospitalization, rehabilitation, and home modifications have been a major financial burden, and he cannot afford to purchase a different wheelchair.

His church is holding a fundraiser for him to modify his bathroom. Now Joe has to decide between a modified bathroom and a different wheelchair so that he can drive. There would be no decision necessary if the therapist prescribing the wheelchair had taken into account, early on, the instrumental activity of daily living of driving by simply involving the consultation of a driver rehabilitation specialist.

— *Anne Hegberg, MS, OTR/L, CDRS*

Of equal concern is that many clients or caregivers discover adaptations through myriad channels, such as the Internet, forgoing the medical expertise and training essential to optimizing safety and success. For example, hand controls purchased from the Internet and attached to a steering column with Velcro® pose a safety concern for the client, the client's family, and the public. The goal of this chapter is to build a beginning knowledge base about the physical factors in driving and how the appropriate equipment can make driving possible.

Occupational therapists are specialists in instrumental activities of daily living (IADLs). They should have a basic knowledge of community mobility, driving, and adaptive driving equipment and the potential they offer for increased independence, safety, and efficiency. Decisions made early in the rehabilitation process, such as the type or model of wheelchair prescribed, can affect the client's ability, affordability to drive, and access to community mobility for years to come (see Practitioner's Reflection 10.1).

This chapter provides an overview of the range of adaptive equipment available to compensate for physical impairments. **Table 10.1** includes **adaptive equipment resources**, which is also provided on the accompanying flash drive to assist with the clinical reasoning process in determining referrals for evaluation and training on equipment.

History of Adaptive Driving Equipment

Adaptive driving equipment has been in existence almost since the invention of motor vehicles. An early account of adaptive driving equipment dates back to 1928, when Judge Quentin Corley lost both hands in a train accident. His goal of independent community mobility prompted him to adapt his vehicle with an early version of an amputee steering ring (Pellerito, 2006).

Like Judge Corley, individuals who were invested in the industry of adapting vehicles either had a physical challenge themselves or had a family member with an impairment that required an adaptation. Because there were no commercially available adaptations, equipment was homemade or, probably more accurate, "farm-made." Many manufacturers started by working out of their own garages

Table 10.1. Adaptive Equipment Resources

Organization	Source	Information Available
Association for Driver Rehabilitation Specialists	www.aded.net	• Directory of certified driver rehabilitation specialists • Diagnosis-specific fact sheets, including common equipment needs
CarFit	www.car-fit.org	• AAA, AOTA, and AARP program; facts and event locations
National Highway Traffic Safety Administration	www.nhtsa.dot.gov	• Booklet, *Adapting Motor Vehicles for Older Drivers* • Laws and regulations for vehicle adaptations
National Mobility Equipment Dealers Association	www.nmeda.org	• Information for consumers and professionals, *Consumer Reference Guide to Purchasing Adaptive Vehicles and Equipment* • Membership directory
Rehabilitation Engineering Research Center on Wheelchair Transportation Safety	www.rercwts.org	• List of crash-tested wheelchairs • Education and research on wheelchair transport, including the "Ride Safe" brochure • WC-19 information

Company	Contact	Equipment (Noninclusive)
Active Forever	www.activeforever.com	Panoramic rearview mirror, swivel seat, cushions, door-frame strap
Adapted Shifter	www.adaptedshifter.com	Adaptation for console shifter handle
Autobarn	www.autobarn.net	Seat and back cushions, arm rests, seat-belt pads
AutoSport Catalog	www.autosportcatalog.com	Back and seat cushion, mirrors, seat-belt covers
B&D Independence	www.bdindependence.com	Transfer seat bases for drivers and passengers
BraunAbility	www.braunability.com	Wheelchair-accessible minivans; wheelchair platform lifts for vans
Bruno	www.bruno.com	Wheelchair and seat lifts; scooter and wheelchair storage devices
Crescent Industries	www.crescentindustries.com	Remotes for secondary controls
Drivemaster	www.drive-master.com	Modified steering and braking systems, hand controls, pedal extensions
Driving Systems, Inc. (Menox)	www.drivingsystems.com	Wide variety of mirrors, hand controls, high-tech driving system
Dynamic Living	www.dynamic-living.com	Swivel seats, mirrors, handybar, key holders, seat-belt aids, cushions
Electronic Mobility Controls	www.emc-digi.com	High-tech driving systems

(Continued)

Table 10.1. Adaptive Equipment Resources *(cont.)*

Company	Contact	Equipment (Noninclusive)
EZ Lock	www.ezlock.net	Wheelchair docking system
GoShichi	www.goshichi.com	Wheelchair-accessible pickup truck
Handybar	www.handybar.com	Assistance in entering and exiting a car
Harmar	www.harmarmobility.com	Wheelchair and scooter lifts and hoists
Howell Ventures	www.suregrip-hvl.com	Hand controls, steering devices, left gas pedal, pedal blocks
International Medical Equipment Company	www.imec-online.com	Upper-torso positioning belts
Mobility Products and Design (Veigel)	www.mobilityproductsdesign.com	Hand controls, steering devices, left gas pedal, pedal blocks
MPS Corporation	www.mps-handcontrols.com	Hand controls, steering devices, left gas pedal, pedal blocks
NorCal	www.norcalmobility.com/vehicle-selection-101	Mobility dealer: chart of accessible minivan dimensions
Patterson Medical	www.pattersonmedical.com	Key holders, seat-belt aids
Permobil	www.permobilus.com	Power wheelchairs and docking systems
Sure-Lok, Q'Straint	www.sure-lok.com www.qstraint.com	Manual wheelchair securement and docking systems
Vantage Mobility International	www.vantagemobility.com	Wheelchair-accessible minivans; wheelchair platform lifts for vans

Note. AOTA = American Occupational Therapy Association.

or machine shops. The commercial manufacturing of adaptive driving equipment began in the 1950s (Stav, Hunt, & Arbesman, 2006). These early manufacturers, many still involved in the industry today, designed components that predated regulations and standards.

The industry has matured and grown tremendously over the years, imposing an emerging matrix of regulations and standards. Some standards are federal, such as disconnection of an air bag for an individual who must be positioned close to the steering wheel to control the vehicle. Other guidelines are associated with the professional organizations involved in the industry, for example, the use of a pedal guard for driving with hand controls. Some states or third-party payers have imposed requirements on drivers, such as requiring the completion of a driver evaluation when adaptive driving equipment is necessary. Finally, some practices are regional, based on the expert judgment of the local mobility dealer or available evaluator, such as mobility dealers who will not install left-foot accelerator pedals because of their concerns for risk and liability.

Multidisciplinary Team: Interconnection of Team in Driver Rehabilitation

Client: A Person Requiring Community Mobility

Every client evaluated by an occupational therapist should have his or her community mobility skills screened. Whether driving is addressed depends on the unique characteristics of the client, but everyone needs to be safe when moving about the community. Typically, occupational therapists think of the *client* as a person who has a disability that affects his or her ability to safely operate a motor vehicle. These clients can range in age from the mid-teens to older adults. Impairments vary greatly. The diagnosis may be a long-standing, congenital condition such as cerebral palsy (CP), or it may be an acquired impairment such as stroke, traumatic brain injury (TBI), or Parkinson's disease (PD).

In some cases, the client is the caregiver or family member of a person with disability who requires assistance for safe transport of that person. For example, what if a parent cannot physically secure a child in a standard, commercially available car seat because he or she has the use of only one hand after a stroke? What about children with physical attributes that preclude the use of a standard car seat? When a client, particularly a child, is in a wheelchair, how can the caregiver ensure that the wheelchair is secured in a vehicle? As developmentally appropriate, how will the child be able to independently move about the community to engage with friends? As the child grows, the parent may continue to require an occupational therapist to assist with safely accessing the community.

A teenager getting a wheelchair before the age of driving will likely use that same wheelchair to determine whether and when he or she can drive. Are driving needs considered when the type of wheelchair is determined? If the person will not be a driver, access to the community through private or public transportation is an area that needs to be addressed. Caregivers cannot afford to be injured while attempting to physically transfer their child, spouse, or parent into a vehicle. It is important for the occupational therapist to have resources available to educate and assist with transfers and safe transportation for all involved in the process.

Evaluator: Evaluating the Driver–Vehicle Fit

In regard to adaptive equipment, the *evaluator* is the person who recommends or prescribes adaptive equipment for the client requiring community mobility. This role varies greatly on the basis of many factors, including, but not limited to, the payer source, availability of a certified driver rehabilitation specialist (CDRS), availability of a knowledgeable occupational therapy generalist, the complexity of the client's needs, and the individual mobility dealer.

Typically, the driving evaluator is an occupational therapist, a driver educator, or a professional with specialized education in driver rehabilitation. The driver rehabilitation specialist (DRS) with a medical background, typically in occupational therapy, evaluates the client in the areas of vision, cognition, and motor function as related to driving and community mobility. Depending on the structure of the given program and the certification of the evaluator, the DRS may work independently or in partnership with a generalist. Typically, the DRS conducts the clinical portion and the on-road evaluation to make a recommendation based on the information from both portions. In some settings, the generalist occupational therapist will evaluate the client's community mobility–related skills, such as accessing public transportation, and will then provide a referral to a DRS who can explore the appropriate adaptive equipment.

As a generalist, it is critical to know about the driving program to which you might refer clients. Not all programs address all aspects of driver rehabilitation. On the basis of staff training, state regulations, and available adaptive equipment, driver rehabilitation programs may address older adults without adaptations, clients with low vision, or novice drivers and teenagers, or they may have a fully adapted van. Contacting and visiting local driver rehabilitation programs will inform you of their assets and capabilities.

In the best of circumstances, a mobility dealer works in conjunction with the CDRS or occupational therapist to design the best equipment to fit the needs of the client. However, some mobility dealers who do not have access to an occupational therapist or DRS may base vehicle adaptation decisions on their own knowledge and expertise. Mobility dealers are well versed in vehicles and available adaptations, but they may not be knowledgeable about the medical conditions underlying the current disability.

Statically (when the vehicle is not in motion), the client may operate adaptive equipment without difficulty. However, when the vehicle is traveling at various speeds, navigating turns, accelerating, or stopping, the dynamics of motion raise a host of issues. For example, consider the client with poor trunk control trying to maintain sitting balance on a turn without the proper chest restraint. It is the CDRS, not the mobility dealer, who takes the client on road to assess the effect of dynamic forces when the vehicle is in motion.

Manufacturers: Vehicles for Individuals With Disabilities

The **National Mobility Equipment Dealers Association (NMEDA)** differentiates manufacturers into two categories: (1) the original equipment manufacturers (OEMs) and (2) the equipment manufacturers (see Chapter 3 for a description of NMEDA). *OEMs* are the manufacturers of the original vehicle, such as Ford, Toyota, or GM. Each OEM has a mobility division dedicated to understanding and addressing the needs of drivers with disabilities. *Equipment manufacturers* are referred to as second-stage manufacturers, alterers, or modifiers. These companies either manufacture components that bolt onto an OEM vehicle, such as hand controls, or perform substantial structural and mechanical alterations to the vehicle (e.g., raising the vehicle's roof or lowering the vehicle floor to accommodate a wheelchair and lift).

Mobility dealers or *retailers* are the companies that provide the local source for adaptive equipment. They either sell components and modifications for an existing vehicle or sell a complete, fully modified vehicle. Mobility dealers are staffed by the representatives and distributors of products from the second-stage manufacturers and equipment manufacturers and employ mobility consultants and technicians who are knowledgeable about vehicles and adaptive equipment. The industry changes quickly, and developing a strong working relationship with the local mobility dealer is invaluable. The mobility dealer can provide information regarding vehicle compatibility with specific equipment. The dealer may offer working displays of equipment or may be able to bring a demonstration vehicle to a client. An important caveat is that if a mobility dealer stocks only a certain manufacturer's product, the dealer may not have all the possible options, and another product might work better for an individual client.

Physical Assessment for Mobility

All occupational therapy evaluations should begin with the client's occupational profile, followed by an analysis of occupational performance related to motor, cognitive, and visual skills. The clinical evaluation results guide the occupational therapist to identify strengths, weaknesses, and the potential to drive. When motor skills are affected, adaptive equipment may be the solution. With experience and knowledge, the therapist formulates an idea of what, if any, adaptive equipment may be indicated. Regardless of whether the client is a caregiver or a person with a disability, as with any recommended activity of daily living (ADL) or IADL equipment, occupational therapists in the generalist setting should have samples of aids that may assist their clients, including aids to assist with ingress, egress, securement, and positioning.

Depending on the diagnosis or need, a referral to an occupational therapy DRS may be warranted. For example, if a client has a spinal cord injury (SCI) and is unable to move his or her foot from the gas to the brake, hand controls of some type will be required, along with training for use. However, because driving is more than the motor and praxis performance skills that can be easily observed and measured, a DRS's decisions and recommendations are often based on an interplay of complex factors. For instance, consider a client with multiple sclerosis (MS) who has difficulty stopping his or her vehicle. The specialist must determine whether this difficulty is related to impairments in cognition, vision, or motor function, or a combination of all three, and, more importantly, determine whether there is a way to compensate.

A host of adaptive equipment options have been designed to compensate for physical impairments. Thus, in addition to the visual and cognitive assessments, the DRS evaluates the client's physical abilities before considering adaptive equipment possibilities. This section reviews some specific guidelines for selecting what physical assessments should be done.

Clearly, active range of motion (ROM), strength, and coordination are important component skills for the driving task. For some impairments, formal manual muscle testing of individual or groups of muscles may be necessary. For other impairments, a functional motor evaluation is sufficient. For example, a client with an SCI requires a more comprehensive physical evaluation than a person with dementia.

The key idea is that *functional* ability is necessary for the driving task. Is the client able to fully turn his or her head to the left and right? Neck rotation is necessary to visually scan intersections, turn when reversing, and look over either

In addition to the visual and cognitive assessments, the DRS evaluates the client's physical abilities before considering adaptive equipment possibilities.

shoulder when performing a blind-spot check during a lane change. Does the client have full range and strength of both shoulders and elbows for turning the steering wheel unassisted?

Grasp and motor coordination of both hands need to be assessed. Hand function is important not only for gripping the steering wheel but also for such motor tasks as inserting and turning the key in the ignition, adjusting mirrors, and regulating the heating and air conditioning controls. The lower extremities are used for ambulation to and from the vehicle and transferring and operation of foot controls, including the accelerator and brake pedals as well as the parking brake in some vehicles. To operate the pedals without adaptation, ankle plantar flexion and dorsiflexion of the right leg are needed. In addition to strength and range, the quality of movement needs to be examined. The presence of associated movements, tremors, or spasms may negatively affect safe vehicle control. Assessment of a client with CP always should include observation for an exaggerated startle reaction.

Sensation and proprioception, particularly of the lower extremities, are critical to evaluate. The client must be able to accurately move his or her foot from the gas to the brake without looking at the feet. Sensation is also important in modulating the amount of pressure on the accelerator and brake pedals. Clients with long-term diabetes either as a primary or a secondary diagnosis often lack full sensation in the lower extremities.

Finally, assessment of balance, both sitting and standing, is important. When seated in a vehicle, the client must have the ability to maintain his or her upright posture at various speeds and with quick turns. Standing balance and the ability to safely use one's mobility device (e.g., cane, walker, wheelchair) can affect the decision on the type of vehicle as well as adaptive driving equipment needed.

Adaptive Equipment and Vehicles

As with all kinds of adaptive equipment, there is a range from the simple to the complex, or *high tech*. As in any area of medicine where there is a range of service, it is critically important that occupational therapists design their program with pathways for referral as needed. The generalist needs to clearly understand the legal liability and ethical responsibility associated with the IADL of community mobility. As a general rule, generalists can demonstrate and recommend equipment that does not interfere with the operation of a moving vehicle. It is important to understand that even a simple aid can affect the interface between driver and vehicle. Instruments and controls are specifically positioned in a vehicle for a reason. Thus, occupational therapists should consider the potential effect of any recommended piece of equipment or aid. For example, an added seat cushion that allows the client to have better visibility and positioning may be good. However, in a crash, if the cushion is too soft or not properly secured, the client could be displaced by the hips sliding forward under the gap created between the lap belt and the cushion. This is called *submarining* under the lap belt, and it places a driver or passenger at a greater risk of injury.

No driver rehabilitation program has all the equipment available on the market, but occupational therapists should use their knowledge about what is available to refer clients elsewhere as necessary. At the most basic level, the **CarFit®** program has increasingly recognized the importance of awareness by generalists and the public as to the challenges facing many drivers as they or their loved ones age with medical conditions. Occupational therapists who are aware of the simple aids that can assist the client or caregiver as driver or passenger make a positive contribution to the client's community mobility.

Vehicle Choice

Many clients may already have access to a vehicle when they begin considering their return to driving. The client, vehicle, adaptive equipment, and mobility device or devices must all balance. If the client is planning to purchase or replace a vehicle, an early initial consultation with a DRS is recommended to ensure that the vehicle purchased is appropriate for the client's needs. Sedans, minivans, trucks, and sport utility vehicles all have pros and cons, and there is no simple list. Not only does the type of vehicle matter, but the year, model, and condition of the vehicle also can affect the success of the purchase.

Vehicle Entry

The first step toward community mobility is entering and exiting a vehicle safely. A simple device such as the "handybar" mobility handle provides added stability for either a driver or a passenger when entering or exiting a vehicle (see Figure 10.1). The handybar is portable and compatible with most vehicles. It attaches to the door

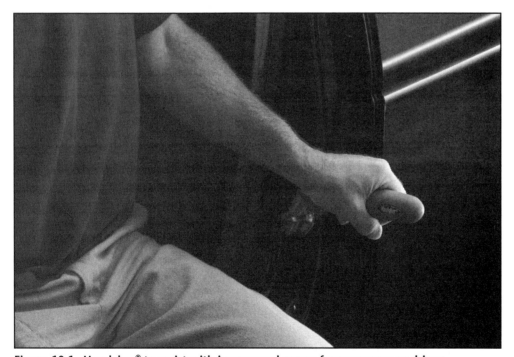

Figure 10.1. Handybar® to assist with ingress and egress for passenger or driver.
Note. Used with permission of Avenue Innovations, Inc., Sidney, British Columbia.

striker (the steel loop that the door latches into when closed). The user pushes down on the bar when moving from sit to stand. A leg lifter may be used for the client who has difficulty positioning his or her lower extremity in the vehicle. Beyond the simple mechanical aids, there are many products to assist with transfers as well as with wheelchair storage. Available for both drivers and passengers, manual and power seat lifts will lift a client from wheelchair level to vehicle seat level (Figures 10.2 and 10.3). These devices also are beneficial to caregivers to decrease the physical demands of transferring a person in and out of the vehicle. There are specific application considerations including, but not limited to, the vehicle, the client's weight, and the client's functioning.

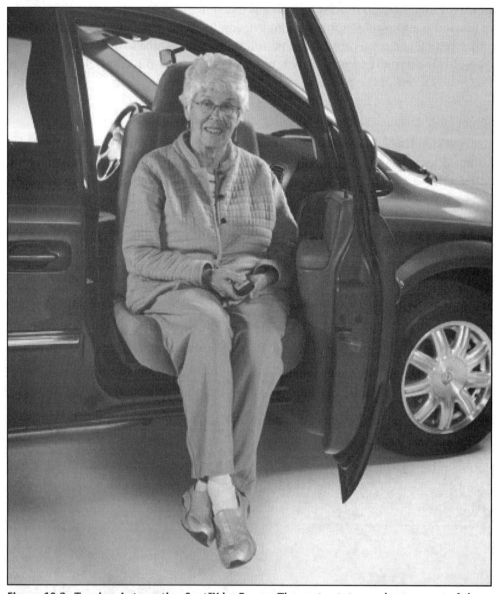

Figure 10.2. Turning Automotive Seat™ by Bruno. The seat rotates and comes out of the vehicle for easier transfer.

Note. Used with permission of Bruno Independent Living Aids, Oconomowoc, WI.

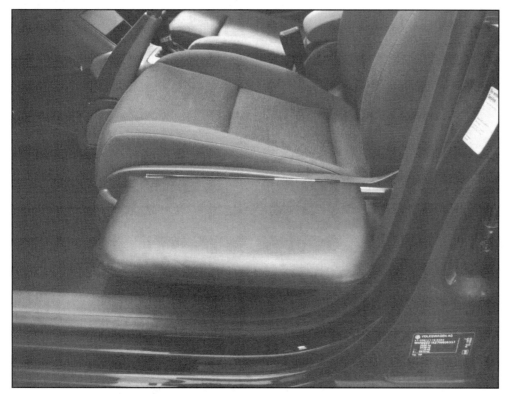

Figure 10.3. Driver-side transfer seat by Veigel bridges the gap between wheelchair and driver's seat.

Note. Used with permission of Mobility Products and Design, Shelby Township, MI.

Mobility Device Storage

Once the client is safely in the vehicle, mobility device storage is next. Is the client able to fold or break down his or her wheelchair, scooter, or walker so that it fits in the vehicle? If it is stored in the trunk or rear hatch, is the person able to independently ambulate to the driver seat? Consider the weather conditions of the area, including snow, ice, or extreme heat. Additionally, consider the ability to perform the action throughout and at the end of the day. For example, a client with MS may be able to ambulate from the trunk to the driver seat in the morning but not on a hot afternoon after a day of work. The physical demands of operating lifts and hoists vary (Figures 10.4 and 10.5). In some cases, the client must have the balance to stand and guide the wheelchair or scooter into the back of the vehicle. Other lifts require the person to roll the scooter or wheelchair onto a platform where it is then lifted and stowed.

A manual wheelchair may be appropriately stored in a sedan. The ability of the client to fold, dismantle, or break down the wheelchair can be a limiting factor. The size and weight of the wheelchair, the balance of the client reaching out of the vehicle to pull the wheelchair into the vehicle, and the room within the vehicle must be considered. How many times per day will the client need to perform the activity? What are the weather conditions? What is the client's stamina? A client who drives as part of his or her job may need to repeat the procedure many times throughout

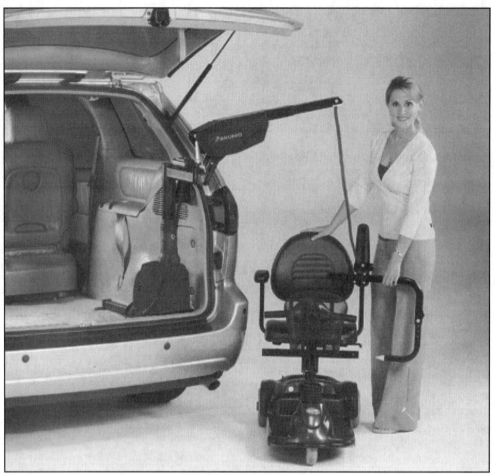

Figure 10.4. Curb-Sider® hoist for unoccupied wheelchair or scooter.
Note. Used with permission of Bruno Independent Living Aids, Oconomowoc, WI.

the day. Other clients drive to work and are in one location for the duration of the day. Wear and tear on shoulders and elbows as well as time needed for the process should be taken into account.

Wheelchair-Accessible Vehicles

A variety of vehicles are available that are accessible and permit a client to remain in a wheelchair. A full-sized van with wheelchair lift was the only option for many years. Often full-sized vans are still used by schools and public transportation sources. However, because of the smaller size, gas mileage, and user-friendliness of minivans, they are vastly more popular for personal transportation than the full-sized van. The great advantage of an accessible van or minivan is that the client can transfer onto a seat or secure a wheelchair within the safety and comfort of the vehicle (Figures 10.6 and 10.7). (See **Appendix 10.A** for a **Wheelchair information form**.)

The modification of an OEM minivan is performed by a second-stage manufacturer (e.g., BraunAbility, Winamac, IN; Vantage Mobility International, Phoenix, AZ), and then the vehicle is sent to the local mobility dealer. The minivan may be new or used, but there are strict parameters regarding year, make, model, and mileage that each manufacturer allows. When modifying the minivan, the floor is lowered 10–14 in., depending

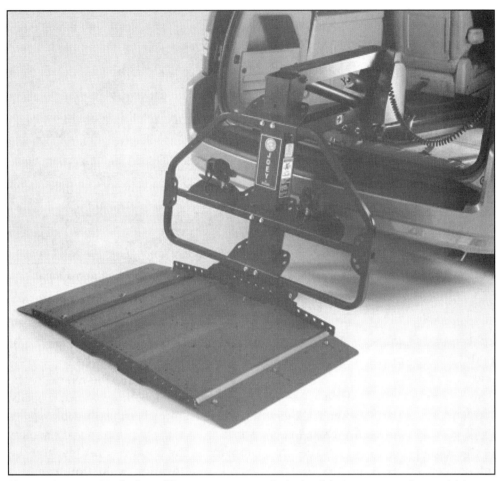

Figure 10.5. Joey™ platform lift to store unoccupied wheelchair or scooter into vehicle.
Note. Used with permission of Bruno Independent Living Aids, Oconomowoc, WI.

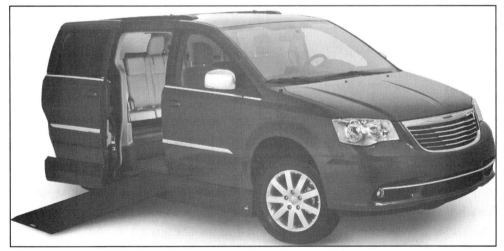

Figure 10.6. Chrysler wheelchair-accessible, lowered-floor minivan by Vantage Mobility International.
Note. Used with permission of Vantage Mobility International, Phoenix, AZ.

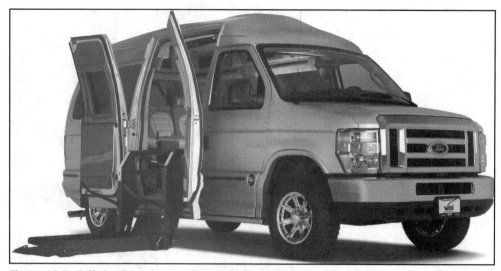

Figure 10.7. Full-sized Ford van with wheelchair lift by Vantage Mobility International.
Note. Used with permission of Vantage Mobility International, Phoenix, AZ.

on the vehicle and the modification. A ramp is installed either on the side or at the rear of the vehicle. An electromechanical kneeling system that further lowers the vehicle and reduces the angle of the ramp is added to allow easier access into the vehicle for the wheelchair user. When the client presses a button on a key fob, the power door opens, the van "kneels down" (lower to the ground), and the ramp automatically deploys.

The make, model, and year of the minivan, as well as the preferences and resources of the second-stage modifier, affect the ramp angle, the doorway opening, and the interior height. (See **Appendix 10.B** for a **vehicle modification evaluation form**.) To compare various available minivan conversions (the changes made to the vehicle itself by a credentialed modifier), see the **NorCal Web site (www.norcalmobility.com/vehicle-selection-101/minivan-estimated-specifications)**.

Entering and exiting by means of a ramp, especially when using a manual wheelchair, can be difficult. Power-assist wheels make it easier for the manual wheelchair user although they add weight and width to the wheelchair. Adding grade aids, also called *hill climbers,* prevents the wheelchair from rolling down the ramp as the client changes hand position when ascending the ramp. Space to maneuver within any vehicle is limited. The client should have the opportunity to try several different vehicles to determine which would best meet his or her needs as well as the needs of others using the vehicle.

Because not everyone wants to drive a minivan (e.g., a 20-year-old man with an SCI), the industry is constantly looking at adapting nontraditional vehicles for wheelchair users such as the Honda Element, the Toyota Scion, and pickup trucks (Figure 10.8). These vehicles also have limitations that need to be considered before purchase. A major consideration is how the client fits in the vehicle, but also the vehicle's compatibility with the adaptive equipment is recommended. Not all modifications are created equal. Many standards and regulations are important for client safety. Before the purchase of any vehicle, it is important to consult with a local mobility dealer. To find a local dealer and as a resource for standards, NMEDA is valuable for both consumers and professionals.

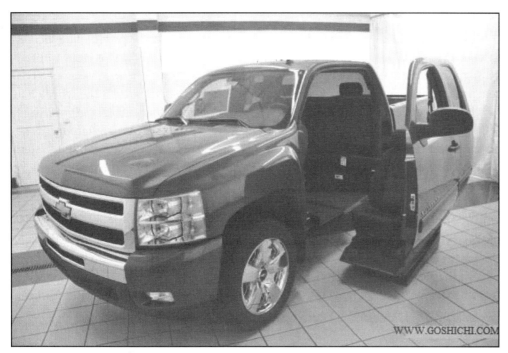

Figure 10.8. GoShichi® wheelchair-accessible pickup truck.
Note. Used with permission of GoShichi 4×4, Fort Wayne, IN.

A distinction needs to be made between a vehicle that will only be used for transportation in the community and one that a client will be driving. Transport vehicles are often less expensive, as they may not have such features as power door openers, kneel systems, or an automatic ramp or fully automatic lift. Unfortunately, often a transporter cannot be converted to a vehicle for a driver with a disability. Factors affecting the selection and ultimate approval of a particular vehicle as viable for adaptation include the adaptive driving equipment required; the year, make, and model of the vehicle; and the funding source's requirements. Most funding sources have requirements as to the age and condition of a vehicle appropriate to warrant the expense of adaptation. It does not make sense to add thousands of dollars of adaptive equipment to a vehicle that will not be reliable and safe for the client. Therefore, occupational therapy generalists should know that if a client has the *potential* to be a driver in the future, it is important to make the client and family members aware of the implications of vehicle choice and to facilitate consultation with a DRS *before* the client's or family's purchase of any vehicle (see Case Example 10.1).

> **Case Example 10.1. Client With Muscular Dystrophy**
> **The client is a 25-year-old with muscular dystrophy** using a power wheelchair. The family was told to purchase a van and then to pursue a driver evaluation. The extended family assisted and pooled their resources and purchased what they could afford: a 4-year-old GM Uplander minivan with low mileage. Unfortunately, because GM has since discontinued the Uplander, no manufacturer will make it wheelchair accessible by lowering the floor and installing a ramp. The family is back to square one.

Securement

It is important that all mobility devices (e.g., wheelchair, scooter, walker) be secured in a vehicle. During a sudden stop or collision, the device could become a potentially hazardous object moving within the vehicle. Additionally, the device needs to remain accessible for the client to retrieve at his or her destination. If the wheelchair or walker is out of the client's reach, that person could be trapped in the vehicle.

A wheelchair tie-down occupant restraint system (WTORS), also referred to as *tie-downs, restraints,* or *securement system,* is a manual or four-point securement system that attaches four points of the wheelchair frame to four points on the vehicle floor with webbed straps (Figure 10.9). The securement system secures the wheelchair only. When the wheelchair is occupied, the client also needs to be secured with a crash-worthy shoulder and lap belt. Attachment points to the wheelchair and positioning of the shoulder and lap belt are critical for safe transport. It is beyond the scope of this chapter to go into detail on the proper use of a WOTRS; for more information, refer to the **Rehabilitation Engineering Research Center on Wheelchair Transportation Safety.** Its Web site (www.rercwts.org) has educational information for both the consumer and the professional, including information on WC19, a voluntary industry standard regarding the use of a wheelchair as a seat in a motor vehicle.

If the client is to drive while seated in a wheelchair, an automatic securement or docking system will be necessary. The most common systems have a specific bracket mounted to the wheelchair frame with a docking pin underneath

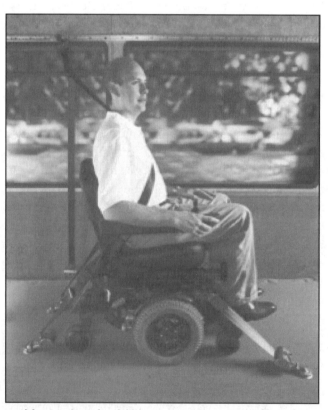

Figure 10.9. Manual four-point wheelchair securement system.

Note. Used with permission of Q'Straint, Fort Lauderdale, FL.

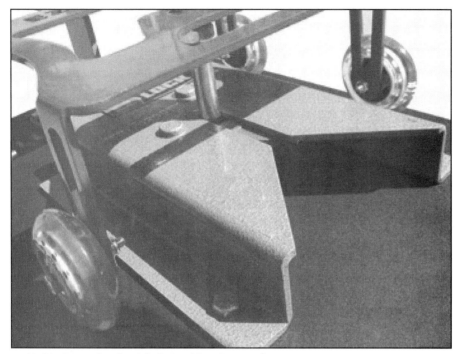

Figure 10.10. EZ Lock Wheelchair Docking System.®

Note. Used with permission of EZ Lock, Inc., Baton Rouge, LA.

(Figure 10.10). The wheelchair user guides the docking pin into a floor-mounted receptacle that automatically latches when the pin is correctly positioned. Docking systems have auditory and visual alarms if the wheelchair is not secured correctly.

It is important to note that the docking systems do not work with all wheelchairs. To determine wheelchair compatibility, check the bracket charts of docking systems with manufacturers such as EZ Lock© (Baton Rouge, LA) or Q'Straint™ (Fort Lauderdale, FL). The bracket and the pin remain on the wheelchair. This does add weight (6–10 lb.) and prevents folding of the manual wheelchair. As the lowest point on the wheelchair, the protruding pin may interfere with mobility on rough terrain and over some surfaces such as curbs and door thresholds. Permobil® (Lebanon, TN) is the first wheelchair company to offer a docking pin that retracts when not in the docking station. It is for use only on specific models of Permobil power wheelchairs and only with the Permolock docking base.

Regardless of the docking system used, it secures only the wheelchair. The occupant still requires a properly positioned, crashworthy lap and shoulder belt to be secured properly. Drivers with minimal dexterity often will drive into a seatbelt that is already fastened in the driver station.

Docking systems are not an option for public transit or school buses because the base and bracket are individualized for one wheelchair user. In personal vehicles, because of the cumbersome task of attaching the four securement straps, manual tie-downs often are not used properly. Although more expensive than the manual four-point system, the docking system cost may be justified for personal transportation if it is used with greater consistency and accuracy. A system that is not used properly will not protect the client or other people in the vehicle.

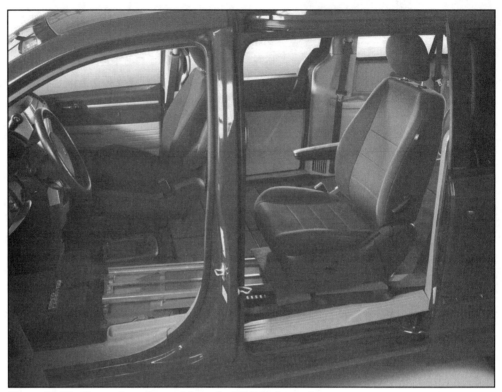

Figure 10.11. Power transfer seat base by B&D Independence.
Note. Used with permission of B&D Independence, Inc., Mount Carmel, IL.

Transfer Seat

With a modification to the driver seat, some clients are able to position themselves to perform a lateral, sliding transfer directly onto the driver's seat. The client secures the wheelchair in the transfer position, typically behind the driver's seat at an angle conducive to an independent transfer. The OEM seat is modified with an additional power seat base installed under it (Figure 10.11). Using toggle switches, the driver has the control to move the seat forward and back, rotate up to 90°, as well as move up and down.

Predrive

Once in a vehicle, add-on straps are available to allow easier access to the seat belt, and padded covers will soften pressure on the neck. In addition to online resources, auto-parts and big-box stores offer a limited variety of these accessories. A seat-belt extension (4- to 6-in. seat-belt webbing with male and female components on each end) is also useful. It is snapped into the original seat-belt buckle, thus extending the buckle so it is easier to access. It changes the angle across the chest, which may be beneficial for the client whose seat belt irritates the neck. These extensions are inexpensive and can be obtained directly through the specific OEM vehicle dealer. Seat-belt extensions are specific to the year, make, and model of a vehicle.

Sitting position is key for visibility of the driving environment. Whether the person is driving from a wheelchair or the vehicle seat, the sitting position goal is for the line of sight to be 3 in. above the steering wheel. There are commercially available cushions for the driver to use, however, some clients may require a custom cushion. To provide stability, the cushion should be firm. Again, to prevent sliding or submarining under the steering wheel, the cushion should be fastened so it does not slide with a sudden stop. For safe air-bag deployment, the **National Highway Traffic Safety Administration (NHTSA)** recommends that 10 in. be allowed from the air-bag cover (at the center of the steering wheel for the driver and in the dashboard for a front-seat passenger) to an individual's breastbone (NHTSA, n.d.). If medically necessary, vehicle modifiers can disconnect or install an on–off switch for the air bag.

Trunk stability is crucial for all clients. Often clients have learned to compensate for weak trunk muscles by "hooking" one arm on the wheelchair cane and using the other arm for the required task. This strategy is not possible when driving. Clients may find that when performing a turn, they lose balance and attempt to regain it by pulling on the hand controls or steering wheel. This practice is unsafe. Additional lateral supports on the wheelchair or an upper-torso positioning belt often are used to provide trunk stability. The upper-torso positioning belt is approximately 5 in. wide and is attached either to the driver's seat or the wheelchair. The Velcro closure allows the client to tighten the strap to provide needed support for decreased trunk balance. The OEM seat belt is not sufficient for trunk support but must be used because the torso belt is *not* a substitute for the seat-belt system.

All vehicles have blind spots or areas on the road that are not visible to the driver. The safe defensive driver will know where the blind spots are on his or her individual vehicle and learn to compensate for them. When a client has limited vision or limited neck mobility, additional mirrors may be indicated to provide the driver with a method for checking traffic at all points around the vehicle. Convex mirrors offer a greater viewing field; however, they may hinder the ability to judge the speed and distance of approaching vehicles. Add-on mirrors may be affixed directly to the side mirrors, either on the mirror itself or on top of the mirror housing (Figure 10.12). The OEM rear-view mirror may be replaced with a panoramic (convex) mirror, a multipanel mirror (3 or 5 panels angled to greatly reduce blind spots), or a combination mirror (sometimes called a *lane-changer* with a standard and convex mirror on top of each other).

Vehicle manufacturers constantly change offerings that can be available on a vehicle. Rear-view cameras, blind-spot alerts for lane changes, and backup sensors are all becoming more common. They are available both as OEM features and as after-market additions, but they help only if the driver knows how to use them. Positioning and practice with any additional equipment are necessary. The role of the generalist can be to inform the client of the potential benefit of these adaptations and to refer him or her to a DRS who can facilitate the installation and provide training in the proper use of the adaptations.

Driving Controls

Primary Controls

Primary controls are engaged while the vehicle is in motion and affect the direction and speed of the vehicle. Primary controls are gas, brake, and steering.

In selecting adaptive equipment for driving, it is critical to consider the safety component related to a driver's ability to learn and physically use the controls.

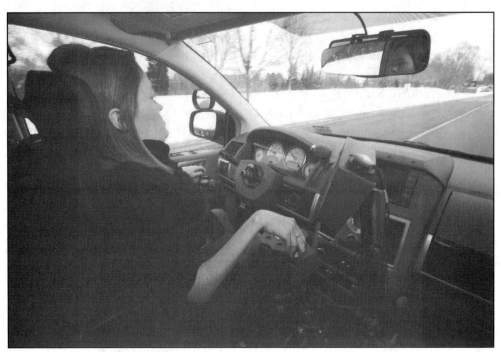

Figure 10.12. Additional mirrors to decrease blind spots.
Note. Provided by A. Hegberg. Used with permission.

Each person's ability to learn new tasks is based on previous experience, motivation for the task, learning ability, and a host of other issues. Any time the primary vehicle controls are to be modified, a qualified mobility dealer should perform the modifications after the client has completed a comprehensive driving evaluation and behind-the-wheel training.

Primary Control Adaptations

Extended pedals for the gas and brake are used for clients of short stature. Some vehicle manufacturers offer adjustable pedals as an OEM option. There also are after-market pedal extensions that attach directly to the pedal. Although many types are available over the Internet for self-installation, this practice is not recommended. Extended pedals are bolted directly to the OEM pedals (the gas and brake pedal) and are available with an extension that would move the pedals up to 10 in. closer to the driver's foot (Figures 10.13 and 10.14). Some pedals have the option to be disconnected or folded down in case there are drivers without disabilities who also use the vehicle. A foot pedestal is recommended to support the feet, increase stability, and decrease fatigue. Depending on the lower-extremity function, two-footed control as well as one-footed control should be examined. Careful attention to the client's sitting position, including proximity to the air bag, is needed. In some instances, a better sitting position may be possible with hand controls.

A *left accelerator pedal* is a device for the client who has lost the use of the right leg. Common reasons for requiring this adaptation are stroke and amputation. On the surface, the left accelerator pedal appears quite simple. The accelerator pedal is to the left of the OEM brake pedal, and the client uses the left foot for both gas

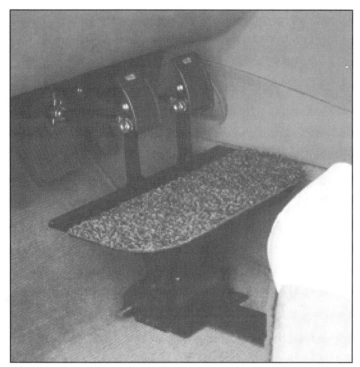

Figure 10.13. Menox Stamp Extensions bring pedals 4–10 in. closer to the client than the original pedals.
Note. Used with permission of Driving Systems, Inc., Van Nuys, CA.

and brake (Figure 10.15). The space and angle of the left pedal should mirror that of the OEM accelerator pedal. In addition to the left pedal, there is a metal plate attached to the device that blocks the right foot, or prosthesis, from accidentally getting under or on the OEM pedal. The device has a quick-release feature for the client to share his or her vehicle with a driver without a disability.

Although simple in concept, this product has been reported to be the cause of many accidents. Several large mobility dealers have opted not to install this device on any vehicle because of liability concerns. Although it can be risky, this device may be the only solution for some clients. Therefore, skill and expertise in the specialist conducting both the comprehensive driving evaluation and the training are a *must*. The experienced driver is more likely to have difficulty than a novice driver because the experienced driver must unlearn years of driving with the right foot. A critical contraindication is a diagnosis that includes cognitive or perceptual impairments (e.g., poststroke, TBI).

Mechanical hand controls allow the client to operate the accelerator and brake without the use of either lower extremity. These controls may be needed as the result of lower-extremity amputation, SCI, or decreased strength and coordination of the lower extremities such as with MS or CP. In the case of a client with a right lower-extremity amputation because of circulation impairment, often diabetes related, hand controls should be considered. The left foot may be functional at the time of the evaluation; however, it is at a higher risk for skin breakdown and neuropathy in the future. Because of a lack of sensation and fine motor control of a prosthesis, using one to operate the gas or brake is not recommended. Some states

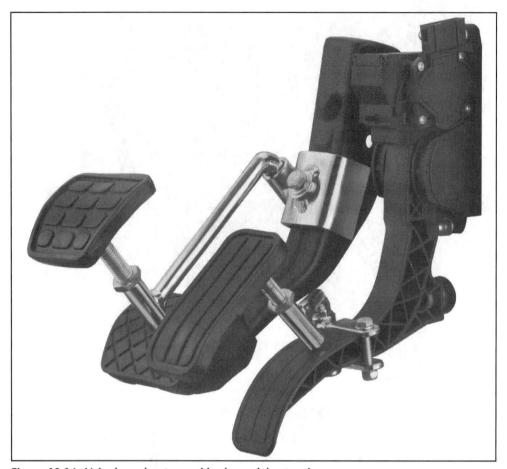

Figure 10.14. Veigel accelerator and brake pedal extensions.

Note. Used with permission of Mobility Products and Design, Shelby Township, MI.

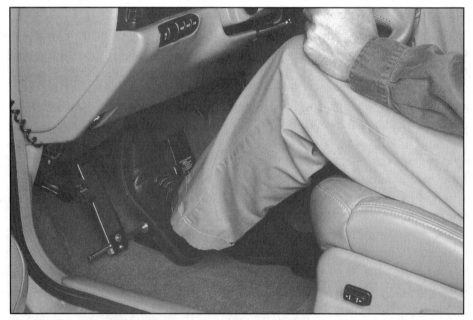

Figure 10.15. Left-foot gas pedal.

Note. Used with permission of MPS Corporation, Escondido, CA.

do not permit drivers to use a lower-extremity prosthesis to operate the gas and brake pedals, and other states do not address the issue.

Hand controls are defined by their action for acceleration because all mechanical hand controls push forward (toward the dash) for braking. Although requiring a similar action, manufacturers do have differences that may or may not affect a specific client. Different hand controls may be mounted under the steering column (left or right) and have adjustability for force and stroke. Typically the stronger, more coordinated, or dominant upper extremity steers, leaving the other to operate the gas and brake. A variety of handles are available such as a knob, a straight foam handle, or a handle with wrist support. Driver rehabilitation programs have several types of hand controls that can be mounted on the evaluation vehicles so that clients can try different hand controls and be trained with the type best for them.

Push right-angle hand controls can be installed under the steering column either to the left or right of the steering wheel. This style of hand control has been in the industry for more than 40 years. Little has changed in that time, and they are the most common type of hand control. Acceleration is activated by pushing the hand control lever toward the knee. Letting off the acceleration brings the lever up to a neutral position that is then pushed forward (at a right angle to the gas action) toward the dash, for braking (Figure 10.16). Client and vehicle space must be kept in mind because the lower extremities can interfere with the action for gas.

Push-rock hand controls are available only for installation on the left side. The handle is L-shaped and the hand placed on the top rocks rearward for gas. Because

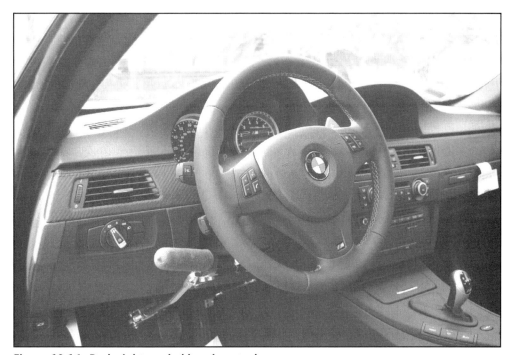

Figure 10.16. Push right-angled hand controls.
Note. Used with permission of MPS Corporation, Escondido, CA.

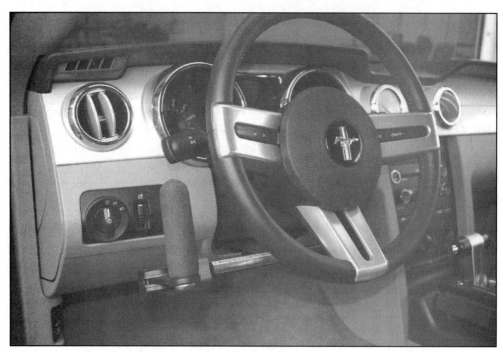

Figure 10.17. Push–rock hand controls.

Note. Used with permission of MPS Corporation, Escondido, CA.

the motion is rearward rather than downward, this control reduces interference with the lower extremities. The upright portion of the handle is pushed forward for braking (Figure 10.17).

Push–twist style controls can be installed on the left or right. The user twists the handle (similar to a motorcycle throttle) to activate the accelerator; it is then released and pushed forward to brake. Hand strength and risk of wrist fatigue can be issues with these controls, but they do allow more space for the lower extremities.

Push–pull hand controls are of two basic styles. They can be mounted under the steering column, similar to the types described earlier, or they can be mounted on the floor (Figures 10.18 and 10.19). Both types can be installed on the right or left. Acceleration is achieved by pulling back; braking is pushing forward. Because the action is opposite, it eliminates the possibility of applying the gas and brake simultaneously, which is a risk with other hand controls. The floor-mounted hand controls offer the advantage of leaving the area under the steering wheel clear, thus maintaining the tilt or telescoping feature of the wheel or column. Left floor-mounted controls may interfere with entry through the driver-side door. For the wheelchair driver, having limited space on the left, because of the door, can make it difficult to achieve a center position behind the steering wheel. Various handles are available, including a tri-pin that allows a client with minimal hand function to use these controls.

Considerations when determining the type of hand controls are based on client function, space within the vehicle, and personal preference. In the case of a client with a progressive disease, it is important to look at his or her current function and the prognosis for the future. If the person is having difficulty with specific controls, he or she will be increasingly difficult and unsafe with the progression of

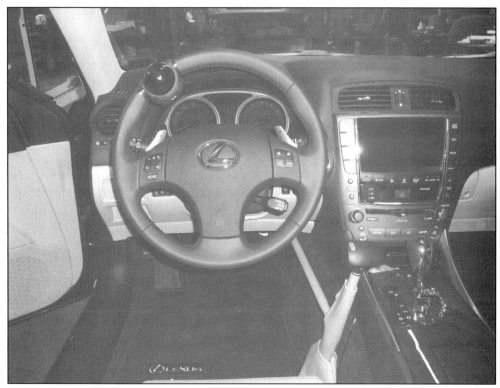

Figure 10.18. Floor-mounted push–pull hand controls, available with different handles.

Note. Used with permission of Driving Systems, Inc., Van Nuys, CA.

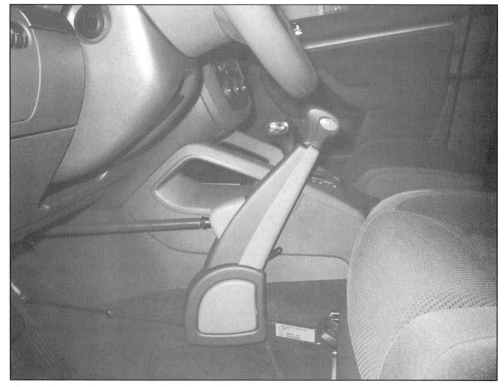

Figure 10.19. Floor-mounted push–pull hand controls.

Note. Used with permission of Mobility Products and Design, Shelby Township, MI.

the disease. Additionally, with diagnoses such as MS, be sure to address the daily variability of strength and fatigue that can accompany the disease.

All hand controls have some inherent amount of adjustability, and so it is imperative that the person prescribing the equipment be present for a final fitting or conformance inspection. This is done with the client at the mobility dealer when the client's vehicle is adapted before he or she takes possession of it. The fitting and inspection include confirming that all equipment prescribed is installed. Additionally, the DRS performs a functional inspection with the client driving the vehicle. Even when all equipment is installed per the manufacturer requirements, adjustments often are required after the drive. The fitting is a cooperative venture among the client, the funding agency, and the mobility dealer. Many state funding agencies also require a rehabilitation engineer inspection, which is an excellent idea because this person will look at the mechanical and electrical components of the installation.

Safety Features

Safety features have come to the forefront over the past few years. When a client is using mechanical hand controls, the OEM pedals still function. If the client's leg spasms or gets out of position, it can interfere with safe driving by landing on the accelerator or brake pedal. Just as dangerous is the possibility of the foot, or prosthesis, going under the brake pedal and preventing it from depressing when the hand control lever is pushed forward. For that reason, a *pedal guard* or block is recommended in most cases. The guard fits over the OEM pedals and has a quick-release mechanism to remove it when others are driving. The guard either covers the gas pedal or the gas and brake pedals (Figure 10.20).

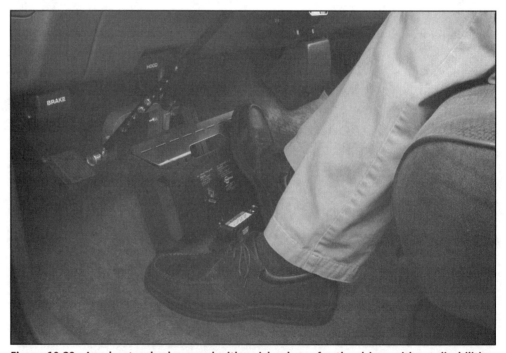

Figure 10.20. Accelerator–brake guard with quick release for the driver without disabilities.

Note. Used with permission of Mobility Products and Design, Shelby Township, MI.

Recently, hand control manufacturers have added *accelerator lockouts* to some of their hand controls. When activated, the lockout prevents the hand control from accelerating to prevent inadvertent activation by driver without disabilities (e.g., valet, mechanic, family member). When the hand control user drives, it is a simple process to inactivate the lockout. Because of the mounting of the hand controls under the steering column, features may be lost, including telescoping and tilting of the steering wheel. If the client shares the vehicle with a family member who is of a significantly different size, the adjustability of the steering wheel may be an important feature. The floor-mounted style of hand controls should be considered.

Steering

Steering is the other primary control. Steering spinners or steering devices are used to enable the client to maintain control of the steering wheel throughout an entire turn with one hand. The device may be needed because of impaired function of one upper extremity, or it may be that one hand is controlling the gas or brake, leaving the other to steer. There are many manufacturers of steering devices, each with subtle differences that may affect their use. Ultimately, the device chosen is based on the client's hand function.

The base is attached to the steering wheel with either metal bands or a clamshell (two separate pieces tightened around the steering wheel). The configuration and dimensions of the client's steering wheel may affect the base used as well as the placement. The steering device attaches and detaches from the base with a quick-release mechanism. This mechanism varies in size and effort required to attach and detach.

If hand function is impaired for the client or other drivers in the family, investigate which device will be most usable. With all steering devices, the base is permanently mounted to the steering wheel. Within one manufacturer's line, the steering devices all go into the same base, but they are not interchangeable between manufacturers.

The most common steering device is a *spinner knob* or *steering knob*. The palm of the steering hand presses on the top of the knob for one-handed steering control. The user of the knob has good hand and wrist function (Figure 10.21). Other common steering devices are the *straight pin, bi-pin* (also called *quad fork, V-grip,* or *U-grip*), *tri-pin, palm grip,* and *amputee ring*. The bi-pin is used for clients with good wrist function but impaired hand function. The hand is placed sideways in the device, and the pins are adjusted accordingly. Using the palm grip (flat-palm spinner), the driver's hand is fitted into the device in either a supinated or pronated position. The amputee ring steering device is designed for those with a hook-style prosthetic device. Tension on the hook is important so that the client does not come out of the device on a quick turn. The tri-pin allows a client with decreased wrist function and poor hand function to control the steering wheel. The three pins are adjustable to secure the hand in position. The tri-pin is often the device of choice for clients with quadriplegia.

When fitting the client with any steering device, watch that the device does not make contact with the client or his or her clothes. If the client wears gloves to push a wheelchair, a decision needs to be made regarding keeping the gloves on or off when in the steering device. At the fitting, the device is adjusted accordingly.

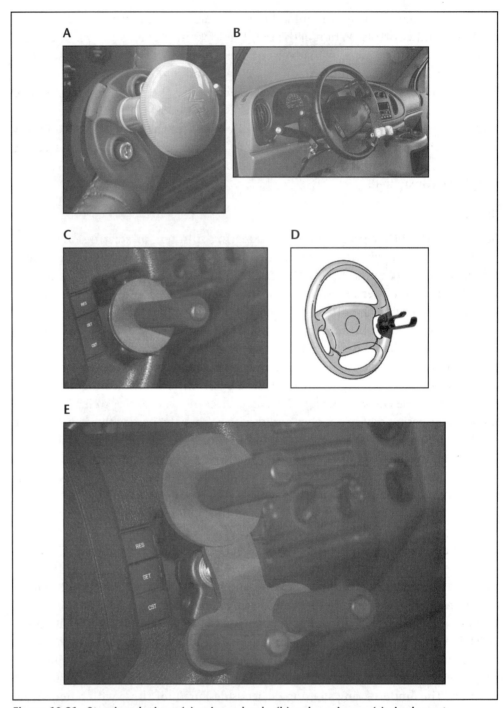

Figure 10.21. Steering devices: (a) spinner knob, (b) palm spinner, (c) single post, (d) quad-fork spinner (bi-pin), and (e) tri-pin spinner.

Note. Used with permission of MPS Corporation, Escondido, CA.

Secondary Controls

Secondary controls, also called *primary auxiliary controls,* are those controls that must be accessible when the vehicle is in motion but do not affect the speed or direction of the vehicle. These controls include the turn signals, horn, dimmer, washer-wiper, and cruise set.

Secondary controls can be adapted either mechanically with extensions of some type or with remote switches to activate them. OEM turn signal levers are universally on the left side of the steering wheel. Other secondary controls may be on the right, on the steering wheel, or on a center console. Extensions may be attached to the turn signal lever either to bring it down closer to the left hand or to cross over the steering column to activate the signals with the right hand (Figure 10.22).

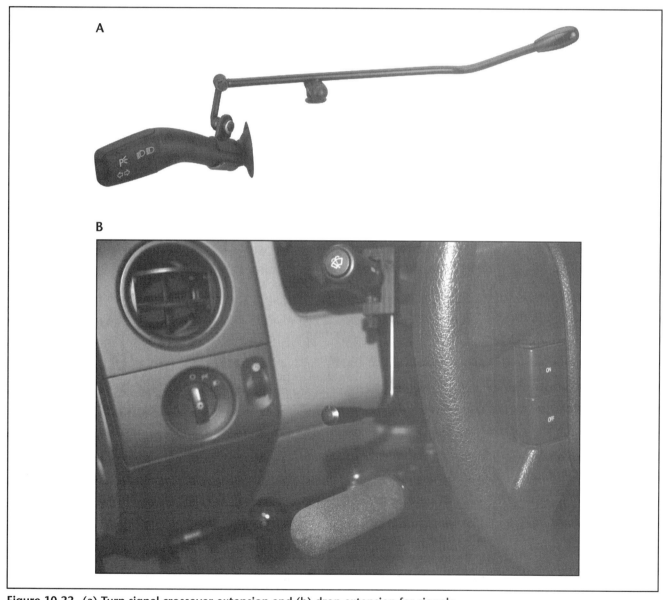

Figure 10.22. **(a) Turn signal crossover extension and (b) drop extension for signals.**

Note. Used with permission of Mobility Products and Design, Shelby Township, MI, and MPS Corporation, Escondido, CA.

Extensions also can be attached to other secondary controls for easier activation; for example, extensions can be added to a wiper lever for easier access.

When mechanical extensions are not sufficient, the activation of controls can be remote. For example, there are soft-touch pads, single or multi-buttons, and toggle switches that can be used for any or all of the secondary functions. The switches can be integrated on a primary control device such as hand controls or a steering device (Figure 10.23). The switch may be activated with an elbow, the head, or a lower-extremity movement. The possibilities are endless and are customized to the individual. The most important feature is that the client can activate the secondary controls while maintaining his or her eyes on the driving environment and maintaining complete control of the vehicle.

Tertiary (or Secondary Auxiliary) Controls

Activation of tertiary controls does not need to be performed when the vehicle is in motion but must be accessible to the client. The tertiary controls, such as ignition, gear shifter, and air conditioner, can be activated either when the client is holding the brake or when the gear shifter is in park.

Because as the configuration of these OEM controls varies widely between vehicles, it is important to know what vehicle the client will be adapting. Gear shifters are a good example of OEM variations, as they may be mounted on the steering column, a center console, or the front dash. Because of placement and the amount of strength and coordination needed, one type of shifter may be more suitable than another for the client. Additionally, many OEM features are available as an option for a specific vehicle so that modifications are not required. For example, some vehicles have a keyless ignition as an option.

When a client is unable to access the OEM controls, then extensions, levers, or other mechanical means of operating controls are investigated (Figure 10.24). Once the mechanical options have been exhausted, the evaluator then would consider remote switches or electronic modifications (Figure 10.25).

Beyond Mechanical Adaptations

When mechanical adaptations are not sufficient, medium- to high-tech modifications are needed.

When mechanical adaptations are not sufficient, medium- to high-tech modifications are needed. For the vehicle's primary controls, devices involving *servomotors* (an electric motor creating mechanical force) would be required to assist with controlling the gas, brake, and steering. Conventional power steering can be modified so that less strength is needed to turn the steering wheel through the entire range. Reduced effort (~50% of OEM effort) or zero effort (~20% of OEM effort) can be installed for a client who has the ROM but not the strength. This adaptation requires a backup system so that if there is a failure, the client could steer the vehicle to the side of the road.

When reduced or zero-effort steering is installed, self-recovery of the wheel after a turn is lost. The driver must steer back out of a turn, which can be fatiguing for some clients. Reduction of steering effort varies among vehicles just as OEM power steering varies. When using zero-effort steering, NMEDA guidelines require the use of a counterbalance weight, which is installed in a steering base directly across from the steering device and should be of equal weight. The counterbalance is used so that the client with limited strength will not be working against the weight of the

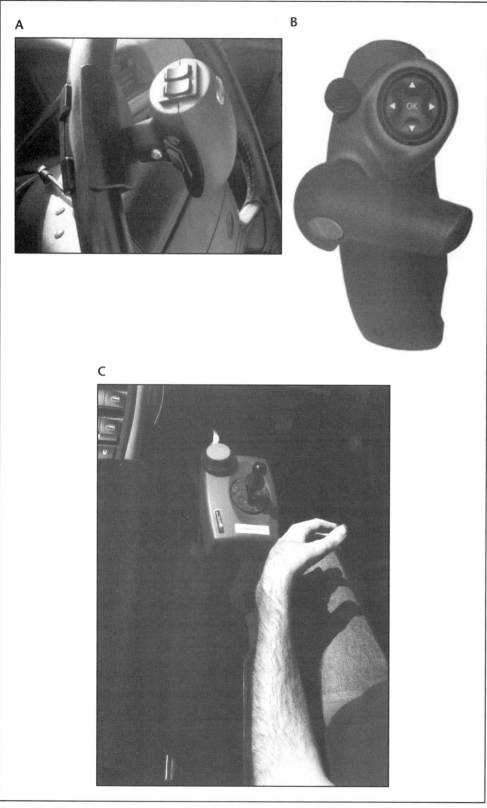

Figure 10.23. (a) Secondary controls mounted on steering device, (b) secondary controls mounted on hand controls, and (c) DigiTone® single button to activate multiple secondary controls.

Note. Used with permission of Driving Systems, Inc., Van Nuys, CA; Mobility Products and Design, Shelby Township, MI; and Electronic Mobility Controls, Augusta, ME.

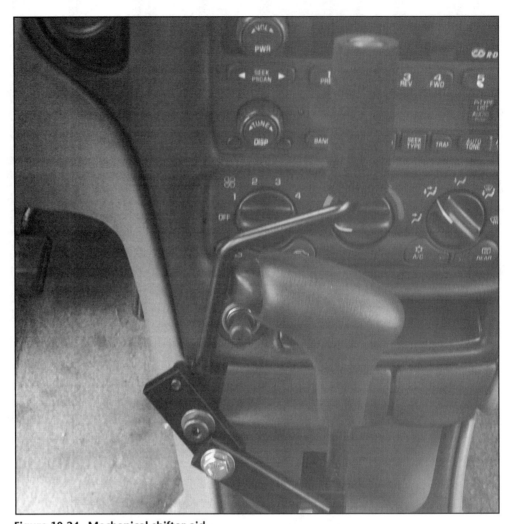

Figure 10.24. Mechanical shifter aid.

Note. Used with permission of Mobility Products and Design, Shelby Township, MI.

steering device as he or she is driving. A client with quadriparesis using a tri-pin at the 4:00 position could easily become fatigued, with the weight of the device pulling toward the 6:00 position, causing the vehicle to go to the right.

If the client has the strength but not the ROM, steering wheels of smaller diameters can be used (10, 12, or 14 in.). Be aware that when the wheel is smaller, greater effort is required. A combination of reduced- or zero-effort steering with a smaller wheel may be the solution for some clients. The plane of steering remains upright with reduced-effort or reduced-diameter steering wheels. Various steering column extensions (2, 4, or 6 in.) can be installed to bring the steering wheel closer to the client driving from his or her wheelchair (Figure 10.26).

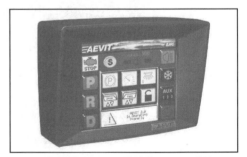

Figure 10.25. Smart-Shift® power shifter for gears.

Note. Used with permission of Electronic Mobility Controls, Augusta, ME.

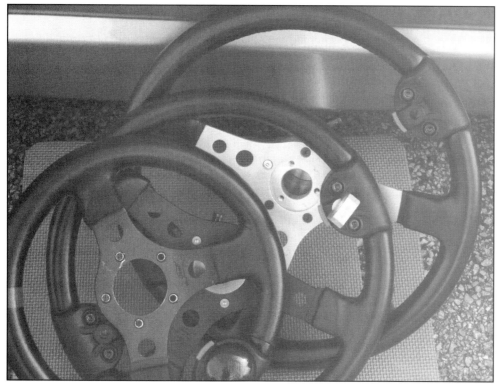

Figure 10.26. Reduced-diameter steering wheel and steering column extensions.
Note. Provided by A. Hegberg. Used with permission.

A horizontal steering column permits steering with a small wheel in a flat plane. The OEM wheel is removed, and the horizontal wheel is centered directly in front of the client. With this modification, the air bag is removed. Steering reduction also is combined with this adaptation (Figure 10.27). Although not common, foot steering is an option for clients who lack function in either upper extremity. The steering plate is mounted on the floor, and the client uses one foot to steer and the other to operate the gas and brake (Figure 10.28).

A technological possibility is available to compensate for significantly impaired motor strength and ROM required for the primary controls. There are several manufacturers of high-tech systems. The client's level of maturity, responsibility, and cognitive competence is important to understand the complexities of the system

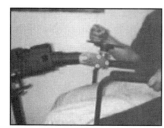

Figure 10.27. Horizontal steering.
Note. Used with permission of Drive Master Co., Inc., Fairfield, NJ.

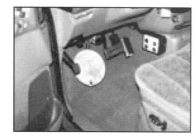

Figure 10.28. Foot-steering system.
Note. Used with permission of Drive Master Co., Inc., Fairfield, NJ.

as well as the risks and limitations associated with them. The advantage of these systems is that the input device for steering can be placed wherever it is most accessible to the client. The device may be a small wheel (~7 in. in diameter) or a joystick, which has a variety of *orthotics* (a device the client interfaces with directly, such as a small ball) and requires minimal strength (~3.2 oz effort) to control.

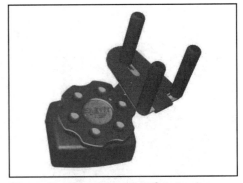

Figure 10.29. AEVIT 2.0–W® (wheel) remote steering system.

Note. Used with permission of Electronic Mobility Controls, Augusta, ME.

This type of steering is commonly used for clients with functional fine-motor coordination but weak proximal strength, such as those with spinal muscular atrophy, muscular dystrophy, or some cases of ontogenesis imperfecta or arthrogryposis. One of these systems may be appropriate for clients with high-level SCIs (C-5). Various orthotic steering devices can be used to interface with the systems such as a tri-pin. Because of the sensitivity of these systems, support for the extremity in use, trunk support, and stability of the wheelchair are crucial for functional control (Figure 10.29).

Often used in conjunction with horizontal, zero-effort, or remote-steering systems is a high-tech system for the primary control of gas or brake. The client controls the gas and brake either with a lever or a joystick, which is positioned within easy reach. A variety of orthotic devices can be used on the basis of the client's function. Secondary controls may be integrated on the system (pin switch or soft-touch button) for activation while maintaining position on the controller (Figure 10.30).

At the end of the driving spectrum is a single joystick controller for the gas or brake and the steering (Figure 10.31). Clients frequently compare the action to that of a power wheelchair; however, it is quite different. When the client pulls

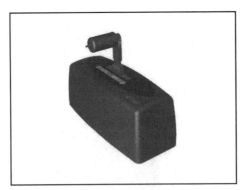

Figure 10.30. AEVIT 2.0–L® (lever) gas–brake steering system.

Note. Used with permission of Electronic Mobility Controls, Augusta, ME.

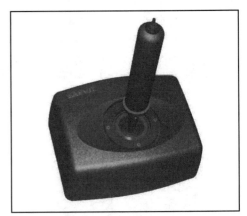

Figure 10.31. AEVIT 2–J® (joystick) for steering, gas, and brake.

Note. Used with permission of Electronic Mobility Controls, Augusta, ME.

back on the wheelchair joystick, the wheelchair reverses. Pulling back on a driving joystick will apply either the gas or the brake, depending on the specific system being used. A 300-lb. power wheelchair at 6 mph has very different dynamics than a 2-ton vehicle at 60 mph. Good trunk stability and stability of the wheelchair are essential. It is important to go back to a basic therapeutic principle: stability before mobility. Many clients using this type of equipment are using a power wheelchair.

The newer power wheelchairs have improved suspension as well as articulating parts for features such as tilt and recline. The wheelchair base is secured in the driving station, but the wheelchair seat may move when the client is braking, resulting in a decreased ability to control the vehicle as the client oscillates forward and back. Increased stability may need to be added to the client's wheelchair to maximize vehicle control. A seating and mobility specialist should be consulted because a change in the seating system may result in unwanted side effects such as pressure sores.

Beyond Equipment

Advances in technology have provided the tools for many clients, even those with severe disabilities, to be able to drive independently. However, there are considerations beyond adaptive equipment that need to be addressed, including licensing, fitting, financial considerations, documentation, and qualified modifiers.

There are considerations beyond adaptive equipment that need to be addressed, including licensing, fitting, financial considerations, documentation, and qualified modifiers.

Licensing

Many funding sources require that clients be licensed with adaptive equipment before adaptation of their personal vehicle; this often is done in the driver rehabilitation training vehicle. State licensing requirements for clients driving with adaptive equipment vary greatly. It is important to know the laws and requirements in the state where one practices. A medical report form of some type may need to be completed and sent to the state licensing agency. The American Medical Association's ***Physician's Guide to Assessing and Counseling Older Drivers*** (Carr, Schwartzberg, Manning, & Sempek, 2010) contains contacts and reporting procedures for all 50 states.

Fitting

A conformance inspection (also called a *fitting*) takes place at the mobility dealer with the client and the DRS. It is an integral part of the driver rehabilitation process. The purpose is to determine whether all equipment has been installed as specified and is functional for this particular client. Installations may follow the manufacturer instructions and appear fine statically, but in the dynamic driving environment, problems may arise that require further adjustment. Obvious problems are brought forward and solutions are discussed. The solution may be a simple adjustment of a piece of adaptive equipment, or it may require major changes and a second fitting.

Ideally, an outside inspector, often a rehabilitation engineer, is also present at the fitting to inspect the vehicle. Some state agencies employ a person who acts in this role; others contract with an individual. The inspector goes beyond the functional inspection performed by the DRS. The inspector not only checks that all equipment was installed per manufacturer's instructions but also scrutinizes wiring, fasteners, leaks, or other potential hazards. Although an invaluable resource, the presence of an inspector is generally based on the payer source. Many, but not all, state vocational rehabilitation agencies require involvement of a rehabilitation engineer for an inspection.

Financial Considerations

Cost of adaptations varies dramatically. Obviously, the more equipment and the more extensive the technology used, the more expensive it will be. The combination of a steering device with mechanical hand controls may run in the $2,000 range. A complete high-tech driving system, with modification for a wheelchair driver, may exceed $100,000. These costs do not include the cost of the vehicle (chassis), which may add another $20,000 to $30,000 to the total cost. Both the vehicle and the adaptations need to be insured. The client's ability to insure and maintain the vehicle is an important consideration.

Financial assistance is available through various funding sources. For the client who is working or plans to return to work, individual state vocational rehabilitation programs offer some funding for transportation. Their goal is obtaining or maintaining employment. Assistance may include driver rehabilitation services, transport services, or vehicle modification. It is the responsibility of the client to supply an appropriate vehicle. No vehicle should be purchased for adaptation without consulting the DRS and the vehicle modifier.

Other sources of assistance for services or equipment include disease-specific organizations such as the Multiple Sclerosis Society. Organizations such as Shriners Hospitals, local independent living facilities, and Area Agencies on Aging sometimes have grants available for driving adaptations. Most vehicle manufacturers offer rebates at some level for newly purchased vehicles that are modified within a specific period of time. Local mobility dealers and the OEM vehicle dealer are resources for these rebates.

Documentation

Documentation is specific to the state, service provider, and payer source. The mobility dealer is using the driver rehabilitation report to obtain information for the cost and installation of the equipment. It is important to have an open relationship established with the mobility dealer because this is a dynamic and changing industry. Questions will arise; it is difficult, if not impossible, to keep up with all the technology changes. A vehicle that was appropriate 6 months ago may have an OEM change that negates its use for a specific modification.

The written prescription specifies what type of adaptive equipment was used for the evaluation and training as well as what follow-up is required. The specific manufacturer of the device may or may not be included. Some state agencies require generic specifications regarding the device that was used (e.g., specific manufacturer). There may be one or several manufacturers that meet the specifications. No driver rehabilitation program has every type and manufacturer of equipment. It is important to know what is available at other facilities to refer clients appropriately.

The client should always drive the specific prescribed equipment. In addition to driving with the specific equipment, if client is to drive from a wheelchair in his or her van, then he or she should drive from his or her wheelchair for the evaluation and training. The dynamics are different from driving from the OEM seat.

Qualified Modifiers

NMEDA has guidelines to provide specific information regarding federal standards and standards established by the mobility industry. The NMEDA Quality Assurance Program (QAP) is the accreditation program for the adaptive mobility equipment industry. Modifiers are required to follow Federal Motor Vehicle Safety Standards (FMVSS) established by NHTSA. Exceptions can be made; however, proper documentation of changes is needed so that the vehicle is in compliance. Beyond inspections for compliance with FMVSS, liability insurance, 24-hour service to customers, and certified technicians and welders are some of the QAP requirements (see www.nmeda.org for a full list of requirements and dealers).

Conclusion

Adaptive equipment for driving and community mobility covers a wide span of information. For generalist occupational therapists, the thought of exploring driving with equipment or modified vehicles or discussing costly modifications for transporting passengers can be daunting. However, the equipment spectrum is broad and begins with basic education, devices for the non–moving vehicle, and referral. Many simple changes can be incorporated into occupational therapy practice to assist clients with community mobility. In some situations, the goal for community mobility may focus on educating family members on transfers into a vehicle and managing equipment in a manner that is safe for both the family and the client. In other situations, the generalist may prepare a client for driving cessation and the transition to alternative forms of transportation.

Most important, know that driver evaluation programs are a resource. Know where these programs are located, and get to know them. Build a referral pathway to ensure that clients have access to specialized services that include preliminary consultation, comprehensive driving evaluation, adaptation and vehicle modification, and the expertise of mobility dealers.

References

Carr, D. B., Schwartzberg, J. G., Manning, L., & Sempek, J. (2010). *Physician's guide to assessing and counseling older drivers* (2nd ed.). Washington, DC: National Highway Traffic Safety Administration.

National Highway Traffic Safety Administration. (n.d.). *Air bags and on–off switches: Information for an informed decision*. Washington, DC: Author.

Pellerito, J. M. (Ed.). (2006). *Driver rehabilitation and community mobility: Principles and practice*. St. Louis, MO: Elsevier/Mosby.

Stav, W. B., Hunt, L. A., & Arbesman, M. (2006). *Occupational therapy practice guidelines for driving and community mobility for older adults*. Bethesda, MD: AOTA Press.

Appendix 10.A. Wheelchair Information Form

Client will be driving from a _____ (wheelchair, transfer seat, original equipment manufacturer seat).

This individual currently _____ (owns, will be getting) a _____ (manual [e.g., folding, rigid-frame wheelchair] , power wheelchair, power scooter). Pertinent wheelchair or scooter information is as follows:

	Measurement, Description, Additional Information
Manufacturer	
Make/model	
Serial #	
Weight: Client	
Weight: Chair	
Overall total weight (chair and client)	
Width: drive wheels	
Width: front wheels	
Width: rear wheels	
Width: armrests	
Width: foot rests	
Overall length (including client's feet)	
Front-to-rear wheel length	
Ground clearance (lowest point)	
Footrest clearance	
Battery clearance	
Height: floor to top of head	
Height: floor to eye ellipse	
Height: floor to seat cushion	
Height: floor to armrests	
Height: floor to knee	
Size and type of seat cushion	
Type of armrests	Swing away, removable, desk or regular length
Type of foot rests	Static, platform, swing away, removable
Size and type of rear wheel	
Size and type of front wheel	
Control site for joystick	Right or left
Additional features	Tilt, standing, reclining, elevating
WC-19 compliant (lockdown points on wheelchair)	Yes or no
Highest part once seat is folded down	
Recommended changes to wheelchair	Lateral supports, stabilizers, back, cushion

Note. Provided by A. Hegberg. Used with permission.

Appendix 10.B. Vehicle Modification Evaluation Form

Application of Adapted Vehicle Modifications | 2009

"Cruisin' for Success" Evaluation Form	Date___/___/__

Name_____DOB:_____Phone_____

Address_____

Referral   Disability

Referral Goals_____

Client Goals_____

Other's Goals_____

Vehicle to Be Adapted

Make_____

Model_____

Year_____

VIN #_____

Mileage_____

Engine_____

Features OPS-OPB-OAuto Tran-OPwind-OPlock
OPcargo door(s),L,R,Rear-Swing/Slide-ORear HVAC

Estimated Monthly Payment
w/Equipment_____

Parking_____

Garage_____

Wheelchair Specifications

Make	
Model	
Serial number	
Style	
Size (W x D x H)	
Width at drive wheels	
Width at widest point	
Length, foot to rear wheel/anti-tip	
Wheelbase	
Seat height w/cushion	
Seat to top of head	
Knee height	
Armrest height	
Eye Height	
Head height	
Ground clearance at footrest	
Footrest style	
Ground clearance at battery box	
Joystick side	
Back height (W/C)	
Back height, folded down (W/C)	
Folded width	
Chair/Client weight w/accessories	
Power positioning components	

(continued)

Appendix 10.B. Vehicle Modification Evaluation Form (*cont.*)

Application of Adapted Vehicle Modifications | 2009

ADAPTIVE EQUIPMENT CHECKLIST

Entry
Exterior switching, lift/doors)
- ❑ Hand held remote (RF)
- ❑ Magnetic switching

Door openers
- ❑ Hand held extension
- ❑ Powered swing doors
- ❑ Powered sliding door
- ❑ Rear hatch
- ❑ **Raised doors**
- ❑ **Raised roofs**
- ❑ **Roof support**
- ❑ **Lowered floor**

Flooring
- ❑ Substrate
- ❑ Carpet
- ❑ Non-slip sheet

Seat lift
- ❑ Full
- ❑ Platform , single/bi-fold

Ramps
- ❑ Manual fold, attached/portable
- ❑ Manual slide
- ❑ Manual extend
- ❑ Power fold
- ❑ Power slide

Platform Lifts
- ❑ Dual post tall
- ❑ Dual post short
- ❑ Single arm
- ❑ Under vehicle

Stowage
- ❑ Trunk hoist, Manual/Scooter
- ❑ Hatch hoist Docking/Platform
- ❑ Side door hoist
- ❑ Roof top hoist
- ❑ Hitch platform
     Manual/Scooter/Power
     base
- ❑ Trailer

Securement
Unoccupied wheelchair
- ❑ Automatic
- ❑ Belting

WTORS passenger
- ❑ Automatic
- ❑ Adjustable belt
- ❑ Retractor belt
- ❑ **WTORS automatic driver**

Adapted belting
- ❑ Latches
- ❑ Length
- ❑ Stanchion
- ❑ Drive in
- ❑ Chest belt

Positioning
Power seat
- ❑ Eight way
- ❑ Six way
- ❑ Four way
- ❑ Two way (swivel)

Inserts
- ❑ Booster
- ❑ Stabilizing
- ❑ **Straps and Handles**
- ❑ **Removable seat base**

Control
Braking/Acceleration
- ❑ Extended pedals,
     Clamp/Linkage
- ❑ Left foot accelerator

Mechanical hand controls
- ❑ Push/Pull right angle
- ❑ Push pull
- ❑ Push twist
- ❑ Push rock
- ❑ Pedestal push pull

Servo hand controls
- ❑ Pneumatic
- ❑ Electric
- ❑ In-line
- ❑ Wheel mount
- ❑ **Reduced effort brakes**
- ❑ **Back up brakes**

Steering
Spinners
- ❑ Knob
- ❑ Dual pin, Flat/Round
- ❑ Tri-pin
- ❑ Flat palm
- ❑ Ring
- ❑ Custom
- ❑ Counter balance

Wheels
- ❑ Smaller diameter
- ❑ Remote/Servo

Columns
- ❑ Extension
- ❑ Horizontal
- ❑ **Reduced effort** low/zero

- ❑ **Back-up**
- ❑ **Foot**
- ❑ **Joystick**
- ❑ **Uni-lever**

Primary Auxiliary Controls
Extensions
- ❑ Turn signal cross over
- ❑ Wiper rotational
- ❑ Straight extension

Remote (multiple switches)
Consoles/Packages
- ❑ Hand control
- ❑ Steering spinner
- ❑ Elbow
- ❑ Head w/power headrest

Multi-function switches
- ❑ Voice menu
- ❑ Tone menu

Secondary Auxiliary
Extensions
- ❑ Parking brake
- ❑ Gear shift, Straight/Crossover
- ❑ Windows, locks, mirrors
- ❑ HVAC
- ❑ Key
- ❑ Radio
- ❑ Lighting

Remote
- ❑ Parking brake
- ❑ Gear shift
- ❑ Windows, locks, mirrors
- ❑ HVAC
- ❑ Ignition/start
- ❑ Lighting
- ❑ Doors and lift
- ❑ Consoles

Vision
Mirrors
- ❑ Exterior convex mirrors
- ❑ Interior wide view rear mirror
- ❑ **Cameras,** back up
- ❑ **Lighting,** Ramp/lift

General safety
- ❑ Air bag switch
- ❑ Pedal blocks
- ❑ Back up battery
- ❑ Fire extinguisher

Appendix 10.B. Vehicle Modification Evaluation Form (*cont.*)

Application of Adapted Vehicle Modifications | 2009

Primary Auxiliary Controls

Item	Activation Method	Switch type	Location
Left turn			
Right turn			
Wiper/wash			
Wiper, slow			
Wiper fast			
Horn			
Dimmer			
Cruise set			

Secondary Auxiliary Controls

Item	Activation Method	Switch type	Location
Gear shift			
Parking brake			
Automatic tie down			
Ignition			
Start			
Driving lights			
Parking lights			
Interior lighting			
HVAC fan			
HVAC temperature			
HVAC mode			
Cruise on			
Window left			
Window right			
Locks			
Hazards			
Mirror left			
Mirror right			
Lift			
Door/s			

Controls Key

Activation Method
LHF	Left Hand/Finger
RHF	Right Hand/Finger
LE	Left Elbow
RE	Right Elbow
H	Head

Switch Type
TS	Toggle Small
TL	Toggle Large
RS	Rocker Small
RL	Rocker Large
PBS	Push Button Small
PBL	Push Button Large
EX	Extension
TP	Touch Pad

Location
F	Factory
DD	Driver's Door panel
D	Dash
CL	Console Left
CR	Console Right
CD	Console Dash
S	Spinner
HC	Hand Control

Notes on Primary/Secondary Auxiliary Controls_____

_____

_____

_____

HVAC = heating, ventilation, and air conditioning; WTORS = wheelchair tie-down occupant restraint system.

CHAPTER 11

Clinical Reasoning Process in the Comprehensive Driving Evaluation

Sherrilene Classen, PhD, MPH, OTR/L, FAOTA, and Desiree N. Lanford, MOT, OTR/L, CDRS

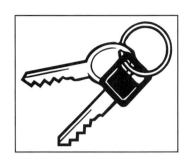

Learning Objectives

At the completion of this chapter, readers will be able to

- Delineate the general data collection process used by the occupational therapist to (1) obtain data through interviews, self-report, clinical tests, and the behind-the-wheel assessment and (2) identify the general strategies to improve fitness to drive;
- Identify the clinical reasoning skills underlying the occupational therapist's ability to make decisions for determining fitness to drive; and
- Delineate, by way of a case study, how the occupational therapist uses the clinical reasoning process to integrate data from all sources (described in the first point) in making final determinations, recommendations, referrals, and consultations about the client's driving fitness.

Key Words

- comprehensive driving evaluation
- clinical reasoning
- conditional reasoning
- fitness to drive
- interactive reasoning
- procedural reasoning

Introduction

Clinical reasoning is the thought process that guides occupational therapy practice. It is a way to start framing one's thought processes with words and explaining the rationale behind one's clinical decisions (Neistadt, 1996). As Joan C. Rogers (1983) described it, "The artistry of clinical reasoning is exhibited in the craftsmanship with which the therapist executes the series of steps that culminates in a clinical decision" (p. 612). This chapter discusses the entire comprehensive driving evaluation process and describes how to collect information and use clinical reasoning to provide recommendations and counseling about driving fitness. A case example provides a relationship to real life and the concepts of this chapter.

Clinical Reasoning

Clinical reasoning is the purposeful and goal-directed thinking process occupational therapists use to analyze information to create a plan of care for their clients

Clinical reasoning **is the purposeful and goal-directed thinking process occupational therapists use to analyze information to create a plan of care for their clients.**

(Mattingly & Fleming, 1994), and it distinguishes the unique service of the occupational therapy driving program. Mattingly and Fleming (1994) described clinical reasoning as using a three-track mind through (1) procedural, (2) interactive, and (3) conditional reasoning. The occupational therapist uses all three types of clinical reasoning in Case Example 11.1 to make the final clinical interpretations on the basis of each of the clinical assessments used.

Procedural Reasoning

Procedural reasoning is used to determine what activities to use to increase the client's level of functional independence when thinking about the disease or disability. For example, procedural reasoning would occur when discussing medication management and alerting the client to drive only when he or she feels "on" (this term is used in conjunction with Parkinson's disease [PD] to indicate that the person is not experiencing dyskinesias or tremors and that he or she feels, according to subjective experience, in his or her best functional state).

Interactive Reasoning

Interactive reasoning is conducted during the face-to-face experience with the client to get the client's perspective about the illness, injury, or disability and to involve him or her in the goal making for the intervention plan. At this point, the therapist gathers information about how the client feels and thinks about the disability and uses it to match treatment aims and strategies and desired outcomes. An example may be to ask the client to complete the Safe Driving Behaviors Measure (Classen et al., 2010; now called the ***Fitness-To-Drive Screening Measure***) and to get the client's opinion on his or her driving ability over the past 3 months.

Conditional Reasoning

Conditional reasoning occurs when the bigger picture is evaluated, meaning that the occupational therapist reviews the client's functional status before the disability and at the present time. The physical contexts and social contexts in which the client lived and lives and the meaning that the illness or disability currently has for the client are all considered. As with interactive reasoning, the therapist also involves the client during the creation of the possible outcomes. For example, the occupational therapist might discuss driving recommendations or restrictions with the client and get his or her feedback, ideas, and agreement to these suggestions.

Data Collection

Data collection is a crucial part of clinical reasoning. It informs the occupational therapist of the client's demographic background, medical history, and driving history and habits, giving the therapist a clearer picture of the client's potential strengths, weaknesses, and potential for safe driving. As part of the evaluation process, data collection helps determine the most appropriate occupational therapy intervention. Ongoing data collection occurs as the occupational therapist monitors how the client responds to intervention, helping the therapist determine whether intervention is working (Kramer & Hinojosa, 2010).

Demographic Data

Data are collected through observation and oral and written interviews, including person, vehicle, and environmental factors. Demographic information such as age, gender, race, ethnicity, education, employment status, disabilities, and mobility is obtained to help create a clearer representation of the life stage, responsibilities, and motivations to drive. Additional information such as living arrangements and marital status may be particularly useful in discerning the person's roles and patterns of driving or in ascertaining whether access and support are available for the use of community mobility.

Medical History

Medical history and health data such as previous or current diseases, illnesses, conditions, comorbidities, medications, and surgeries, provide rich information about the driver's capabilities in, potential impairments in, and limitations to the task of driving. The occupational therapist routinely obtains a listing of all prescribed or over-the-counter medications, herbal products, vitamins, and nutraceuticals to help understand the potential impact of drugs on the functional performance that may affect driving.

Driving History and Habits

The person's driving skills initially are assessed through interviews and questionnaires, as discussed in Chapter 9 (Owsley, Stalvey, Wells, & Sloane, 1999). The occupational therapist is encouraged to always obtain the person's driver's license status and history of driving habits, roles, and routines. A person's history of being reported to the state driver license authority, or having driven with a suspended or revoked driver's license, will certainly alert one to concerns about the person's driving ability or behaviors. Asking about previous citations, crashes, violations, or near misses will provide one with indications of poor or unsafe driving performance. The frequency of driving, places traveled to, preferred times of driving, distances driven, and modes of transportation used will provide a context from which the occupational therapist can understand the person's needs, motivations, requirements, and demands to drive.

Collecting information on driving history also provides a basis for exploring the person's willingness or openness to use other mobility options such as shuttles, buses, or commuter trains. The self-report may uncover avoidance behaviors, such as not driving on highways or at night, and compensatory strategies, such as using low-traffic-density roads instead of interstate roadways. To ascertain a person's insight into his or her own safe driving ability, it is a good idea to query the driver's self-perception on safety and ability to perform a variety of driving maneuvers (e.g., driving during rush-hour traffic).

> **Collecting information on driving history also provides a basis for exploring the person's willingness or openness to use other mobility options such as shuttles, buses, or commuter trains.**

Self-Report or Refresher Course and Driving

Completing a self-report questionnaire or a driving refresher course is a good indicator that the driver is proactively seeking information to learn about or understand the aging process and how it relates to his or her driving performance. The driver's newfound knowledge and awareness may improve his or her openness and participation during the comprehensive driving evaluation and goal planning.

Vehicle

There are many vehicle factors, which may include the type of vehicle, automatic or standard transmission, size of vehicle; number of doors; crashworthiness and presence of airbags; a brake-assist system; and dynamic stability control. The condition of the vehicle and the usability of equipment (e.g., lights, horn, windshield wipers, tires) must sustain the principle of safe driving. Standard equipment such as head restraints, visors and extendable visors, knobs for controls (e.g., climate, audio), and mirrors should be in good working condition. Adjustable controls such as the steering wheel must be adjusted for optimal positioning, functionality, and safety. Doorway space and head room must accommodate drivers adequately.

In more modern cars, the availability of smart in-vehicle features is becoming standard in the manufacturing process, and the occupational therapist should be knowledgeable of the use of and reliance on these features, such as navigation, heads-up display, adaptive cruise control, rear camera–collision avoidance systems, lane deviation prevention systems, adjustable foot pedals, and tilt and telescoping steering wheels. Likewise, it is important for the occupational therapist to have knowledge of after-market products and adaptive vehicle equipment, such as adaptive mirrors that may be larger and angled, hand controls, a left-foot accelerator, steering devices, a wheelchair tie-down system, steering-wheel covers, cushions, lumbar supports, lifts, carriers, door openers, and any specialized adaptive driving equipment.

To optimize person–vehicle fit experiences, the occupational therapist observes the person in his or her own vehicle and ensures the following:

- The seat belt is worn with the chest strap crossing though the mid-clavicle and across the sternum, and the lap belt is positioned low across the hip bones;
- The chest is at least 10 in. from the center of the steering wheel, which is angled toward the chest for optimal seat positioning;
- The seat height is raised to where the eyes are at least 3 in. above the steering wheel;
- The head restraint is positioned with the middle of the back of the head 2.5 in. away or closer and to the middle of the head restraint;
- The driver's feet reach the pedals without the driver reaching or pointing the toes; and
- Mirrors are positioned to maximize visibility and reduce blind spots.

Environment

Environmental factors include the chosen routes and roadways, traffic density, frequency of road trips, passengers in the vehicle during the trips, and exposure to other road users. When inquiring about the routes and types of roadways traveled, the occupational therapist must gather information on the characteristics of the roads, such as whether they are residential, rural, or highway, and on the characteristics of roadways, such as whether they include stop signs, traffic lights, unprotected turns, school zones, or construction sites. Clearly, such elements can increase environmental complexity and will require more visual, cognitive, and psychomotor reserves than simply driving—which itself requires simultaneous use of visual, cognitive, and motor skills.

Understanding the individual driver's attention to environmental characteristics contributes to the assessment of the person's capacity to safely (or conversely unsafely) negotiate the complex driving environment. Obtaining details on the presence and roles of passengers and pets may provide useful information related to driver–passenger (in)dependence or environmental distracters. For example, the driver may be dependent on the "way-finding" cues given by a passenger to effectively negotiate roadways. Such passenger copiloting functions are not desired behaviors and may be indicative of the driver's declining cognitive or visual functions.

Functional Limitations That May Affect Driving

Limitations in vision, cognitive functioning, and physical functioning can significantly affect a client's ability to safely drive or move about the community. It is important for occupational therapists to accurately assess these three particular areas during the evaluation process.

Vision Functioning

Eye-related diseases that affect driving may include macular degeneration, glaucoma, diabetic retinopathy, or functional visual impairments (e.g., inability to see objects in the driving environment that leads to near misses, poor lane keeping, inability to read road signs). Discussing each of the eye conditions is beyond the scope of this chapter; see Chapter 8 for a detailed description of interventions associated with vision-related diseases.

The occupational therapist must focus on assessing and interpreting functional impairments as a result of the underlying disease process. Such limitations may include decreased visual acuity that may hinder the ability to read road signs; impaired depth perception that may make objects seem closer or farther away than their actual position and therefore lead to tailgating, hitting or running over curbs, or making turns too wide; and impaired contrast sensitivity that may interfere with the ability to see low-contrast structures such as medians during dusk and nighttime driving.

Cognitive Functioning

Many neurological disorders and chronic diseases, currently on the rise with the aging of the baby boomers, may impair cognitive functions. For a detailed discussion of cognitive diseases, please refer to Chapter 7. Key cognitive skills necessary for driving are orientation; attention; memory; processing speed; and visual–cognitive functions, such as visual attention. Related driving skills affected by such cognitive limitations may be decreased way finding, impaired road sign recognition, impaired dual-task driving, and distracted driving.

Not having the desired cognitive skills may have deleterious effects on safe driving. For example, slowed processing time may affect reaction time, which may lead to delayed braking responses and potentially result in rear-ending a car. Poor divided or selective attention disrupts one's ability to attend to multiple road, vehicle, and environmental stimuli, which often occur simultaneously in the driving environment (Uc, Rizzo, Anderson, Shi, & Dawson, 2004; Uc et al., 2006, 2007). Memory loss may lead to forgetting driving destinations, getting lost in familiar areas, or even being at risk for further adverse events as a result of getting lost (Hunt, Brown, & Gilman, 2010).

Physical Functioning

Age-related physical conditions such as arthritis or chronic pain may impair the physical skills underlying driving performance. For example, adequate range of motion, strength, coordination, gait, static and dynamic balance, postural control, proprioception, stereognosis, and kinesthesia are necessary, but not essential, physical skills required for safe driving. If these skills are not intact, problems may arise in the driver's ability to execute control over the vehicle or to safely maneuver the vehicle in the driving environment. For example, poor coordination skills may lead to the inability to manipulate vehicle equipment effectively, such as under- or overshooting while trying to adjust or manipulate the vehicle controls. Impaired upper-body strength may result in problems with maneuvering the vehicle safely, evidenced in poor execution of lane keeping or making turns too wide. Decreased strength and range of motion (ROM) may cause problems with ingress and egress, such as difficulty lifting feet into or out of the vehicle, or with safe handling of the vehicle, such as displaying jerkiness during steering or accelerating erratically.

Strategies to Compensate for Functional Limitations

In deciding on strategies to compensate for visual, cognitive, and physical limitations, the planning process is done in conjunction with the client and family members, when appropriate, to ensure a client-centered approach in prioritizing the goals for continued safe mobility. The intervention plan must take into consideration the array of programs and resources available in the community. The occupational therapist may teach the client compensatory strategies, such as visual search or scanning, or may refer the client to a vision specialist such as an ophthalmologist or functional optometrist. Examples of these processes are clearly described in Case Example 11.1.

Behind-the-Wheel Assessment and On-Road Performance

The on-road portion of the comprehensive driving evaluation offers the real-world context of the client's interface with both the vehicle and the driving environment. By observing the environmental context while on-road, the driving rehabilitation specialist (DRS) uses his or her clinical reasoning skills and theoretical perspective to critically observe, analyze, and describe the client's driving performance.

The occupational therapist will recapitulate the errors made. For example, the therapist will take into consideration the amount of errors, type of errors, location of errors, and whether the errors are a result of the person's driving habits or deficit as determined from the previous clinical information. The occupational therapist also will discern how critical the errors are. For example, the therapist will determine whether a particular error is critical, such as the client driving at high speed

Case Example 11.1. Mr. P. G.: Idiopathic Parkinson's Disease

Personal History

Mr. P. G. is a 67-year-old White man living in the community with his wife; he has a driver's license in Florida. He had some college education after high school graduation. He was referred by a neurologist with specialty training in movement disorders from the Movement Disorders Center with a concern about his continued safe driving.

Medical History

The client's primary diagnosis, made 17 years ago, is idiopathic Parkinson's disease. He self-reports that he has high blood pressure (5 years), Type II diabetes (6 years), thyroid disorder (8 years), sleep apnea (10 years), and arthritis in the bilateral knees and neck (3 weeks). He has had deep brain stimulation (DBS), implanted with a single lead 3 months before his comprehensive driving evaluation, and his stimulator has been adjusted for optimal functioning once out of the four scheduled times. He wears eyeglasses with trifocal lenses. At the time of the evaluation, he was cooperative but appeared to have a flat affect.

Medications

All medication information was obtained from the *Clinical Pharmacology* 2010 Web site (www.clinicalpharmacology-ip.com) and is documented in Table 11.1. The table represents all the medications that Mr. P.G. is currently taking.

Table 11.1. Mr. P. G.'s Medications

Drug	Dosage	Class	Action	Potential Side Effects to Driving
Stalevo	75 mg, 1 tab 5 times per day	Neurological agent	Combination product for the treatment of idiopathic Parkinson's disease	Sleepiness, hyperkinesias, dyskinesia
Synthroid	0.1 mg, 1 tab per day	Hormone and hormone modifier	Exhibits actions of endogenous thyroid hormone	Mental status changes
Singulair	30 mg, 1 tab per day	Respiratory agent	Respiratory anti-inflammatory agent	Drowsiness, disorientation
Sinemet	25/100 mg, 2 tabs 6 times per day	Neurological agent	Antiparkinsonian agent	Sudden sleep, dyskinesia, sporadic movements, anxiety, confusion, dizziness
Celebrex	200 mg, 1 tab per day	Nonsteroidal anti-inflammatory drug, COX-2 inhibitor	Musculoskeletal anti-inflammatory agent	Increased risk of serious cardiovascular thrombotic events, myocardial infarction, and stroke
Nexium	20 mg, 1 tab per day	Gastrointestinal agent	Anti-ulcer agent	None
Benicar	20 mg, 1 tab 2 times per day	Cardiovascular agent	Antihypertensive agent	Dizziness, syncope
Metformin ER	500 mg, 2 tabs per day	Hormone or hormone modifier	Anti-diabetic agent	None
Toviaz	4 mg, 1 tab per day	Genitourinary agents	Bladder antispasmodic	Insomnia, stomach pain, chest pain, back pain
Nasonex	2 sprays each nostril per day	Respiratory agents	Respiratory anti-inflammatory agent	Chest pain, musculoskeletal pain

(Continued)

Case Example 11.1. Mr. P. G.: Idiopathic Parkinson's Disease (*cont.*)

Summary of Medications and Their Potential Effect on Driving

A drug interaction report for all 10 medications places this person at Level 3, which is considered a moderate level of risk for experiencing adverse events from drug–drug interactions. Alterations in the drug therapy may be required by the physician. Therefore, the client should be monitored for possible symptoms of interactions. The drug interactions may result in additive hypotensive effects, gastrointestinal effects, and changes in glycemic control and blood glucose. (see www.clinicalpharmacology-ip.com/Default.aspx. Note: This Web site requires membership. To identify potentially driver-impairing prescription drugs, also see www.drivinghealth.com/PDIdrugindex.html.)

The combination of all of these drugs indicates that there may be times when this person should not be driving, especially when having an off day because of PD symptoms and adverse reactions to medication. This patient should be retested periodically (at least once per year or more often if changes in medication or declines in medical status, performance skills, or client factors take place).

The occupational therapist must ask questions about the client's medication intake and compliance, including the following: What medications is the person consuming? Any new medications? Prescribed and over-the-counter medications, herbs, or supplements? Do medications pose side effects to driving? If so, how do the medications affect driving? Are there contraindications?

Conclusion on Medications

The occupational therapist determined that the client is on 10 medications, representing a variety of classes, which are listed in Table 11.1. The side effects (e.g., sudden sleep, confusion or dyskinesias, dizziness, syncope) may affect driving performance, because the medications potentially alter levels of alertness, orientation, mentation, and motor performance. From the theoretically derived interaction report, the occupational therapist determined that the interaction effects of the medications score at a moderate risk level, putting the client at a potential risk for unsafe driving performance. The occupational therapist should consider consulting with the referring physician to address driving-related concerns and recommend annual retesting to the client or caregiver.

Driving History

Mr. P. G. drives a 2007 Buick Century. He usually drives about 5 times per week in the community to access goods (e.g., shopping and services, doctor appointments). His main passenger is his wife. He does not use alternative forms of community mobility. He self-reports that he has not been in any crashes in the past 3 years, nor did has he received any citations or violations within the same time period. Before the DBS he drove minimally, but after the improvement in function resulting from the DBS he increased his frequency of driving again. He reports taking a driving education class more than 3 years ago but did not elaborate on the type or content. The driving evaluator suspects that he had been pulled over by a law enforcement officer and that the driving education class was a mandatory defensive driving class. He uses no adaptive equipment in his car and has not had a prior comprehensive driving evaluation.

Conclusion on Driving History

Mr. P. G. is dependent on his automobile as his primary source of transportation and seems to be actively involved in driving-related activities. He is still driving 5 times per week and seems to be a safe driver but is suspected of perhaps having had a citation for a moving violation.

Self-Report

Upon asking the client, his wife, and the neurologist whether the client will pass or fail the on-road evaluation, the client responded "pass," his wife responded "pass," and the neurologist responded "fail."

The occupational therapist scored him 297/340 on the Safe Driving Behaviors Measure (Classen et al., 2010), the client scored himself 336/340, and his wife scored him 300/340. The client and wife both reported that he is very good at determining whether he is having a good or bad day as relates to Parkinson's disease and medication-related symptoms. They both said that he does not drive at all when he has recognized increased sleepiness, tremors, or extreme discomfort.

Conclusion on Self-Report

The self-report gives the occupational therapist a perspective on how the person views himself as a driver and the level of awareness of his strengths and limitations. In this case, the client and his wife display insight into his driving performance. Interestingly the client overrates his safe driving ability level compared with his wife and the occupational therapist.

Clinical Tests

Mr. P. G. completed the battery of visual, cognitive, and motor clinical tests from the driving center. The tests, scores, results, and interpretation are presented in Table 11.2.

Case Example 11.1. Mr. P. G.: Idiopathic Parkinson's Disease (*cont.*)

Table 11.2. Summary of the Battery of Clinical Tests

Clinical Tests	Score	Results	Interpretation
Vision: Optec 2500 visual analyzer			
Peripheral visual field: tested at 85°, 70°, 55°, and 35° in each eye	Intact when all are correct, impaired when one or more fields are not seen	Intact for all degrees	WFL
Static acuity for distance: both eyes, right eye, left eye	State requirement is ≤20/70 with or without corrected lenses	20/70 both eyes, 20/40 right eye, 20/40 left eye; skipping around, missing letters and adding letters	Impaired binocular vision, intact monocular vision in the left and right eye; WFLs for the state requirement
Color discrimination	2 or more incorrect = impaired	2 incorrect	Mildly impaired
Depth perception	Any floating circles missed = impaired	Missed 5/9	Severely impaired
Contrast sensitivity[a]	5 slides (A, B, C, D, E) representing different visual structures in the CNS with response options varying from sharp contrast to low contrast across for each of the 9 options per slide, rated as WFLs or impaired	All responses were within functional limits, with D and E being in the low range of normal, implying that the client may have some difficulty in unfamiliar environments with limited contrast, such as streets not well lit	WFL
Lateral phorias	Identify an object from a variety of objects on the horizontal level	Only 1 correct object should be identified in a range of objects	Impaired, as the client identified an object outside the range
Vertical phorias	Identify an object from a variety of objects on the vertical level	Only 1 correct object should be identified in a range of objects	Intact, as the client identified an object within the range
Saccades	Intact when both eyes are moving smoothly	Noticeable strabismus of both eyes horizontally	Impaired
Glare recovery[a]	Self-report	Deny	WFL
Cognition			
Mini-Mental State Examination (Folstein et al., 1975)	≤26 = mild cognitive impairment	30	Intact
Trail Making, Part B (Reitan, 1958)	Complete test in <3 min (180 s)	3 min, 27 s; skipped letters and required verbal cuing to complete test as per protocol	Impaired
Uttl letter cancellation (Uttl & Pilkenton-Taylor, 2001)	Two timed trials and omissions and commissions are counted	Trial 1: 1 min, 7 s; 1 omission, 0 commissions; Trial 2: 1 min, 5 s; 0 omissions, 0 commissions	WFL

(Continued)

Case Example 11.1. Mr. P. G.: Idiopathic Parkinson's Disease (*cont.*)

Table 11.2. Summary of the Battery of Clinical Tests (*cont.*)

Clinical Tests	Score	Results	Interpretation
Visual attention			
UFOV 1	500 ms	56.7 ms	Intact
UFOV 2	500 ms	159.9 ms	Impaired
UFOV 3	500 ms	280.1 ms	Intact
UFOV risk index	Category 1–5, with 5 being very high risk for motor vehicle crashes	Category 3	Moderate risk
Motor			
ROM: Trunk and neck, left and right	WFL or impaired	Impaired	Impaired
ROM: Upper extremity, left and right	WFL or impaired	WFL	WFL
ROM: Lower extremity, left and right	WFL or impaired	WFL	WFL
Strength: Upper extremity, left and right	WFL or impaired	WFL	WFL
Strength: Lower extremity, left and right	WFL or impaired	WF	WFL
Coordination: Upper extremity, left and right	Intact or impaired	Intact	Intact
Coordination: Lower extremity, left and right	Intact or impaired	Intact	Intact
Grip strength	WFL or impaired	WFL	WFL
Ambulation or gait	WFL or impaired	WFL	WFL
Transfers	Independent, assisted, dependent	Independent	Independent
Rapid-pace walk	>7 s has a risk for motor vehicle crash involvement	6.15 s	WFL
Other sensory			
Proprioception: Upper extremity, left and right; lower extremity, left and right	WFL or impaired	WFL	WFL

Case Example 11.1. Mr. P. G.: Idiopathic Parkinson's Disease (*cont.*)

Table 11.2. Summary of the Battery of Clinical Tests (*cont.*)

Clinical Tests	Score	Results	Interpretation
Stereognosis: Upper extremity, left and right	WFL or impaired	WFL	WFL
Kinesthesias: Upper extremity, left and right; lower extremity, left and right	WFL or impaired	WFL	WFL
Sensation: Upper extremity, left and right; lower extremity, left and right	WFL or impaired	WFL	WFL
On-road test			
Global rating score	Pass, pass with recommendations, fail with remediation potential, fail	Pass with recommendations: • Plan for driving retirement • Driver education • Driving reevaluation every year • Driving restrictions. Some suggestions: no highway driving; do not drive on off days when experiencing limiting Parkinson's symptoms; have someone drive with client periodically; no long-distance driving; limit noise in car	Pass with recommendations and restrictions
Sum of maneuvers score	0–273, with 273 = perfect driving; driving center's cut-off for failing ≤230	252	Pass with recommendations to avoid complex driving, such as highway driving and driving in rush-hour traffic
SDBM (Classen et al., 2010)	336 (by client self-report)	Driver reported no difficulty with most behaviors and moderate difficulty with driving when talking to passengers and with complex drives	Client is potentially not safe with passengers in the vehicle who may cause distraction and when negotiating very complex driving situations, for example, driving in peak traffic hours or having to negotiate multiple road stimuli such as busy intersections; therapist made a strong recommendation to restrict driving to avoid these situations

Note. CNS = central nervous system; SDBM = Safe Driving Behaviors Measure; ROM = range of motion; UFOV = Useful Field of View; WFL = within functional limits.

[a]Assesment is discussed in Chapter 9.

(Continued)

Case Example 11.1. Mr. P. G.: Idiopathic Parkinson's Disease (*cont.*)

Summary of Performance on the Visual Test

Questions that stimulate the clinical reasoning process: Does the client have any visual impairments? If so, is he aware of the problem and does he understand how it affects driving? Should there be a recommendation to see an eye-care specialist?

Conclusion on Visual Test

The client will be referred to an eye care specialist for the limitations with his lateral phorias (procedural reasoning). This client will be educated on his visual impairment and how the limitations in his depth perception and binocular vision may influence his driving. In this case, the client experienced objects appearing farther away than where they really were (procedural reasoning). A compensatory strategy will be to discuss executing a maneuver, for example, stopping at a stop sign, by watching environmental cues such as being able to see the lane markings of the white line in front of the vehicle and the stop sign to the front corner of the vehicle (conditional reasoning); see Figure 11.1.

Summary of Performance on the Cognitive Tests

Questions that stimulate the clinical reasoning process: Does testing reveal cognitive impairment? Has the person been diagnosed with an impairment? Is this the first time this driver has received feedback? Is a referral to the primary care physician or neurologist appropriate? Does the occupational therapist need to give specific examples and explain what cognition is and how it affects thinking and driving?

Conclusion on Cognitive Tests

This client had poor divided attention skills (procedural reasoning). He is counseled by the occupational therapist on strategies to avoid distractions in his vehicle, such as eating, drinking, or having a conversation during driving (procedural reasoning).

Summary of Performance on the Physical Tests

Questions that stimulate the clinical reasoning process: What physical impairment affects driving and the ability to transfer in and out of the person's vehicle? Are there adaptive equipment needs? If so, what would be appropriate? Is cognition sufficient for new learning about the equipment? Does the person need to be referred to occupational or physical therapy to increase endurance, strength, movement, or coordination?

Conclusion on Physical Tests

This client has moderate stiffness in his neck and is limited in his trunk rotation (procedural reasoning). He understands how these limitations can affect his driving, for example, not seeing objects in his blind spots because doing so requires turning the head and upper trunk to look to the left (interactive reasoning). The occupational therapist will further recommend flexibility training, obtaining blind-spot mirrors, and receiving instruction on positioning of the side mirrors and the client's position in his car to optimize his field of view (conditional reasoning).

<u>Stop at a stop sign so car stops completely before the marked line and the stop sign is to the front corner of the vehicle</u>

Correct   Incorrect

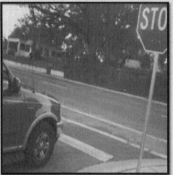
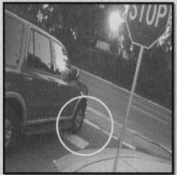

Figure 11.1. Example of a compensatory strategy taught to a patient with depth perception and binocular vision problems as it pertains to stopping at a stop sign.

Case Example 11.1. Mr. P. G.: Idiopathic Parkinson's Disease (*cont.*)

Summary of Performance on the Visual, Cognitive, and Physical Tests

Questions that stimulate the clinical reasoning process: Is there a medical diagnosis of a progressive disease? Where is this person in the stages of disease progression? Are medication effects or interactions impairing the person? Does the occupational therapist need more information from the client's health care professionals, family, or caregivers? Which are the major and minor areas impairing the client's ability to drive safely and independently? Where can the occupational therapist assist to improve independence? What referrals can the occupational therapist make to improve the client's overall health and well-being?

Conclusion on All Tests

Mr. P. G. is an older man with a diagnosis of Parkinson's disease made 17 yr ago and is functioning with the use of a DBS and the use of 10 medications (procedural reasoning). He is well medicated and verbalizes how the side effects of his medications affect his functioning and driving performance (interactive reasoning). The client is experiencing impairment in lateral phoria and has visual–perceptual problems. His main cognitive impairment pertains to divided attention deficit. According to the client and his caregiver, his physical functioning has improved significantly after the DBS implant, but he has impairments with left-sided coordination and is limited in his neck and trunk flexibility (interactive reasoning). The occupational therapist recommended client education, compensatory strategies, and referral to an eye care specialist, as well as vehicle adaptation strategies, to address his visual, cognitive, and physical limitations (conditional reasoning).

Summary of Performance on the On-Road Evaluation

Questions that stimulate the clinical reasoning process: What types of errors were made? How often were those errors made? Were they common errors (e.g., rolling stops)? Were they critical errors (e.g., running a red light)? What may be causing the errors? Does this person need specialized or adaptive vehicle equipment? What is the person's financial status? Who will pay for behind-the-wheel training or equipment?

Conclusion on On-Road Evaluation

The client made common errors, such as not coming to a complete stop or stopping over the white line. He drifted to the left twice during the drive, but no vehicles were approaching. He had speed regulation errors, mostly going slower than the posted speed limit. He had 4 vehicle positioning errors and 2 signaling errors. The occupational therapist's findings were that he probably made the common errors as a result of the visual–perceptual deficits and that he generally drives slower than the posted speed limit, perhaps because of his divided attention deficits (procedural). The client mentioned that he knew when he had an off day and that he did not drive on those days (interactive reasoning). The client did not, as such, engage in any dangerous driving behaviors. The client did not need any adaptive equipment (conditional reasoning).

Final Summary of Decision for Continued Driving

Questions that stimulate the clinical reasoning process: Will behind-the-wheel training increase safety and independence? Does the person have cognition of and insight into his deficits? If not, then training will be difficult. If the client cannot acknowledge a problem, it will be challenging to get the person to understand the meaning and purpose of the training. Is comprehension and retention of new learning a problem? If so, it will be frustrating for the person to learn how to use new equipment. Should the client retire from driving? What is the time frame for this transition? Is it appropriate to discuss community mobility and transportation options? Should the person be reported?

Final Conclusion

The occupational therapist recommended that Mr. P. G.

- Continue to drive, with strong recommendations for driving in low-traffic, low-speed roadways; avoiding driving on off days or driving longer distances (more than 15 mi), and limiting noise, conversation, and activity (e.g., eating, drinking) in the vehicle;
- Return for yearly comprehensive driving evaluations, or sooner if there is a decrease in medical or functional status;
- Always come to a complete stop at a stop sign and stay behind the white line;
- Return for 6 to 8 hr of behind-the-wheel training to help him compensate for the visual, cognitive, and physical limitations;

(Continued)

Case Example 11.1. Mr. P. G.: Idiopathic Parkinson's Disease (*cont.*)

- Consider seeing an eye care specialist for a comprehensive vision evaluation to determine whether intervention is necessary (e.g., prism glasses);
- Invite his wife periodically to drive with him to check his driving and to provide feedback on his driving behaviors; she will look for driving errors such as driving out of his lane and other hazardous driving behaviors; if her feedback does not assist in correcting errors, a comprehensive driving evaluation should be scheduled immediately;
- Consider driving retirement planning and the use of transportation options in the event that he can no longer drive safely; and
- Visit the Florida Senior Safety Resource Center (finding transportation options that meet a list of 5 transportation priorities identified in this comprehensive driving evaluation process or some manner of structuring this exploration, allowing him to explore the pros and cons, to enhance success) and consider alternative transportation options via the Web site http://fssrc.phhp.ufl.edu.

The results of the report were discussed with the client, his caregiver, and the referring physician at the Movement Disorders Center. The occupational therapist used a client-centered and family-centered approach to discuss Mr. P. G.'s deficits and how his limitations may affect his continued independence and safety in driving and community mobility. Both the client and his caregiver acknowledged how his medical condition, his deficits, and his medications affected his driving ability. Mr. P. G. and his wife were open to the recommendations made by the occupational therapist and spontaneously provided suggestions on how to integrate these recommendations. Both Mr. P. G. and his wife acknowledged that they needed to start the planning process for his driving retirement and articulated their plan to start exploring the use of alternative transportation options.

and endangering himself or herself and other road users, or whether the driving error is common, such as not turning on a signal (Shechtman, Awadzi, Classen, Lanford, & Joo, 2010).

Virtual Reality Driving Simulator

The interactive driving simulator is used to observe driving habits, behaviors, and errors in a more protected environment, free from real contact with other roadway users. The term *simulator* describes machines that may range from very simple to highly complex. Occupational therapists must take caution to understand the machine (the model and characteristics of the simulator) and its capabilities when interpreting descriptions of interactive driving simulation–based programs and promised outcomes. For example, some simulators offer a single-screen monitor with a gas–brake pedal box placed on the floor and a table-mounted joystick to "drive" the car through obstacles, and others may place a driver in a vehicle cab projecting immersive video on screens surrounding the vehicle. Each simulator measures driver responses of vehicle control and evasive maneuvers. The therapist must take the ethical responsibility to understand the strengths and limitations of the performance observed and the data gathered.

Similar to the on-road evaluation, data are collected on the type, frequency, and location of driving errors, understanding that these errors are programmatically defined and gathered. If the driver hits an object during the simulated drive, no (actual) injuries or damage occurs. Data can be collected about driving behaviors while conducting particular maneuvers, such as the time between visual display of a hazard (e.g., simulated car enters roadway from the right) and the driver's response such as applying the brake (commonly described as *speed of response*). Simulation offers the graded opportunity to modify the driving scenarios to tailor the assessment and on-road experience to address assessment and training goals.

Table 11.3. Michon's Behavior Model

Domain	Definition	Example of Activity for Therapist to Use
Strategic	Reflects general goal formation including trip planning and selecting a route and its alternatives	Planning a trip or deciding to drive with or without a passenger
Operational	Involves the ability to control the vehicle given the environmental or situational influences (Ranney, 1994)	Teaching the client to safely execute a driving maneuver such as coming to a complete stop
Tactical	Reflects the navigational influences of the selected route, such as turns, curves, and traffic planning	Teaching the client, by using a virtual reality driving simulator, rapid responses to avoid collisions

Understanding driver limitations after the road evaluation (on-road or via simulation) helps occupational therapists to determine why particular errors are made and to assist in the development of recommendations for driving status or in developing a community mobility plan. For example, if a client drives too closely to vehicles (tailgates) and hits curbs while turning, a judgment can be made that poor depth perception (data obtained during clinical testing) might be interfering with the ability to make accurate assessments with distance of other vehicles and curbs. However, for a different client who hits the curb, this error might be associated with binocularity problems or visual–spatial deficits. It is the therapist's responsibility to do a comparative analysis of the clinical testing results with the actual or simulated driving behaviors.

Behind-the-Wheel Performance

Strategies may include general recommendations addressing each of the driving domains (strategic, operational, and tactical) as identified by Michon (1985; Table 11.3).

The effectiveness of performance skills and patterns may further be enhanced through on-road training. For example, if the client is making wide turns and touching the shoulder of the road, behind-the-wheel training is useful, as the therapist can point out errors and teach the client compensatory strategies. This training may involve instructing the client to gauge the turn on the basis of the position from the midline of the vehicle to the road. In follow-up sessions with the client, the occupational therapist establishes safe behaviors through repetition, feedback, and practice.

Adaptive Vehicle Equipment and Training

In some cases, the occupational therapist will use an evaluation vehicle equipped for evaluation and training (Exhibit 11.1). For example, if the client cannot use his or her right foot to drive because of an amputation, decreased ROM, or strength or coordination limits, the occupational therapist will provide options to train the client to use a left-foot accelerator or hand controls with the appropriate steering device or equipment. The occupational therapist will allow the person to test both options and then initiate training with the client, according to his or her preferred method, in a test vehicle. Usually the training will start in a low-traffic situation, such as a parking lot, and then progress to low-speed public roads, and finally expose the client to higher-speed demands and higher-traffic roadways. A good

---

Exhibit 11.1. The Evaluation Vehicle

The vehicle used to evaluate a client's ability to drive is equipped with an assortment of models of driving controls (e.g., gas, brake, steering) to allow the therapist to evaluate which control system will best meet the client's needs. The systems typically used include steering column–mounted hand controls for left-hand use; a left-foot accelerators; and a floor-mounted, push–pull hand-control system for right-hand use. The driving controls can be easily swapped out by the therapist by using a system of quick-disconnect mounting bases permanently installed in the vehicle. The steering wheel has a base to accept a steering knob, a single post, or a specialized orthotic cuff. This base can be relocated anywhere on the steering wheel to optimize the client's strength and ROM. The evaluation vehicle will also require an instructor brake on the passenger side to allow the therapist to stop or slow the vehicle if needed.

---

resource has been developed by the AAA Foundation in collaboration with the University of Florida, called *Smart Features for Mature Drivers*, and this brochure, with practical hints and tips for older adults to use enhanced vehicle features, is available from AAA (2008).

Referrals to Other Health Care Professionals or Services

The occupational therapist addressing driving and community mobility will build a network of adjunctive professional services, and referring clients to other health care professionals (e.g., neuro-ophthalmologist, physical therapist) is always considered where and if appropriate. Additionally, the occupational therapist should consider other services, such as those provided by **Eldercare** (www.eldercarelink.com, www.eldercare.gov/Eldercare.NET/Public/Index.aspx), to get the client assistance for meal delivery or other assistance in community mobility (see Chapter 2). A primary aim in recommending these services is to increase the client's general health, independence, and well-being, which are determinants of fitness to drive.

Stakeholder Education

The occupational therapist views the client as an entity who is intrinsically involved with and influenced by other stakeholders, such as caregivers, family members, other clinicians, court officials, or the state licensing authority. It is of utmost importance that the occupational therapist be knowledgeable of various resources (both local and national) and communicate with all interested and appropriate stakeholders to ensure a high standard of care and continuity in the delivery of services. As such, the necessary information from the evaluation, interventions, or derived outcomes must be shared, with the client's consent, with other stakeholders.

Driving Cessation

When planning for transition to driving retirement or driving cessation, the occupational therapist will provide education to the client and his or her family members or caregivers (see **Appendix 11.A** for resources). The therapist may suggest and facilitate options for driving retirement (e.g., locating a senior retirement community that offers transportation). The therapist also may assist the person with the process when the recommendation is driving cessation (to stop driving). The therapist should promote planning for driving retirement so that driving cessation is not abrupt. In some cases, abrupt cessation is unavoidable, and the therapist may immediately help the person to find alternative transportation sources.

The client may be introduced to new resources, including the availability of community services such as accessible and affordable alternative transportation options (see Chapter 2). For examples of how specific states are addressing the importance of making these resources available to the public, see up-to-date resources in Florida at http://fssrc.phhp.ufl.edu, and in California at www.dmv.ca.gov/about/senior/senior_top.htm.

The client also will be introduced, through consultation, to services provided by the community for ease of access to goods. Such services may include those delivered by Eldercare (e.g., assistance with medication delivery or grocery shopping). Finally, the occupational therapist may assist the client in becoming proficient, through education and training, in the use of public transportation. Community mobility training may entail teaching the client to read a bus or a train schedule, how to purchase tickets, and how to manage successful entry to and egress from public modes of transportation.

Recommendations for Determining Fitness to Drive

Discussion, treatment planning, and follow-up will be initiated with the client and the consenting caregiver or family member, initially and throughout the occupational therapy process by means of oral and written documentation. The occupational therapist will make recommendations via report writing to the referral sources (e.g., primary referring physician, health care specialist). Appendix 11.B provides an example of a summary report (on the basis of client Mr. P. G.'s performance during the comprehensive driving evaluation) prepared for a referring health care provider.

If necessary, the occupational therapist will be in contact with the Department of Highway Safety and Motor Vehicles (DHSMV), Division of Drivers Licenses, or the equivalent licensing authority (the name of the authority varies by state) by submitting a report of test results and recommendations. **Appendix 11.C** provides an example of the **Florida DHSMV medical reporting form**, a summary report prepared for the Medical Advisory Board of the Florida DHSMV. (This form can be retrieved from http://www.flhsmv.gov/forms/72190.pdf and is also on the flash drive.)

Summary

The goal of this chapter was to familiarize occupational therapists with the data collection and clinical reasoning processes to determine fitness to drive by way of a comprehensive driving evaluation, discussing how to collect relevant data about driving perceptions and skills and make recommendations on the basis of data. The occupational therapist must account for the person, vehicle, and environment factors as they relate to driving. It is essential that the therapist accurately incorporate all of the information to make sound clinical decisions and recommendations regarding the client's driving fitness and community mobility.

References

American Automobile Association. (2008). *Smart features for mature drivers*. Retrieved August 6, 2009, from www.aaaexchange.com/Main/Default.asp?CategoryID=3&SubCategoryID=38&ContentID=363

Classen, S., Winter, S. M., Velozo, C. A., Bédard, M., Lanford, D., Brumback, B., et al. (2010). Item development and validity testing for a safe driving behavior measure. *American Journal of Occupational Therapy, 64*, 296–305. doi:10.5014/ajot.64.2.296

Folstein, M. F., Folstein, S. E., & McHugh, P. R. (1975). Mini-Mental State: A practical method for grading the cognitive state of patients for the clinician. *Journal of Psychiatric Research, 12*, 189–198.

Hunt, L. A., Brown, A. E., & Gilman, I. P. (2010). Drivers with dementia and outcomes of becoming lost while driving. *American Journal of Occupational Therapy, 64*, 225–232. doi:10.5014/ajot.64.2.225

Kramer, P., & Hinojosa, J. (2010). Philosophical and theoretical influences on evaluation. In P. Kramer & J. Hinojosa (Eds.), *Evaluation: Obtaining and interpreting data* (3rd ed., pp. 21–39). Bethesda, MD: AOTA Press.

Mattingly, C., & Fleming, M. H. (1994). *Clinical reasoning: Forms of inquiry in therapeutic practice*. Philadelphia: F. A. Davis.

Michon, J. A. (1985). A critical view of driver behavior models: What do we know, what should we do? In E. L. Evans & R. Schwing (Eds.), *Human behavior and traffic safety* (pp. 485–520). New York: Plenum.

Neistadt, M. E. (1996). Teaching strategies for the development of clinical reasoning. *American Journal of Occupational Therapy, 50*, 676–684. doi:10.5014/ajot.50.8.676

Owsley, C., Stalvey, B. T., Wells, J., & Sloane, M. E. (1999). Older drivers and cataract: Driving habits and crash risk. *Journals of Gerontology, Series A: Biological Sciences and Medical Sciences, 54*, M203–M211.

Ranney, T. A. (1994). Models of driving behavior: A review of their evolution. *Accident Analysis and Prevention, 26*, 733–750.

Reitan, R. M. (1958). Validity of the Trail Making test as an indicator of organic brain damage. *Perceptual and Motor Skills, 8*, 271–276.

Rogers, J. C. (1983). Clinical reasoning: The ethics, science, and art [Eleanor Clarke Slagle lecture]. *American Journal of Occupational Therapy, 37*, 601–616. doi:10.514/ajot.37.9.601

Shechtman, O., Awadzi, K. D., Classen, S., Lanford, D., & Joo, Y. (2010). Validity and critical driving errors of on-road assessment for older drivers. *American Journal of Occupational Therapy, 64*, 242–251. doi:10.514/ajot.37.9.601

Uc, E. Y., Rizzo, M., Anderson, S. W., Shi, Q., & Dawson, J. D. (2004). Driver route-following and safety errors in early Alzheimer disease. *Neurology, 63*, 832–837.

Uc, E. Y., Rizzo, M., Anderson, S. W., Sparks, J. D., Rodnitzky, R. L., & Dawson, J. D. (2006). Driving with distraction in Parkinson disease. *Neurology, 67*, 1774–1780.

Uc, E. Y., Rizzo, M., Anderson, S. W., Sparks, J. D., Rodnitzky, R. L., & Dawson, J. D. (2007). Impaired navigation in drivers with Parkinson's disease. *Brain, 130*(Pt. 9), 2433–2440.

Uttl, B., & Pilkenton-Taylor, C. (2001). Letter cancellation performance across the adult life span. *Clinical Neuropsychologist, 15*, 521–530.

Appendix 11.A. Clinical Reasoning–Related Resources

- **ElderCarelink:** http://www.eldercarelink.com
ElderCarelink is a public service of the U.S. Administration on Aging that connects services for older adults and their families, assisting families in finding such services as assisted living, nursing homes, adult day care, private-duty nursing, care management, and home care. With participating providers in all 50 states, ElderCarelink identifies qualified elder-care service providers and product suppliers that meet the specific needs for each family's individual situation. Transportation-related resources may include options for assistance with meal delivery or transportation options.

- **ElderCare Locator:** http://www.eldercare.gov/Eldercare.NET/Public/Index.aspx
The ElderCare Locator is very useful for clinicians and consumers. It provides a means to search for resources by zip code.

- **DriveWell Toolkit:** http://www.nhtsa.gov/Driving+Safety/Driver+Education/Senior+Drivers/Drive+Well+Toolkit:+Promoting+Older+Driver+Safety+and+Mobility+in+Your+Community)
The DriveWell Toolkit was developed under an NHTSA-funded cooperative agreement with the American Society on Aging. This multifaceted speaker's toolkit offers a range of resources available online. All materials can be used, printed, and distributed free of charge. Credit needs to be offered to the authors, but official permission is not required.

- **Toolkit for Professionals:** http://www.aota.org/Older-Driver/Professionals/CE/Toolkit/Professional.aspx
The Toolkit for Professionals was developed as part of a cooperative agreement between AOTA and NHTSA. The toolkit contains numerous resources and templates for expanding programs and services that address driving and community mobility. Each resource (e.g., how to develop a brochure, conducting an educational seminar for varied audiences, how to estimate costs when proposing the development of a driving rehabilitation program) was developed by the recipients of the mini-grant funding.

- **CarFit:** http://www.car-fit.org
CarFit is a community education program that offers older adults the opportunity to see how well their personal vehicles "fit" them. The CarFit program also provides information and materials on community-specific resources that could enhance safety for drivers or increase their community mobility options.

Appendix 11.B. Summary Report Based on Mr. P. G.'s Performance During the Comprehensive Driving Evaluation

Date: _____

Dear Dr. X. Y.:

RE: Results of Comprehensive Driving Evaluation: Mr. P. G.

Your patient, Mr. P. G., underwent a comprehensive driving evaluation on 4/7/11. I administered a battery of clinical assessments and an on-road evaluation. The clinical tests were used to examine his vision, cognition, and motor performance. The on-road evaluation was used to assess his vehicle positioning and handling of the vehicle, visual scanning, speed control, lane maintenance, signaling, yielding, and adjustment to environmental stimuli.

The results of the evaluation are representative of the client's performance level at the time of the evaluation and may not be predictive of unanticipated medically related issues, roadway conditions, or interactions with other roadway users. Please refer to the clinical summary, on-road summary, and recommendations below.

Clinical Assessment Summary

Physical performance: A physical screen revealed that Mr. P. G.'s overall muscle strength, sensation, and coordination were within functional limits. Neck and trunk rotation to the left and right were moderately impaired. He reported no pain.

Vision: Mr. P. G.'s vision was screened using the OPTEC 2500 vision testing machine. His peripheral vision was normal on both right and left sides. Distance acuity was 20/40 with the right eye and 20/40 with the left eye. He had difficulty reading the eye chart with both eyes. Color discrimination tests noted a mild impairment. Depth perception testing revealed a severe impairment because he could identify only 3 of the 9 "floating objects." He performed within normal limits on the contrast sensitivity test, which examines the ability to see during low-light conditions and at night. *Lateral phoria* (ability for eyes to work together side to side) was impaired, and *vertical phoria* (ability for eyes to work together up and down) were normal. Strabismus was noted during the scanning test. The client denied glare recovery problems, and no further formal testing was pursued.

Cognition: Mr. P. G. scored a 30/30 on the Mini-Mental State Exam (MMSE), indicating no cognitive deficits. It took him 3 minutes and 27 seconds, to complete the Trail Making Part B test, a test of set shifting; this score is considered failing compared with normative data. The test must be completed in 3 min or less to be considered normal. Trails B examined mental flexibility and scanning skills. On the Uttl letter cancellation test, a test of scanning and visual perception abilities, he scored within normal limits.

Visual information processing (intersection of vision and cognition): The Useful Field of View (UFOV) Risk Index score (a score indicative of risk for crash involvement) placed Mr. P. G. in Category 3, which is considered a moderate risk for crash involvement (1 indicates a *low risk of being crash involved* and 5 indicates a *very high risk of being crash involved*). The UFOV sub tests revealed normal visual processing speed (Subtest 1), impaired divided attention skills (Subtest 2) and within normal limits for selective attention.

Appendix 11.B. Summary Report Based on Mr. P. G.'s Performance During the Comprehensive Driving Evaluation (*cont.*)

On-Road Assessment Summary

Mr. P. G. was assessed behind the wheel in the test vehicle, a 2007 Buick Century, equipped with dual brakes. I assessed basic parking lot maneuvers (e.g., parking and backing up) and progressed to a more complex environment, including higher speed and higher traffic roadways. He had noticeable deficits during the on-road assessment. For example, he tended not to come to complete stops at stop signs, did not consistently use his turn signal, occasionally drove under the posted speed limit, and crossed the white line during stopping. He performed poorer on the highway, for example, he drove too slowly when merging on the highway and drifted toward the left, requiring verbal cues to move the car toward the right. He was able to safely maneuver the car off of the highway and back to the assessment office.

The results of each component of the evaluation and the recommendations were discussed with Mr. P. G. and his wife. They both seemed to understand the feedback and recommendations. We talked in great detail about his disease progression as it pertains to Parkinson's and its effects on driving abilities. They are both aware that Mr. P. G. may need to retire from driving in the future. We have discussed a plan for continued community mobility and the use of alternative transportation options.

I have provided the following recommendations:

- Do not drive high-traffic or high-speed roadways (e.g., highways).
- Driving reevaluation every year or as needed if medical condition changes.
- Limit talking and restrict other distractions while driving.
- Do not drive during rush hour.
- Plan for driving retirement.
- Begin to seek and explore alternative transportation options via www.fssrc.phhp.ufl.edu.

Thank you for the opportunity to provide this service. Please contact me at xxx-xxx-xxxx if you have any questions.

Sincerely,

_____   _____
A. B., MOT, OTR/L, CDRS   Date
Occupational Therapist
Certified Driving Rehabilitation Specialist

Appendix 11.C. Sample State Medical Reporting Form

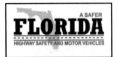

**STATE OF FLORIDA
DEPARTMENT OF HIGHWAY SAFETY
AND MOTOR VEHICLES
DIVISION OF MOTORIST SERVICES**

Medical Reporting Form

Section 322.126 (2), (3), Florida Statutes, provides that "Any physician, person, or agency having knowledge of any licensed driver's or applicant's mental or physical disability to drive...is authorized to report such knowledge to the Department of Highway Safety and Motor Vehicles... The reports authorized by this section shall be confidential... No civil or criminal action may be brought against any physician, person or agency who provides the information herein."

When reporting an individual whose driving ability is questionable due to some physical or mental impairment, please complete as much of the information listed below as possible:

Name:_____   Date of Birth:_____

Address:_____   City:_____

☐   Male   ☐   Female   Zip Code:_____

Driver License Number:_____   State:_____

Physical or Mental Handicaps Noted:

☐   Seizures   ☐   Severe Cardiac Condition   ☐   Stroke

☐   Loss of Consciousness   ☐   Uncontrollable Diabetes   ☐   Dementia/Memory Defects

☐   Psychiatric Disturbance   ☐   Drug/Alcohol Addiction   ☐   Severe Visual Defect

☐   Other

Comments: _____

_____

_____

_____

_____

(Continued)

Appendix 11.C. Sample State Medical Reporting Form (*cont.*)

Originating Source

Date of Report:_____

Name:_____ Signature_____

Address:_____ City:_____

Zip:_____ Telephone:_____

Note: The name and signature of the reporting person is required to investigate the report.

Mail this completed form to:

Division of Motorist Services
Attn: Medical Review Section
Neil Kirkman building, MS 86
Tallahassee, Florida 32399-0500

Fax   (850) 617-3944
Telephone   (850) 617-3814

CHAPTER 12

Behind the Wheel: Driver Rehabilitation Intervention

*Anne Dickerson, PhD, OTR/L, FAOTA,
and Donna Stressel, OTR/L, CDI, CDRS
With Michael D. Justiss, PhD, OTR, and
Michele Luther-Krug, COTA/L, SCADCM, CDRS, ROH*

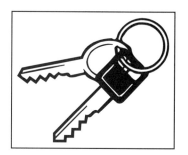

Learning Objectives

At the completion of this chapter, readers will be able to

- Delineate driver education and driver rehabilitation program models so as to use the unique driver interventions effectively,
- Identify appropriate remedial and compensatory intervention strategies for driving based on assessment findings, and
- Delineate the use of remedial and compensatory interventions with appropriate populations.

Key Words

- **closed course**
- **competence**
- **driver rehabilitation program**
- **driver–vehicle fit**
- **fixed route**
- **on-road**
- **performance skills**
- **variable route**

Introduction

Driving assessments, screenings, and evaluations are critically important in ascertaining whether medically at-risk individuals are safe to return to driving, need further intervention to return to driving, or need to consider driving cessation. Current research, particularly in aging, is focused on determining the appropriate and efficient combination of assessment tools, cutoff scores for assessments, and appropriate protocols for specific diagnostic categories (Bédard, Weaver, Dārziņš, & Porter, 2008; Classen et al., 2008; Dickerson et al., 2007; Dickerson, Reistetter, Schold Davis, & Monahan, 2011).

What needs to be just as important to the occupational therapist is intervention. Because driving is one of the most valued instrumental activities of daily living (IADLs; Dickerson, Reistetter, & Gaudy, in press), returning to driving or finding alternative methods of transportation is imperative for a client's well-being. What is the point of assessment unless the therapist uses the information to improve the client's occupational performance and quality of life? This chapter discusses driver rehabilitation intervention. As with many performance-based assessments, the on-road experience can be discussed as both an assessment and an intervention. Different models of driver programs will be described as well as a variety of intervention strategies.

As with all daily living tasks, intervention aimed at achieving the ability to drive can be at the component level (e.g., motor, cognitive, perceptual skills) or at the functional level (e.g., actual driving task), or both. Presently, most driver rehabilitation specialists (DRSs) effectively evaluate the component and functional skill levels through the clinical evaluation and the on-road evaluation. However, intervention by DRSs primarily has aimed at the functional level (behind the wheel), which is reasonable considering the cost of specialized intervention and the fact that there are few DRSs. What may not be addressed are deficits at the component skill level that might be improved through intervention by an occupational therapy generalist before or after a driving evaluation.

Thus, a major objective of this chapter is to consider intervention needed for clients to improve the chances of a positive driving evaluation outcome. As IADLs, community mobility and driving are essential areas of occupation in the occupational therapist's domain of practice. General-practice occupational therapists should address these areas of occupation through improving performance skills for driving and community mobility and determining the appropriate time for referral to a DRS.

Performance Skills for Driving

One way of considering the skills of driving is Michon's (1985) Hierarchy of Driving Behavior. Michon categorized driving into three levels of behavior: (1) strategic, (2) tactical, and (3) operational. The higher-level decision-making process is the *strategic* level of driving behavior, which includes determination of trip goals and mode of traveling, navigation or mapping to where one is going, and related personal factors. Decisions at this level affect all aspects of driving, including the decision of competency to perform driving tasks. The *tactical* level pertains to decisions made during driving maneuvers, including slowing to accommodate weather conditions, deciding whether to pass a vehicle, or making a left-hand turn. The third level, *operational*, captures the human–machine interaction necessary to control the vehicle safely and contains the visual–motor skills or coordination needed to fulfill the tactical-level decisions.

> **Michon categorized driving into three levels of behavior: (1) strategic, (2) tactical, and (3) operational.**

Using Michon's model, one can consider different outcomes at each level. An individual with an intact strategic level of driving may be able to plan a route but needs to have someone with intact operational skills actually drive because of significant physical impairment. The more difficult case is the client with early dementia who still has good operational-level skills but demonstrates impairment in the tactical- and strategic-level skills. The question would be whether there are enough strategic-level skills to compensate for restricted driving that would enable the individual to avoid making risky decisions at the technical level.

For generalist occupational therapists, it may be sufficient to know that the act of driving requires performance skills in the areas of vision, cognition, and physical functioning, and any impairment in any of these areas may affect the ability to drive. One must have adequate skills or the ability to compensate for deficits in any of these areas to operate a motor vehicle and interact with other motor vehicles safely. Previous chapters have individually addressed each of these three areas and the relationship to driving. To provide remedial intervention at the component or skill level of physical, cognitive, visual, or perceptual abilities, generalists can use their usual intervention strategies in each of these areas. Compensation strategies, however, are different because compensation is embedded in the functional performance of the task (see Table 12.1).

Table 12.1. Compensatory Strategies for Driving and Community Mobility

Performance Skills	Performance Implications for Community Mobility	Performance Implications for Driving	Compensatory Strategies for Driving
Acuity • Contrast sensitivity • Night vision • Glare recovery	Depending on degree of impairment, may affect the ability to walk down hallways, sidewalks, or stairs. Can prevent safe crossing at intersections or cause difficulties with uneven terrain. May limit independence in shopping centers or use of public transportation. Orientation and mobility training would benefit individuals with substantial impairment for training with mobility guides and devices.	State minimum requirements will need to be met. Slow to recognize signs and has delayed responses to the environment. Difficulties increase with speed or in low-light situations such as bad weather or entering a tunnel. Difficulty adapting to the dark or bright lights from other vehicles.	Use corrective lenses. Drive on roadways with reduced speed limits and increase following distance. Keep eyes moving and diverted away from glare. Avoid areas or times of day with poor illumination or contrast. May need to restrict driving on cloudy and overcast days, at dusk and dawn, or at night.
Visual field • Peripheral vision • Field cut • Scotomas	Increases probability of bumping into objects or hazards and causing falls. Difficulty in unfamiliar surroundings or crowded areas. Ability to effectively scan decreases with speed or complexity of environment.	May cause random and inefficient eye movements. May miss streets or stimuli on the impaired side. May affect lane position or timing of turns. May not see vehicles on quick glance at intersections or lane changes. May miss hazards. Difficulties increase with complexity of the environment, increased speed, and in the dark.	Use prism lenses to increase field of vision. Compensate with extra head turns and frequent eye movements. Properly adjusted and additional or larger mirrors may be beneficial. May need to have speed-limit or night-driving restrictions. If unable to adequately compensate, will need to refrain from driving.
Visual attention • Neglect	Depending on extent of deficit, can impair ability to safely ambulate within the home and community. May bump into door jambs or other obstacles. Increases potential for falls. Difficulty increases with unfamiliar areas or complexity of environment. Powered mobility (e.g., bicycles, lawn mowers, scooters) should be considered prudently.	May miss important information while attending to other details. May be slow to respond to signs and signals. Disregards signs or hazards to right or left side. May drift out of lane and too close to other objects with little or no improvement when cued.	Insight regarding deficit and impact on driving is usually limited. Deficiency most often prevents safe driving.
Ocular–motor skills • Pursuits • Saccades • Scanning	May have difficulty scanning intersection and safely crossing street. Could prevent ability to ride a bicycle or other form of propelled mobility such as skateboard, scooter, lawn mower, or golf cart. May have difficulty navigating in unfamiliar areas.	May stare at road scene or move eyes randomly and be distracted by any movement. May have difficulty with lane position and keeping track of other vehicles and may miss signs or hazards. May have difficulty sequencing mirror use and blind-spot checks. Will likely miss the most important information and have difficulty dealing with intersections or cross-traffic.	Instruct in proper visual search patterns and efficient scanning. Inability to effectively locate, track, and scan may prevent safe driving.

(Continued)

Table 12.1. Compensatory Strategies for Driving and Community Mobility *(cont.)*

Performance Skills	Performance Implications for Community Mobility	Performance Implications for Driving	Compensatory Strategies for Driving
Stereopsis or depth perception	Difficulty navigating up stairs and curbs. May create problems in crowded or congested areas by colliding with other people or objects.	May have difficulty judging distance, which can affect stopping distance, timing of turns, following distance, gap acceptance, passing, merging, and parking. May have difficulty estimating speeds of other vehicles.	Learn to use environmental cues (e.g., stop lines, crosswalks, tires of car ahead). Instruction in 3-, 6-, 9-second rule for following distance and gap acceptance. May need to limit night driving.
Color perception	Should not impair functional mobility or community mobility.	Difficulty identifying signs based on color only. May have difficulty with horizontal traffic lights. May be slow to respond to brake lights or turn signals.	Learn the sequence of traffic lights and the shapes of signs. Increase following distance.
Visuo-cognition • Visual discrimination • Visual closure • Figure–ground • Spatial relations • Visual memory	Could cause problems with independent travel in school or a shopping mall. May have difficulty navigating from place to place or following a map. May prevent independent use of fixed-route public transportation.	May have difficulty recognizing signs, dealing with intersections, or recognizing hazards. May have difficulty interpreting signs or traffic control devices that are partially occluded. May not be able to interpret a traffic scene or anticipate developing hazards. Inability to distinguish signs, signals, and vehicles from insignificant background. Will have increasing difficulty as traffic increases or the road scene increases in complexity. May have difficulty finding controls or dashboard information quickly. May have difficulty positioning vehicle in center of road or for turns. May have difficulty performing lane changes or merging and may come close to other vehicles or hazards. May have difficulty operating vehicle in reverse or while parking. May impair ability to cross or turn into traffic at intersections. Can impair topographic orientation.	Specific instruction in interpretation of environment and available cues such as waiting to turn the wheel for a turn until the tires are past the curb or using the back of the stop sign facing the opposite direction to identify a stop sign partially occluded by a tree branch. Drivers who are able to compensate may need to limit driving to familiar areas during non–rush hours, reduce speed, and increase following distance. Use of navigational devices may prove beneficial. Significant impairment may prevent safe interaction with other traffic and driving will not be permissible. Restrict driving to familiar areas during non–rush hours.
Visual information processing speed	Could raise safety concerns with other means of powered mobility (e.g., bicycles, lawn mowers, go-carts, power wheelchairs).	Slow to recognize signs, signals, or traffic scene. May drive too slowly. Difficulty increases with complexity of traffic situation or speed.	Limit driving to familiar areas and to roads with reduced speed limits. Avoid peak traffic times or complicated intersections.

(Continued)

Table 12.1. Compensatory Strategies for Driving and Community Mobility *(cont.)*

Performance Skills	Performance Implications for Community Mobility	Performance Implications for Driving	Compensatory Strategies for Driving
Attention • Sustained • Selective • Alternating • Divided	May raise safety concerns with regards to ambulating within the community (e.g., crossing streets, attending to vehicles, being aware of dangers). May have difficulty using modes of public transportation such as buses, subways, and shuttles. May have navigational problems, especially in complex or unfamiliar areas.	May have difficulty maintaining lane integrity or speed control. May miss signs or signals. May be easily distracted and unable to efficiently monitor environment for signs and signals. May miss red arrow below solid green ball at traffic light or the sign for no right on red. May cause delayed braking. May have difficulty maintaining vehicle control while observing mirrors and blind-spot checks when preparing for a lane change or merge. May have difficulty attending to traffic light while waiting for a safe gap to turn. Difficulty attending to signs, signals, other vehicles, and hazards at the same time. May fail to notice pedestrian crossing street while making a left turn at a light and waiting for a safe gap from oncoming traffic. May have problems driving when engaging in a non-driving task such as talking, eating, or looking at a map.	Significant deficit will prevent safe driving. If able to drive, should limit driving to familiar areas and avoid peak traffic times. Limit distractions in vehicle such as eating or drinking, radio play, conversations, electronic devices, and small children or pets.
Memory	May forget or improperly use mobility aids and safety devices such as canes, walkers, brakes on wheelchair, or bike helmets. May have difficulty with navigation and getting lost. May need supervision because of an inability to adhere to restrictions (e.g., assisted transfers, no stairs) or wandering. May not be independent and safe using fixed-route public transportation. Will have difficulty in new or unfamiliar environments and with new routines or schedules.	Difficulty remembering and applying rules of the road. May signal for turn and then fail to make turn, or may stop for stop sign and forget to go when safe. May have difficulty remembering traffic to the left when looking right. May get lost in familiar areas or forget where the car is parked.	Minor deficits may be compensated for by limiting driving to familiar and local areas in daylight hours only. Navigational systems and vehicle locator devices may be useful. Individuals with notable deficits or diagnoses with progressive declines may need to cease driving and be assisted with appropriate alternative transportation options.
Information processing	May have difficulty with other forms of powered mobility.	Slow to react to signs and signals. Has delayed braking in response to other vehicles and hazards. Slow to decide right-of-way and gap acceptance. May brake excessively or unnecessarily. Difficulty increases with speed and complexity of traffic environment.	Limit driving to familiar areas and to roads with reduced speed limits. Avoid peak traffic times or complicated intersections. Minimize distractions and conversations. Deficit may prevent safe driving.

(Continued)

Table 12.1. Compensatory Strategies for Driving and Community Mobility *(cont.)*

Performance Skills	Performance Implications for Community Mobility	Performance Implications for Driving	Compensatory Strategies for Driving
Decision making or judgment	May need assistance transitioning to public transportation. There are safety concerns in public (e.g., trusting strangers, walking in unsafe areas).	Trouble adhering to rules of the road and right-of-way. Difficulty judging safe gap at intersections or when changing lanes. Unable to appropriately respond to errors by other vehicles.	Poor decision making and judgment most likely will prevent safe driving as well as the capability to recognize the dangers of continued driving.
Executive function	May have difficulty with transitioning to alternative transportation or using public transportation.	May be unpredictable with regard to right-of-way and safe gap, being either too hesitant or too hasty. May indicate poor planning for upcoming maneuvers such as observing for a lane change or merge or moving to the left lane to prepare for a left turn. Inability to control emotions causing indecisive or "road rage" responses.	Education and retraining may improve ability to respond to situations appropriately. If unable to correct behaviors and consistently interact with traffic safely, will need to refrain from driving.
Small body size • Height • Lower extremities • Upper extremities	Likely will not directly impair functional mobility or community mobility.	May prevent adequate sitting position for visibility and distance away from air bag. May have poor or uncomfortable fit of seat belt. May have difficulty reaching accelerator and brake. May have difficulty turning steering wheel or reaching dashboard controls.	Careful selection of vehicle and features (i.e., adjustable seat and seat belt, telescoping steering wheel, adjustable pedals). May benefit from seat or back cushion or both. May require adaptive equipment.
Flexibility, strength, endurance, sensation, and pain • Neck and trunk rotation • Upper extremities • Lower extremities	May require a mobility device for long distances or community mobility. May have difficulty using fixed-route public transportation. Can limit ability to manage a mobility aid into and out of vehicle without a loading device.	May have difficulty entering and exiting a vehicle or reaching for seat belt. May have problems turning to observe traffic at intersections or when backing up and parking. May be unable to check blind spots when preparing for lane changes or merging. May have problems reaching to adjust mirrors or accessing gear selector, ignition, directional, or other secondary controls. May have difficulty turning steering wheel. May have difficulty moving foot between accelerator and brake or maintaining pressure on pedal(s). May be unable to set or release a foot-operated parking brake. May be unable to drive for extended periods of time.	Impact of limited neck and trunk rotation is greater when peripheral vision also is reduced. Education on proper adjustment of mirrors and auxiliary or larger mirrors to decrease blind spots. Devices designed to assist with transfers. Vehicle design considerations or driving aids such as a seat belt handle. Power or reduced-effort steering. Location or modification of parking brake. May consider modification to primary or secondary controls. Automatic transmission, power brakes, and cruise control. Adaptation of parking brake. May need to consider hand controls.

Table 12.1. Compensatory Strategies for Driving and Community Mobility *(cont.)*

Performance Skills	Performance Implications for Community Mobility	Performance Implications for Driving	Compensatory Strategies for Driving
Coordination	May prevent individual from learning how to run, ride a bike, or skate. Will affect ability to control other means of powered mobility.	Difficulty operating vehicle with standard transmission. May have difficulty coordinating steering for turns or parking. May have difficulty operating secondary controls on one side or the other.	Use vehicle with automatic transmission. May benefit from adaptive driving equipment designed for use with either right or left extremities if hemiparetic or have problems with integrated coordination (i.e., spinner knob, left foot accelerator).
Reaction time		Slow or delayed responses to signs, light changes, stopping or turning vehicles, or other hazards. Problems intensify with increased speed or traffic congestion.	Drive on roads with reduced speed limits and avoid peak traffic times or congestion. Increase following distance and drive defensively.

Sources. Eby, Molnar, & Shope (2000); Eby, Trombley, Molnar, & Shope (1998).

Driver–Vehicle Fit

Physical Considerations

As part of discharge planning, occupational therapists should ensure that the client is able to access his or her motor vehicle and manage mobility devices. At some health care facilities, getting in and out of a motor vehicle may be a mobility issue that the physical therapist addresses. However, as an IADL, community mobility is within the occupational therapist's domain, including the driver–vehicle fit. There are many vehicle choices whose design in terms of seat or wheel height, visibility, and location of controls supports or impedes the driver–vehicle interaction. The national program CarFit (www.car-fit.org) has identified basic guidelines that allow trained volunteers to assist an older driver with familiarization of driver–vehicle fit. Occupational therapy generalists should be familiar with these guidelines and be able to assist their clients with making vehicle adjustments both as passengers and as drivers, if returning to driving.

If there is an impediment to an appropriate fit, a generalist should know that resources are available and a referral to a DRS may be warranted. For example, an older adult with a lower-extremity amputation from diabetes may not have to cease driving if he or she can learn how to use hand controls. A DRS should then be contacted for assessment and training with the specific design of hand controls for the client's particular vehicle so that the client can compensate for his or her physical impairment.

Cognitive Considerations

Intervention for the client with cognitive impairment may be at the initial level of in-vehicle assessment, ascertaining the client's understanding of basic vehicle controls and features for both operation and safety. For an experienced driver, these skills should transfer even in an unfamiliar vehicle. Identification and understanding of primary control features (e.g., steering wheel, brake, accelerator) should transfer to any vehicle with minimal to no prompting. Although original equipment manufacturers (OEMs) such as Ford or General Motors pride themselves on being able to offer consumers a unique product, they must abide by certain safety and design standards related to human–machine interface with primary vehicle controls. Secondary control features such as windshield wipers, lights, and mirror controls can vary widely among OEMs, requiring more orientation to an unfamiliar vehicle. However, basic concepts such as putting on a seat belt, adjusting the mirrors, or positioning oneself in relation to the steering wheel and pedals can provide important information to therapists observing functional tasks so they can evaluate the status of a client.

Behind the Wheel

As described in previous chapters, the evaluation of motor, cognitive, vision, and perception in the clinical portion of the driving assessment is a familiar process for occupational therapists. Most of the tools in driver rehabilitation programs are known to practitioners, although some are unique to this practice area, and thus practitioners may need to learn the process to administer and interpret specific tools.

It is the on-road evaluation that is considered distinctive to the practice of driver rehabilitation and demands the specialized skills of an occupational therapist as a DRS. However, the on-road evaluation is essentially the same as other IADL assessments in that the best evaluations of IADLs are done within the natural context of the client. For example, to determine if cooking can be done safely by a client, the therapist observes the client making a meal in a kitchen. Thus, to get the best picture of the performance of driving, the practitioner must observe the individual driving a motor vehicle in the driving environment. The on-road evaluation has been described as the most ecologically valid method for determining driving safety or competence (Hunt et al., 1997; Justiss, Mann, Stav, & Velozo, 2006; Odenheimer et al., 1994).

What makes the on-road evaluation different from evaluation of other IADLs is that the natural driving environment is dynamic and complex and cannot be completely controlled by the therapist. There is often an inverse relationship between control of the environment and ecological validity when evaluating driving performance. The DRS has to balance providing an environment in which to fairly evaluate the client and selecting a safe environment to reduce the risk of potential collisions. The challenge is providing enough real-life driving opportunity to determine driving competence while maintaining a level of control through specific strategies (e.g., dual-brake systems) to ensure safety for the driver, the DRS, and others. This is true for both on-road evaluation and intervention. On-road intervention requires the DRS to spend significant time with the client behind the wheel.

Steps of the On-Road Evaluation or Intervention

Stationary In-Vehicle Assessment and Orientation

DRSs typically have several steps in providing an on-road evaluation or providing intervention. The first step is the stationary in-vehicle assessment and orientation. Similar to vehicle fit, the evaluator orients the client to the vehicle. Although all vehicles are different, the primary controls are so similar that for the experienced driver, it should not take a lot of time to adjust to driving a different vehicle. It

> ## Practitioner's Reflection 12.1. Orientation
>
> I have had clients who reach between the seats to shift the vehicle into another gear despite the gear selector being located on the steering column, or they continue to turn the headlights on and off when attempting to adjust the windshield wipers. These errors reflect variations in vehicle design and do not suggest a cognitive impairment that would affect driving safety. However, I have had clients tell me that their accelerator pedal is located on the other side of the brake (not a modified vehicle) or have difficulty understanding the meaning of "P-R-N-D" on the gear selector indicator. This confusion is more concerning and indicates a cognitive decline that interferes with driving safety.
>
> —*Donna Stressel, OTR/L, CDI, CDRS*

may not *feel* right, but the essential functions remain the same (see Practitioner's Reflection 12.1). The evaluator makes sure that the client adjusts the seat, puts on the seat belt, and adjusts the mirrors. Some evaluators purposely knock mirrors out of line so the drivers have to adjust them for themselves. For the novice driver, vehicle orientation is a new experience, and much more time needs to be spent in this first step as the client gets used to the vehicle's components.

Closed-Course or Off-Road

The next step is to start the on-road evaluation within a protected environment. This may be a restricted area (closed course) or a quiet neighborhood. A *closed-course* or *off-road* environment means an environment that does not have other vehicles, traffic control devices, objects, or pedestrians, which limits the exposure of both driver and evaluator to unpredictable driving and confounding behaviors. It allows basic vehicle maneuvering in a controlled environment so the DRS can concentrate on closely observing the client to determine if he or she is able to continue with the on-road evaluation. It also allows the DRS to work more closely with the client when assessing the need for or training in the use of adaptive equipment (see Practitioner's Reflection 12.2).

On-Road

Although the closed course provides a safe environment, it limits the ability for a driver to respond in a real-world or potentially hazardous situation. If the client demonstrates basic skills and awareness of the environment, the next step

> ## Practitioner's Reflection 12.2. Adaptive Equipment
>
> Many individuals are reluctant or resistant to driving with adaptive equipment. I have worked with several clients with multiple sclerosis or incomplete spinal cord injury (SCI) who were not convinced that driving with hand controls was a better alternative than driving with their feet. I recall a 26-year-old man with an incomplete SCI who was ambulating with a walker, but despite poor sensation in his lower extremities, he felt he could drive without adaptive equipment. He was taken to a residential area and allowed to drive with his foot. After a few stops and starts he was concentrating on a garbage truck when his foot got stuck behind the brake pedal. He began to panic when he realized he did not have control of the vehicle and could not stop. After this incident he was eager to try the hand controls.
>
> I firmly believe that if he was not allowed to attempt driving without hand controls, he would have done so on his own and the consequences could have been devastating. Because of the dual brake in the training vehicle, I was able to intervene at any time and was in control of the vehicle the entire time, but it allowed the client to experience what might have happened if he had lost control of the vehicle on his own.
>
> —*Donna Stressel, OTR/L, CDI, CDRS*

is to proceed to the *on-road* component or public roadway. The typical procedure is to gradually increase the level of complexity including other vehicles, traffic signals, and various maneuvers. On the basis of the client's driving habits and home environment, the evaluator decides if a highway component is necessary for assessment or intervention. On-road methodologies use a *fixed* or *variable* course design.

Whether to use a fixed or a variable route will continue to be debated by both licensing entities and driver rehabilitation programs. Some states' licensing programs have kept their testing procedures for new or renewed licensing the same for years, whereas others are attempting to meet the needs of their older citizens by doing specialized evaluations in and around an individual's home. Fixed and variable routes have their advantages and disadvantages, and it is a question that needs research before there is enough evidence to make a definitive statement about which to use, with what kind of driver, and when to use a particular kind of route.

Fixed Route. The fixed-route option has been identified as a foundation for reliable and valid assessment of driving performance (Galski, Bruno, & Ehle, 1993; Hunt et al., 1997; Justiss et al., 2006; Odenheimer et al., 1994). A *fixed-route* design includes a variety of traffic situations that progress from basic maneuvers to maneuvers of increased complexity. A progressively complex, fixed-route course of approximately 45–60 minutes usually provides adequate environmental exposure for a driving evaluator to determine driver competence (Stephens et al., 2005). The course should be designed to encompass most traffic scenarios that a driver is likely to encounter, including varying speeds, types of roadways, intersections with varied traffic signs and signals, and situations necessitating knowledge of rules of the road and right-of-way.

In a fixed route, most of the maneuvers at intersections are directed with the intention of requiring the driver to make judgments about right-of-way and safe gap. Frequently, the driver's unfamiliarity with the route necessitates the evaluator to give navigational assistance. However, evaluators can require more decision making on the part of the driver by asking him or her to "choose any street on the left and turn before the next light" or "follow the signs to the hospital." The familiarity of a fixed-route model affords the evaluator opportunities to allow the driver to make errors under manageable conditions. For example, there may be an intersection controlled by stop signs that has the necessary visibility that allows the evaluator to let the driver run the stop sign without consequences. The evaluator's knowledge and comfort with the fixed route is its greatest advantage and cannot be underestimated. Giving explicit directions (e.g., turn right, make a left turn at the next intersection) for all turns can be avoided by considering ways to challenge those clients who can follow directions but otherwise might easily get lost (see Practitioner's Reflection 12.3).

Variable Route. The *variable route* is when the DRS evaluates the client in the client's community. The variable-route option is unavoidable when the evaluator travels to the client's geographic area. Certainly the variable route has the advantage of being more occupation centered, as it allows the driver to be assessed navigating to those businesses or activities to which he or she needs or wants to go. The variable route is

---

Practitioner's Reflection 12.3. Fixed Routes

Part of the route I developed has a 2-mile section in which the only instruction that is provided is to "keep going straight until you cannot go straight any further," which requires the driver to attend to stop signs (two-ways and all-ways), traffic lights, and lane markings (e.g., showing which lane allows traffic to proceed straight). This ensures that the driver will be exposed to various situations that will assess how any clinical deficits affect driving competency and safety. Cognitive functioning also can be challenged by requesting a driver to locate a particular business or turn the vehicle around for a "missed" turn.

—Donna Stressel, OTR/L, CDI, CDRS

I ended my fixed route in a neighborhood where I asked my clients, at a stop sign, to go straight but return to the same intersection. This would require 3 short-block right turns, but cognitively challenged drivers would drive straight and forget the direction or make the first right turn and get completely lost.

—Anne Dickerson, PhD, OTR/L, FAOTA

---

particularly useful to see the client in his or her natural setting. However, the disadvantage is that it significantly increases the demands on the DRS to anticipate environmental factors.

Although the DRS may start out on a fixed route for training and intervention, when possible, the variable route or home area should be incorporated into the behind-the-wheel intervention. A component of the intervention is to find the areas that may pose more risk and assist the client in route planning to avoid problematic intersections or to reduce risks such as left turns (see Practitioner's Reflection 12.4).

Vehicles Equipped for Driver Rehabilitation Programs

The most commonly selected vehicle purchased for use in driver rehabilitation programs is a two- or four-door sedan with automatic transmission, power steering, and power brakes. Another sedan feature that will assist the client with access to a vehicle is a split front bench seat. All program vehicles should have a right-side brake pedal and an instructor's mirror.

Practitioner's Reflection 12.4. Variable Routes

We do most of our training with equipment or novice drivers around the hospital parking lots and driveways. For the individuals needing equipment, familiarity is not an issue; they just need practice driving. For the novice driver, I have specific areas that I go to when I want to work on a specific skill. For example, there is a stretch of highway that has different kinds of entrance–exit ramps for working on merging, or there are a variety of two-way versus all-way stops. My colleague and I often share particular spots with a good teaching layout. This is one of the advantages to having clients come to our center for training: I have a plan, and I know where to go to provide the challenges that are needed for specific training that I might not be able to find if I go to the client's home area.

The real advantage for driving in someone's area would be to assess and train older clients—not only to see how they navigate but also to make suggestions on route restructuring. I do this when folks live close by; the cost would be prohibitive on a regular basis. I have lived in the area most of my life and know the majority of areas that people are talking about, and when needed I have gone on Google maps to see the areas to assist if I cannot drive with them in those areas.

—Donna Stressel, OTR/L, CDI, CDRS

Exhibit 12.1. Useful Intervention Vehicle Adaptations for Program Vehicles

- *Mechanical gas–brake control.* Adaptations are necessary for clients who have lost lower-extremity function. The adaptive equipment will assist the user with an option for compensation through equipment designed to allow access by the upper extremity or an opposite leg, and it includes hand controls and left-foot accelerators.

- *Steering devices.* These devices are necessary to assist those with decreased grasp because of neurological changes, spinal cord injury, orthopedic impairments, or other impairments that affect grasp and operation of the steering wheel. The different kinds include spinner, single post, tri-pin, amputee ring, palmer cuff, and V grip.

- *Mirrors.* Many types of mirror options should be available to assess the driver's ability to compensate for visual or cervical rotation problems. Some to consider are the lane-changer mirror, smart-view mirror, panel mirror, and panoramic mirror.

- *Postural supports.* Some clients may have decreased trunk control as a result of spinal cord or neurological conditions, which may affect trunk muscles and balance. It is critical to secure trunk balance for optimal upper-extremity function to facilitate the best control of adaptive equipment for the primary controls using torso supports or chest straps and various sizes of cushions.

- *Key extensions.* These devices are used to improve pincher or lateral grip to help with inserting a key into an ignition or door lock. A key is held by the extended handle, allowing the user increased leverage when inserting and turning the key.

- *Turn-signal crossover.* For the person who has an impaired upper extremity on the side of the vehicle where the turn signal indicator lever is located, this device provides an extended lever that allows the user access on the opposite side of the steering column where the other extremity is more functional.

- *Door latch levers.* These are various manufactured or custom-made devices that enable the person with decreased hand function to grasp and open the door handle of a car with an extended hook.

- *Easy Reach™ seat-belt handle or seat-belt loops.* These devices enable users to reach and grasp the seat belt in spite of their limitations with shoulder, elbow, or hand function.

- *Swivel Seat Cushion.™* This cushion assists users with decreased trunk mobility to rotate their hips to aid with transfers in and out of the vehicle.

- *Handy Bar.™* This device is helpful because it can be hooked into the vehicle's door latch loop and be used as a grabber handle to assist with entry and exit from either the driver side or passenger side of the vehicle.

- *Car Caddie.™* This device is a sewn nylon strap that attaches at varying heights of the vehicle's window. It enables the user to get assistance by pulling up and lifting oneself when trying to stand and exit the vehicle.

- *Gas Cap Wrench.™* This device enables the user with decreased grasp to rotate the gas cap to fuel the vehicle.

If the program works primarily with individuals who are functioning at the wheelchair level, a lowered-floor minivan with ramp entry or a lowered-floor, full-sized van with platform lift entry should be selected. A program then should establish a collaborative relationship with a local National Mobility Equipment Dealer–certified vehicle modifier. This vehicle modifier will be the dealer or dealers with whom the program will work when having the program vehicle adapted. See Exhibit 12.1 for a list of typical adaptations that driving rehabilitation programs use on their vehicles.

Models of Driver Rehabilitation Programs

There are different models of driver rehabilitation programs with varying approaches for assessment and intervention for addressing driver competency and community mobility needs. In considering each of the models, it is important to keep in mind that one is not better than the other and that each practice catchment area should have the full scope of services, that is, from screening to intervention as well as transitioning to alternative transportation options.

Comprehensive Driver Rehabilitation Program

Typically, when a program considers itself a *comprehensive* driver rehabilitation program, the DRSs provide

1. All components of the driving evaluation, including clinical and on-road evaluations;
2. Vehicle or equipment evaluations, recommendations, and "checkout";
3. In-vehicle training for novice drivers or vehicle modification training;
4. Licensing assistance, including using the program's modified vehicle for specialized testing; and
5. Transportation counseling.

These kinds of programs usually are associated with a comprehensive rehabilitation facility within a hospital system, are a free-standing rehabilitation system, or are an independent private practice. Many states have requirements for providing a driving program that include guidelines for appropriate vehicles and qualified staff for the populations served. Most comprehensive programs include modified vehicles for all levels of clients, including high-tech vans and minivans.

As with any comprehensive program, the advantage is a one-stop shopping service. This is particularly advantageous when there is not a clear concept of the needs or requirements of service by the client, referring physician, or other referral source such as state vocational rehabilitation services. The DRS will be able to address any issue. The continuity of care is also an advantage with a comprehensive program.

Unfortunately, many times comprehensive programs are in one location, so clients in the regional area must travel more distance to be served by a comprehensive program. Another issue is that clients may appreciate more than just one program's perspective or service. Another disadvantage of a private practice comprehensive driver rehabilitation program may be a lack of a referral network to send clients to direct occupational therapy services for remediation of component skills. This can be an issue even with programs associated with health care facilities. The need for such a referral network should be recognized and reinforced so that clients can receive the most cost-effective interventions as needed.

Driver Assessment Program

Some hospital systems or rehabilitation centers understand the need to address driving as a functional outcome and provide a smaller scope of services than the comprehensive programs described earlier. These types of programs may have one or two vehicles and one or two therapists who may or may not be addressing driving full-time. The focus may be only on assessment or training with vehicle modifications limited to hand controls. The limitation of services is typically demand driven, and for that facility, this limited service may be adequate. For occupational therapists either in the driving program or providing referrals, it is critical to know when to make a referral to more specialized services (for higher-technology equipment), to ensure that adequate training is done, and to provide the transitional information or counseling needed if cessation is necessary.

Driver Rehabilitation Program Linked With Driving School

Another model for driving programs is the cooperative program between DRSs and driving schools. Typically, with this type of program, the clinical assessment of skills is done by the occupational therapy DRS, and the certified driving instructor or driving educator provides the behind-the-wheel vehicle and evaluation. Some programs have the occupational therapist observing the client's driving competence from the back seat while the driving instructor is in the front monitoring the driving environment for safety. An alternative model is the driving instructor completing the evaluation independently and reporting back to the professional about the behind-the-wheel performance. The occupational therapist and the driving instructor typically discuss the results of both assessment components, and a recommendation is made about the client's driving performance.

This dual-evaluator model is the chosen model with programs that choose not to have their occupational therapy DRSs doing the on-road component. For some settings this model works because the facility does not have the means to maintain a program vehicle or does not feel the cost is justifiable for its client census. There are inherent challenges with this model, including the fact that driving instructors may not have the medical and science background to adequately evaluate medically at-risk clients. Another challenge is the communication of findings. The therapist and the driving instructor must build a feasible system and build a trust relationship to make justified decisions. Finally, the responsibility for conveying recommendations or providing additional services such as training or licensing needs to be clearly delineated. Although the dual-evaluator model has challenges, when these challenges are addressed, this model of practice can work well in rural or smaller communities, particularly if evaluation in a client's home environment is possible.

Referral-Based Driver Rehabilitation Program

The referral-based driver rehabilitation program is a relatively new model of providing services. In this model, occupational therapy generalists are identified as the appropriate professionals to make referrals for driving evaluation. Either all the therapists in the general setting may make referrals, or one is identified as having a more specialized skill set but not at the level of a DRS. This generalist with the skill set evaluates the client using selected screening and assessment tools. Assessment results or cutoff points, jointly agreed upon by the generalist and the DRS, are used to make a determination. The generalist may recognize the client as not being ready for a comprehensive driving evaluation, discuss driving cessation, or refer to a DRS for a full driving evaluation, including behind the wheel.

With this collaborative model, the DRS can use the results of the generalist assessment and decrease the time of the clinical assessment or further investigate unusual or suspect results. In addition to being a cost-effective model for facilities, this model can address the issue of DRS shortages by using their services more efficiently (see Exhibit 12.2). This model also may assist the client as the generalist can use information gained from working directly with the client as well as work on intervention strategies that the DRS might suggest after evaluation.

Community-Based Driving Program

There are several kinds of driving schools or programs established in communities that address the needs of the novice driver (typically teenagers, but not necessarily). These programs may have educational components that include driver safety or established curricula for school-based instruction. Driver instructors are

Exhibit 12.2. Genesis Rehabilitation Program

Genesis Rehabilitation is piloting a Driving Champions program. The American Occupational Therapy Association (AOTA) and Genesis Rehabilitation Services have created a framework that addresses the IADL of driving and community mobility as a part of occupational therapy practice across the continuum of care. There are four major issues when considering driving competence: (1) finding the appropriate mix of screens and assessments to identify those at risk, (2) determining which clients require the service of a driver rehabilitation evaluator, (3) ascertaining the availability of driving evaluators, and (4) obtaining reimbursement for driving evaluations. This model starts with occupational therapists who do not specialize in driving and community mobility, known as *generalists*. The generalists, however, understand the activity analysis of driving and community mobility. Their responsibility is to identify the medically at-risk client while in the general setting, optimize his or her skills needed for the identified goal of driving, enhance client and family awareness of risk factors, ensure that a referral when deemed beneficial to the client is justified and defendable, and prepare for the necessary transitions. Through optimized communication and referral systems, the generalist can identify strengths and weaknesses in relation to driving, building criteria on which to base the decision to refer to a highly trained DRS.

This project seeks to identify the criteria that warrant and justify the comprehensive driving evaluation (e.g., performance in the context of behind the wheel or adaptive equipment) to successfully refer to the DRS. To accomplish the task, the language and terminology must be consistent, the reimbursement areas appropriately identified, effective referral networks created, and educational support systems developed to ensure appropriate education and training for the generalists and other health care professionals. Through the resources of AOTA, the outcomes of the process and the findings of the educational component will contribute to the goal of creating a framework that can be duplicated within other settings and communities to increase the capacity to address driving and community mobility with all medically at-risk individuals.

---

experienced trainers and experts on the rules of the road. For the older adult who needs a refresher driver safety course, requires assistance with new technology, or is returning to driving after not driving for nonmedical reasons, the community based-programs are reasonably priced and widely available. The disadvantage of these programs is that driving instructors do not have the medical knowledge background to evaluate individuals with medical conditions.

Decision of Competence

Survey research results indicate that most DRSs rely heavily on the outcome of the behind-the-wheel component of the comprehensive driving evaluation over other assessments when determining fitness to drive (Dickerson, 2011; Korner-Bitensky, Bitnesky, Sofer, Man-Son-Hing, & Gelinas, 2006). Researchers concur, using the on-road evaluation as the gold standard of measurement in outcomes research (Langford et al., 2008; Wheatley & Di Stefano, 2008). The difficulty lies in the fact that there is not one standardized method of performing an on-road evaluation; no universal standardized scale; and, because of the contextual differences of environments, no one level of difficulty. The decision of a client's fitness to drive is a subjective clinical judgment made on the basis of a snapshot of performance.

However, there are some common practices with most DRSs. For example, most DRSs use a program vehicle with safety features to protect the client, evaluator, and others. The driving evaluations usually start in a relatively safe environment such as a parking lot and progress slowly to increasingly complex and dynamic environments. Evaluations generally last about 1 hour and include various maneuvers, neighborhoods, speeds, and types of intersections. Most evaluators include or eliminate a highway portion depending on the history or needs of the client (Dickerson, 2011).

The key to the on-road evaluation is the keen observation of performance skills used to control the vehicle safely along routes of increasing complexity. Some DRSs use established checklists or create their own checklists; some use self-notes; and others are vigilant, with eyes on the road observing the skills, and note the errors later. Regardless of the system, all DRSs expect certain behaviors or combinations of behaviors under certain environmental circumstances. For example, as a driver approaches an intersection for a left turn across oncoming traffic, the driver is expected to stop, observe traffic, and make a calculated judgment before turning. Deviations from expected behavior are documented as part of the assessment or intervention process. There may be minor errors that can be corrected with education, such as not making a full stop at a stop sign. A critical error may be poor judgment about the gap in traffic and pulling out in front of a vehicle, requiring the DRS to take over control of the vehicle.

DRSs report that they use the clinical assessment results to target characteristics that they want to specifically look for during the on-road evaluation (Dickerson, 2011). For example, if the client does poorly on the processing-speed tasks, the evaluator will want to make sure that there are intersections that require the individual to respond to environmental changes quickly, such as judgment of a gap in traffic for a left-hand turn. The question for the evaluator will be whether the slower processing speeds are (1) not evident during the on-road evaluation because of overlearning and the practice of driving skills; (2) too slow for compensation strategies and necessitate driving cessation; or (3) slowed, but maybe not critically, so that compensation strategies such as avoiding left-hand turns or yield signs will probably be sufficient.

Outcomes of the on-road evaluation are generally grouped as *pass, pass with restrictions, needs training,* or *fail.* Within each of these categories, there are nuances for specific states, driving evaluators, and interpretations unique to some clients. It should be noted that the DRS is usually rendering a *recommendation,* as it is the state licensing agency that grants or takes away the license.

Generally a recommendation of a *pass* is made for a driver with no specific restrictions or reevaluations established who can return to driving or the novice driver who can proceed with establishing experience. A *pass with restrictions* is for an individual who is considered fit to drive with some specific limitations or restrictions. This may be a restriction of daytime driving only for the diagnosis of glaucoma, specific equipment for an amputee with hand controls, or a restriction of speed for a client with cognitive impairment. The restriction may be permanent or temporary, and often a driver with restrictions will be required to have reevaluations at set times, such as 6 or 12 months. For example, an individual with early Parkinson's disease may be evaluated and considered safe to drive in familiar areas but will need to be reevaluated every 12 months because of the disease progression. The individual who has an impairment that may improve over time may initially be considered unsafe to drive but has the potential for improvement or can benefit from vehicle modification, and he or she might get a *needs training* recommendation.

Finally, the DRS who observes critical errors that endanger the driver or others on the road is ethically obligated to recommend *driving cessation*. The challenge may be with the cognitively impaired experienced driver who seems to follow all the rules of the road, but the on-road evaluation has not presented enough risk to tax the ability of his or her overlearned skill. Many experienced DRSs will extend evaluations with these clients to ensure that the challenges of day-to-day driving have been met.

For training and intervention, errors should decrease as experience on the road increases. There are differences in training times and techniques between a novice driver and an experienced driver using adaptive equipment, but regardless, there comes a time when the DRS needs to determine if the intervention has been successful. That is, not only does the novice need to pass the state driver licensing test, but the DRS must determine if the driver is competent after an adequate number and range of experiences.

Some disability populations, such as clients with low vision, may require advanced in-vehicle training, requiring a team of experts to ensure competency. For example, the driver diagnosed with low vision may be able to use optometric interventions to qualify for driving in accordance with his or her individual state driver licensing requirements.

In the event that a client is unable to drive an automobile successfully, either temporarily or long-term, alternative transportation and community mobility options must be considered. The occupational therapist may provide individualized assistance to the client and family to locate and identify options available in the community to help the client select options that meet his or her personal needs.

Accordingly, using expertise in activity analysis to individualize and evaluate needs for community mobility based on assessments of vision, hearing, cognition, balance, and mobility needs, the occupational therapist generalist can address which mobility options are safe for individual clients' level of functioning. Pedestrian safety, endurance, use of a mobility device, and the ability to negotiate these devices safely through the community are all a part of an individualized plan. Through this individualized approach, the client is provided with solutions that are user-friendly and address fall prevention and safe community mobility independence (see Chapters 2 and 3).

Behind-the-Wheel Interventions

State licensing agencies will always have driver examiners who take the novice or a questionable driver out for a driving test ending in an outcome of pass or fail. However, in some states, the agencies have recognized that seniors may be at a disadvantage in testing because of the unfamiliarity of the test environment and actually test seniors around the community in which they will drive. Driving schools have driving instructors with years of on-road training with novice and senior drivers.

So, what is it that the occupational therapist with expertise in driver rehabilitation offers? In addition to the science background knowledge of medical conditions, the occupational therapist considers the evaluation the beginning point,

The DRS who observes critical errors that endanger the driver or others on the road is ethically obligated to recommend *driving cessation.*

not the end point! Even when performing a comprehensive driving evaluation, the occupational therapist begins the educational process for the client, family members, and other health care providers with discussion of the community mobility needs of the client, what training is needed, and what equipment should be installed. It is the *process of intervention* that is the unique contribution of the DRS.

In the following case examples (12.1–12.5), we illustrate outcomes of the comprehensive driving evaluation, but more importantly we highlight the critical process of intervention by a DRS who collaborates with his or her clients, their families, and the occupational therapy generalists. None of these cases depict actual individuals but illustrate what might typically occur with individuals.

Case Example 12.1. Mr. Weathers: Driving Cessation

Don Weathers was introduced in Chapter 6 with his occupational profile completed by a general-practice occupational therapist. Mr. Weathers is 75 years of age, and although his daughter felt that he had some problems with finances and managing household tasks, she thought that his driving was fine. After the performance analysis, the occupational therapist suspected that his cognitive impairment may affect the safety of his driving and referred him to the DRS for a comprehensive driving evaluation. The generalist shared the results of his cognitive performance with the DRS, including Mr. Weathers' ability to follow directions, his attention, and his memory.

Appendix 12.A illustrates Mr. Weathers' community mobility clinical assessment with CDRS Donna Stressel. Over her years of experience, Donna has created an assessment form to summarize some of the essential information she needs for the clinical component. Rather than using all the same assessments for each client, Donna selects from a toolkit of assessment resources on the basis of the diagnosis, medical history, referral, or the report from Mr. Weathers' occupational therapy. In this case, the referring therapist was able to give ample information on Mr. Weathers' cognitive status so that further evaluation in this area was not indicated. Based on the given information, a behind-the-wheel assessment was required to make a determination of fitness to drive. Appendix 12.A shows the completed on-roads (functional) evaluation as well as Mr. Weathers' community mobility recommendations.

Mr. Weathers's cognitive impairment was affecting many aspects of his IADL, including driving. All of the information obtained needed to be reviewed for integration to make a suitable recommendation and plan for his community mobility. He and his daughter were unaware of how his "cautiousness" was putting him at risk for a crash. His slow rate of speed and excessive braking for green lights put him at greater risk for a rear-end collision and could have been a contributing factor to his crash 2 years earlier. His intermittent use of his left foot to brake while parking and his tendency to depress both pedals at the same time placed him at risk for pedal confusion.

When first confronted with the recommendation to quit driving, Mr Weathers was surprised and angry. He could not remember the mistakes he had made on the road, and when confronted with the errors, he minimized the safety concerns. When he was allowed to express his concerns about becoming a burden and how not driving would affect his daily routine, he became upset and tearful. He was reassured by his daughter that she was more concerned for his well-being and that she would be devastated if anything happened to him or if anyone else was ever hurt.

Mr. Weathers was advised that he could take control of the situation and decide to quit driving on his own, or the state would most likely become involved and suspend his license if he continued to drive. He decided that he wanted to make this decision and agreed that his daughter could have his car. His transportation needs were addressed by trying the following: One of his long-time friends at church could pick him up for his biweekly services; he would use the senior bus to go to the grocery store; and he and his daughter would use his car to go to doctor appointments and to garage sales every other weekend. He could still wash his car every Sunday afternoon after church. His daughter also was provided with information on home services and contact information for help in discussing his current and future living arrangements. (See **algorithm depicting the occupational therapy process for driving and community mobility for programs** [Dickerson et al., 2011].)

Case Example 12.2. Mrs. Tidd: Driving Restrictions

Mrs. Tidd is an 82-year-old woman who was referred to Donna Stressel for a comprehensive driving evaluation after her daughter expressed concerns about her driving. There were not any specific medical conditions, so it was a self-referral, not from a health professional. The daughter did not identify any specific driving issues but was concerned because her mother did not have much driving experience until her father had a stroke. Now her mother needs to drive for all of their appointments and errands. Mr. and Mrs. Tidd live in an area that has little to no transportation options available, and if her mother is not safe to drive, the daughter feels they will need to move.

Mrs. Tidd has no significant health problems but does have the beginning of cataracts and had a right total-knee replacement 8 years earlier because of degenerative joint disease. The clinical assessment indicated all areas to be within functional limits despite some normal age-related changes (minimally decreased distant acuity, depth perception, and peripheral vision, and slightly slower reaction time). An on-road evaluation revealed good vehicle control, and Mrs. Tidd obeyed all signs, signals, and rules of the road. She had safe interaction with other traffic observed throughout the assessment but did have some difficulty maintaining and getting up to speed and observing when changing lanes and merging onto the highway. She reported that she was nervous while driving and that it took a lot of concentration to attend to all that was going on.

After the behind-the-wheel evaluation, Donna completed the compensatory strategies handout (Appendix 12.B) with Mrs. Tidd and her daughter, and her recommendation was for Mrs. Tidd to be allowed to continue driving but to limit her driving to familiar and local areas, daylight hours, and no peak traffic times and to limit distractions. Donna continued her intervention by discussing routes that Mrs. Tidd should take and how to modify her routes to avoid highway driving. Donna demonstrated how additional mirrors could be used to assist with lane changes and merging. Mrs. Tidd also was provided with information on defensive driving courses in her community and encouraged to take a driving lesson from a local driving school to develop her comfort level and confidence. This recommendation is an excellent example of how the DRS can refer the right type of client to practice skills to the driver instructor, which is a more affordable option and located near the client's home. The topic of driving cessation was introduced to Mrs. Tidd and her daughter so that both of them could explore options for their future living arrangements and transportation needs.

Case Example 12.3. Mr. Mitchell: Evaluation and Training

Mr. Mitchell is a 67-year-old man with a right below-knee amputation. In addition to hypertension controlled by medicine, he also has a 20-year history of insulin-dependent diabetes mellitus, well controlled by insulin, and he checks his blood sugar 3 times daily. He has no diabetic retinopathy or any other eye-related diseases and has his eyes checked every 6 months by his ophthalmologist. Mr. Mitchell was referred by his physiatrist to Donna Stressel for an evaluation of driving and training in the use of a left-foot accelerator. He was an experienced driver and is eager to return to driving, but he has had not been driving since his amputation.

The clinical assessment indicated significant neuropathy in the left lower extremity and an inability to move the left foot between the pedals on the reaction timer without looking at his foot. As a result, the on-road evaluation was completed using hand controls and not a left-foot accelerator. As training started, this evaluation became intervention on using hand controls on the program vehicle. Initially there was a lot of confusion with the accelerator and brake of the hand controls, and his first instinct was to attempt to use his left foot to stop the vehicle. He would become so preoccupied with differentiating between the accelerator and brake that he would forget to steer, and Donna would need to gain control of the vehicle. However, after about 20 minutes he was demonstrating good vehicle control and was able to progress into more traffic situations.

At the end of the session, Mr. Mitchell again began to show confusion between the accelerator and brake, especially when asked to back up and park, letting go of the steering knob and thus losing control of the vehicle. Donna recommended that additional training was needed for Mr. Mitchell to demonstrate competency with the new equipment. She could have considered referring Mr. Mitchell to a driving school for training, but with Mr. Mitchell's medical condition, Donna felt her expertise was still needed to determine which type of hand controls and spinning knob he would perform with best; she also felt that he would achieve competency in all areas.

Using the Driver Rehabilitation On-Road Program Goals and Flow Sheet (Appendix 12.C), Donna started training with Mr. Mitchell. After 4 hours of training in the use of hand controls and a right steering knob, he demonstrated proficient use of the adaptive equipment in all traffic situations and was able to select the style of hand control that he preferred. Donna provided assistance in obtaining a restricted license from the New York Department of Motor Vehicles, and information was provided on area vendors to modify Mr. Mitchell's current vehicle. Additional information on vehicle selection and manufacturers' rebates for adaptive equipment was given in the event that Mr. Mitchell decides to purchase a new vehicle in the future.

Case Example 12.4. Ms. Wells: Fail, Intervention, Reassess

Ms. Wells is a 27-year-old woman who sustained a traumatic brain injury as the result of a fall while ice skating. She had a 2-week stay at a rehabilitation hospital and was finishing up with her outpatient therapy, including vision therapy for deficits in the areas of vergence, stereopsis, and visual inattention. Although it was only 2 months postinjury, Ms. Wells was anxious to return to work as an office manager. She was referred to Donna for a comprehensive driving evaluation by her physician and indicated that she was cleared to return to work once she successfully passed the comprehensive driving evaluation.

During the clinical assessment, Ms. Wells complained of continued photosensitivity issues and frequent headaches. Although improved over her initial rehabilitation results posttrauma, she demonstrated continued decreased divided attention, slow processing speed, and some mild short-term memory deficits. She was easily frustrated with difficult tasks and showed significant anxiety regarding the need to return to work to keep her job. During the behind-the-wheel assessment, Ms. Wells, an experienced driver, demonstrated good vehicle control but showed inconsistent attention to signs and signals. She made a right turn on red at an intersection in which it was prohibited, needed a cue to get into the left-turn lane to make a turn, and demonstrated delayed braking for light changes and slowing vehicles. Although she completed the on-road evaluation, she complained that she had a headache and was fatigued following the 60-minute drive.

Based on both the clinical and on-road evaluations, Donna explained to Ms. Wells that she was not ready to return to driving and recommended that she continue to work on her vision therapy exercises. In this case, Donna's intervention strategies included the referral back to the generalist occupational therapists so that Ms. Wells could continue working on her rehabilitation goals. To make sure Ms. Wells could understand that this also would be working toward driving, Donna described several additional in-vehicle activities that she could work on as a passenger. This included road sign or vehicle scavenger hunts to assist in improving visual attention. Donna also explored colored ultraviolet filters that were able to reduce the photo-sensitivity.

Donna referred Ms. Wells to vocational rehabilitation to assist with her transition back to work and to psychology for coping with her anxiety in dealing with life changes. With communication from Donna to the physician, Ms. Wells' physician agreed to clear her to return to work with the support of vocational rehabilitation and public transportation. A reevaluation was scheduled for 3 months to assess her progress and driving skills.

When Donna reevaluated Ms. Wells, there was a marked improvement in all areas in the clinical assessment and the behind-the-wheel evaluation. Ms. Wells still complained of headaches and fatigue when under stress or after a hectic day, but she reported on most days that she was symptom-free. After this session, there was a recommendation to allow the resumption of driving with supervision to monitor her ability to consistently attend to details in a variety of traffic situations and under varying conditions, both environmental and physical. A follow-up driving evaluation was scheduled for 6 weeks to assess the need for continued supervision and any additional restrictions.

Case Example 12.5. Mr. Miller: Intervention for Caregivers or Families

As with many clients with dementia, the occupational therapist is not using intervention strategies with the client but is educating caregivers or family members on how to structure the environment to provide a safe and comfortable setting for the client. Such is the case with Mr. Miller and his DRS.

Mr. Miller is a 77-year-old man with a diagnosis of dementia of the Alzheimer's type. When he was diagnosed the previous year, he was seen by Donna for a comprehensive driving evaluation that resulted in a recommendation to make a plan for driving retirement. Mr. Miller and his wife were provided with information on transportation options in their area, but Mrs. Miller indicated that as a driver, she would be able to meet all of their transportation needs. When Donna received a new referral for evaluation, she contacted the physician's office to clarify the need for a new evaluation as Mr. Miller was already advised to cease driving. The nurse manager explained that Mrs. Miller was distraught and frustrated because her husband would continue to sneak out and drive when she was not home despite his license being medically suspended. She tried hiding the keys, but Mr. Miller would demand the keys and become aggressive when she refused. Several times Mrs. Miller had to retreat into a locked bedroom in fear for her safety. Mrs. Miller was in crisis. Although the physician did know it was best for Mr. Miller not to drive, he did not know what to do except to consider reevaluation.

Mr. Miller was scheduled for reevaluation and intervention with the DRS. Donna discussed the legal implications of Mr. Miller driving without a license with both Mr. and Mrs. Miller. Mr. Miller was adamant that he was a safe driver and that he wanted to get his license back. Donna made an agreement to help him get a temporary removal of the suspension that would allow him to be

> **Case Example 12.5. Mr. Miller: Intervention for Caregivers or Families** *(cont.)*
>
> reevaluated. As part of that agreement, he would consent to having his wife remove his car from the property and surrender all keys to the vehicle, and he would abide by the outcome of this final recommendation. A "contract" was signed and a copy given to the Millers along with information on area support groups. Donna contacted the physician's office describing the plan, indicating that it would be a slow process, which would hopefully calm the situation at home.
>
> It took slightly over a year to get the authorization needed to reevaluate Mr. Miller. As expected, Mr. Miller's skills and performance had continued to decline, and the outcome was again to not drive. His response to this was matter of fact, and his wife reported that during the year he had adjusted to not driving and only rarely brought the matter up. She had used the contract as a tool to manage her husband's behavior as he adjusted to the change in his life.

Summary

This chapter's focus was on intervention. However, as every occupational therapist knows, intervention and assessment are often interwoven. Thus, in this chapter, we have described the relationship among the clinical assessment for driving, the behind-the-wheel assessment, and the driving intervention for the client.

As stated previously, the DRS who is also an occupational therapist is different from the driving evaluator because of the intervention process. A driving decision is not and should not be the outcome measure of DRSs. The success of the client–therapist interaction is when the client has the ability to get to where he or she wants and needs to go, by whatever means. In other words, if a client comes in for a driving evaluation because he wants to be able to get to work, visit his family, or buy groceries, an occupational therapist should not just inform him that he cannot drive for the next 2 months until he recovers from a medical condition. The goal has always been listen to the needs of the client, to work collaboratively with him or her to meet that need, and to work with the client and family for successful outcomes.

If driving is not a viable strategy, if even for a short time, the occupational therapist is obligated to find the means to meet the IADL for that client. Using the profession's considerable knowledge about health conditions and an understanding of the occupational profile of clients, possible remedial strategies or methods of compensation should be debated.

This chapter also highlights some examples of models of program structures that might vary across settings, in a city, or between states. There is no one model for all communities, as generalists and DRSs collaborate to develop systems that work in their communities.

References

Bédard, M., Weaver, B., Dārziņš, P., & Porter, M. (2008). Predicting driving performance in older adults: We are not there yet! *Traffic Injury Prevention, 9,* 336–341.

Classen, S., Horgas, A., Awadzi, K., Messinger-Rapport, B., Shechtman, O., & Joo, Y. (2008). Clinical predictors of older driver performance on a standardized road test. *Traffic Injury Prevention, 9,* 456–462.

Dickerson, A. E. (2011, April). *Identify the most critical determinants of whether a client is fit-to-drive.* Paper presented at the American Occupational Therapy Conference Institute, Philadelphia.

Dickerson, A. E., Molnar, L., Eby, D., Adler, G., Bedar, M., Berg-Weger, M., et al. (2007). Transportation and aging: A research agenda for advancing safe mobility. *Gerontologist, 47,* 578–590.

Dickerson, A. E., Reistetter, T., & Gaudy, J. (in press). The perception and meaningfulness and performance of instrumental activities of daily living from the perspectives of the medically-at-risk older adult and their caregiver. *Journal of Applied Gerontology.*

Dickerson, A. E., Reistetter, T., Schold Davis, E., & Monahan, M. (2011). Evaluating driving as a valued instrumental activity of daily living. *American Journal of Occupational Therapy, 65,* 64–75. doi:10.5014/ajot.2011.09052

Eby, D. W., Molnar, L. J., & Shope, J. T. (2000). *Driving decisions workbook.* Ann Arbor: University of Michigan Transportation Research Institute.

Eby, D. W., Trombley, D. A., Molnar, L. J., & Shope, J. T. (1998). *The assessment of older drivers' capabilities: A review of the University of Michigan Transportation Research Institute.* Ann Arbor: University of Michigan Transportation Research Institute.

Galski, T., Bruno, R. L., & Ehle, H. T. (1993). Prediction of behind-the-wheel driving performance in patients with cerebral brain damage: A discriminant function analysis. *American Journal of Occupational Therapy, 47,* 391–396. doi:10.5014/ajot.47.5.391

Hunt, L. A., Murphy, C. F., Carr, D., Duchek, J. M., Buckles, V., & Morris, J. C. (1997). Reliability of the Washington University Road Test: A performance-based assessment for drivers with dementia of the Alzheimer type. *Archives of Neurology, 54,* 707–712.

Justiss, M. D., Mann, W. C., Stav, W. B., & Velozo, C. (2006). Development of a behind-the-wheel driving performance assessment for older adults. *Topics in Geriatric Rehabilitation, 22,* 121–128.

Korner-Bitensky, N., Bitensky, J., Sofer, S., Man-Son-Hing, M., & Gelinas, I. (2006). Driving evaluation practices of clinicians working in the United States and Canada. *American Journal of Occupational Therapy, 60,* 428–434. doi:10.5014/ajot.60.4.428

Langford, J., Braitman, K., Charlton, J., Eberhard, J., O'Neill, D., Staplin, L., et al. (2008). TRB Workshop 2007: Licensing authorities' options for managing older driver safety— Practical advice from the researchers. *Traffic Injury Prevention, 9,* 278–281. doi:10.1080/15389580801895210

Michon, J. A. (1985). A critical view of driver behavior models: What do we know, what should we do? In E. L. Evans & R. Schwing (Eds.), *Human behavior and traffic safety* (pp. 485–520). New York: Plenum.

Odenheimer, G. L., Beaudet, M., Jette, A. M., Albert, M. S., Grande, L., & Minaker, K. L. (1994). Performance-based driving evaluation of the elderly driver: Safety, reliability, and validity. *Journal of Gerontology, 49*(4), M153–M159.

Stephens, B. W., McCarthy, D. P., Marsiske, M., Shechtman, O., Classen, S., Justiss, M., et al. (2005). International Older Driver Consensus Conference on Assessment, Remediation and Counseling for Transportation Alternatives: Summary and recommendations. *Physical and Occupational Therapy in Geriatrics, 23,* 103–121. doi:10.1300/J148v23n02_07

Wheatley, C. J., & Di Stefano, M. (2008). Individualized assessment of driving fitness for older individuals with health, disability, and age-related concerns. *Traffic Injury Prevention, 9,* 320–327. doi:10.1080/15389580801895269

Appendix 12.A. Mr. Weathers's Community Mobility Recommendations

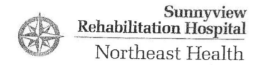

Sunnyview Rehabilitation Hospital
Northeast Health

1270 Belmont Avenue
Schenectady, New York 12308

ON-THE-ROAD (FUNCTIONAL) EVALUATION

Name: Don Weathers   Date: 10/11/11

ID#: 04295   Start Time: 10:00   End Time: 11:00

Areas Covered: Residential: ✓ Rural: ✓ Light Business: ✓ Heavy Business ✓
Highway: ✓

Weather Conditions: Clear: ✓ Rain: ___ Fog: ___ Snow: ___ Ice: ___

I. Preparation and Vehicle Operation

Operation	Independent	Comments
Open/Close Door	✓	
Transfers	✓	
Mobility Aid Management	NA	
Adjusts Seat	✓	
Fastens Seat Belt	✓	needed cue to put on
Adjusts Mirrors	✓	cued to adjust prior to moving
Key Insertion	✓	
Ignition	✓	
Parking Brake	NA	
Gear Selector	✓	
Brake Pedal	✓	Drove with two feet (left foot braking) while in parking lot. Did not fully release brake while accelerating to back out of parking space.
Accelerator Pedal	✓	
Steering Wheel	✓	
Turn Signal	✓	
Windshield Wipers	NA	
Head Lights	NA	
High/Low Beams	NA	
Dashboard Controls	NA	
Windows	NA	

(Continued)

Appendix 12.A. Mr. Weathers's Community Mobility Recommendations (cont.)

Name: Don Weathers   ID: 04295

II. Vehicle Control	Adequate	Comments
Steering Control	✓	
Smooth Acceleration	✓	
Controlled Braking	⇒	Several occasions would brake for no apparent reason. Excessive braking for green lights
Centered Lane Position	⇒	In center of road on residential streets. Did not cross over roads with center yellow line.
Maneuvers Turn (road position and speed)	⇒	One wide right turn and three short left turns.
Complete Stop	✓	
Appropriate Stopping Distance	✓	
Appropriate Speed Control	⇒	usually 5mph below posted speed limit. more than 10 mph below on roads with speed of 55mph
Proper Following Distance	✓	
Backing Up	⇒	Decreased observations while backing up. Excessive manuvering and time to get in or out of space. On accelerator and brake at same time while parking
Parking	⇒	

III. Turns and Intersections	Adequate	Comments
Signals For Turn	✓	
Positions in Propper Lane For Turn	✓	
Checks Traffic	✓	
Yields Right of Way	✓	
Appropriate Gap in Traffic	⇒	Due to slow speed of turns needs to allow more gap for left turns.
Appropriate Speed Adjustment	⇒	
Turns Into Proper Lane	✓	

Appendix 12.A. Mr. Weathers's Community Mobility Recommendations *(cont.)*

Name : Don Weathers   ID: 0429S

III. Turns and Intersections
(Continued)

	Adequate	Comments
Obeys Traffic Signs and Signals	⟹	After stopping for one stop sign was beeped at from car behind to go. Said he was waiting for the light to change
Anticipates Light Changes	✓	
Timely Decision Making	⟹	hesitant to take turn at all way stops.

IV. Lane Changes and Merging

	Adequate	Comments
Signal for Lane Change/Merge	✓	
Checks Rear View Mirror	✓	
Checks Side View Mirror	⟹	Inconsistent and does not use Right side view mirror at all.
Checks Blind Spot	no	Failed to check even after cues to do so.
Maintains Good Lane Position	⟹	Speed drops and drifts in lane when checking rear view mirror and waiting for traffic to pass.
Appropriate Speed Adjustment	⟹	
Appropriate Gap in Traffic	✓	
Appropriate Use of Acceleration/Deceleration Ramp	⟹	Slow to get up to speed and observe. Pulls into faster lane of traffic more than 10 mph below speed of traffic
Merges Safely	⟹	

(Continued)

Appendix 12.A. Mr. Weathers's Community Mobility Recommendations (cont.)

Name: Don Weathers   ID: 04295

V. Driver Interaction Skills	Adequate	Comments
Handles Distractions	⇒	minimal conversation while driving. at times distracted by his own thoughts
Maintains a Safe Space Cushion	✓	
Plans Ahead for Maneuvers	⇒	cues given for all navagation needed directions repeated or would forget to make turns
Demonstrates Good Decision Making and Judgment	no	slow speeds, excessive braking, + hesitant decisions make him the hazard.
Adjusts Speed and Position for Potential Hazards	no	appears unaware of possible situations developing around him. unable to
Responds Quickly to Changing Conditions and Unexpected Events	no	make changes to driving behaviors even after cues.
Communicates and Interacts with Other Drivers Safely	no	

Additional Treatment Required: no

Frequency of Treatment: _____ sessions per week of _____ minutes, for _____ weeks.

Recommendations:

Patient demonstrated fair vehicle control but unsafe driving behaviors. Slow processing speed, decreased attention, decreased memory, and increased reaction time are major areas of concern. Deficits present while driving and cause poor speed management, inconsistent attention to signs, difficulty with right-of-way, and an inability to make improvements to driving behavior when cued. Patient advised not to drive. Patient's daughter present for discussion and provided with information on alternative transportation options

Therapist Signature: _____ Date: _____ Time: _____

Appendix 12.A. Mr. Weathers's Community Mobility Recommendations *(cont.)*

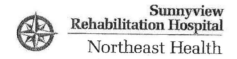

Sunnyview
Rehabilitation Hospital
Northeast Health

1270 Belmont Avenue
Schenectady, New York 12308

COMMUNITY MOBILITY RECOMMENDATIONS

Name: Don Weathers   ID #: 04295   Date: 10/11/11

Driving Recommendations:

_____ Demonstrates adequate skills for safe driving while driving in;

_____ residential _____ rural _____ light business _____ heavy business _____ highway

_____ Limit driving to:

_____ daylight hours
_____ familiar areas
_____ local areas (_____ mile radius of home)
_____ single lane roadways
_____ roads with speed no greater than _____ mph.
_____ no rush hour or peak traffic times
_____ reduced distractions (eating, conversations, radio play, young children in vehicle, etc.)
_____ supervised by a licensed driver
_____ other _____

_____ Additional training required
_____ Attend a defensive driving course
_____ A re-evaluation recommended in approximately_____ to re-assess skills and safety.
_____ Driving not recommended at the present time. A re-evaluation may be performed at a later date (approximately _____).
__✓_ Driving not recommended. Advised to use alternative means of transportation.

Reasons: Inconsistent attention, slow processing and reaction time, decreased memory and diminished road sign recognition and knowledge of rules of the road.

Vehicle/Equipment Restrictions:

_____ automatic transmission
_____ power brakes/steering
_____ left foot accelerator, with quick release pin and pedal guard over right accelerator pedal
_____ left/right steering knob at_____ position
_____ hand controls

_____ push/pull   _____ push/rock   _____ right angle push
mounted on _____ side of steering column

_____ pedal guard, with quick release pin, over right accelerator pedal
_____ other: _____
_____

(Continued)

Appendix 12.A. Mr. Weathers's Community Mobility
Recommendations *(cont.)*

Name: *Don Weathers*   ID #: *04295*

Patient/Family Education:

_____ Provided information on area vendors of adaptive driving equipment.

_____ Informed of the need to report to the Department of Motor Vehicles for restrictions to be placed on drivers license.

Provided the following handouts:

- ☐ compensatory strategies
- ☐ tips for safe driving
- ☐ driving strategies
- ☐ six tips for driving wellness
- ☐ medications and driving
- ☐ defensive driving courses
- ☐

- ☐ vehicle design considerations
- ☐ manufacturers' rebate programs
- ☐ adaptive vehicle rentals
- ☐ fitting the car to the driver
- ☐ adjusting/setting your mirrors
- ☐ CarFit gadgets

- ☒ alternative transportation options
- ☐ The Hartford: We need to talk...
- ☐ The Hartford: At the Crossroads
- ☒ getting by without driving
- ☒ DMV: medical conditions of a driver and accident re-examination

Acknowledgement:

The above recommendations have been reviewed with me and I understand them. I am aware that my physician will make the final decision regarding my driving status. The results and recommendations included in this report are based on the patient's performance during the period of the evaluation and should not be relied on as absolute predictors of future performance. The conclusions reached and recommendations made in this report are based, in part, upon medical information available at the time this report was written. If subsequent to the issuance of this report, the patient's medical status changes in such a manner that may compromise the patient's abilities as a driver, this report can no longer be relied upon as valid.

_____	_____	_____
Patient Signature	Date	Driver Rehabilitation Specialist

_____	_____	_____
Witness	Date	Relationship to Patient

Patient's Comments: _____

_____

_____

Note. Provided by Sunnyview Rehabilitation Hospital, Schenectady, NY. Used with permission.

Appendix 12.B. Compensatory Strategies Handout

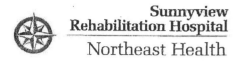

Sunnyview
Rehabilitation Hospital
Northeast Health

1270 Belmont Avenue
Schenectady, New York 12308

COMMUNITY MOBILITY RECOMMENDATIONS

Name: Tidd, J.   ID #: 2234   Date: 10/1/11

Driving Recommendations:

___✓___ Demonstrates adequate skills for safe driving while driving in;

___✓___ residential ___✓___ rural ___✓___ light business ___NO___ heavy business ___NO___ highway

___✓___ Limit driving to:

    ___✓___ daylight hours

    ___✓___ familiar areas

    ___✓___ local areas (__10__ mile radius of home)

    _____ single lane roadways

    _____ roads with speed no greater than _____ mph.

    ___✓___ no rush hour or peak traffic times

    ___✓___ reduced distractions (eating, conversations, radio play, young children in vehicle, etc.)

    _____ supervised by a licensed driver

    _____ other _____

_____ Additional training required

___✓___ Attend a defensive driving course

_____ A re-evaluation recommended in approximately_____ to re-assess skills and safety.

_____ Driving not recommended at the present time. A re-evaluation may be performed at a later date (approximately _____).

_____ Driving not recommended. Advised to use alternative means of transportation.

    Reasons: _____

    _____

    _____

Vehicle/Equipment Restrictions:

_____ automatic transmission

_____ power brakes/steering

_____ left foot accelerator, with quick release pin and pedal guard over right accelerator pedal

_____ left/right steering knob at_____ position

_____ hand controls

    _____ push/pull   _____ push/rock   _____ right angle push

    mounted on _____ side of steering column

    _____ pedal guard, with quick release pin, over right accelerator pedal

___✓___ other: Auxiliary mirrors, extended rearview mirror

    _____

(Continued)

Appendix 12.B. Compensatory Strategies Handout *(cont.)*

Name: Tidd, J   ID #: 2234

Patient/Family Education:

_____ Provided information on area vendors of adaptive driving equipment.

_____ Informed of the need to report to the Department of Motor Vehicles for restrictions to be placed on drivers license.

Provided the following handouts:

☒ compensatory strategies	☐ vehicle design considerations	☒ alternative transportation options
☐ tips for safe driving	☐ manufacturers' rebate programs	☐ The Hartford: We need to talk…
☒ driving strategies	☐ adaptive vehicle rentals	☐ The Hartford: At the Crossroads
☐ six tips for driving wellness	☐ fitting the car to the driver	☐ getting by without driving
☐ medications and driving	☒ adjusting/setting your mirrors	☐ DMV: medical conditions of a
☒ defensive driving courses	☐ CarFit gadgets	driver and accident re-examination

☒ information about mirrors

Acknowledgement:

The above recommendations have been reviewed with me and I understand them. I am aware that my physician will make the final decision regarding my driving status. The results and recommendations included in this report are based on the patient's performance during the period of the evaluation and should not be relied on as absolute predictors of future performance. The conclusions reached and recommendations made in this report are based, in part, upon medical information available at the time this report was written. If subsequent to the issuance of this report, the patient's medical status changes in such a manner that may compromise the patient's abilities as a driver, this report can no longer be relied upon as valid.

J. Tidd   10/1/11
_____   _____   _____
Patient Signature   Date   Driver Rehabilitation Specialist

_____   _____   _____
Witness   Date   Relationship to Patient

Patient's Comments: _____
                           _____
                           _____

Appendix 12.B. Compensatory Strategies Handout *(cont.)*

Tidd, S.

SUNNYVIEW HOSPITAL AND REHABILITION CENTER
1270 Belmont Avenue, Schenectady, New York
OCCUPATIONAL THERAPY DEPARTMENT

Compensatory Strategies

Your driver evaluation indicates that you scored below the standard or may have difficulty in one or more of the following areas (see checks). For each area checked there are recommendations to guide you in your return to driving

1. _____ Visual Acuity:
   Good acuity allows you to read traffic signs, street names and addresses at a distance that gives you time to respond safely to conditions. New York State requires 20/40 vision with or without correction. If you do not meet the standard, you should consult an eye care specialist before you drive.

2. __✓__ Night Vision/Glare Recovery:
   Age as well as many eye conditions can affect your ability to see at night. Reduce the amount of night driving you do, or stop altogether. If you must go out at night, try to drive on well-lit streets. The more light there is, the easier it is to read signs, and the less head light glare there is. Before starting out, give your eyes at least 5 minutes to adjust to the darkness. Avoid wearing tinted glasses or sunglasses. Make sure that your car's windshield, window, mirrors, and headlights are clean. Avoid looking directly into the headlights of other cars.

3. __✓__ Contrast Sensitivity:
   The ability to see objects of reduced contrast can be impaired by a wide variety of eye diseases. Low contrast can make distinguishing cars or pedestrians against back ground scenery difficult. Avoid driving at dusk and dawn or when it is foggy and over-cast.

4. __✓__ Field of Vision/Peripheral Vision:
   Age as well as eye disease can affect the ability to see to the sides, up and or down. New York State requires a visual field of 140° with certain eye conditions. If you have a decrease in field of vision it may effect lane position, or the ability to see vehicles on quick glances for lane changes. Move your head and eyes often while driving. Adjust existing mirrors on your car to increase your range of vision. Use additional mirrors that are designed to give a larger field of view.

5. __✓__ Depth Perception:
   This allows you to judge distances between yourself and other vehicles, pedestrians, and objects, as well as judging speed. We use depth perception to

(Continued)

Appendix 12.B. Compensatory Strategies Handout *(cont.)*

merge with and to cross traffic, as well as for parking. These abilities may decline with age. Allow more distance between your car and the car in front of you (three or more seconds). Stop so you can see the tires of the car in front of you, or the stop lines or cross walk. Use regulated intersections when ever possible. Choose parking spaces that have additional space. Avoid driving at night.

6. _____ Color Perception:
The ability to discriminate different colors or shades of the same color diminishes with age due to the yellowing of the eye's lens. Recognizing brake lights or turn signals of the vehicles in front of you may become delayed. Some traffic lights might become hard to see. Slow down and allow more distance between you and the car in front of you. Approach traffic lights cautiously.

7. _____ Visual Perception:
This is the ability to analyze, interpret and make use of the incoming visual information in order to interact with the environment. Visual perception includes the following sub skills;

> Visual Discrimination: The ability to be aware of the distinctive feature of forms including shape, orientation, size and color. Deficits may cause problems with; recognizing signs, dealing with intersections, or recognizing hazards.

> Figure Ground: The ability to distinguish an object from background or surrounding objects. Deficits may cause difficulty finding signs among other stimuli of the environment. Will have increasing difficulty as traffic increases and/or road scene increases in complexity. May have difficulty finding controls or dashboard information quickly in the vehicle.

> Visual Closure: The ability to perceive a whole figure when only fragments are visible. Visualizing missing information is important to safe driving because it allows you to recognize a whole object when only part of it is in view. Deficits may cause difficulty recognizing signs or other traffic control devices that are partially covered by trees or other objects. May not be able to look ahead and see what's happening in the whole environment, or perceive the safety threat represented by a vehicle or pedestrian that is partially obstructed at the side of the road, and may be about to move into the driver's path.

> Visual Memory: The ability to recognize one stimulus item after a very brief interval. May impair ability to cross or turn into traffic at intersections. Can create difficulty with navigation or mapping skills.

> Spatial Relationships: The ability to orient one's body in space and to perceive the positions of objects in relation to oneself and to other objects.

Appendix 12.B. Compensatory Strategies Handout *(cont.)*

May cause trouble staying in lane, or orienting vehicle when in curves or coming out of turns. Difficulties increase at complex and/or angled intersection. May have trouble backing up and parking.

Perceptual Time: The speed at which perception takes place. How quickly visual information is interpreted. Slower perceptual time will cause a delay in responding to signs, signals and traffic situations. May cause the driver to drive too slowly in traffic.

Deficits in any or all of these areas may prevent safe driving altogether. If driving is still possible limit driving to familiar areas and do not drive in busy or congested areas.

8. _____ Attention Skills:
The ability to stay focused on a task for a sustained period of time, to ignore what is not important while focusing on what is important, and the ability to do two things at once are all functions of attention. As attention abilities decline, the chance of being in an accident increases. Research shows that attention abilities become harder as we age. Many medical conditions can also affect attention. If you have diminished attention, drive in familiar areas, avoid driving in busy traffic situations, and reduce distractions such as talking, playing the radio, or trying to eat while driving.

9. _____ Processing Time:
The speed of your thinking and decision making declines with age and other medical conditions. This change can lead to slow or hesitant driving, unexpected lane changes, and slowed reactions to driving situations. All of these things combine to increase the chance of being in a traffic accident. To reduce your risk while driving, drive in familiar areas, avoid busy traffic situations, take routes that are less crowded, and drive on roadways with slower speeds.

10. _____ Memory:
Memory helps us use a familiar traffic route, and to remember and consistently apply traffic rules and regulations. It is particularly important to remember when traffic rules change, for example when the speed or direction on a street changes from one time of day to another, or when permission to turn is different from one intersection to the next. Our memory is also important in problem solving and decision making. If you have memory difficulties limit driving to a select few places that are in familiar areas and use fixed routes. Make a habit of parking in the same place or writing down where you have parked.

11. _____ Reduced Knowledge of Rules of The Road:
Many drivers have not had formal driver training, and may not have properly learned the rules of the road. Many drivers also become "rusty" or complacent with following them. Stay current on rules of the road and become familiar with new lane markings and traffic signals and signs. Consider taking a driving

(Continued)

Appendix 12.B. Compensatory Strategies Handout *(cont.)*

refresher course. Communicate your intentions by positioning your car in the proper lane and consistently signaling. Know where you biggest dangers are and drive defensively.

12. ___✓___ Physical Fitness:
Drivers may have several minor physical or medical problems, each of which taken separately may not affect their driving ability very much, but when taken together, could make driving dangerous. Flexibility can be reduced, making it harder to do certain driving tasks. Decreased neck flexibility makes it hard to turn our heads leading to difficulty backing up, checking for traffic at intersections, and changing lanes. Depending on how your mirrors are adjusted, and the kind of car you drive, there are usually several blind spots around your vehicle. Discomfort in joints can slow reaction time and reduce our ability to turn the steering wheel or step on the brake. Lack of strength in our arms or legs may interfere with our ability to accelerate, brake, or steer while driving. Fortunately physical fitness can often be improved through exercise. Begin a fitness program; it's never too late to start. Make sure you have a good fitting vehicle with an adjustable seat, steering wheel and seat belt. Use a seat cushion or back support for better position and comfort. Power steering and brakes require less strength and stamina. Fit your car with adaptive equipment such as special mirrors, steering wheel covers and grips or devices recommended by your driver rehabilitation specialist. Avoid long periods of driving without a break. Avoid driving when muscle or joint pain is increased.

13. ___✓___ Reaction Time:
A delay in how fast you can move from the accelerator to the brake can cause you to travel many extra feet before stopping. Slow down, maintain extra distance between yourself and other cars, and avoid heavy traffic situations.

14. _____ Medication Use:
Both prescription and over-the-counter medications can slow reflexes, blur vision and cause drowsiness or dizziness. How a drug will affect an individual is difficult to predict. When one or more drugs are taken in combination, it may cause serious adverse effects. As we age, our body chemistry changes and drugs have stronger effects than when we were younger. Make sure to read medication labels and follow directions carefully. Check with your doctor or pharmacist about the possible side effects of the drug(s) you are taking, especially effects that could impair driving abilities. Also ask what, if anything, you can do to counter the side effects that affect driving. Never stop your medication or change the dosage without checking with your doctor. Do not drive when using medications that make you sleepy or affect your ability to drive.

Note. Provided by Sunnyview Rehabilitation Hospital, Schenectady, NY. Used with permission.

Appendix 12.C. Driver Rehabilitation On-Road Program Goals and Flow Sheet

Sunnyview Rehabilitation Hospital
Northeast Health

Driver Rehabilitation Program Progress Report

Name: Mitchell, R.
ID #: 21749

Insurance: ☒ Medicare ☐ Medicaid ☐ Worker's Comp ☐ Self Pay ☐ Other
☐ ACCES-VR

Diagnosis: RBKA, OLE Neuropathy

Date: 9/5/11   Start Time: 1:00   End Time: 3:00   Tx: 97537   Minutes: 120   Units: 8   Session #: 1 - Evaluation
Client's Comments: Pt has not driven since RBKA 7/11
Response to Treatment: No significant DM other than RBKA, and decreased proprioception + kinesthesia in OLE Due to sensory loss, Pt assesses with hand controls + not OLE foot accelerator. Pt demonstrates the ability to drive w/ hand controls but additional training required. Pt being patient in the use of ada drive equipment.

☐ current medical diagnoses and medications reviewed/updated.   ☐ continue current treatment
Signature: _____   Date: 9/5/11   Time: 3:30

Date: 9/12/11   Start Time: 10:00   End Time: 11:00   Tx: 97537   Minutes: 60   Units: 4   Session #: 2
Client's Comments: Pt reports less nervous now about hand controls that to expect
Response to Treatment: Pt drove w/ push/pull style of hand controls. No attempts to use OLE foot to brake but frequently would brake just to reassure himself he could stop the vehicle. Pt advised of the risk for a rear-end collision if no brakes unexpectedly.

☐ current medical diagnoses and medications reviewed/updated.   ☐ continue current treatment
Signature: _____   Date: 9/12/11   Time: 11:00

Date: 9/14/11   Start Time: 10:00   End Time: 11:00   Tx: 97537   Minutes: 60   Units: 4   Session #: 3
Client's Comments: Pt eager to practice backing up and parking
Response to Treatment: Good control of vehicle w/ backing up + parking. Good judgment of driveways at parking spaces and confusion of gas or brake. Good number of all speeds and traffic conditions. Able to carry a conversation while driving + solving road signs.

☐ current medical diagnoses and medications reviewed/updated.   ☐ continue current treatment
Signature: _____   Date: 9/14/11   Time: 11:00

Date: 9/16/11   Start Time: 10:00   End Time: 11:00   Tx: 97537   Minutes: 60   Units: 4   Session #: 4
Client's Comments: Pt eager to resume driving and "return to living his life"
Response to Treatment: Pt assessed in different style of hand controls (push/rock). Pt demonstrated good control w/ Pt expressed all signals + rules of the road safe interaction w/ other traffic. No further training.

☐ current medical diagnoses and medications reviewed/updated.   ☐ continue current treatment
Signature: _____   Date: 9/16/11   Time: 11:00

Page: 1

(Continued)

Appendix 12.C. Driver Rehabilitation On-Road Program Goals and Flow Sheet *(cont.)*

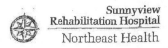

Sunnyview
Rehabilitation Hospital
Northeast Health

Name: mitchell, R.
ID #: 21749

Driver Rehabilitation On-Road Program Goals and Flow Sheet

Goals Addressed:

Vehicle Control:

	Date: 9/5/11	Date: 9/12/11	Date: 9/14/11	Date: 9/19/11
Able to coordinate acceleration/braking and steering simultaneously.	✓	✓	✓	✓
Signals for turns in a timely manner.	✓	✓	✓	✓
Good lane position and speed for right and left turns.	✓	✓	✓	✓
Good lane position and speed on roads with speeds up to 30 mph.	✓	✓	✓	✓
Complete stops including appropriate stopping distance.	✓	✓	✓	✓
Demonstrated appropriate following distance and maintains safe space cushion.	✓	✓	✓	✓
Good lane position and speed on roads with speeds up to 55 mph.		✓	✓	✓
Adjusts speed and position for hazards.	✓	✓	✓	✓
Good observations, speed control, and steering when backing up.	✓	✓	✓	✓
Good skills and observations with angular and perpendicular parking.			✓	✓
Consistently signals and checks over shoulder prior to leaving curb.			✓	✓
Good technique and observations when performing 3-point turns.			✓	✓
Good technique and observations when parallel parking.				

Intersection Management:

	Date: 9/5/11	Date: 9/12/11	Date: 9/14/11	Date: 9/19/11
Recognizes 2 way versus all way stops and takes turn accordingly.	✓	✓	✓	✓
Obeys traffic signs.	✓	✓	✓	✓
Obeys traffic signals and anticipates light changes.	✓	✓	✓	✓
Positions in proper lane for turn.	✓	✓	✓	✓
Checks traffic and is aware of prevalent threat(s)/danger(s).	✓	✓	✓	✓
Yields right of way.	✓	✓	✓	✓
Appropriate gap in traffic for manuvers.	✓	✓	✓	✓
Turns into propper lane.	✓	✓	✓	✓
Utilizes shared left turn lane appropriately.		✓	✓	✓

Lane Changes and Merging:

	Date: 9/5/11	Date: 9/12/11	Date: 9/14/11	Date: 9/19/11
Signals for lane change/merge.		✓	✓	✓
Checks rear view mirror.		✓	✓	✓
Checks appropriate side view mirror		✓	✓	✓
Checks blind spot and adequately observes.		✓	✓	✓
Maintains good lane position.		✓	✓	✓
Appropriate speed adjustment.		✓	✓	✓
Appropriate gap in traffic.		✓	✓	✓
Appropriate use of acceleration/decceleration ramps.		✓	✓	✓
Merges safely.		✓	✓	✓
Appropriate and safe use of toll lanes/booths.				✓

Driver Interaction Skills:

	Date: 9/5/11	Date: 9/12/11	Date: 9/14/11	Date: 9/19/11
Utilizes an organized visual search pattern and adequate visual lead time.		✓	✓	✓
Manages time and space appropriately.		✓	✓	✓
Plans ahead for manuevers.		✓	✓	✓
Responds quikly to changing conditions and unexpected events.		✓	✓	✓
Communicateds and interacts with other drivers safely.		✓	✓	✓
Appropriately controls emotions and impulses.		✓	✓	✓

Appendix 12.C. Driver Rehabilitation On-Road Program Goals and Flow Sheet *(cont.)*

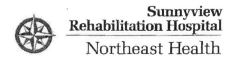

Sunnyview Rehabilitation Hospital
Northeast Health

1270 Belmont Avenue
Schenectady, New York 12308

COMMUNITY MOBILITY RECOMMENDATIONS

Name: mitchell, R.   ID #: 2749   Date: 9/19/11

Driving Recommendations:

✓ Demonstrates adequate skills for safe driving while driving in;

____ ✓ residential ____ ✓ rural ____ ✓ light business ____ ✓ heavy business ____ ✓ highway

____ Limit driving to:

____ daylight hours

____ familiar areas

____ local areas (_____ mile radius of home)

____ single lane roadways

____ roads with speed no greater than _____ mph.

____ no rush hour or peak traffic times

____ reduced distractions (eating, conversations, radio play, young children in vehicle, etc.)

____ supervised by a licensed driver

____ other _____

____ Additional training required

____ Attend a defensive driving course

____ A re-evaluation recommended in approximately_____ to re-assess skills and safety.

____ Driving not recommended at the present time. A re-evaluation may be performed at a later date (approximately _____).

____ Driving not recommended. Advised to use alternative means of transportation.

Reasons: _____

_____

_____

Vehicle/Equipment Restrictions:

✓ automatic transmission

✓ power brakes/steering

____ left foot accelerator, with quick release pin and pedal guard over right accelerator pedal

✓ left/right steering knob at 4'.00 position

✓ hand controls

✓ push/pull   ____ push/rock   ____ right angle push

mounted on left side of steering column

✓ pedal guard, with quick release pin, over right accelerator pedal

____ other: _____

(Continued)

Appendix 12.C. Driver Rehabilitation On-Road
Program Goals and Flow Sheet *(cont.)*

Name: Mitchell, R.   ID#: 2749

Patient/Family Education:

✓ Provided information on area vendors of adaptive driving equipment.

✓ Informed of the need to report to the Department of Motor Vehicles for restrictions to be placed on drivers license.

Provided the following handouts:

☐ compensatory strategies	☐ vehicle design considerations	☐ alternative transportation options
☐ tips for safe driving	☑ manufacturers' rebate programs	☐ The Hartford: We need to talk…
☐ driving strategies	☑ adaptive vehicle rentals	☐ The Hartford: At the Crossroads
☐ six tips for driving wellness	☐ fitting the car to the driver	☐ getting by without driving
☐ medications and driving	☐ adjusting/setting your mirrors	☐ DMV: medical conditions of a
☐ defensive driving courses	☐ CarFit gadgets	driver and accident re-examination
☐ _____		

Acknowledgement:

The above recommendations have been reviewed with me and I understand them. I am aware that my physician will make the final decision regarding my driving status. The results and recommendations included in this report are based on the patient's performance during the period of the evaluation and should not be relied on as absolute predictors of future performance. The conclusions reached and recommendations made in this report are based, in part, upon medical information available at the time this report was written. If subsequent to the issuance of this report, the patient's medical status changes in such a manner that may compromise the patient's abilities as a driver, this report can no longer be relied upon as valid.

R. Mitchell	_9/19/11_	_____
Patient Signature	Date	Driver Rehabilitation Specialist

_____	_____	_____
Witness	Date	Relationship to Patient

Patient's Comments: _____

_____

_____

Note. Provided by Sunnyview Rehabilitation Hospital, Schenectady, NY. Used with permission.

CHAPTER 13

Assessing, Treating, and Preparing Youth With Special Needs for Driving and Community Mobility

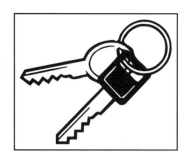

Miriam Monahan, MS, OTR/L, CDRS, CDI

Learning Objectives

At the completion of this chapter, readers will be able to

- Identify how youth with special needs may be at risk for being ill prepared for driving because of a lack of participation in predriving activities;
- Identify driving situations that challenge social and executive function skills;
- Identify evaluation considerations for youth with cognitive or physical limitations for driving; and
- Identify intervention concepts to develop a student's executive function skills for managing intersections, maneuvers, and roadway hazards.

Key Words

- **driving school instructor**
- **independence**
- **life skills**
- **passenger activities**
- **plan of care**
- **social capital**

Introduction

As they approach driving age, most adolescents are interested in attaining their license to move to a new level of independence. They want to go places without adults; go and come as they please; and expand their social, leisure, and vocational opportunities. Not everyone is ready to drive at the age at which it is legal to drive in their state. In fact, some adults would argue that all youth should not be able to obtain a driver's license until 18 or 21 years of age.

Scientific evidence indicates that the frontal lobe is not fully developed at the age most people are considering learning to drive. Much of the research on the developing adolescent brain has been done with magnetic resonance imaging scans. The scans indicate increased myelination in the frontal cortex of 20- to 23-year-olds as compared to 12- to 16-year-olds (Sowell, Thompson, Holmes, Jernigan, & Toga, 1999). The increase in myelination "likely relates to the maturation of cognitive processing and other 'executive' functions" (National Institute of Mental Health [NIMH], 2010, p. 2). The adolescent brain presents a unique challenge when it comes to identifying the readiness to drive of a youth with special needs who may have executive function deficits.

During the natural maturation process, a young person typically is engaged in activities that prepare him or her for driving. Riding bikes, operating motorized recreational vehicles (e.g., boats, all-terrain vehicles [ATVs]), playing basketball, jumping rope, skateboarding, and other activities help to develop visual, motor, and cognitive skills for operating a car. These activities directly stimulate the neurological pathways that enable a driver to scan the environment, process what he or she sees, make a plan, and physically react—all in a timely manner.

In addition, as they age, youth are gaining independence at home and in the community. They may be responsible for younger siblings, pets, household chores, or jobs in the community. They may be traveling alone in the community—walking as pedestrians, riding bikes, or using public transportation. As youth mature, they interact with strangers without the support of familiar adults. Independence in all of these activities indicates that the youth has the cognitive and behavioral skills needed to be a responsible driver.

The youth with special needs may not have engaged in many of these predriving activities for several reasons. Whether an occupational therapist is a generalist or a driver rehabilitation specialist (DRS), the therapist has the capacity to analyze the task of driving and the activities a student is currently engaged in to determine if those necessary predriving skills have been developed. If driving is not an appropriate goal, the practitioner can identify what means of community mobility is appropriate for a particular youth as well as provide strategies to help that individual compensate for deficits.

All therapists working with youth with special needs should address activities that prepare students for driving or community mobility from an early point in development. The school, home, and the community are all great settings to develop these skills.

This chapter provides an overview of essential evaluation components for assessing a student's readiness to learn to drive and to independently access the community. The skills used in driving and community mobility are broad and are incorporated in all facets of life, so information gathered from the assessments is valuable for creating a student's vocational, academic, and independent living goals. The chapter also introduces principles that are essential for driver training when working with youth with special needs. Although it can be very challenging to work with the adolescent population, it also can be greatly rewarding.

This chapter focuses on the needs of young people, but it is also applicable to older individuals who are learning to drive for the first time. In this chapter, youth may be referred to as *students,* because they are individuals learning to drive.

Before Working With New Drivers

The occupational therapist who desires to provide driver training to youth with special needs should strongly consider becoming a certified driving school instructor. (*Note.* State requirements vary as to whether an occupational therapist needs to be a driving school instructor. Required or not, obtaining this education is recommended.) Teaching any novice how to drive can be complicated. For example, think about instructing someone on when to return the steering wheel after initiating a right or left turn. The steering wheel is returned just before the turn is complete and the car is straight in the lane. This is an action most of us do multiple times a day, but most of us could not articulate the position of the car in the lane when the steering wheel is returned.

Now think about teaching someone with visual–perceptual deficits or bilateral coordination deficits on when and how to return the wheel. In addition to the inherent physical, visual, and cognitive deficits that may be present because of an individual's condition, teaching a new driver with a disability may be further complicated by the youth's lack of experience participating in the activities that help prepare him or her for driving. As mentioned earlier, riding a bike, a skateboard, or a motorized ATV, among many other activities, can support learning how to maneuver a vehicle. Students with special needs may not have participated in these or similar activities.

A driving school instructor's background provides the occupational therapist with the skills needed to break down the task of driving into teaching units that build on themselves. Occupational therapists have the ability to add appropriate strategies or break down the task further to aid the student with special needs. Occupational therapists who seek the additional education to understand how to teach driving, by fulfilling the requirements to be a driving instructor, are well equipped to serve this population.

Every state's program for training driving school instructors is unique. If the state's requirements for driving school instructors are minimal, the therapist should seek out other educational opportunities. The therapist should become familiar with the state's motor vehicle driver requirements for youth and novice operators. The therapist should determine the requirements for attaining a learner's permit, maintaining the permit, and acquiring a license with or without a disability. Some states have instituted junior operator's permits and licenses that have specific requirements.

Common Diagnoses Typically Seen in Students With Special Needs

Students who come to driver rehabilitation seeking an evaluation for driving typically have a condition that is either congenital or acquired. A physical impairment may have caused limited range of motion or strength. A vision impairment may cause low acuity, ocular–motor limitations, or visual field defects. A cognitive impairment may cause challenges with visual perception, cognitive-processing speed, attention, executive functions, or social and behavioral skills. A student may have a combination of visual, physical, and cognitive deficits. The following diagnoses are commonly seen in adolescents seeking driver rehabilitation services:

- Spina bifida (SB)
- Cerebral palsy (CP)
- Muscular dystrophy
- Low intelligence quotient (IQ)
- Autism spectrum disorders (ASDs)
- Traumatic brain injury (TBI)
- Spinal cord injury (SCI).

Physical Impairments

When physical impairments prevent students from driving with standard driving equipment, the clinical assessment is the same as for experienced drivers with a physical disability. Therapists should be concerned about a student's ability to drive safely, even when the physical disability may appear mild. If the therapist is uncertain whether the identified physical limitations will interfere with the student's ability to drive safely, he or she should refer the student and the student's family to a certified DRS.

The outcome of the DRS's evaluation should provide a list of adaptive equipment and vehicle recommendations. Obtaining funding for that equipment can be difficult for some families. If cost is a significant concern, then the function of the driver rehabilitation program would be to direct the student and family to potential funding resources. Sometimes the funding sources do not want to fund a student until that individual can manage the expenses to maintain and insure the equipped vehicle. For example, the funding source might not be willing to fund a 16-year-old to obtain a $100,000 van but would be willing to fund the same van for a 24-year-old who graduated from college and has an income to manage the costs incurred to operate such a vehicle.

Setting up a vehicle for an individual with a congenital impairment is typically more challenging than working with an individual with an acquired injury such as a SCI. For example, individuals with conditions such as arthrogryposis, dwarfism, and SB have unique physical presentations and require creativity when selecting and positioning the driving equipment.

Setting up a vehicle for someone with a congenital disability is a trial-and-error process that takes patience and perseverance.

It is important to realize that setting up a vehicle for someone with a congenital disability is a trial-and-error process that takes patience and perseverance. Compared to other youth, students with physical limitations typically have very little or no experience with vehicles such as ATVs, snowmobiles, toy ride-on cars, and bicycles. Therefore, students with physical impairments may not have experience controlling gas, brake, and steering. During the on-road assessment for driving equipment, the therapist is teaching the student to steer and control the gas and brake while assessing the student's ability to operate the equipment. The therapist will be determining whether observed problems are because of novice driving skills or because of the driving equipment. The more complicated cases often take multiple sessions to select the right equipment and position of the equipment.

In addition to attending to the setup of the vehicle, the therapist should attend to the big picture. Remember that driving will enable many of these young people to be alone in the community for the first time. The therapist will need to evaluate the ability of the student to be alone in the community. Can the student take care of toileting, do appropriate pressure relief, and drink fluids, or will that person require a personal care attendant (PCA)? It may be time to relook at how the individual is taking care of himself or herself and to update some of the self-care skills, because abilities and technology may have changed since the last therapist's evaluation. If the student requires a PCA, driving will not enable independence in the community. External funding sources may be reluctant to support such cases.

Training

The training of new drivers on equipment is more extensive than training the experienced driver to drive with adaptive equipment. The student must learn how to drive in addition to learning how to use the adaptive equipment; the more complex the equipment, the longer the learning curve. Most youth observe adults driving standard driving equipment and, through that observation, learn how to operate a vehicle. The student driving with adaptive equipment may never have observed someone driving with those particular aids.

The therapist or instructor can provide training in different ways to consider the needs of the client. Driver's education may be provided in the high school as part of the academic curriculum, or it may be available through privately run driver education schools. The curriculum may take place both in the classroom and behind the wheel. For the student whose primary deficit is a physical disability, receiving the classroom education from a standard driver's education program in the public school or through a private driver training school is typically a very effective way for the student to learn and is a conservative financial approach.

When a therapist provides on-road training, the basic curriculum should be what is required by the state's licensing authority for any new driver. Exhibit 13.1 provides a sample of a **progression of driving skills** that can be incorporated with the individual state's requirements.

Driver training for these students should incorporate other life skills. Remember that these adolescents are emerging to independent living, and it's a great opportunity to address transitional life skills. The therapist may need to teach advocacy skills in the context of driving and for negotiating with strangers at a level the student may not have encountered before (see Practitioner's Reflection 13.1).

Students need to be educated on any laws that pertain to them for accessing fuel and other roadway assistance that may be applicable to them. Some states have laws that allow for full-service fueling without a service charge when the driver has a physical impairment. If the student is driving a van, he or she will need to learn how best to position the vehicle when parking to avoid other vehicles parking too close to the van's ramp or lift. Students who use manual wheelchairs need to learn how to transfer the chair in and out of the vehicle. It is likely that others have been providing this assistance. Many of these students never have had an occasion to dismantle the manual chair to its components for transfers.

Preparing for Driving

Preparing students with physical impairments for driving can begin long before they reach driving age. All therapists working with youth can address passenger transportation on multiple levels. The therapist should address safety when the youth is traveling in a wheelchair or riding in a vehicle where the standard seat belt and seating are inappropriate for the youth's needs. Just as custom seating

---

Practitioner's Reflection 13.1. Intervention Strategy for Self-Advocacy

I have had students enter parking garages with the adaptive van. Upon retrieving the ticket from the automated machine that opens the gate when the ticket is removed, several students have dropped the ticket on the ground. Obviously, they are not going to get out of the van in the wheelchair to retrieve it for many reasons, including that there is no space between the van and the machine for the wheelchair. Upon exiting the garage they have come in contact with people who don't understand why they don't have the ticket. I intentionally don't pick up the ticket because it is a great time to work on self-advocacy.

—*Miriam Monahan, MS, OTR/L, CDRS, CDI*

Exhibit 13.1. Example of a Progression of Driving Skills

Skills to Be Incorporated	Dates Addressed by Therapist			
Motor skills:				
Maneuvering for accelerating, braking, and steering in residential area				
Four-scan patterns for intersections (right and left turns from a stop, right and left turns from a moving position)				
Emphasize recognizing line-of-sight restrictions; practice in residential area				
Regulating speed for hills and curves (25–40 mph roadways)				
Lane position and speed regulations for hazard management (25–40 mph roadways)				
Making right and left turns onto 25–40 mph roadways from a stop (no light)				
Perpendicular parking and backing*				
Visual skills:				
Visual search for critical information—computer and on-road				
Checking rear when braking and approaching intersections				
Simple traffic circle				
All-way-stop intersections				
Scanning for left turn at multilane intersections (blind-spot hazards)				
Scanning parking lots and unstructured areas (shopping malls, pulling away from gas pumps, drive-through banks, and restaurants) with proper merging into other traffic				
Lane changes on an interstate and merging on the interstate				
Lane changes in business traffic				
Maneuvers for Department of Motor Vehicles exam:				
Turning around ("K" turn, three-point turn)				
Parallel parking				
Hill start				
Executive function skills:				
Car breaks down—where to stop the vehicle and who to get to help (rural, city, interstate environments)				
How best to turn around if you've gone past your destination; evaluating the best exit and entrance in parking lots				
Navigation: Using a computer program or map when traveling to an unfamiliar location; what to do if you get lost, and where to go for help				

Note. *Parking and backing are introduced at this level for the student to achieve confidence moving forward, mastering pedal orientation, and understanding the importance of visual scanning and line-of-sight limitations.

is needed for wheelchairs, it also can be needed in vehicle seats. Therapists can intervene with seating aids to allow youth with short stature to see out the window when riding in a vehicle. Too often, youth with short stature don't see what is happening on the roadway and lose valuable opportunities to understand traffic rules, driver behaviors, and potential solutions for driving problems and emergencies.

Therapists should address community independence with these youth as a possible means to reach independence as a driver. Youth must be able to function without a PCA and be able to self-advocate when in the community.

Cognitive Impairment

It is important for therapists working in the school systems, driver rehabilitation clinics, and outpatient rehabilitation programs to determine whether a student may be at risk if he or she becomes a driver, or whether the student shows the potential to be a safe driver (see Case Example 13.1). This section addresses cognitive assessment components that should be considered when evaluating a student's potential to drive. The therapist's skills, the practice setting, and the student's abilities and problems guide the selection of appropriate tools in the evaluation process. A therapist may initially administer some assessments and then refer a student to a DRS if the student possesses the necessary predriving skills. If, however, a therapist identifies a student as being at significant risk if he or she pursues driving, the therapist should advise the youth's team (e.g., parents, school officials, physician) of those concerns. Properly evaluating an individual's driving skills is rooted in understanding his or her condition and how that condition can affect driving skills.

Occupational therapists often work with students who have been diagnosed with an ASD, attention deficit hyperactivity disorder (ADHD), nonverbal learning disability (NVLD), or low IQ that may affect the ability to learn to drive safely. The following sections provide information specific to each of these categories.

Autism Spectrum Disorders

Among the ASDs, typical candidates for driving are students diagnosed with Asperger's syndrome (AS) or high-functioning autism (HFA). The following are characteristics of individuals with AS or HFA:

- IQ is typically normal to gifted
- Anxiety interferes with activities of daily living and overall performance
- Performance can be erratic.

Information processing:

- Takes in too much information
- Interprets what he or she hears literally

Case Example 13.1. Identifying Risk

Therapists in the school system can often identify whether a student is at risk if he or she pursues learning to drive. An occupational therapist in a school system was asked to consult on a student's handwriting. The therapist identified visual–perceptual and executive function challenges. The therapist appropriately became concerned that the student had signed up for driver's education the next semester.

The occupational therapist in the school system used her knowledge of the task of driving to determine that this student was at risk and acted by getting a referral from the school to driver rehabilitation. (The student's family also was kept informed.) The occupational therapy DRS's evaluation identified that the same deficits identified by the school occupational therapist would negatively affect the student's ability to safely drive. The occupational therapy certified DRS recommended that the student receive occupational therapy driver rehabilitation services to complete driver's education instead of completing driver's education through the school system.

- Considers all information to have equal importance and therefore has difficulty prioritizing
- Has sensory integration impairments.

Motor skills:

- Has eye–hand coordination difficulties.

Executive functions:

- Has time management skill deficits
- Has difficulty initiating tasks because of problems with planning and organization
- Has difficulty with mental flexibility
- Has slow attention-shifting skills
- Has limitations in self-monitoring
- Has deficits in problem-solving skills.

Social skills:

- Has difficulty interpreting verbal and nonverbal information
- Is overly confident and will lead you to believe that the individual understands even if he or she does not (Kowalski, 2007).

The skills that are affected by AS and HFA are used in daily driving situations. The therapist needs to carefully evaluate skills, because often these students' good verbal abilities and performance on standardized clinical tests may cause the therapist to overestimate the student's ability to drive. This situation may lead to serious consequences for the student.

To understand the effect on driving, analyze the driving task in the context of the skills that are affected by the condition. Picture a typical roadway scene with a multilane intersection in a business district. There is a tremendous amount of visual information to sift through to find critical information. Individuals with HFA or AS may have difficulty prioritizing information. They may think that the person walking on the sidewalk is as important as the vehicle braking in front of them. Drivers need to prioritize information because if they see all information as equal, they will misdirect their attention at critical moments, thus impairing reaction speed.

For individuals with AS and HFA, reaction speed can be further complicated by a slow rate of attention shifting. Individuals with ASDs have a tendency to perseverate, which inhibits the ability to shift attention (Hill, 2004). Driving demands quick attention shifting; a driver can only momentarily check the traffic light and check the actions of the other drivers who may be braking, signaling, or entering his or her path.

Individuals with AS or HFA tend to be rule based. They expect everyone else to follow the rules of the road to the letter. However, drivers don't always follow the rules, which makes it difficult for individuals with AS or HFA to anticipate the actions of other drivers. In addition, individuals with AS or HFA have difficulty interpreting nonverbal cues; this is an underlying skill that most drivers use to anticipate the actions of drivers who don't follow the rules. For example, individuals with AS or HFA may not anticipate that another driver who is tailgating them and not using a turn signal is about to pass them. In the same situation, a neurotypical driver may anticipate that the other driver is likely to pass because of the tailgating behavior. The neurotypical driver is able to interpret the nonverbal cue of tailgating as the other driver is aggressive and in a hurry and therefore likely to pass at any moment. Thus, the neurotypical driver does not require a turn signal to anticipate the actions of the other driver.

Problem solving in an emergency situation can be a challenge for someone with HFA or AS. Drivers routinely encounter problems on the roadway: getting lost, the vehicle breaking down, being stopped by police, road closures and detours, or a passing emergency vehicle. The individual with HFA or AS may not be able to plan, organize, and sequence a solution to resolve a driving problem.

Attention Deficit Hyperactivity Disorder

ADHD is a disorder characterized by serious and persistent difficulties in attention span and behavior. There are three subtypes of ADHD: (1) predominantly hyperactive–impulsive, (2) predominantly inattentive, and (3) combined hyperactive–impulsive and inattentive (NIMH, 2008). One in 10 children in the United States are estimated to be diagnosed with ADHD (Visser, Bitsko, Danielson, Perou, & Blumberg, 2010). The following are characteristics of individuals with ADHD:

Information processing:

- Is easily distractible
- Does not process internal signs such as fatigue, distractibility, or hunger.

Executive functions:

- Has poor attention to detail in planning the timing, monetary funds, and sequence of steps to complete a task
- Has difficulty organizing tasks
- Is forgetful in daily activities.

Social skills:

- Often talks excessively
- Blurts out answers before questions are completed
- Does not listen when directly spoken to (Centers for Disease Control and Prevention [CDC], 2010; ERIC Clearinghouse on Disabilities and Gifted Education, 1998; NIMH, 2008).

All drivers have experienced the dangers of inattention when driving. Talking on a cell phone can result in delayed reactions to a driving situation or, even worse, a crash. Most drivers can recall situations that caused them to be momentarily inattentive: a conversation with a passenger, a crying baby, a bee or wasp in the car, or a spilled drink. In fact, 20% of the vehicle crashes that result in injury involve a distracted driver (National Highway Transportation Safety Administration [NHTSA], 2010).

The age group with the greatest proportion of distracted driving crashes is under age 20 (NHTSA, 2010). If teen drivers at large are at risk for distraction, it is easy to understand that youth with ADHD are at greater risk for a crash because of their inattentive tendencies.

The impulsivity and hyperactivity characteristics of ADHD may cause the individual to enter intersections or make lane changes before fully assessing the traffic situation. In the first 2–5 years of driving, individuals with ADHD are involved in four times as many automobile accidents as to their peers without ADHD. They are more likely to cause bodily injury in accidents and receive three times as many citations for speeding as compared to their peers without ADHD (Jerome, Segal, & Habinski, 2006). The stakes are high. Identifying when the student with ADHD is ready to learn to drive should be a critical function for the occupational therapist.

Youth with ADHD tend to be immature. The youth with ADHD may not have the necessary respect for the inherent responsibilities that come with driving (Snyder, 2001). Being a responsible driver includes taking prescribed medications to improve ADHD inattention symptoms. Without medications, some students with ADHD may not be able to drive safely (Snyder, 2001; Weafer, Camerillo, Fillmore, Millich, & Marczinski, 2008). Of those with ADHD, 66.3% are prescribed medication treatment to manage their ADHD symptoms (CDC, 2010). Medication adherence for individuals with ADHD has been studied, and the adherence estimates vary from 13% to 64% of children, adolescents, and adults (Adler & Nierenberg, 2010). One can conclude that some individuals with ADHD may not be taking prescribed medications while driving, and performance maybe impaired.

The occupational therapist should assess the attitude and behaviors toward medications (if prescribed) of students with ADHD and their day-to-day responsibilities at home and in the community. For example, Do the students break rules at home or at school that endanger themselves or others? Do they break rules that endanger other people's property (Snyder, 2001)? Is the student's attitude about medications different from that of his or her parent? In other words, does the parent perceive that the student needs medications to be a safe driver, and the student does not share this perception?

It may be appropriate to interview the student's psychologist or psychiatrist to achieve a better understanding of the student's level of maturity, because family dynamics may make this challenging to assess. In addition to assessing life skills and maturity, the therapist should assess cognitive skills, particularly sustained attention and executive functions.

Nonverbal Learning Disability

Individuals with NVLD have outstanding verbal skills compared to their performance skills (Stein & Kalyani, 2007). The following are characteristics of individuals with NVLD:

Information processing:

- Has poor visual recall
- Has impaired visual–spatial perception
- Has limited visual attention
- Has good attention to detail, but at the consequence of understanding the larger meaning.

Motor skills:

- Has difficulty with motor planning.

Executive functions:

- Has difficulty in generalizing information
- Has difficulty with problem solving
- Has difficulty in anticipating consequences
- Has difficulty with abstract reasoning.

Social skills:

- Has deficits in social judgments
- Tends to be concrete and literal, interfering in social interactions
- Has deficits with regulating behavior, emotions, and impulse control (Stein & Kalyani, 2007; Tanguay, 2002).

NVLD presents a host of challenges for driving. These students have highly developed verbal skills that often mask their performance skill deficits. Functional tasks are very challenging for students with NVLD, and driving can be exceptionally so. It is critical that the occupational therapist conduct functionally based assessments and not rely on an interview to truly understand the student's abilities.

The physical abilities of individuals with NVLD are characterized as awkward, which can make learning basic vehicle control challenging. For example, bilateral coordination deficits can impede progress in learning how to turn the steering wheel.

Individuals with NVLD also have visual–spatial deficits that interfere with managing time and space. Drivers rely on visual–spatial skills for executing roadway maneuvers and managing roadway hazards. For example, the management of *space* is integral when parking in a single space between two cars. Management of *time* (as well as space) is required for appropriate deceleration when approaching a red light.

Visual–spatial deficits also can interfere with more advanced driving skills such as managing roadway hazards. For example, if a neurotypical driver encounters a disabled vehicle in the right lane on a multilane roadway, he or she anticipates needing to change lanes in advance (i.e., management of space) and possibly slowing down (i.e., management of time). The driver with NVLD may not anticipate the need to make a lane change or decelerate.

In addition, the individual with NVLD has difficulty interpreting the actions of others. In this same example, the student with NVLD may have difficulty anticipating that the drivers in front of and behind him or her also may be planning to move into the other lane.

Reading a map requires spatial skills to orient oneself to a location. This can be a very challenging task for someone with NVLD. Even in a familiar shopping mall parking lot, the person with NVLD may have difficulty using landmarks to orient his or her direction of travel.

Low IQ

Intelligence is the ability to learn new information, to understand it, and to apply the knowledge to manipulate one's environment or to think abstractly (Merriam-Webster, 2011). The Wechsler Intelligence Quotient is a common measure of an individual's IQ (Wechsler, 1939). For educational IQ classifications, normal or average intelligence is a score of 90–109. Low average is an IQ of 80–89. Borderline is an IQ of 70–79. Extremely low is an IQ of 65 and below (Benet, 2011).

Although IQ and driving have not been directly studied, there is research investigating IQ and cognitive skills that are used in driving. Several studies have addressed reaction speed and speed of cognitive processing. These studies concluded that reaction times and cognitive processing are slower for individuals with lower IQ scores (Bates & Stough, 1997; Jensen, 1979; Lindley, Smith, & Thomas, 1988). In addition, children with borderline IQs have pervasive deficits in visual–spatial, working-memory, and executive function skills compared to those with IQs of over 95 (Alloway, 2010).

Delayed cognitive processing speed and impaired executive functions can be the most limiting factors for these students to learn to drive. These students may not be able to drive simply because they cannot process what they see at the pace of the traffic environment. It may be too challenging for them to analyze what they see and think abstractly to identify a plan of action for routine and nonroutine driving situations. The inherent deficits in cognitive-processing speed and higher executive function are likely to prevent them from benefiting from remediation and strategies to learn to drive safely.

Students With Multiple Challenges

CP and SB are examples of congenital conditions that may impair visual, cognitive, and physical skills. Acquired brain injury and TBI, although not discussed in this chapter, also can affect these skill areas. These students may require a combination of approaches used for students with cognitive and physical limitations.

Cerebral Palsy

The occupational therapist needs to evaluate the cognitive, visual, and motor skills of a student with CP to determine if the student has the underlying skills necessary for driving. The therapist will need to direct specific attention to primitive reflexes, muscle tone and coordination during operation of adaptive driving equipment, ocular motor skills, cognition, and visual perception.

Primitive reflexes such as asymmetric tonic neck reflex (ATNR) need to be assessed: Are they fully integrated, or will these reflexes interfere with driving? For example, during a lane change, the individual who has an ATNR may inadvertently turn into the lane when looking over his or her shoulder to identify whether the lane is clear. An individual with an exaggerated startle reflex may have an involuntary motor response when startled. The reflex could occur from a bump in the road, from an emergency vehicle's siren, or when another driver uses the horn. If these reflexes are severe enough, they may prohibit the individual from safely driving.

When assessing the driving equipment for an individual with CP, it is important to understand the classification of the CP in terms of limb involvement and muscle tone. Primary driving controls should be operated by the uninvolved limbs or the least involved limbs. For example, the student with right-side hemiplegia may benefit from a spinner knob for the left upper extremity and a left foot accelerator. The student's muscle tone should be assessed to determine whether there is evidence of hypertonia or hypotonia. The driving equipment may need to be adjusted to manage the tone difference. Hypertonia, for example, may require more resistance on the hand controls, whereas hypotonia may require less.

When adaptive equipment is needed, the careful selection of equipment is essential for success. Students with CP often present with coordination deficits. Multiple hand controls may need to be assessed before finalizing the vehicle prescription. For example, the push–pull style hand controls may be easier for some students with coordination deficits, whereas others will do better with the rock–push style.

A vision assessment is also necessary for students with CP, with particular attention paid to ocular–motor skills. It is important to assess whether the student has *strabismus* (in which the eyes are not properly aligned with each other), *diplopia* (simultaneous perception of images, often known as "double vision"), or *amblyopia* (central vision impairment in one eye, often known as "lazy eye"). These students can have ocular misalignments that may cause them to suppress one eye or to alternate the suppression between the eyes. This suppression can cause havoc with maintaining a lane position, making lane changes, and identifying appropriate gaps in traffic.

Students with CP can have cognitive impairments and difficulty processing visual information. An assessment of cognitive skills and visual perception should be completed, even for the student who has no academic challenges. Visual–perceptual deficits can make learning basic vehicle control very challenging, even for the honors student. These students may require an extended period of time to learn to drive.

Spina Bifida

The most common type of SB is myelomeningocele. Hydrocephalus may affect as many as 90% of the individuals with myelomeningocele (National Center for Biotechnology Information, 2011). Hydrocephalus can cause cognitive involvement in the areas of attention span, concentration, memory, and social skills (Reed, 1991). Specific areas that need to be assessed are visual perception, ocular–motor skills, trunk stability, primitive reflexes, muscle tone, muscle strength, stature, and cognition (Reed, 1991).

For some students with SB, the perceptual aspects of driving can be the greatest challenge when learning to drive. For example, the students may have difficulty with timing when to initiate turning the wheel and returning the wheel when making basic right and left turns. For some students, perceptual deficits may be far too great to enable them to drive.

Students with SB may be ambulatory with a device or may require a wheelchair for functional mobility. The therapist should assess if adaptive equipment is necessary. Commonly used driving devices for individuals with SB include hand controls, a spinner knob, and a chest strap for trunk stability. The student may require modified seating to drive because of the short stature typically seen with this condition. Ultimately, some individuals with SB will require a modified van because of limitations with transferring and dismantling the wheelchair.

However, for evaluating and training, a car is an ideal vehicle. The smaller vehicle allows for graduating the learning process to manage vehicle space, which can be challenging for these individuals given the potential for visual–perceptual deficits. For the student who uses a wheelchair, sensation may be impaired; the student may need advice regarding pressure relief when sitting for prolonged periods while driving.

Integrating Life Skills and Passenger Activities Into the Occupational Therapy Evaluation

Although there are many standardized tools available for assessing driving-related skills (as outlined in earlier chapters), not all clinical assessments include norms for adolescents. There is limited research on this population and driving. Therefore, in addition to the comprehensive driving evaluation described in earlier chapters, this author has identified two areas as useful data in determining the readiness of young students to develop driving-related skills:

1. *Life skills* assessment to determine maturity and readiness to drive
2. *Passenger activities* that use the cognitive and visual skills of a driver.

Life Skills

In the years leading up to driving age, young people typically engage in activities and occupations that develop the skills needed to drive and interact in the community. Students with cognitive and social limitations may not have developed these necessary skills. The following are examples of life skills that should be independent or be emerging to an independent level before a student considers learning to drive:

- Select appropriate clothing for the weather or an activity.
- Safely move through a public parking lot, negotiate pedestrian and vehicle traffic, and cross a busy street as a pedestrian.
- Be alone at home for several hours.
- Plan and prepare a simple meal on the stove or in the oven without complications.
- Be responsible for someone or something else (e.g., home chores, vocational responsibilities, younger sibling, pet).
- Be able to interact with strangers such as asking where the public restroom is located.
- Be fiscally responsible (e.g., can the student save gift money or earnings over time to purchase a ticket for a trip or a desired item, or does he or she act on impulse with money?).
- Plan and prepare for a familiar recreational task (e.g., if going to the beach is a routine family event, does the youth plan ahead and pack a bathing suit, sunscreen, sunglasses, and appropriate footwear, or does he or she need cues?).
- Be able to manage a simple household problem (e.g., leaking faucet, plugged toilet, burnt-out light bulb).
- Be responsible for medications—taking medication should not require constant reminders and is particularly important when the student takes medications to treat attention or seizures, for example (Monahan & Patten, 2009).

The occupational therapist is in a great position to identify whether the life skills are deficient, are able to be achieved with intervention, or are appropriate for driving. Parents, medical providers, and school systems may not be able to comprehend why a therapist may advise that a student not pursue driving when clinical tests alone are used to evaluate. However, when the therapist reports on the life skills status and correlates the skills to driving, the student's team is more likely to understand. For example, if a student cannot select the appropriate clothing for the weather conditions, he or she will not be able to identify when weather conditions make driving unsafe. The student who is unsafe in the kitchen leaving food cooking unattended is not able to attend to the driving task. The student who cannot problem solve a simple home repair such as replacing a light bulb or managing a power outage is unlikely to manage a roadside emergency or a road detour.

A standardized life skills assessment for adolescents is the Adaptive Behavior Assessment System (Harrison & Oakland, 2003). A student's life skills are reported by parents and teachers by means of a checklist that can be scored, and the student's skill level is compared to his or her peers.

Appendix 13.A includes a nonstandardized life skills assessment tool, the **Adolescent Skills Checklist**. When using this tool, have a parent or guardian complete the form. Interview this person to understand why the student is or is not independent with a particular skill. The interview questions should be open so that they do not lead the parent or guardian down a path and maintain the quality of the assessment. For example, ask the parent or guardian the following:

- "Give me an example of something your daughter cooked recently, and tell me what happened."
- "What gave you cause to not leave your son home alone anymore? Was there a particular incident?"
- "When your daughter is involved in a disagreement, how does she manage her feelings?"

Don't underestimate the motivation of parents to want their child to succeed. Parents often view the ability to drive for their special needs child as a means to "normalize" the child with his or her peers as well as to help their child to have opportunities as an emerging adult. They see driving as a means to open doors to self-reliance and vocational and social opportunities, and they may overlook the obvious signs that their child is not ready.

The nonstandardized life skills assessment also can be appropriate for the student to complete. Some students develop insight into what skills they need to have developed before driving or living alone in their own apartment.

Passenger Activities

Passenger activities in a vehicle provide the occupational therapist with a means to identify whether a student's performance skills are intact for learning to drive. The passenger activities are functional tasks that incorporate the visual and cognitive skills used in driving without incorporating the rules of the road. A parent or guardian typically rides in the back of the vehicle while the student rides in the front passenger seat. The therapist drives the vehicle and introduces one activity at a time.

The following four examples of passenger activities include (1) lane position, (2) scanning, (3) judging gaps, and (4) problem solving in an emergency.

Lane Position

The occupational therapist gives the student a diagram of five different lane positions (Mottola, 2003) while the vehicle is stationary (Figure 13.1). After the student is instructed on the activity and expectations, the therapist drives the car randomly into the five different lane positions on the roadway as traffic allows.

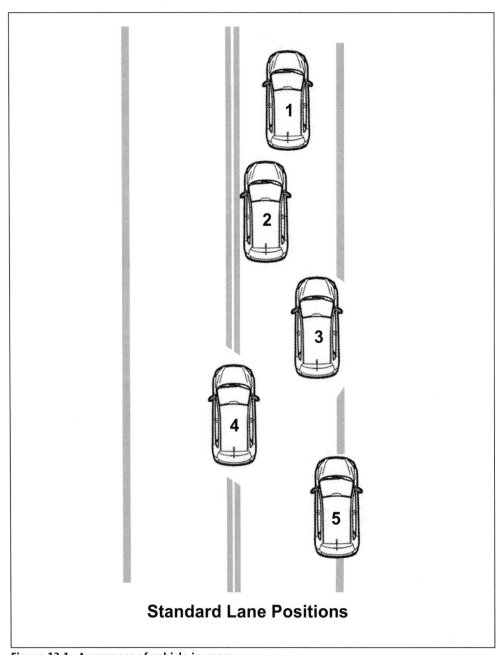

Standard Lane Positions

Figure 13.1. Awareness of vehicle in space.

Note. Provided by M. Monahan. Used with permission.

The activity allows the therapist to assess visual–perception and processing speed. A student who is not aware of the location of the vehicle, or is slow to recognize the location of the vehicle as a passenger, is likely to have difficulty as a driver with maintaining a lane position or making an adjustment in the lane position when there is a change in traffic conditions that requires an adjustment in lane position. Situations that require drivers to make lane position changes are broad but can include a pedestrian, a cyclist, construction, or a parked vehicle.

Scanning

The purpose of scanning is to have the student identify stimuli on the roadway to simulate how the driver scans the environment. The occupational therapist adds one stimulus at a time: streets on the right and left, traffic light colors, speed-limit signs, brake lights, turn signals of the vehicle directly in front, and regulatory signs such as stop signs and one-way signs.

In addition to seeing if the student is able to identify the information, the therapist is measuring how quickly the student recognizes information. Does the student recognize the brake lights or red light before the therapist initiates braking, or does the student tell the therapist after he or she stops the vehicle or is nearly stopped? The therapist also can identify additional executive function skills for driving. For example, can the student discern a parking lot from a side street (Figure 13.2)?

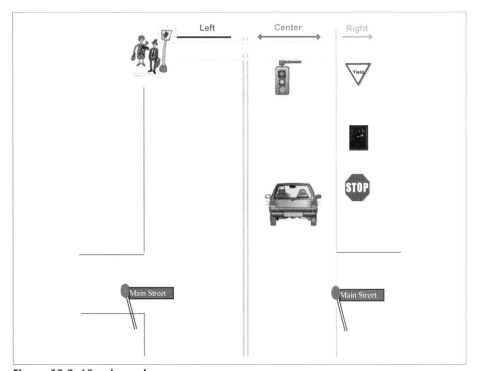

Figure 13.2. Visual search.
Note. Provided by M. Monahan. Copyright © 2009. Used with permission.

Judging Gaps

The purpose of the judging gaps passenger activity is to identify whether the student can judge safe gaps in traffic when the occupational therapist drives to a stop-sign intersection or a business exit. The student is asked to tell the therapist when it is safe to enter the intersection. The therapist can observe the student's speed in scanning the intersection in terms of the pace of traffic and whether the student takes into account the line of sight restrictions and traffic flow.

Problem Solving in an Emergency

The purpose of the problem-solving task is to determine whether the student is able to problem solve a roadside emergency. The occupational therapist tells the student, "Pretend that the vehicle we are driving has a flat tire." While the therapist drives, the student creates a solution for a roadside emergency scenario. The therapist explains that the solution should be within the context of the specific environment such as, "Tell me which parking lot you want me to turn into, such as 'the Salad Bowl restaurant,' instead of 'turn into a parking lot.'" The therapist should observe whether the student can identify solutions at an appropriate pace, in the context of the driving environment, or whether the student provides only general solutions.

Finalizing a Driving or Community Mobility Plan of Care

Making a final decision about whether a youth has the potential to drive needs to be based on the evaluation components described earlier. The therapist needs to conclude whether deficits can be remediated with strategies and whether the student has the insight to be aware of his or her deficits so as to incorporate the strategies. If the answer is yes, the therapist needs to decide whether an occupational therapy driver rehabilitation program is necessary or if a traditional driver's education program is appropriate. Using an occupational therapy driver rehabilitation program is critical if the student has executive function limitations, because he or she will require specific strategies and activities to succeed.

If the student is not ready to pursue driving, the therapist should develop an appropriate plan of care to develop the skills that are deficient. If the deficits have the potential to be remediated and developed, the therapist should recommend occupational therapy services to promote independence in life skills. Recommendation for services is particularly important if the student has not reached the mid-20s and his or her brain is still developing (Sowell et al., 1999). Depending on the student, it may be appropriate for the therapist to counsel the student and his or her team that driving may be a possibility in the future, as there is a natural phase of brain development.

The therapist's understanding of the diagnosis and clinical course can guide clinical reasoning. For example, a student with a low IQ demonstrating delayed information processing speed is unlikely to significantly improve over time; the therapist should address other forms of community mobility. Based on the assessments, the therapist can identify what forms of community mobility would be most appropriate.

Whether a therapist is a DRS in driving or is working with the youth in a school system or in an outpatient clinic, addressing the life skills that are the foundation

Practitioner's Reflection 13.2. Intervention Strategy for an Individualized Driving Program

It is not unusual for me to treat a student with a cognitive impairment for 16–24 sessions over 1 to 2 years. I request that parents provide supervised driving practice 4–5 hours per month or between driver rehabilitation sessions.

—Miriam Monahan, MS, OTR/L, CDRS, CDI

for community access is essential, whether a student drives or not. The therapist can use the life skills assessment in combination with the clinical evaluation in any setting to identify what types of community mobility goals are within a student's capabilities. Developing the skills for a student to be potentially safe as a pedestrian, a cyclist, or a user of public transportation can be an outcome of the evaluation.

Driver Training for Youth With Cognitive Limitations

Students with ASDs, ADHD, NVLD, or cognitive challenges from congenital conditions such as CP and SB typically will need an occupational therapist who is also a driving school instructor to learn how to drive. Each student will require an individualized approach for learning to drive. However, there are some generalizations about the components that need to be incorporated in the training.

Overview of the Individualized Driving Program

Plan 1 to 2 years to complete training, because students with cognitive limitations require multiple experiences to be able to generalize skills to different intersections and driving environments. The student's progress is often inconsistent. Look for a positive progression of skills over a period of time versus progress at each session. If the therapist is planning to have family members provide practice between sessions, have the parent or guardian observe the training session so that everyone understands the specific goal for the session as well as for practice, what environment is appropriate, and what verbal language is being used (see Practitioner's Reflection 13.2). This provides consistency with instruction. These students often don't have the capacity to manage significant differences in instruction.

Gradually introduce skills: Realize that these students can have a combination of motor, visual, and physical skill deficits. Break down skills to their basic elements. Let the student master a skill before adding another dimension to the skill or another driving skill (see Practitioner's Reflection 13.3).

> **Students with cognitive limitations require multiple experiences to be able to generalize skills to different intersections and driving environments.**

Practitioner's Reflection 13.3. Intervention Strategy for Breaking Down Tasks

When I begin teaching a student to drive, I begin in a quiet residential area. I find a residential area to be better than an open parking lot as it allows for some structure. My focus is to develop the motor skills needed for operation of the vehicle. I provide total assistance for scanning intersections and making a decision on when to enter the intersection. I add the other dimensions to the intersection when the student masters the motor aspects. By breaking down the task, I can also reduce the anxiety level and improve the potential to learn. I carry on the concept of breaking down the task as I progress into more advanced skills.

—Miriam Monahan, MS, OTR/L, CDRS, CDI

Practitioner's Reflection 13.4. Intervention Strategy for Scanning Intersections

When I first introduce scanning intersections, I explain why I look a particular direction just before I enter the intersection. My reasoning for looking a particular direction may be due to line of sight restriction or traffic flow such as an intersection where vehicles could enter with limited notice.

—*Miriam Monahan, MS, OTR/L, CDRS, CDI*

Executive Functions

Infuse executive function training from the beginning of training. The obvious is not always obvious to these students. The therapist should explain why certain steps are important. The following are activities that are particularly useful for developing executive function:

- Route-planning activities are for making decisions about what entrance or exit to use out of a parking lot when there are multiple choices. Some exits could be more challenging based on the desired direction of travel.
- Other route-planning activities incorporate getting and following directions to an unfamiliar destination.
- Driving environments that are less structured such as parking lots require practice to understand traffic flow to know where to search. Traffic flows at large stores, at gas stations, and at drive-through banks are all very different (see Practitioner's Reflection 13.4).

Interacting Socially in the Driving Environment

For students who have social skills challenges, interpreting the actions of other drivers can be difficult. The therapist should explain the social components and identify patterns and rules to help the student anticipate and interpret the actions of other drivers. Some driving situations require more social skills than others. The following are examples of critical driving skills and strategies that should be addressed in training (see also Practitioner's Reflection 13.5):

- *Tailgating:* Students will not necessarily be aware that another driver is tailgating them. Provide a rule that if they can't see the front bumper of the car behind them, the other driver is too close. It is essential that they can recognize a tailgater before they learn how to manage the situation.
- *All-way stop intersection:* The flow of traffic does not follow typical rules. Drivers enter the intersection before the intersection is clear. Give students a rule to enter the intersection when their path of travel is clear.
- *Multilane roadway:* Anticipating the actions of other drivers can be complex because drivers don't always signal their intentions to pass and may be traveling too fast for the speed limit.

A great place to practice categorizing drivers is on the interstate while the student is driving in the right lane. A student can observe the actions of other drivers without incorporating the steps of a lane change.

Practitioner's Reflections 13.5. Intervention Strategy for Driving Behaviors

I teach students to categorize drivers to anticipate their actions when traveling on multilane roadways. I give the students three types of driving behaviors and give those drivers a name:

1. A *zoomer* is a driver who is in the lane directly behind and coming up very fast. The zoomer is likely to make a lane change without signaling. When a student identifies a zoomer, he or she knows it is not a good time to make a lane change in the other lane.

2. *Tailgaters* will likely pass the first chance they get, and therefore, don't attempt a lane change.

3. A *pauser* is a driver in the adjacent lane who sees your turn signal and knows you want to make a lane change and is willing to let you move over. Pausers will not wait for long, so it is necessary to move over once you are sure that they are letting you into the other lane.

—*Miriam Monahan, MS, OTR/L, CDRS, CDI*

Management of Self

Many students struggle with poor awareness of internal signs, such as hunger, fatigue, and poor attention. The student may have minimal insight on how these internal signs affect his or her driving performance. The therapists interventions should include activities that help the student develop awareness and insight.

For example, a customized **self-monitoring log** (Exhibit 13.2) that includes driving performance along with hours slept can be helpful for a student with poor sleep hygiene to understand the impact of insufficient sleep on driving performance. Videorecording a student's drive and having the student review it may help that individual to be more aware of the impact of inattention on his or her driving performance. The therapist also should plan ahead for when the student eventually attains his or her driver's license. A family plan should be made in the event that a student realizes that he or she has not taken medications after beginning to drive, is too tired, or is distracted. A "no questions asked" policy to help the student feel comfortable calling home and asking for a ride may be appropriate.

Exhibit 13.2. Example of a Self-Monitoring Log

Date	Duration of Drive	Type of Driving Environment	Destination	Problems During Drive (describe, if any)	Were You Tired, Distracted, or Hungry?	How Many Hours Did You Sleep?	Other Comments
2-1-12	20 minutes	Rural and city	Walmart	I did not stop soon enough for the stop sign; I parked too close to the car to my right	No	7	Mom said I was not concentrating well
2-5-12	30 minutes/ 30 minutes	Rural roads and interstate	Uncle John's	I had difficulty getting on the highway	I was hungry, and told we were not eating until we got to Uncle John's	10	I was scared about the interstate
2-7-12	40 minutes	Rural roads and downtown	Errands	I missed a stop sign; I was late to stop for a red light; I did not see a car	Distracted	9	I forgot my meds

Conclusion

Driving and community mobility are essential for accessing vocational, academic, recreational, and social opportunities, goods (e.g., food, bank, drug store), and medical services. In addition, driving and community mobility enable adolescents to begin to develop social capital. *Social capital* refers to the relationships and social connections that an individual has within his or her community (Condeluci, 2008). These connections are established and grow at work, church, school, and community events and are strengthened through interactions with neighbors, friends, relatives, and business relations.

Community mobility is essential to establish and maintain social capital. Without community mobility, an individual has diminished social capital. Conversely, increased social capital increases an individual's options and leads to an increased quality of life (Gotto, Calkins, Jackson, Walker, & Beckmann, 2010).

Youth with special needs are at risk for not developing social capital if their community mobility skills are inadequate.

Youth with special needs are at risk for not developing social capital if their community mobility skills are inadequate. When a therapist can identify the correct means of community mobility, he or she also is addressing social relationships; vocational, academic, and recreational opportunities; and access to services.

As important as driving is to the development of social capital for teens with disabilities, the decision to drive needs to be considered carefully for each individual. The CDC (2008) reported that motor vehicle crashes are the leading cause of death for U.S. teens, accounting for more than one in three deaths in this age group—more than drugs, guns, or any disease. The risk of motor vehicle crashes is higher among 16- to 19-year-olds than in other age groups. Per mile driven, teen drivers 16 to 19 years of age are four times more likely than older drivers to crash (CDC, 2008).

Teen drivers are already at high risk, and adolescents with special needs are potentially more at risk. It is essential that occupational therapists address the instrumental activity of daily living (IADL) of driving with youth with special needs, as they are uniquely qualified to identify an individual's risk factors and how they impact the specific tasks of driving. No IADL claims more lives of adolescents than driving. Therapists working with this population simply cannot ignore their responsibility to address it.

References

Adler, L. D., & Nierenberg, A. A. (2010, January). Review of medication adherence in children and adults with ADHD. *Postgraduate Medicine, 122,* 922–927.

Alloway, T. P. (2010). Working memory and executive function profiles of individuals with borderline intellectual functioning. *Journal of Intellectual Disability Research, 54,* 448–456.

Bates, T., & Stough, C. (1997). Processing speed, attention, and intelligence: Effects of spatial attention on decision time in high and low IQ subjects. *Personality and Individual Differences, 23,* 861–868.

Benet, W. E. (2011). IQ classifications. *Assessment Psychology Online.* Retrieved November 18, 2011, from http://www.assessmentpsychology.com/iqclassifications.htm

Centers for Disease Control and Prevention, National Center for Injury Prevention and Control. (2008). *Teen drivers: Fact sheet.* Retrieved January 7, 2009, from http://www.cdc .gov/ncipc/factsheets/teenmvh.htm

Centers for Disease Control and Prevention. (2010). *Facts about ADHD.* Retrieved November 12, 2011, from http://www.cdc.gov/ncbddd/adhd/data.html

Condeluci, A. (2008). *Best practices in brain injury service delivery XVI.* Des Moines: Brain Injury Association of Iowa.

ERIC Clearinghouse on Disabilities and Gifted Education. (1998). *Teaching children with attention deficit/hyperactivity disorder* (ERIC Digest E569). Retrieved January 7, 2009, from http://www.ericdigests.org/1999-2/attention.htm

Gotto, G. S., Calkins, C. F., Jackson, L., Walker, H., & Beckmann, C. (2010). *Accessing social capital: Implications for persons with disabilities* [White Paper]. Retrieved March 16, 2012, from http://www.aucd.org/docs/Accessing%20Social%20Capital%20Implications%20 for%20Persons%20With%20Disabilities,%20Final.pdf

Harrison, P. L., & Oakland, T. (2003). *Adaptive Behavior Assessment System–Second edition manual (ABAS–II).* San Antonio, TX: Harcourt Assessment.

Hill, E. L. (2004). Evaluating the theory of executive dysfunction in autism. *Developmental Review, 24,* 189–233.

Jensen, A. R. (1979). Outmoded theory or unconquered frontier? *Creative Science and Technology, 2,* 16–29.

Jerome, L., Segal, A., & Habinski, L. (2006). What we know about ADHD and driving risk: A literature review, meta-analysis and critique. *Journal of the Canadian Academy of Child and Adolescent Psychiatry, 15*(3), 105–125.

Kowalski, T. (2007). *Asperger's syndrome: Assessment and intervention strategies from preschool to adulthood.* Eau Claire, WI: Medical Educational Services.

Lindley, R., Smith, W. R., & Thomas, J. T. (1988). The relationship between speed of information processing as measured by timed paper-and-pencil tests and psychometric intelligence. *Intelligence, 12,* 17–25.

Merriam-Webster. (2011). Intelligence. In *Merriam-Webster dictionary.* Retrieved February 10, 2012, from http://m-w.com/cgi-bin/dictionary?book=Dictionary&va=intelligence

Monahan, M., & Patten, K. (2009). *Creating successful transitions to community mobility independence for adolescents: Addressing the needs of students with cognitive, social, and behavioral limitations* [CEonCD]. Bethesda, MD: American Occupational Therapy Association.

Mottola, F. R. (2003). *Your car is a monster: Ten habits that will keep it caged.* Cheshire, CT: National Institute for Driver Behavior.

National Center for Biotechnology Information. (2011). Myelomeningocele. In *A.D.A.M. medical encyclopedia.* Retrieved February 10, 2012, from http://www.ncbi.nlm.nih.gov/ pubmedhealth/PMH0002525/

National Highway Transportation Safety Administration. (2010). *Statistics and facts about distracted driving.* Retrieved November 12, 2011, from http://www.distraction.gov/stats-and-facts/index.html

National Institute of Mental Health. (2008). *Attention deficit hyperactivity disorder (ADHD).* Retrieved November 12, 2011, from http://www.nimh.nih.gov/health/publications/ attention-deficit-hyperactivity-disorder/complete-index.shtml

National Institute of Mental Health. (2010). *Teenage brain: A work in progress* (Fact sheet). Retrieved February 8, 2010, from https://docs.google.com/viewer?url= http%3A%2F%2Fwww.isu.edu%2Firh%2Fprojects%2Fbetter_todays%2FB2T2VirtualPacket %2FBrainFunction%2FNIMH-Teenage%2520Brain%2520-%2520A%2520Work%2520in% 2520Progress.pdf

Reed, K. L. (1991). *Quick reference to occupational therapy.* Gaithersburg, MD: Aspen.

Snyder, M. J. (2001). *AD/HD and driving: A guide for parents of teens with ADHD.* Whitefish, MT: Whitefish Consultants.

Sowell, E. R., Thompson, P. M., Holmes, C. J., Jernigan, T. L., & Toga, A. W. (1999). In vivo evidence for post-adolescent brain maturation in frontal and striatal regions. *Nature Neuroscience, 2,* 859–861.

Stein, J. A., & Kalyani, K. (2007). Nonverbal learning disability and executive function: The challenges of effective assessment and teaching. In L. Meltzer (Ed.), *Executive function in education, from theory to practice* (pp. 123–149). New York: Guilford Press.

Tanguay, P. (2002). *Nonverbal learning disabilities at school: Educating the student with NLD, Asperger syndrome, and related conditions.* London: Jessica Kingsley.

Visser, S. N., Bitsko, R. H., Danielson, M. L., Perou, R., & Blumberg, S. J. (2010). Increasing prevalence of parent-reported attention-deficit/hyperactivity disorder among children— United States, 2003 and 2007. *Morbidity and Mortality Weekly Report, 59,* 1439–1444.

Weafer, J., Camarillo, D., Fillmore, M. T., Milich, R., & Marczinski, C. A. (2008). Simulated driving performance of adults with ADHD: Comparisons with alcohol intoxication. *Experimental and Clinical Psychopharmacology, 16*(3), 251–263.

Wechsler, D. (1939). *The measurement of adult intelligence.* Baltimore: Williams & Wilkins.

Appendix 13.A. Adolescent Skills Checklist

Driving involves, among other things, being able to be alone, to follow rules and instructions, to solve problems as they emerge out in the community, to manage time to safely reach destinations on time, and to manage the financial and maintenance aspects of caring for and owning a vehicle. All these skills have their foundation in earlier common activities that young people typically master in the years leading up to the driving age.

Although young drivers don't need to have *all* of these skills in place when learning to drive, it *is* very beneficial that they be working toward these skills and that they be able to realistically attain them in the future.

Parent/guardian/case manager: Please complete this entire checklist to the best of your knowledge based on the youth's activities and performance *over the last 6 months*. After each item, place a check in the box of the column that most appropriately describes the youth's abilities in that area. If appropriate, have the youth fill out a separate checklist for himself or herself. You can use it later to compare answers and to promote discussion and goal setting.

Name and relation of person completing this checklist:			Name of the youth:		
	Does do ...		Does *not* do ...		
Kitchen	*Without* assistance or supervision	*With* some assistance or supervision	Due to difficulty or problems	Due to preference or opportunity	Not sure or not applicable
Example: **Operates appliances (stove, oven, microwave, toaster, dishwasher)**		✔			
Operates kitchen appliances safely (stove, oven, microwave, toaster, dishwasher)					
Uses common kitchen tools (can opener, knife, measuring cups and spoons, grater, timer)					
Helps to plan and prepare meals					
Follows a recipe accurately on a box or out of a book					
Puts away leftovers; checks for spoiled food					
Makes own lunch for school or work					
Sets the table					
Washes the dishes					
Shows familiarity and basic understanding of packaged food contents and ingredients					

Comments:

Appendix 13.A. Adolescent Skills Checklist *(cont.)*

Family responsibilities	Does do ...		Does *not* do ...		Not sure or not applicable
	Without assistance or supervision	*With* some assistance or supervision	Due to difficulty or problems	Due to preference or opportunity	
Shows interest in others' activities and perspectives					
Helps take care of siblings or other children					
Participates in family decisions					
Plans activities with friends or family					
Obeys the established family rules					
Answers the phone and takes messages for others					
Negotiates a compromise during a conflict					
Takes care of a pet					

Comments:

Home responsibilities	Does do ...		Does *not* do ...		Not sure or not applicable
	Without assistance or supervision	*With* some assistance or supervision	Due to difficulty or problems	Due to preference or opportunity	
Cleans and maintains own room					
Makes and changes the bed					
Gets involved in room or home organization and decor					
Minor repairs (change light bulb, repair or assemble toys)					
Takes out the trash and recycables					
Cleans up after self in the bathroom or kitchen					
Performs simple errands in the neighborhood					
Basic sewing or mending skills					

Comments:

Laundry	Does do ...		Does *not* do ...		Not sure or not applicable
	Without assistance or supervision	*With* some assistance or supervision	Due to difficulty or problems	Due to preference or opportunity	
Puts dirty clothes in hamper					
Sorts clothes for washing					
Operates the washer and dryer					
Reads clothing labels					
Takes care of all of own laundry					
Folds clothes and puts them away					
Plans ahead for when needs clothing					

Comments:

(Continued)

Appendix 13.A. Adolescent Skills Checklist *(cont.)*

Gardening, workshop	Does do ... Without assistance or supervision	With some assistance or supervision	Does *not* do ... Due to difficulty or problems	Due to preference or opportunity	Not sure or not applicable
Involved in planning or designing a garden or yard project					
Mows and maintains a yard					
Weeds and waters the garden or flower beds					
Uses simple tools or power tools (drill, sander, paint brush and paint, screwdriver)					
Follows a schematic or instructions to put together a simple piece of furniture or gadget					
Takes appropriate precautions to avoid cuts, burns, or injury					
Uses yard, garden, hobby, and workshop chemicals and tools appropriately					

Comments:

Safety and emergencies	Does do ... Without assistance or supervision	With some assistance or supervision	Does *not* do ... Due to difficulty or problems	Due to preference or opportunity	Not sure or not applicable
Can follow emergency procedures to exit home in a fire					
Knows where emergency supplies are kept (candles, flashlights, fuses)					
Knows how to use a fire extinguisher					
Knows community emergency telephone numbers or can locate them					
Reads labels before using chemicals or household products					
Knows where extra house key is located					
Can be at home alone for several hours at a time					
Can unclog a stopped-up sink or toilet					

Comments:

Appendix 13.A. Adolescent Skills Checklist *(cont.)*

	Does do ...		Does *not* do ...		
Community skills	*Without* assistance or supervision	*With* some assistance or supervision	Due to difficulty or problems	Due to preference or opportunity	Not sure or not applicable
Uses public transportation, taxi					
Gets around on city streets as a pedestrian					
Crosses busy streets and manages complex intersections					
Organizes and pursues leisure and recreation activities in the community with others					
Rides a bike or scooter (please comment below regarding level of traffic)					
Goes shopping for personal needs or gifts					
Creates a shopping list for a few items					
Can find and purchase items on a grocery list					
Finds public restrooms, information, or asks for help					
Uses a map or follows directions to plan a local trip					
Gets to an unfamiliar location using a map or directions					
Knows how to recognize and avoid scam artists					
Uses the post office					
Gets a library card and checks out books					

Comments:

	Does do ...		Does *not* do ...		
Health care skills	*Without* assistance or supervision	*With* some assistance or supervision	Due to difficulty or problems	Due to preference or opportunity	Not sure or not applicable
Understands personal health status and diagnoses					
Prepares questions for doctor or therapist					
Responds to questions from doctor or therapist					
Knows personal and common medications and what they are for					
Anticipates when a prescription needs to be refilled					
Knows personal vital information					
Knows how to use and interpret a thermometer					
Understands personal role in maintaining good health (diet, exercise, regular doctor visits)					
Discusses alcohol and drug use issues with family					
For females, takes care of menstrual needs					
Asks for help when facing difficulties with medical, psychological, social, or spiritual matters					

Comments:

(Continued)

Appendix 13.A. Adolescent Skills Checklist *(cont.)*

Personal skills	Does do ...		Does *not* do ...		Not sure or not applicable
	Without assistance or supervision	*With* some assistance or supervision	Due to difficulty or problems	Due to preference or opportunity	
Obtains messages from the answering system					
Carries a house key; remembers to lock the door					
Manages personal grooming (shampoo, bath, shower, nails, oral care)					
Makes necessary appointments					
Chooses appropriate clothes to wear for weather or activity					
Initiates, organizes, and pursues leisure and recreation activities at home or in neighborhood					

Comments:

Financial skills	Does do ...		Does *not* do ...		Not sure or not applicable
	Without assistance or supervision	*With* some assistance or supervision	Due to difficulty or problems	Due to preference or opportunity	
Can write cash or deposit a check					
Uses an ATM to get a balance or cash					
Balances checkbook or savings account					
Budgets personal spending or has a savings account					

Comments:

Time management	Does do ...		Does *not* do ...		Not sure or not applicable
	Without assistance or supervision	*With* some assistance or supervision	Due to difficulty or problems	Due to preference or opportunity	
Gets to classes on time					
Wakes up in time for school, work, or plans					
Anticipates the time it will take for morning self-care routine					
Turns in school assignments in a timely manner					
Anticipates the time it will take to complete school assignments					
Anticipates the time it will take to complete a recipe or project					
Gets out the door or to the bus stop on school days					
Keeps a planner or calendar of activities					

Comments:

Note. Modified with permission from the Adolescent Health Transition Project at the Washington State Department of Health.

Advocating for Change: Community Mobility Across the Lifespan

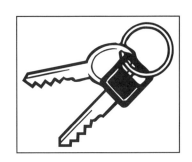

Wendy B. Stav, PhD, OTR/L, SCDCM, FAOTA

The time has come for occupational therapists to become advocates of change regarding issues related to community mobility across the lifespan. With relatively little effort, the area of driving and community mobility could undergo substantial transformation through awareness efforts, infusion of community mobility services into existing programs, development of expertise among practitioners, and advocacy efforts both inside and outside the profession. Advocacy can take many forms ranging from increasing a coworker's awareness through education to formal political lobbying. Whatever shape advocacy efforts take, they should include the steps outlined by the International Council of Nurses (2008; Table E.1).

The International Council of Nurses (2008) defines *advocacy* as the following: "Blending science, ethics and politics, advocacy is self-initiated, evidence-based, strategic action that health professionals can take to help transform systems and improve the environments and policies which shape their patients' behaviors and choices, and ultimately their health" (p. 5). Although this definition can seem overwhelming, addressing one or two steps at a time will help practitioners accomplish their advocacy goals. Table E.1 outlines the steps and actions to shape any advocacy efforts.

Advocating Within the Profession

Practitioners can initiate their advocacy efforts within their own profession and practice settings, which serve as a familiar context to advocate to known entities. Successful advocacy efforts in a comfortable environment and observation of outcomes will increase practitioner confidence to advocate outside of the profession.

Understanding the Role of Occupational Therapy

The first area of focus within one's own profession is increasing understanding of the role of occupational therapy in driving and community mobility. This area of concentration may seem obvious; however, a large portion of the occupational

Table E.1. 10-Step Advocacy Framework

Step	Action
Taking action	Overcoming obstacles to action
Selecting your issue	Identifying and drawing attention to an issue
Understanding your political context	Identifying the key people you need to influence
Building your evidence base	Doing your homework on the issue and mapping the potential roles of relevant players
Engaging others	Winning the support of key individuals or organizations
Elaborating strategic plans	Collectively identifying goals and objectives and the best ways to achieve them
Communicating a message and implementing plans	Delivering your message and counteracting the efforts of opposing interest groups
Seizing opportunities	Timing intervention and actions for maximum impact
Being accountable	Monitoring and evaluating process and impact
Catalyzing health development	Building sustainable capacity throughout the process

Note. From *Promoting Health: Advocacy Guide for Health Professionals,* by the International Council of Nurses, 2008, p. 11. Copyright © 2008, by the International Council of Nurses. Used with permission.

therapy profession recognizes driving and community mobility solely as a specialty area of practice. As mentioned in Chapter 1, driving and community mobility are well within the scope of all areas of occupational therapy practice, as defined by *Occupational Therapy Practice Framework: Domain and Process, 2nd Edition* (American Occupational Therapy Association [AOTA], 2008) as an instrumental activity of daily living (IADL). In addition, driving and community mobility are critical areas of occupational performance for occupational therapy clients, as they serve as the conduit for engagement in several other areas of occupation in their role as occupation enablers.

Thus, it is a matter of best practice to address the community mobility concerns of clients if the practitioner is enhancing health and wellness through optimized occupational engagement. Advocacy within our own profession serves to disseminate the understanding that occupational therapy is the ideal and qualified discipline to address community mobility concerns in clients of all ages and conditions.

Increasing Recognition, Optimizing Attention, and Establishing Expertise

These advocacy efforts should aim toward achieving three goals: (1) increase recognition of the importance of driving and community mobility in daily life, (2) optimize the attention to driving and community mobility needs in existing services, and (3) establish expertise in occupational therapy departments specific to the client populations served. Advocacy toward the first goal began almost a decade ago when AOTA formalized efforts to increase recognition of the practice area and community mobility issues. Those efforts have resulted in a considerable amount of resources, including an older driver expert panel, an AOTA (2010) official statement, fact sheets, a portion of the association Web site dedicated to the practice area, continuing education resources, this textbook, a staff member dedicated to driving and community mobility, and educational campaigns identifying driving as an IADL. There are several other tangible results from these efforts reaching outside of the profession, which will be addressed in the next section.

Although AOTA has demonstrated consistent commitment to advocacy within the profession, these advocacy efforts need to be supplemented by individual members of the profession to fully achieve success. Practitioners use the numerous resources to advocate for the development of community mobility services within programs, educate therapists at the entry and postprofessional levels, and train fieldwork students in the importance of community mobility in daily life.

Practitioners can engage in several activities to optimize attention to driving and community mobility needs in existing services. Although some of the activities are aimed at building the infrastructure within a program or department, others are focused on professional development. Exhibit E.1 lists activities to increase services.

The final focus area for advocacy within the profession is the establishment of expertise in a department specific to the client population. There are several areas in which occupational therapists can obtain specialized training or certifications that would enhance the existing menu of services offered in a department. Many of the options are population-specific and should be selected based on the needs of the program clientele.

Practitioners working in pediatric settings can become certified in child passenger safety through Safe Kids USA (cert.safekids.org) and provide a valuable supplemental service for children of all ages to ensure that they are traveling safely as passengers. Additional areas of expertise for practitioners working with pediatric clients include bicycle helmet fittings, pedestrian safety, bike and wheeled sports safety, predriving skills, and travel training in the use of transit. Therapists working with adult physical rehabilitation clients also might develop expertise in bicycle helmet fitting, in addition to car transfers, travel training in the use of transit, paratransit eligibility evaluations, and transit accessibility. Clients with mental health conditions might benefit from practitioners with expertise in medication effects on driving, travel training in the use of paratransit, knowledge of transit and community resources, and cultural and sensitivity training for transit employees. Establishing and promoting expertise in any of these areas will increase recognition and

---

Exhibit E.1. Advocacy Activities to Optimize Attention to Community Mobility Needs in Existing Programs

Infrastructure Building
- Modify program documentation forms to include an inquiry about driving and community mobility status
- Create a mechanism to gather information related to history of driving and community mobility habits and routines
- Establish a referral pathway to direct clients with needs to driving and community mobility specialists
- Generate a list of community mobility options and service delivery for distribution to clients
- Write departmental policies specific to referrals, recommendations, and medical reporting

Professional Development
- Build a condition-specific evidence library with literature to support and guide client education and recommendations
- Establish a case study review program and incorporate community mobility issues
- Host in-services from community mobility and driving rehabilitation specialists (DRSs)

attention to driving and community mobility services and contribute to changes in the profession to ultimately grow the practice area beyond just a specialty area.

Advocating Outside the Profession

Advocacy outside of the profession is also a necessity, as other disciplines and service recipients are part of the context that influences the recognition and use of occupational therapy services for community mobility needs. Before advocating outside the profession, an occupational therapist needs to make preliminary efforts to identify the key stakeholders in community mobility issues. This identification will ensure that advocacy efforts are aimed at interested and influential parties to yield the most change. Once the stakeholders are identified, a therapist should assess the circumstances and the scope of the issue to determine the level of advocacy necessary. The most basic level of advocacy is at the clinical or individual level and is reserved for meeting the needs of an individual client. Case Example E.1 shows this level of advocacy.

Other circumstances might call for advocacy at the professional or service level, which targets a driving or community mobility issue profession-wide. This level of advocacy may be related to scope of practice, reimbursement for services, or role delineation. Case Example E.2 shows advocacy at the service level.

On a larger scale, a driving or community mobility issue might necessitate advocacy at the organizational, programmatic, or community level. This level is useful when the advocacy is in favor of change that will benefit individuals and also support the occupational engagement of a larger group of people or an entire community. Case Example E.3 shows what community-level advocacy might look like.

The highest level of advocacy is at the policy or societal level. This level of advocacy involves the broadest-reaching efforts to affect the largest number of people. Practitioners who advocate on the policy or societal level are often doing so at state or national levels. Case Example E.4 shows advocacy at the policy level.

In addition to formal advocacy activities outside of the profession, practitioners can advocate their role to other disciplines by establishing a formal "place at the table" on committees to increase the role visibility and contribution of occupational therapy to the external community. A wide range of existing committees, groups, and task forces are charged with addressing transportation issues of the community, most of which are looking for more volunteer members to share the work of the committee. Occupational therapists should look for committees and task forces to join in state, county, and local agencies that focus on safety, transportation, aging, children and youth, and community design. Other types of committees that

Case Example E.1. Clinic- or Individual-Level Advocacy

A 16-year-old student is enrolled in a school system that provides driver's education for all students. This particular student has special learning needs and will not be able to learn from the traditional high school driver's education teacher, who does not have experience in grading the learning activity and separating the task of driving into components for easier learning. The occupational therapist might advocate on behalf of the student for the school system to provide skilled driver's education programming from a DRS rather than pay for the student to participate in school-based driver's education.

may increase visibility include research consortia; community or municipal planning boards; policy-making bodies for health care facilities and school systems; and boards of directors for transit companies, community associations, and retirement communities.

Once occupational therapists have the attention of key stakeholders or have gained entrée to a constituency group, they should work to increase awareness of what occupational therapy can do for clients in that setting or circumstance. This awareness can be accomplished by providing in-services or presenting a case study. Advocating verbally can be very personal and effective but only reaches people who were present at the time of the presentation. Advocates wishing to produce a lasting impact may want to create printed materials or publish in another discipline's trade magazine.

Opening the Door to Public Understanding

A form of advocacy that can have a very significant impact is providing new or innovative services that can open the door and broaden public understanding and awareness of occupational therapy's role beyond traditional rehabilitation. Occupational therapists can offer innovative services in the area of community mobility with an injury prevention or participation support agenda. These programs can serve to start the conversation to facilitate lifelong mindfulness about community mobility issues, supports for community mobility, the need to transition between modes of mobility, injury prevention, and health and wellness. Innovative programs to open the door to public understanding might include the following:

- Child passenger safety seat–check events
- Bike helmet–check events
- Bicycle rodeos
- Safe Routes to School programming

Case Example E.4 Policy-Level Advocacy

A DRS has seen numerous clients transition in and out of her state of residence across her career for the purpose of residing and obtaining a driver's license in a state with more lenient medical requirements. The therapist is concerned about this phenomenon because the driver's health impairments are the same regardless of the state of residence, putting other road users at risk. This practitioner collaborates with her U.S. representative to propose a bill to the U.S. House of Representatives' Transportation and Infrastructure Committee in support of national driver licensure for all citizens to standardize the health and performance requirements from state to state.

- Walk-to-school days
- CarFit events
- Transit training
- Walking clubs
- Bike clubs
- Automobile dealer partnerships
- Transit trips to the theater for older adults.

Conclusion

Advocating for change is an important task required of all members of the profession if there is hope of growing the practice area, advancing attention to community mobility as an IADL, and supporting community-level engagement for occupational therapy clients. There is a full range of advocacy options in terms of the target audience, the purpose, the level of advocacy, and innovative programs—none more important than the others. Most vital to the change and evolution of driving and community mobility in occupational therapy practice is that each therapist engage in some type of advocacy, at some level, to some audience, for some purpose.

References

American Occupational Therapy Association. (2008). Occupational therapy practice framework: Domain and process (2nd ed.). *American Journal of Occupational Therapy, 62*(6), 625–683. doi:10.5014/ajot.62.6.625

American Occupational Therapy Association. (2010). Driving and community mobility [Statement]. *American Journal of Occupational Therapy, 64,* S112–S124. doi:10.5014/ajot.2010.64S112

International Council of Nurses. (2008). *Promoting health: Advocacy guide for health professionals.* Retrieved April 11, 2011, from http://www.whpa.org/PPE_Advocacy_Guide.pdf

APPENDIX A

Driving as a Valued Occupation

Anne Dickerson, PhD, OTR/L, FAOTA

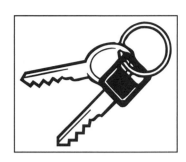

As the U.S. population shifts from a current median age of 34 to 43 years by 2025 (Rand Corporation, 2011), occupational therapy services will also need to shift to deal with the increasing numbers of older adults living longer. On the basis of these demographic characteristics and the importance of individuals engaging in their community, I believe that driver rehabilitation warrants more investment from occupational therapists, and the need is urgent. At this point in time, driving and community mobility should not be categorized as an *emerging area* of practice but instead considered as one of the *essential* instrumental activities of daily living (IADLs) that all occupational therapists should address with their clients.

How Occupational Therapy Can Contribute to Society Through Driver Rehabilitation

Personally, there are many reasons I have embraced driver rehabilitation. For one, it combines my developmental psychology doctoral knowledge with my occupational therapy research on the functional performance of older adults. It is an exciting practice area that requires innovative occupational therapists willing to take on challenges in the real-world community. However, the most significant factor about driver rehabilitation is the recognition of what occupational therapy can contribute to society in this practice arena.

At any meeting, conference, or seminar, transportation leaders and researchers specifically identify occupational therapy as the profession that should provide both evaluation and intervention services. Interdisciplinary national associations (e.g., Gerontological Society of America, Transportation Research Board, American Society on Aging), government agencies (e.g., National Highway Traffic Safety Administration [NHTSA], National Center for Senior Transportation), and other influential groups (e.g., Hartford Insurance, AARP, AAA) understand the role of occupational therapy in transportation and are seeking and begging for our services.

With the "silver tsunami" under way, occupational therapy has an opportunity to be the nationally recognized profession meeting the needs of driving and community mobility—one of the most valued IADLs for young and old adults. So, what is the problem?

There are not enough occupational therapists addressing driving and community mobility. Nationally, there are approximately 600 driver rehabilitation specialists (DRSs), with 80% of those being occupational therapists (Dickerson, Reistetter, Schold Davis, & Monahan, 2011). Over the past 10 years, the American Occupational Therapy Association (AOTA) has maintained the Older Driver Safety Initiative, supporting workshops, mini-grants, initiatives such as CarFit, and a Web site dedicated to increasing program growth in this area. Although there has been significant success with the initiative, it is not enough. I believe that unless a substantial change takes place in addressing the IADL of driving, the occupational therapy profession will lose this area of practice. Action is needed now to avoid the loss of this practice niche.

We must make transportation a national priority for occupational therapy. The 2005 White House Conference on Aging's top three issues to address were (1) the reauthorization of the Older Americans Act of 1965 (P. L. 89–73), (2) long-term care, and (3) transportation (U.S. Administration on Aging [AOA], 2005). Consider for a moment what that means. First, the Older Americans Act funds older adult services for all states thus is critically important. Second, occupational therapists are partners in long-term care, but only a fraction of older adults are living in long-term care (4.1% of the 65-and-older population; AOA, 2010). Third, transportation underlies many other IADLs (e.g., shopping, banking, community outings, medical services) and touches everyone, young and old, with and without disabilities. Now is the time and opportunity, to paraphrase one of our great leaders of occupational therapy, Mary Reilly: Occupational therapy can be one of the great ideas of *21st* (instead of 20th) century *society* (instead of medicine; Reilly, 1962, p. 104).

Every occupational therapist needs to address driving and community mobility. The pediatric occupational therapist needs to ensure that his or her young clients are safely traveling in vehicles with their parents or guardians. Therapists can prepare the families of teenagers with autism spectrum disorders for what to expect in developing independent transportation. Adults with traumatic brain injuries, spinal cord injuries (SCIs), or neurological conditions need their transportation issues addressed so they can return to work or to school or engage in other important tasks of daily life that require getting around the community. Does that mean every occupational therapist needs to become a DRS? No, but we need to use the smaller number of DRSs more efficiently and effectively.

Furthermore, we need to make sure that generalists seek information to improve their understanding of driving and community mobility in terms of activity analysis, resources, and stakeholders so that, as practitioners, they can offer options and opportunity to *all* their clients.

Consider an analogy in medicine. If you think you have a broken arm, you go to your family practice physician to determine if the arm is broken and what to do. Most of the time, the general practitioner will screen, determine a diagnosis, cast the broken arm, and send you home with instructions about managing with the broken arm. The advice includes not getting the cast wet, being careful in activities, not driving until the cast is off, and exploring how else you might manage with the use of only one arm. Only occasionally, the X-ray may show something unusual, and the physician may send you for more evaluation (e.g., magnetic resonance imaging) or a specialist (e.g., orthopedic specialist). We need to build a similar foundation for occupational therapy. When a client presents with a condition requiring occupational therapy services, all activities of daily living and IADLs need to be addressed and intervention offered if appropriate. In the case of driving, the actual activity of driving may need to be revisited when the client develops or recovers the required skill sets, but in the meantime, the client and family may require intervention to move around the community.

Changing Roles of Occupational Therapy Generalists and Specialists

In 2010, my colleagues and I presented an algorithm for the IADL of driving (Dickerson et al., 2011). The purpose of the algorithm is to specify the clinical reasoning process for determining occupational therapy services for community mobility and when to refer to a DRS. Following a step-by-step process on the basis of the *Occupational Therapy Practice Framework: Domain and Process, 2nd Edition* (AOTA, 2008), the occupational therapy generalist can use his or her observation of performance skills, especially of complex IADL tasks, to determine if there are impairments that may trigger problems with driving. The algorithm was developed as a result of a research study illustrating that a standardized IADL assessment tool was able to differentiate between those older adults who passed and those who failed a behind-the-wheel driving evaluation. We argued that although the assessment is an excellent tool, the skilled observation of performance by occupational therapists is the key for facilitating appropriate referrals to DRSs.

What becomes quickly evident with the algorithm is that clients referred to the DRS who do not return to driving often do not receive additional intervention to assist with community mobility options. Because of the DRS's demanding schedules, his or her practice may not bring back the client for additional appointments. Typically, the DRS informs the client and family that driving is not an option on the basis of the evaluation results. Many times the client and caregiver may not be ready to receive additional information, even if available. Thus, it should fall to the generalist either to work with the client on the skills needed for driving or to assist with education or alternative methods of transportation.

Although the research evidence is based on older adults, the algorithm pathway for referral can be used with any population. DRSs have used the algorithm to educate their occupational therapy general practice colleagues about their specific driver rehabilitation programs and adapted the flow chart to work within their specific setting (M. Sweeney, personal communication, August 19, 2011).

Driving and the Baby Boomers

As identified in several chapters of this book, the baby boomers bring the issue of driver assessment to the forefront of public awareness and, thus, occupational therapy. State licensing agencies are struggling with the staggering numbers of older adults and the evidence that although older drivers are safe drivers, aging individuals have more risk of medical conditions that will affect driving (Carr & Ott, 2010). Consider an NHTSA report that analyzed data from the Fatality Analysis Reporting System and National Automotive Sampling System–General Estimates System to identify specific driving behaviors that are performance errors as well as characteristics associated with crash involvement of older adults (Stutts, Martell, & Staplin, 2009).

The data supported that drivers 60–69 years of age have crash rates similar to those of middle-age drivers. However, drivers 70–79 years of age have increased risk, particularly with navigating higher speeds and multiple-lane roadways with junctions, as in suburban areas. For individuals ages 80 years or older, the risk is significantly higher. In fact, of 27 crashes, 26 were fatal errors at intersections with flashing signals or yield signs (Figure A.1). At a yield sign, a driver does not stop but has to make a split-second decision about whether there is enough space (gap acceptance) to merge onto the roadway. We know that the processing speed slows as one ages, and we also know that one in seven individuals over the age of 71 years has some type of cognitive impairment (Plassman et al., 2007).

Does this mean that all people over 80 years old should stop driving? Absolutely not. The evidence clearly shows that driving decisions should be based on function, not age (Barrash et al., 2010; Dickerson et al., 2007). However, with slowed processing, the older driver may still be able to retain his or her mobility by learning to avoid difficult intersections or complex driving situations (e.g., rush hour, inclement weather). The point is that occupational therapists are in the best position to work with physicians, state licensing agencies, older drivers, caregivers, and other

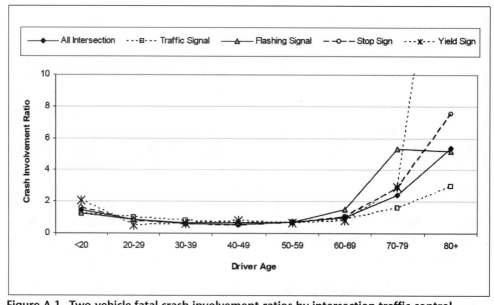

Figure A.1. Two-vehicle fatal crash involvement ratios by intersection traffic control.

Note. From Stutts, J., Martell, C., & Staplin, L. (2009). *Identifying behaviors and situations associated with increased crash risk for older drivers* (Report No: DOT-HS-811-093). Available at http://www.nhtsa.gov/DOT/NHTSA/Traffic%20 Injury%20Control/Articles/Associated%20Files/811093.pdf

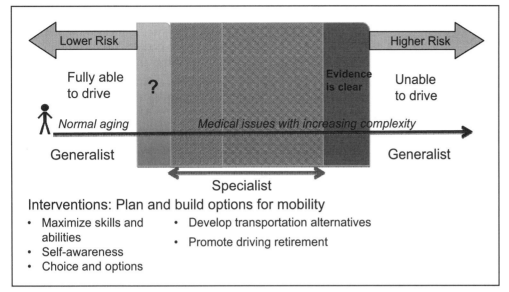

Figure A.2. Occupational therapy intervention: Clinical judgment, evidence, and risk.
Copyright © 2011, by Anne Dickerson and Elin Schold Davis. Used with permission.

stakeholders to assist in determining functioning capabilities, especially for those individuals with medical conditions that might impair driving.

I would argue that all occupational therapists working in settings with adults should have driving and community mobility on their evaluations with the intention of planning and building options for mobility. As shown in Figure A.2, occupational therapy intervention for driving is a combination of the practitioner's clinical judgment and evidence from occupational performance to determine risk. The occupational therapy generalist working with community-living older adults with normal aging processes needs to use opportunities to maximize skills and abilities to prolong their driving lives. This is the optimal time to discuss choices and options as a self-awareness process, understanding that women will outlive their driving ability by 11 years and men by 7 years (Foley, Heimovitz, Guralnik, & Brock, 2002).

Similarly, the generalist working with older adults with medical issues that are exceedingly complex or with an individual with moderate to severe dementia does not need to refer to a DRS. If the practitioner recommends eliminating daily tasks of cooking, financial management, or other complex IADLs, driving will need to be addressed, as it is the most complex of IADLs. The occupational therapist's role is to promote driving retirement and develop transportation alternatives with caregivers or other collaborators. It is those individuals within the gray or middle area who need the DRS's skill set with specialized tools and observation of the client in the vehicle to get an accurate evaluation within the context of the real world.

Summary

In summary, when we consider occupational therapy's brand of *living life to the fullest*, few individuals in the United States would not list driving as an activity that symbolizes independence and is needed to achieve that goal. Even individuals with high-level SCIs, who depend on attendants to assist with the daily tasks of bathing and dressing, desire to drive independently with high-tech vehicles. Young adults with developmental disorders want to be like other teenagers and be driving.

AOTA's Older Driver Initiative has done much to bring the tools and resources to the forefront, but it is now dependent on educators to ensure that every occupational therapy student graduates with a firm understanding of this IADL as well as practitioners to educate themselves and their colleagues. Community mobility is a right of all individuals, and occupational therapists are in demand in this area, but the IADL of community mobility, and driving in particular, is a dynamic, moving target, and unless we step forward, it will be an area of practice lost to another professional group or service providers.

References

American Occupational Therapy Association. (2008). Occupational therapy practice framework: Domain and process (2nd ed.). *American Journal of Occupational Therapy, 62,* 625–683. doi: 10.5014.ajot.62.6.625

Barrash, J., Stillman, A., Anderson, S. W., Uc, E. Y., Dawson, J. D., & Rizzo, M. (2010). Prediction of driving ability with neuropsychological tests: Demographic adjustments diminish accuracy. *Journal of the International Neuropsychological Society, 16,* 679–686.

Carr, D. B., & Ott, B. R. (2010). The older adult driver with cognitive impairment: "It's a very frustrating life." *JAMA, 303,* 1632–1641.

Dickerson, A. E., Molnar, L. J., Eby, D. W., Adler, G., Bédard, M., Berg-Weger, M., et al. (2007). Transportation and aging: A research agenda for advancing safe mobility. *The Gerontologist, 47,* 578–590.

Dickerson, A. E., Reistetter, T., Schold Davis, E., & Monahan, M. (2011). Evaluating driving as a valued instrumental activity of daily living. *American Journal of Occupational Therapy, 65,* 64–75. doi:10.5014/ajot.2011.09052

Foley, D. J., Heimovitz, H. K., Guralnik, J. M., & Brock, D. B. (2002). Driving life expectancy of persons aged 70 years and older in the United States. *American Journal of Public Health, 92,* 1284–1289. doi:10.2105/AJPH.92.8.1284

Older Americans Act of 1965, P.L. 89-73, 42 U.S.C. 3001.

Plassman, B. L., Langa, K. M., Fisher, G. G., Heeringa, S. G., Weir, D. R., Ofstedal, M. B., et al. (2007). Prevalence of dementia in the United States: The aging, demographics, and memory study. *Neuroepidemiology, 29,* 125–132. doi:10.1159/000109998

Rand Corporation. (2011). *Global shifts in population.* Retrieved March 18, 2012, from http://www.rand.org/pubs/research_briefs/RB5044/index1.html

Reilly, M. (1962). Occupational therapy can be one of the great ideas of 20th-century medicine [Eleanor Clarke Slagle Lecture]. *American Journal of Occupational Therapy, 16,* 87–105.

Stutts, J., Martell, C., & Staplin, L. (2009). *Identifying behaviors and situations associated with increased crash risk for older drivers* (Report No. DOT-HS-811-093). Retrieved March 18, 2012, from http://www.nhtsa.gov/DOT/NHTSA/Traffic%20Injury%20Control/Articles/Associated%20Files/811093.pdf

U.S. Administration on Aging. (2005). *2005 White House Conference on Aging: Report to the President and the Congress: The booming dynamics of aging, from awareness to action.* Washington, DC: U.S. Department of Health and Human Services.

U.S. Administration on Aging. (2010). *A profile of older Americans: 2011.* Retrieved February 10, 2012, from http://www.aoa.gov/aoaroot/aging_statistics/Profile/2010/6.aspx

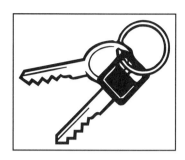

Subject Index

Citation Index

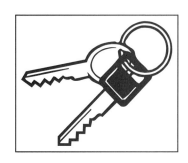